Fundamentals of Nursing

made Incredibly Easy!

Third Edition

Fundamentals of Nursing

made Incredibly Easy!®

Third Edition

Clinical Editors

Keelin Cromar, MSN-Ed, RN
Assistant Professor
Wilson School of Nursing
Midwestern State University
Wichita Falls, Texas

Casey Moebius, DNP, RN
Assistant Chair, RN to BSN Program
Associate Professor
Department of Nurse Education
Del Mar College
Corpus Christi, Texas

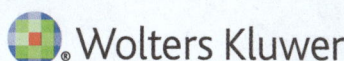 Wolters Kluwer

Philadelphia • Baltimore • New York • London
Buenos Aires • Hong Kong • Sydney • Tokyo

Vice President and Segment Leader, Health Learning & Practice: Julie K. Stegman
Director, Nursing Education and Practice Content: Jamie Blum
Senior Acquisitions Editor: Joyce Berendes
Senior Development Editor: Meredith L. Brittain
Editorial Coordinator: Varshaanaa SM
Marketing Manager: Amy Whitaker
Editorial Assistant: Sara Thul
Manager, Graphic Arts & Design: Stephen Druding
Art Director, Illustration: Jennifer Clements
Production Project Manager: Frances Gunning
Manufacturing Coordinator: Bernard Tomboc
Prepress Vendor: TNQ Tech

3rd edition

Library of Congress Cataloging-in-Publication Data

ISBN-13: 978-1-975236-00-7

Cataloging in Publication data available on request from publisher.

shop.lww.com

Dedication

Thank you, Jason, Brynn, and Teagan, for supporting this adventure, and for my Mom and Dad, who always fostered my dreams. I love you all to infinity and beyond.

Keelin

Thank you, Tim and JT, you bring me sunshine and happiness! Love you both with my whole heart. To my grandma, you are my inspiration; and to my family, thank you for your encouragement.

Casey

Contributors

Stephanie Baker, DNP, MSN, APRN-CNP, PMHNP-BC
Assistant Professor
Wilson School of Nursing
Midwestern State University
Wichita Falls, Texas

Keelin Cromar, MSN-Ed, RN
Assistant Professor
Wilson School of Nursing
Midwestern State University
Wichita Falls, Texas

Tracie Fulton, DNP, MSN-Ed, BSN, RN
Assistant Professor
Wilson School of Nursing
Midwestern State University
Wichita Falls, Texas

Darla Green, DNP, RN, FNP-C
Associate Professor
Del Mar College
Corpus Christi, Texas

Sandra Groth, DNP, MSN-Ed RN, CNE
Assistant Professor
Wilson School of Nursing
Midwestern State University
Wichita Falls, Texas

Robin Lockhart, PhD, MSN, RN
Chair, Nursing Program
Assistant Professor
Wilson School of Nursing
Midwestern State University,
Wichita Falls, Texas

Casey Moebius, DNP, RN
Assistant Chair, RN to BSN Program
Associate Professor
Del Mar College
Corpus Christi, Texas

Catherine Pankonien, DNP, MSN-Ed, RNC-NIC
Associate Professor
Wilson School of Nursing
Midwestern State University
Wichita Falls, Texas

Rachel Reitan, DNP, FNP, MSN-Ed, CWS
Division of Infectious Disease and
   Antimicrobial Stewardship
United Regional Hospital
Wichita Falls, Texas
Adjunct Faculty
Wilson School of Nursing
Midwestern State University
Wichita Falls, Texas

Melody Skinner, DNP, APRN, CPNP
Associate Professor
Del Mar College
Corpus Christi, Texas

Sean Skinner, DNP, APRN, cFNP
Urgent Care FNP
CHRISTUS Spohn Hospital
Corpus Christi, Texas

Lisa Vaira, MSN, RN, CNE, CHSE-A
Adjunct Assistant Professor
Bachelor of Science in Nursing (BSN)
   Online
Unitek Learning
Newport Beach, California

Sarah Wedel, DNP, APRN, FNP-BC, AGPCNP-BC
Nursing Subject Matter Expert
Independent Consultant
Victoria, Minnesota

Laura M. Willis, DNP, APRN-CNP
Family Nurse Practitioner/Lead APC
Bon Secours Mercy Health
Wittenberg University Health Center
Springfield, Ohio

Preface

Fundamentals of nursing are traditionally taught in the first order of courses, because these concepts and knowledge are essential to the support and structure of nursing education. As a nurse progresses through the levels of their education, fundamentals serve as the foundation, which provides the basis for the application and synthesis of all nursing knowledge. For the practicing nurse, reviewing fundamentals serves to strengthen understanding and skills. *Fundamentals of Nursing Made Incredibly Easy!*, Third Edition, is a quick resource for the nurse, the nursing student, *and* the instructor to review the foundational knowledge and skills of nursing.

The content is explained in an easy-to-understand manner and is logically organized into three parts. The first part, "Foundational concepts," provides an overview of nursing and information on health care, ethical and legal considerations, and the nursing process. The second part, "General nursing skills," covers communication, health assessment, vital signs, infection, and key medication information. Finally, the third part, "Physiologic needs," contains information on oxygenation, patient self-care, mobility, skin integrity, pain management, nutrition, and urinary and bowel elimination.

Each chapter in *Fundamentals of Nursing Made Incredibly Easy!* starts by briefly listing the topics that will be covered in the chapter, which lets readers quickly determine where they should focus. Questions at the end of each chapter challenge readers, allowing them to see how much information they absorbed. Colorful illustrations and cartoons make learning fun, which is the surest way to keep readers interested!

In addition, icons draw the reader's attention to important issues:

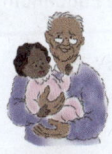 *Ages and stages*—identifies areas and procedures in which age could impact the nurse's care.

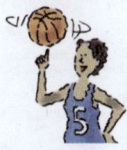 *Stay on the ball*—focuses on critical areas involving possible dangers, risks, complications, contraindications, or ways to ensure safety.

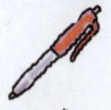 *Take note!*—offers tips on documentation.

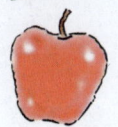 *Education corner*—provides patient-teaching tips on such topics as procedures, equipment, and home care.

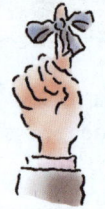

Memory joggers—offer mnemonics and other aids to help you understand and remember difficult concepts.

Important topics of this edition include:
- *Healthy People 2030*
- Nutrition and MyPlate.gov
- Social media relating to the profession of nursing
- Wound care current practice
- Medication and bar code scanning

Fundamentals of Nursing Made Incredibly Easy! is a helpful addition to the *Made Incredibly Easy* series, serving as a handy reference for newly graduated and experienced nurses and also as a valuable guide for nursing students as they prepare for their nursing careers.

Keelin Cromar, MSN-Ed, RN
Assistant Professor
Wilson School of Nursing
Midwestern State University
Wichita Falls, Texas

Casey Moebius, DNP, RN
Assistant Chair, RN to BSN
   Program
Associate Professor
Department of Nurse Education
Del Mar College
Corpus Christi, Texas

Contents

Appendices and index

Part I

Foundational concepts

Chapter 1

Overview of nursing

Just the facts

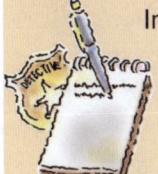

In this chapter, you'll learn:

♦ the historical roots of nursing and its emergence as a profession
♦ practice guidelines and the educational background required for nursing
♦ functions and roles of nurses in various care settings
♦ the guiding principles behind nursing theories and patient care.

Historical evolution of nursing

Since the first part of the 21st century, the role of the nurse has continued to expand. The practice of nursing has become increasingly complex due to a shortage of nurses, reliance on technology, public health issues, and financial stress on systems.

The birth of nursing

The nursing profession's origins lie in religious and military traditions that demanded unhesitating obedience to authority. Florence Nightingale challenged these traditions by emphasizing nursing education, critical thinking, attention to patient needs, and respect for patient rights (Akers & Mauk, 2023).

Go with Flo

Nightingale proposed that schools of nursing be independent of hospitals to provide nursing education without the constant pressure of the hospital environment. She insisted that her schools accept only qualified candidates and that the students learn to teach as well as provide care.

The first schools of nursing based on Nightingale's model opened in the United States in 1873 (Akers & Mauk, 2023). Her ideas were

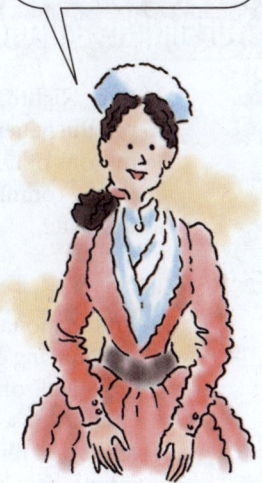

Florence Nightingale challenged traditional views of nursing by emphasizing critical thinking, patient needs, and respect. Way to go, Flo!

soon abandoned when nursing schools realized that they couldn't survive without the hospitals' financial support. At the same time, hospitals recognized that nursing students were a major source of cheap, disciplined labor. They began to hire student nurses instead of more experienced—and more expensive—graduate nurses.

Nurse specialization

After World War II, major scientific discoveries and technological advancements altered the nature of hospital care. Increasingly, the care of hospitalized patients required experienced, skilled nurses. The development of intensive and coronary care units gave rise to the concept of the advanced clinician: a nurse qualified to give specialized care and the forerunner of today's clinical nurse specialist.

After the war, nursing responded to an increased level of public interest in health promotion and disease prevention by creating a new role: the nurse practitioner. Using advanced knowledge and skills, the nurse practitioner helps promote health and prevent illness while caring for health concerns of patients.

Question, analyze, and advocate

Another essential change in nursing stemmed from a mid-20th century shift in attitudes about education for women. The shift that encouraged extending full educational opportunities to women significantly altered the role that nurses play in today's health care system. Armed with a strong educational base, nurses have the confidence necessary to question, analyze, and advocate for patient-centered health care—and to secure a major role for nursing in delivering that care.

Nursing as a profession

Florence Nightingale (1860) believed that a nurse's goal should be "to put the patient in the best condition for nature to act upon him." Definitions of nursing have changed over time, but nursing has retained a common focus: providing humanistic and holistic care to each patient.

Focus, focus

The International Council of Nurses' definition of nursing shares this focus: "Nursing encompasses autonomous and collaborative care of individuals of all ages, families, groups and communities, sick or well and in all settings. Nursing includes the promotion of health, prevention of illness, and the care of ill, disabled and dying people" (International Council of Nurses, 2022).

We've got the power

Nursing practice has seen a significant amount of growth in autonomy in the last 100 years. The nursing profession exercises control over its education and practice, and it has achieved legal recognition through national licensure—every state and Canadian province requires nurses to pass the National Council Licensure Examination for Registered Nurses (NCLEX-RN). In addition, each state and Canadian province has a nurse practice act that regulates the scope of nursing practice. Nursing also has a code of ethics, which is regularly updated to reflect current ethical issues (American Nurses Association, 2015).

Independence is key

The key to professional nursing autonomy is to function independently from any other profession or external force. For many nurses, this remains a goal to be achieved. As employees of large, sometimes inflexible organizations, nurses seldom enjoy full latitude in deciding on patient care within the defined scope of nursing practice. However, by striving for individual excellence, each nurse can help the nursing profession become more autonomous.

Educational preparation

Undergraduate student nurses have three options for nursing education: a baccalaureate of science in nursing (BSN), an associate degree in nursing (ADN), or a hospital-operated diploma program. Regardless of the chosen path, a graduate of any of these three programs is eligible to sit for the NCLEX-RN.

Graduate level

After the nurse receives a baccalaureate degree, they may choose to advance their education at the graduate level. They can choose from a number of graduate fields. Graduate degree options include a Master of Arts (MA) in nursing, Master in Nursing (MN), or Master of Science in Nursing (MSN). These degrees qualify a nurse to serve as a nurse educator, clinical nurse specialist, nurse leader, nurse informaticist, or nurse practitioner.

Doctorate and beyond

Doctoral education in nursing is expanding. Most doctoral programs in nursing lead to a Doctor of Philosophy (PhD) degree or a doctorate in nursing practice (DNP). A nurse with a doctoral degree can assume a leadership position in a practice setting, as an educator, or they can contribute to research endeavors.

Practice guidelines and standards of care

The practice of nursing is guided by two sets of care documents: standards of nursing care and nurse practice acts. The standards of nursing care are administered by the American Nurses Association (ANA), and the nurse practice acts are administered by individual states or provinces.

Standards of nursing care

The *Standards of Professional Nursing Practice* (ANA, 2021) set minimum criteria for job proficiency, enabling nurses to judge the quality of care provided. These standards provide registered nurses with a description of the actions and behaviors they are expected to competently perform (ANA, 2021). Government entities, hospital systems, nurses, and patients refer to these standards. They help to ensure high-quality care, and in the legal arena these documents serve as criteria to help determine whether adequate care was provided to a patient.

The *Standards of Professional Nursing Practice* are divided into the standards of practice, which provide a description of competent nursing practice translated through the nursing process, and standards of professional performance, which define behaviors that exhibit competence in the professional nursing role:

- **Standards of professional performance:** include guidelines for quality of care, performance appraisal, education, collegiality, ethics, collaboration, research, resource utilization, and leadership.
- **Standards of practice:** outline professional responsibilities in assessment, diagnosis, outcome identification, planning, implementation, and evaluation.

Some states refer to standards in their nurse practice acts. Unless included in a nurse practice act, professional standards aren't laws; they're guidelines for sound nursing practice.

Pie in the sky?

Some nurses regard standards of nursing care as pie-in-the-sky ideals that have little bearing on the reality of working life. This opinion is a dangerous error. All nurses are expected to meet standards of care for each task they perform.

Nurse practice acts

Every state sets laws to govern the practice of nursing. These laws are defined in the nursing practice act for each state. The nursing practice act defines the legal scope of practice for professional nurses. Nurse practice acts are broadly worded and vary from state to state. Understanding the general provisions of your state's nurse practice act will help you stay within the legal limits of nursing practice. The emergence of more autonomous and expanded roles for nurses has encouraged states to revise their nurse practice acts to reflect the increased responsibility associated with current nursing practice.

Not an easy task

Interpreting your state's nurse practice act isn't always easy. Because each state has its own version, professional nurses should review and be familiar with the guidelines of the state in which they are practicing. Nurses are responsible for knowing the laws, because those laws are designed to protect the public from unsafe practice (Boehning & Haddad, 2022). The state legislative body gives the state board of nursing the power to regulate, enforce, and discipline nurses who violate nursing laws and regulations. The nursing practice acts are statutory laws; therefore, any amendments must be accomplished through the legislative process. This can be a slow and cumbersome process because development, drafting, and enacting laws is time-consuming. Passing amendments to nursing practice acts may lag behind needs and changes.

It's not enough to know just your state nurse practice act . . . today's nurses need to keep up-to-date with policies, procedures, and nursing trends.

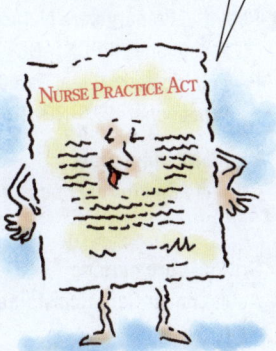

A nursing dilemma

You may be asked to perform tasks that seem to be within the accepted scope of nursing but actually violate your state's nurse practice act. Your state's nurse practice act isn't a word-for-word checklist on how you should do your work. This means you must rely on your education and your knowledge of your facility's policies and procedures.

Limits of practice

Make sure you're familiar with the legally permissible scope of your state's nurse practice act. This legal document is used to govern safe nursing practice, with the ultimate goal of providing safe, competent nursing care to those who need it (National Council of State Boards of Nursing [NCSBN], 2023).

Licensure and certification

All nurses must be licensed in the state in which they practice. All Registered Nurse (RN) candidates must take and pass the NCLEX-RN, which is exactly the same in all states.

The practicing nurse may choose to be certified in a specialty area in which they work. Each certification has minimum requirements, such as education and current work experience. After the nurse has met these requirements and passed an examination, they maintain the certification by continuing education and clinical or administrative practice. (See *Nursing specialty certifications*, pages 8 and 9.)

Nursing specialty certifications

This list includes some of the nursing specialty certifications and their appropriate credentials.

Addictions nursing
Certified Addictions Registered
  Nurse (CARN)

Advanced practice nursing
Acute Care Nurse Practitioner
  (ACNP-BC)
Adult Nurse Practitioner (ANP-BC)
Family Nurse Practitioner (FNP-BC)
Gerontological Nurse Practitioner
  (GNP-BC)
Pediatric Primary Care Nurse
  Practitioner (PPCNP-BC)
Psychiatric and Mental Health Nurse
  Practitioner (PMHNP-BC)

Childbirth educators
Certified Childbirth Educator
  (ICCE)

Critical care nursing
Adult Critical-Care Registered Nurse
  (CCRN)
Cardiac Medicine Certification
  (CCRN-CMC)
Cardiac Surgery Certification
  (CCRN-CSC)
Neonatal Critical-Care Registered
  Nurse (CCRN)
  Pediatric Critical-Care Registered
Nurse (CCRN)
Progressive Care Certified Nurse
  (PCCN)

Diabetes educators
Certified Diabetic Educator (CDE)

Emergency nursing
Certified Emergency Nurse (CEN)

Flight nursing
Certified Flight Registered Nurse
  (CFRN)

Gastroenterology nursing
Certified Gastroenterological
  Registered Nurse (CGRN)

Genetic nursing
Advanced Genetics Nursing
  Certification (AGN-BC)
Genetics Nursing Certification
  (RN-BC)

Health care quality nursing
Certified Professional in Healthcare
  Quality (CPHQ)

HIV-AIDS nursing
AIDS Certified Registered Nurse
  (ACRN)

Holistic nursing
Holistic Nurse–Board Certified
  (HN-BC)

Hospice and palliative nursing
Certified Hospice and Palliative
  Nurse (CHPN)

Infection control nursing
Certified in Infection Control (CIC)

Infusion nursing
Certified Registered Nurse of
  Infusion (CRNI)

Lactation consultant
International Board Certified
  Lactation Consultant (IBCLC)

Legal nurse consulting
Legal Nurse Consulting Certification
  (LNCC)

Managed care nursing
Certified Managed Care Nurse
  (CMCN)

Maternal–neonatal nursing
Inpatient Antepartum Nurse
  (RNC-IAP)
Inpatient Obstetric Nurse
  (RNC, OB)
Low Risk Neonatal Nurse
  (RNC, LRN)
Maternal Newborn Nurse
  (RNC, MNN)
Neonatal Intensive Care Nurse (RNC,
  NIC)

Medical-surgical nursing
Certified Medical Surgical
  Registered Nurse (CMSRN)

Nephrology nursing
Certified Nephrology Nurse (CNN)

Neuroscience nursing
Certified Neuroscience Registered
  Nurse (CNRN)

**Nurse administration: Long-term
care**
Certified Director of Nursing,
  Administration in Long-Term Care
  (CDONA/LTC)

Nurse anesthetist
Certified Registered Nurse
  Anesthetist (CRNA)

Nursing specialty certifications *(continued)*

Nurse midwifery and midwifery
Certified Nurse Midwife (CNM)

Nutrition support nursing
Certified Nutrition Support Nurse
     (CNSN)

Occupational health nursing
Certified Occupational Health Nurse
     (COHN)
Certified Occupational Health Nurse/
     Case Manager (COHN/CM)

Oncology nursing
Certified Oncology Nurse (OCN)

Ophthalmic nursing
Certified Registered Nurse
     Ophthalmology (CRNO)

Orthopedic nursing
Orthopedic Nurse Certified (ONC)

Pediatric nursing
Certified Pediatric Nurse
     (CPN)
Certified Pediatric Nurse Practitioner
     (CPNP)

Pediatric oncology nursing
Certified Pediatric Oncology Nurse
     (CPON)

Perianesthesia nursing
Certified Post Anesthesia Nurse
     (CPAN)
Certified Ambulatory Perianesthesia
     Nurse (CAPA)

Perioperative nursing
Certified Nurse Operating Room
     (CNOR)
RN, First assistant (CRNFA)

Rehabilitation nursing
Certified Rehabilitation Registered
     Nurse (CRRN, CRRN-A)

School nursing
National Certified School Nurse
     (NCSN)

Urology nursing
Certified Urologic Registered Nurse
     (CURN)
Certified Urologic Nurse Practitioner
     (CUNP)

Women's health nursing
Women's Health Care Nurse
     Practitioner (WHNP-BC)
A more complete list of certifications
     can be found at https://nurse.org/
     articles/nursing-certifications-
     credentials-list/.

Professional organizations

Professional organizations are an important part of the nursing profession. They provide current information and resource materials and
give you a voice in your profession. Nursing organizations include
the ANA, the National League for Nursing, the International Council
of Nurses, and the National Student Nurses Association. Nurse
specialty groups include the Association of Critical Care Nurses,
Sigma Theta Tau, the American Association of Nurse Anesthetists,
and the Academy of Medical-Surgical Nursing, to name just a few.
Additionally, each state has its own nursing association that's a
subdivision of the ANA. (See *Individual state and territory nurses'
associations*.)

Individual state and territory nurses' associations

Contacting your state nurses association is only a click away. Can you find the website for your state's association in this list?

Alabama State Nurses Association (ASNA)
https://alabamanurses.nursingnetwork.com/

Alaska Nurses Association (AaNA)
www.aknurse.org.

Arizona Nurses Association (AzNA)
www.aznurse.org.

Arkansas Nurses Association (ARNA)
www.arna.org.

ANA/California (ANA/C)
www.anacalifornia.org.

Colorado Nurses Association (CNA)
http://www.coloradonurses.org/

Connecticut Nurses Association (CNA)
www.ctnurses.org.

Delaware Nurses Association (DNA)
www.denurses.org.

District of Columbia Nurses Association (DCNA)
www.dcna.org.

Florida Nurses Association (FNA)
www.floridanurse.org.

Georgia Nurses Association (GNA)
www.georgianurses.org.

Guam Nurses Association (GNA)
http://guamnursesassociation.org/

Hawaii Nurses Association (HNA)
http://hawaii-ana.nursingnetwork.com/

ANA/Idaho (ANA/ID)
http://idahonurses.nursingnetwork.com/

ANA/Illinois (ANA/IL)
https://www.ana-illinois.org/

Indiana State Nurses Association (ISNA)
http://indiananurses.nursingnetwork.com/

Iowa Nurses Association (INA)
www.iowanurses.org.

Kansas State Nurses Association (KSNA)
http://www.ksnurses.com/

Kentucky Nurses Association (KNA)
http://kentucky-nurses.nursingnetwork.com/

Louisiana State Nurses Association (LSNA)
www.lsna.org.

ANA/Maine (ANA/ME)
http://anamaine.nursingnetwork.com/

Maryland Nurses Association (MNA)
http://mna.nursingnetwork.com/

Massachusetts Nurses Association (MNA)
https://www.massnurses.org/

ANA/Michigan (ANA/MI)
http://www.ana-michigan.org/

Minnesota Organization of Registered Nurses (MNORN)
https://www.mnorn.org/

Mississippi Nurses Association (MNA)
www.msnurses.org.

Missouri Nurses Association (MONA)
www.missourinurses.org.

Montana Nurses Association (MNA)
http://mtnurses.nursingnetwork.com/

Nebraska Nurses Association (NNA)
http://www.nebraskanurses.org/

Nevada Nurses Association (NNA)
www.nvnurses.org.

New Hampshire Nurses Association (NHNA)
http://nhnurses.nursingnetwork.com/

New Jersey State Nurses Association (NJSNA)
www.njsna.org.

New Mexico Nurses Association (NMNA)
http://nmna.nursingnetwork.com/

ANA/New York (ANA/NY)
https://anany.nursingnetwork.com/

North Carolina Nurses Association (NCNA)
www.ncnurses.org.

North Dakota Nurses Association (NDNA)
https://ndna.nursingnetwork.com/

Ohio Nurses Association (ONA)
www.ohnurses.org.

Oklahoma Nurses Association (ONA)
https://oklahomanurses.org/

Oregon Nurses Association (ONA)
www.oregonrn.org.

Pennsylvania State Nurses Association (PSNA)
http://www.psna.org/

ANA/Rhode Island (ANA/RI)
http://risna.nursingnetwork.com/

South Carolina Nurses Association (SCNA)
www.scnurses.org.

Individual state and territory nurses' associations *(continued)*

South Dakota Nurses Association (SDNA)
http://sdnursesassociation.nursing-network.com/

Tennessee Nurses Association (TNA)
www.tnaonline.org.

Texas Nurses Association (TNA)
www.texasnurses.org.

Utah Nurses Association (UNA)
http://www.utnurse.org/

ANA/Vermont (ANA/VT)
http://anavermont.nursingnetwork.com/

Virgin Islands State Nurses Association (VISNA)
https://visna.nursingnetwork.com/

Virginia Nurses Association (VNA)
www.virginianurses.com.

Washington State Nurses Association (WSNA)
www.wsna.org.

West Virginia Nurses Association (WVNA)
www.wvnurses.org.

Wisconsin Nurses Association (WNA)
www.wisconsinnurses.org.

Wyoming Nurses Association (WNA)
www.wyonurse.org.

Functions of nurses

Nursing care changes are based on the patients and populations being served. The functions of the nurse have broadened in response to these changes. The Future of Nursing 2020-2030 report focuses on the nurse's role in leadership and necessary actions to promote health care equity. The report explains the emerging role of nurses as care coordinators in a variety of settings working to address the root cause of poor health, to promote health, and to improve health equity (National Academies of Sciences, Engineering, and Medicine, 2021). Nurses are caregivers, but now they are also educators, advocates, leaders and managers, change agents, and researchers.

Caregiver

Since the beginning, nurses have been considered caregivers, but the activities this role encompasses changed dramatically in the 20th and 21st centuries. Improved education of nurses, expanded nursing research, and recognition that nurses are autonomous and informed professionals have caused a shift in the role of the nurse from a dependent one to one of collaboration and independence.

A model of independence

Medical-surgical nurses now conduct independent assessments and implement patient care based on their knowledge and skills. They also collaborate with other members of the health care team to implement and evaluate that care.

Educator

With greater emphasis on health promotion and illness prevention, the nurse's role as educator has become increasingly important. The nurse assesses learning needs, plans and implements teaching strategies to meet those needs, and evaluates the effectiveness of the teaching. To be a successful educator, the nurse must have effective interpersonal skills and be familiar with the principles of adult learning. Along with teaching come the responsibility of understanding the referral process, identifying community and personal resources, and arranging for necessary equipment and supplies for home care.

Advocate

As an advocate, the nurse helps the patient and their family interpret information from other health care providers and make decisions about their health-related needs. The nurse must accept and respect a patient's decision, even if it differs from the decision the nurse would make.

Coordinator

Nurses manage time, people, resources, and the environment in which they provide care. They carry out these tasks by directing, delegating, and coordinating activities.

All health care team members, including the nurse, provide patient care. Although the health care provider is usually considered the head of the team, the nurse plays an important role in coordinating the efforts of all team members to meet the patient's goals and may conduct team conferences to facilitate communication among team members.

Change agent

As a change agent, the nurse works with the patient to address health concerns and with staff members to address organizational and community concerns. This role demands knowledge of change theory, which provides a framework for understanding the dynamics of change, human responses to change, and strategies for effecting change.

In the community, nurses serve as role models and assist people in bringing about changes to improve the environment, work conditions, or other factors that impact health. Nurses also work together to bring about change through legislation. Some real-life examples include helping to shape and support the laws that mandate the use of car safety seats and motorcycle helmets.

Researcher

The primary tasks of nursing research are to promote growth in the science of nursing and to develop a scientific basis for nursing practice. Each nurse should make an effort to be informed about nursing research and to apply research to their nursing practice.

Although not all nurses are trained in research methods, each nurse can participate in the research process by remaining alert for nursing problems and asking questions about care practices. Many nurses who give direct patient care are able to identify problems, which then serve as a basis for research. Nurses can improve nursing care by incorporating research findings into their practice and communicating the research to others.

Roles of nurses

Nurses have the opportunity to play one of many nursing roles on the health care team. They may be staff nurses, nurse educators, nurse managers, case managers, clinical nurse specialists, nurse practitioners, or nurse researchers.

Staff nurse

The staff nurse functions as a primary caregiver by independently assessing, planning, and implementing direct patient care. For example, a staff nurse may make clinical observations and execute interventions, such as administering medications and treatments and promoting such activities of daily living as bathing and toileting.

Nurse educator

As the emphasis on health promotion and illness prevention has increased, the nurse educator role has become increasingly important. Students of the nurse educator include patients and family members as well as other health professionals.

Many hats, one nurse

The nurse assesses learning needs, plans and implements teaching strategies to meet those needs, and evaluates the effectiveness of the teaching. To be an effective educator, the nurse must have excellent interpersonal skills and be familiar with the appropriate developmental stages of children, adolescents, and adults, as well as the principles of learning for each age group.

Nurse manager

The nurse manager acts as a staff nurse and an administrative representative of the unit, ensuring that effective and quality nursing care is being provided in an environment that is efficient and economical.

Case manager

The role of case manager was developed to counter the trend toward fragmented, depersonalized nursing care. This role enables the nurse to manage the complex and comprehensive care of an individual patient.

Case management is a systematic approach to delivering total patient care within specified time frames and economic resources. It encompasses the patient's entire illness episode, crosses all care settings, and involves the collaboration of all personnel who care for the patient. The case manager is also involved in planning for discharge, making referrals, identifying community and personal resources, and arranging for equipment and supplies needed by the patient on discharge.

Being a case manager means coordinating every aspect of my patient's care and staying on top of all the details—from start to finish!

Clinical nurse specialist

Clinical nurse specialists are advanced practiced registered nurses who have obtained an MSN and have acquired expertise for a specific population, including adult, pediatric, or neonatal (National Association of Clinical Nurse Specialists, 2022). The clinical nurse specialist provides evidence-based nursing care by participating in education and direct patient care, consulting with patients and family members, and collaborating with other nurses and health care team members to deliver high-quality patient care.

Nurse practitioner

A nurse practitioner is a nurse who has completed a master's (MSN) or doctoral degree (DNP) in nursing and has advanced clinical training that surpasses initial nursing preparation. The nurse practitioner can provide primary, acute, and specialty health care to patients and families based on the type of education and training received and can function independently. Nurse practitioners can obtain histories and conduct physical examinations, order laboratory and diagnostic tests and interpret results, diagnose disorders, treat patients, counsel and educate patients and family members, and provide continual follow-up care after patients are discharged (American Association of Nurse Practitioners, 2023).

Nurse researcher

The nurse researcher promotes the science of nursing by investigating problems related to nursing. Developing and refining nursing knowledge and practice is the goal of the nurse researcher. Staff nurses participate in nursing research by reading the current nursing literature, applying the information in practice, and then collecting data. Advanced practice nurses can assist staff nurses by conducting the research study and serving as a consultant to the nurses during the implementation of a research study. Lastly, nurses who hold terminal degrees like a Doctor of Nurse Practice (DNP) or Doctor of Philosophy in Nursing (PhD) are able to institute different types of implementation and theoretical research that impact all realms of nursing practice.

Nursing theories

Many nursing leaders believe that the profession must establish itself as a scientific discipline to enhance its reputation. To do that, nursing needs a theoretical base that simultaneously shapes and reflects its practice.

Concepts common to nursing theories

Four themes guide the development of nursing theory:
- **Person:** principles and laws that govern life processes, well-being, and the optimal functioning of people—sick or well
- **Environment:** patterns of human behavior that describe how people interact with the environment in critical life situations

- **Health:** processes for bringing about positive changes in the health status of individuals
- **Nursing:** the key role nursing has as the central focus of all nursing theories

Nursing theorists

Theorists and researchers are now collaborating with practicing nurses in the development, testing, and refining of nursing theory. (See *Comparing nursing theories*, pages 16 and 17.)

Comparing nursing theories

Nursing theories differ in their assumptions about patients and health, the goals of nursing, and the methods for research and practice. Together, the theories help define nursing's domain. A nursing theory is expressed as a conceptual model, which usually includes a definition of nursing; a statement of nursing's purpose; and definitions of person, health, and environment. This chart describes seven theory-based models.

Theory/ Model	Definition of nursing	Purpose of nursing	Definition of person	Definition of health	Definition of environment
Florence Nightingale: Environmental Theory	• A profession for women that seeks to discover and use nature's laws governing health to serve humanity	• To put the person in the best condition for nature to restore or preserve health • To prevent or cure disease and injury	• A being composed of physical, intellectual, and metaphysical attributes and potentials	• To be free from disease and able to use one's own powers to the fullest	• External elements that affect the healthy or sick person
Myra Estrin Levine: Conservation Model for Nursing	• A human interaction incorporating scientific principles into the nursing process	• To provide human interaction, relying on the idea that humans depend on other humans to subside	• A complex individual who interacts with internal and external environments and adapts to change	• To possess a pattern of adaptive change • To be whole	• Internally, the person's physiology • Externally, perceptual, operational, and conceptual components
Dorothea Orem: Self-Care Deficit Theory	• A human service designed to overcome limitations in health-related self-care	• To make judgments responding to a person's need for self-care in order to sustain life and health	• A person who functions biologically, symbolically, and socially	• A state of wholeness or integrity of the individual, his or her parts, and modes of functioning	• A subcomponent of the person (Together, they compose an integrated system related to self-care)

Comparing nursing theories *(continued)*

Theory/ Model	Definition of nursing	Purpose of nursing	Definition of person	Definition of health	Definition of environment
Sister Callista Roy: Adaptation Model of Nursing	• An analysis and action related to the care of an ill or potentially ill person	• To facilitate adaptation through helping patients have a positive response to stimuli	• A biopsychosocial being in constant interaction with a changing environment • An open, adaptive system	• Part of the health–illness continuum, a continuous line representing states or degrees of health or illness that a person might experience at a given time	• All conditions, circumstances, and influences surrounding and affecting the development of an organism or group of organisms
Betty Neuman: Neuman Systems Model	• A profession concerned with the variables that affect the person's response to stressors	• To reduce a person's encounter with stressors • To mitigate the effect of stressors	• A physiologic, psychological, sociocultural, and developmental being • A person who must be viewed as a whole	• A state of wellness or illness determined by physiologic, psychological, sociocultural, and developmental variables that are relative and on a continuum	• Internally, the state of the person in terms of physiologic, psychological, sociocultural, and developmental variables • Externally, all that exists outside the person
Imogene King: Theory of Goal Attainment	• A human interaction between nurse and client	• To exchange information with the patient and take action together to attain mutually set goals	• A social being who is rational and perceptive • An open system with permeable boundaries that permit the exchange of matter, energy, and information with the environment	• Dynamic adjustment to stressors in the internal and external environment • To make optimal use of resources to achieve maximum potential for daily living	• A background for human interaction • An open system with permeable boundaries that permit the exchange of matter, energy, and information with human beings
Rogers: Science of Unitary Human Beings	• A learned profession that promotes and maintains health and that includes professionals who care for and rehabilitate the sick and disabled	• To promote harmonious interaction between the environment and person	• A being with a four-dimensional energy field identified by pattern and organization and manifesting characteristics and behaviors that differ from those of its parts and that cannot be predicted from knowledge of the parts	• A value word broadly defined by cultures and individuals to describe behaviors considered to be of high or low value	• A four-dimensional energy field identified by pattern and organization and encompassing all that exists outside any given human field

Source: Wayne, G. (2023). *Nursing theories and theorists: The definitive guide for nurses.* https://nurseslabs.com/nursing-theories/

Nonnursing theories

Many theories not specifically developed for nursing have been adopted by the nursing profession to provide guidelines for practicing high-quality patient care.

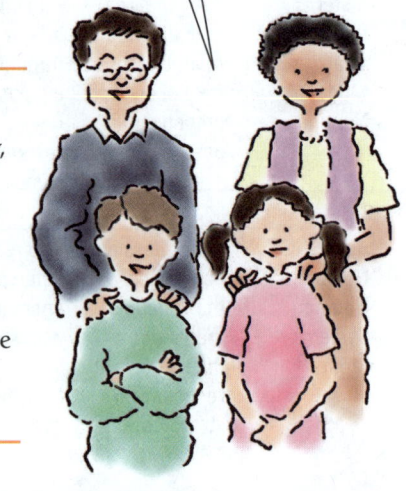

A system can be an individual, a family, or a community.

Systems theories

Systems theories define the system as an individual, a family, or a community. In general, systems theories include a purpose (or goal), content (the information obtained from the system), and a process used to achieve the goal. The whole (be it an individual, family, or community) is broken down, and all of the parts are examined. System theories integrate each part of the whole and examine how each part affects the whole.

Human needs theories

Human needs are the physiologic or psychological factors that must be met for an individual to have a healthy existence. Maslow (1943) categorized these basic needs according to importance when he created *Maslow's Hierarchy of Needs.* This model described that lower-level physiologic needs, such as the need for oxygen, food, elimination, temperature control, sex, rest, and comfort, must be met before higher-level needs, such as a sense of self-worth and self-respect, can be met. These theories are useful when planning and organizing nursing care. (See *Maslow's hierarchy of needs.*)

According to one developmental theory, I'm working on developing my sense of autonomy by banging this bottle on the table right now.

Developmental theories

Developmental theories classify an individual's behavior or tasks according to their age or development. These theories use categories to describe characteristics associated with the majority of individuals at periods when distinctive developmental changes occur. However, they don't consider individual differences. These types of theories focus on only one type of development, such as cognitive, psychosocial, psychosexual, and moral or faith development. Even so, developmental theories allow the nurse to describe typical behavior within a certain age-group, which can be helpful during patient teaching and counseling.

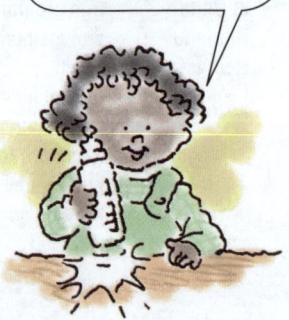

Maslow's hierarchy of needs

To formulate nursing diagnoses, you must know your patient's needs and values. Of course, physiologic needs—represented by the base of the pyramid in the diagram—must be met first.

Self-actualization
Recognition and realization of one's potential, growth, health, and autonomy

Self-esteem
Sense of self-worth, self-respect, independence, dignity, privacy, and self-reliance

Love and belonging
Affiliation, affection, intimacy, support, and reassurance

Safety and security
Safety from physiologic and psychological threat, protection, continuity, stability, and lack of danger

Physiologic needs
Oxygen, food, elimination, temperature control, sex, movement, rest, and comfort

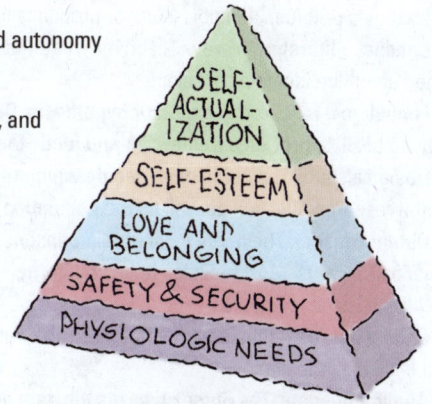

(Adapted from Maslow A. H. (1943). A theory of human motivation. *Psychological Review*, 50 (4), 370–396. This material is in the public domain.)

Nursing research

Research is the foundation on which all sciences are based. Its reliance on observations made in a controlled setting limits confusion over which factors actually produce outcomes and results. Health care professionals have long recognized the importance of research in the laboratory setting but recently have begun to develop ways to make research information more useful in the clinical setting.

Supported by evidence

The goal of research is to improve the delivery of care and, thereby, improve patient outcomes. Nursing care is commonly based on evidence that's derived from research. Evidence can be used to support current practices or to change practices. (See *Research and nursing*.)

The best way to get involved in research is to be a good consumer of nursing research. You can do this by reading nursing journals and understanding the elements of quality research and reported results.

Research and nursing

All scientific research is based on the same basic process.

Research steps

The research process consists of these steps:

1. **Identify a problem.** Identify issues or problems in nursing and nursing care.
2. **Conduct a literature review.** Discover what has already been examined and published about the identified problem.
3. **Formulate a research question or hypothesis.** Develop a strong research question or hypothesis to provide a framework and focus for research efforts.
4. **Design a study.** The nurse must decide which research design is most appropriate for the research question as well as the population being studied.
5. **Obtain consent.** The nurse must obtain consent to conduct research from the study participants. Most facilities have an internal review board that must approve such permission for studies.
6. **Collect data.** After the study is approved, the nurse can begin conducting the study and collecting the data.
7. **Analyze the data.** The nurse analyzes the data and states the conclusions derived from the analysis.
8. **Share the information.** Lastly, the conclusions and results are shared through publications and presentations.

Source: Villegas F. (2023, June 12). *Research process steps: What they are + how to follow.* QuestionPro. https://www.questionpro.com/blog/research-process-steps/

Sharing is caring

Don't be afraid to share research findings with colleagues. Sharing promotes sound clinical care, and all involved may learn about new safe, efficient ways to care for patients.

Evidence-based care

One of the best ways to make research results more useful in clinical practice is by delivering evidence-based care. Evidence-based care isn't based on traditions, customs, or intuition; instead, it's derived from various concrete sources, including

- formal nursing research
- clinical knowledge
- scientific knowledge

An evidence-based example

Research results may provide insight into the treatment of a patient who, for example, doesn't respond to a medication or treatment that seems effective for other patients.

In this example, the care team may believe that a certain drug should be effective for pain relief based on previous experience with that drug. The trouble with such an approach is that other factors can contribute to pain relief, such as the route of administration, dosage, tolerance, and concurrent treatments.

> Providing evidence-based care brings research to the bedside.

First, last, and always

Regardless of the value of evidence-based care, you should always use professional clinical judgment when dealing with patients and their families. Remember that each patient's condition ultimately dictates treatment.

Quick quiz

1. Professional nursing practice should be guided by which of the following? (Select all that apply.)
    A. Nursing educational preparation
    B. The Joint Commission
    C. State nurse practice acts
    D. ANA standards for professional nursing care

Answer: A, C, and D. Professional nursing practice begins with a solid education. After graduation, the professional nurse should utilize their state nurse practice act and the ANA standards for professional nursing care to guide practice.

2. A nurse is helping a patient and their family understand and interpret information that they received from a neurologist. Which nursing function is this nurse fulfilling?
    A. Coordinator
    B. Advocate
    C. Change agent
    D. Researcher

Answer: B. A nurse advocate helps patients and family members interpret and understand information to make informed decisions about their care.

3. Which of the following nurse theorists challenged traditional nursing views by emphasizing nursing education, patient needs, and critical thinking?
    A. Dorothea Orem
    B. Betty Neuman
    C. Imogene King
    D. Florence Nightingale

Answer: D. Florence Nightingale is considered the "mother of modern nursing" because she challenged the nursing profession to adopt professional standards as well as to place an emphasis on education, patient care, and critical thinking.

4. Which of the following nurses has the proper education and credentials to obtain histories, conduct physical examinations, order laboratory and diagnostic tests, interpret results, diagnose disorders, and treat patients?
    A. Nurse practitioner
    B. Case manager
    C. Staff nurse
    D. Nurse manager

Answer: A. The nurse practitioner may obtain histories, conduct physical examinations, order laboratory and diagnostic tests, interpret results, diagnose disorders, and treat patients.

5. The easiest way for a nurse to participate in research is to
    A. be a good consumer of research.
    B. complete a literature review.
    C. conduct a research study.
    D. participate on their institution's internal review board (IRB).

Answer: A. The easiest way to begin to understand and integrate research into practice is to be a good consumer of research. This includes reading and critically appraising research to determine its value in practice.

Scoring

☆☆☆   If you answered all five questions correctly, fantastic! You are building a good nursing foundation.

☆☆   If you answered three or four questions correctly, super! Your foundation is getting strong.

☆   If you answered fewer than three questions correctly, don't worry! With a little review, your foundation will be strong before you know it.

References

Akers S., & Mauk K. (2023). Nursing education's dynamic history: Challenging, creative, and courageous. *Journal of Christian Nursing, 40*(2), 102–109. https://doi.org/10.1097/CNJ.0000000000001048

American Association of Nurse Practitioners. (2023). *What is a nurse practitioner?* https://www.aanp.org/about/all-about-nps/whats-a-nurse-practitioner

American Nurses Association (ANA). (2015). *Code of ethics for nurses: With interpretive statements.* https://www.nursingworld.org/practice-policy/nursing-excellence/ethics/code-of-ethics-for-nurses/

American Nurses Association (ANA). (2021). *Nursing scope and standards of practice* (4th ed.). https://www.nursingworld.org/nurses-books/nursing-scope-and-standards-of-practice-4th-edit/

Boehning A., & Haddad L. (2022). *Nursing practice act.* https://ncbi.nlm.nih.gov

International Council of Nurses (ICN). (2022). *Nursing definitions.* https://www.icn.ch/nursing-policy/nursing-definitions

Maslow A. H. (1943). A theory of human motivation. *Psychological Review, 50* (4), 370–396.

National Academies of Sciences, Engineering, and Medicine. (2021). *The future of nursing 2020-2030: Charting a path to achieve health equity.* The National Academies Press. https://doi.org/10.17226/25982

National Association of Clinical Nurse Specialists. (2022). *What is a CNS?* https://nacns.org/about-us/what-is-a-cns/

National Council of State Boards of Nursing (NCSBN). (2023). *Nurse practice act toolkit.* https://www.ncsbn.org/policy-gov/npa-toolkit.page

Nightingale F. (1860). *Notes on nursing: What it is, and what it is not.* D. Appleton and Company.

Nurse.org. (2023). *Complete list of common nursing certifications.* https://nurse.org/articles/nursing-certifications-credentials-list/

Villegas F. (2023, June 12). *Research process steps: What they are + how to follow.* QuestionPro. https://www.questionpro.com/blog/research-process-steps/

Wayne G. (2023). *Nursing theories and theorists: The definitive guide for nurses.* https://nurseslabs.com/nursing-theories/

Chapter 2

Basics of health and illness

Just the facts

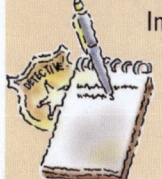

In this chapter, you'll learn:

◆ definitions of health and illness

◆ common factors affecting health and illness

◆ the effects of illness on the family and aging

◆ the national goals established in *Healthy People 2030*.

The health–illness continuum

The definition of health is affected by how people view themselves, as individuals and as part of the environment. At one end of the continuum are health and wellness, which are the highest level of function; at the other end of the continuum are illness and death. All people are somewhere on this continuum, and as their health status changes, their location on the continuum also changes.

Health defined

Throughout history, the definition of health has changed depending on the knowledge and beliefs of the time. Some cultures have regarded health and disease as reward or punishment for their actions. Others have viewed health as soundness or wholeness of the body.

What is it?

Health is a commonly used term, although no single definition is universally accepted. One common definition describes health as a state of being free from illness or injury, but this indicates health is an either-or situation—either a person is healthy or ill.

> The term *health* is commonly used, though the word has many definitions!

WHO says. . . ?

The World Health Organization (WHO) (2023) calls health "a state of complete physical, mental, and social well-being and not merely the absence of disease or infirmity." The word "complete" does not allow for any degree of health or illness and fails to reflect the concept of health as constantly changing (van Druten et al., 2022).

Health and culture

Cultural beliefs impact how people think and feel about health. Culture influences how people view health, healing, wellness, illness, and disease (National Institutes of Health, 2021). Understanding and respecting culture, beliefs, and customs is important when engaging with patients to develop a plan of care consistent with the patient's values (Agency for Healthcare Research and Quality, 2020).

Levels of wellness

Health is often viewed within levels of wellness. Many concepts of health focus on a person's ability to attain their full potential, which is a more holistic and subjective way to define health. Considering health as levels of wellness allows those with chronic illness or disability to achieve their own level of well-being (van Druten et al., 2022).

Factors affecting health

Assisting patients to reach an optimal level of wellness is one of the primary functions of a nurse. When assessing patients, nurses must be aware of factors that influence health and tailor interventions accordingly. Such factors include

- genetics (biological and genetic makeup that causes illness and chronic conditions)
- cognitive abilities (may impact a person's view of health and ability to seek out resources)
- demographic factors, such as age and gender (because certain diseases are more prevalent for a particular gender or age group)
- geographic locale (predisposes a person to certain conditions)
- culture (influences a person's perception of health, the motivation to seek care, and the types of health practices performed)
- lifestyle and environment (such as diet, level of activity, and exposure to toxins)
- health beliefs and practices (can affect health positively or negatively)
- previous health experiences (may influence reactions to illness and the decision to seek care)
- spirituality (may impact a person's view of illness and health care)
- support systems (may affect the degree to which a person adapts and copes with a situation).

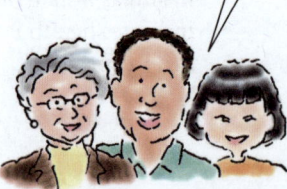

Because so many factors have a bearing on health, interventions need to be tailored accordingly.

Illness defined

Nurses must understand the concept of illness, particularly how illness may affect the patient. Illness can be defined as a sickness or deviation from a healthy state and is considered a broader concept than disease. Disease commonly refers to a specific biological or psychological problem that's supported by clinical manifestations and results in a body system or organ malfunction. (See *Disease development*.) Illness, on the other hand, occurs when a person is no longer in a state of perceived "normal" health. A person may have a disease but not be ill all the time because their body has adapted to the disease.

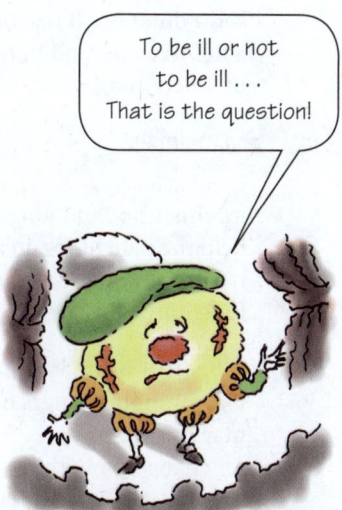

To be ill or not to be ill . . . That is the question!

What does it mean to you?

The meaning of illness also depends on how the patient interprets the source of the disease, its importance, and how the illness or disease impacts their behavior and relationships with others. Also significant is how the individual copes and identifies with the experience of being ill.

Disease development

A disease is usually detected when it causes a change in metabolism or cell division, which, in turn, causes signs and symptoms. How the cells respond to disease depends on the causative agent and the affected cells, tissues, and organs. In the absence of intervention, resolution of the disease depends on many factors functioning over a period of time, such as the extent of disease and the presence of other diseases. Manifestations of disease may include hypofunction, hyperfunction, or increased or decreased mechanical function.

Disease stages

Typically, diseases progress through these stages (Parker et al., 2021):
- *exposure or injury*—target tissue exposed to a causative agent or injury
- *latency or incubation period*—no evident signs or symptoms
- *prodromal period*—generally mild, nonspecific signs and symptoms
- *acute phase*—disease at its full intensity, possibly with complications; called the *subclinical acute phase* if the patient still functions as though the disease wasn't present
- *remission*—second latency phase that occurs in some diseases and is commonly followed by another acute phase
- *convalescence*—progression toward recovery
- *recovery*—return to health or normal functioning, no remaining signs or symptoms of disease.

Types of illness

Illness may be acute or chronic. *Acute illness* usually refers to a disease or condition that has a relatively abrupt onset, high intensity, and short duration. If no complications occur, most acute illnesses end in a full recovery, and the person returns to the previous or a similar level of functioning.

Regain and maintain

Chronic illness refers to a condition that typically has a slower onset, less intensity, and longer duration than acute illness. The goal is to help the patient regain and maintain the highest possible level of health, although some patients fail to return to their previous level of functioning.

Effects of illness

One or more changes occur that signal the presence of illness. These may include
- changes in body appearance or function
- unusual body emissions
- sensory changes
- uncomfortable physical manifestations
- changes in emotional status
- changes in relationships.

Ch–ch–ch–ch–changes . . .

Most people experience a mild form of some of these changes in their daily lives. However, when the changes are severe enough to interfere with usual daily activities, the person is usually considered ill.

Perception and reaction

How people react to feeling ill varies. Some people seek support immediately, and others take no action. Some may overstate their symptoms, and others may deny that their symptoms exist. A patient's perception of and reaction to illness are unique and are usually based on culture, knowledge, view of health, and previous experiences with illness and the health care system.

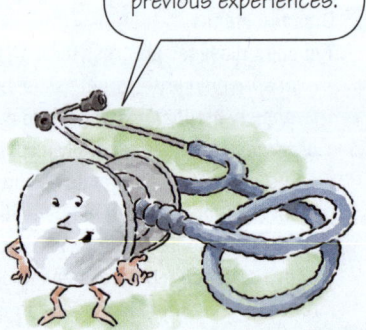

Reactions to illness are often based on previous experiences.

Effects of illness on family

The presence of illness in a family can have a dramatic impact on how the family unit functions. The significance of the impact depends on these factors:
- which family member is ill
- the seriousness and duration of the illness

- the family's social and cultural customs (each member's role in the family and the tasks specific to that role).

Which family member?

Depending on which member of the family is affected by illness, role changes may occur. For example, if the primary financial supporter is ill, other members may need to seek employment to supplement the family income. As the primary financial supporter assumes a dependent role, the rest of the family must adjust to new roles. As another example, if a working single caregiver becomes ill, serious economic and childcare problems may result. The caregiver may have to seek out and depend on additional support systems or face additional stress.

Health promotion

Research shows that poor health practices contribute to a wide range of illnesses, a shortened life span, and increased health care costs. Good health practices have the opposite effect: fewer illnesses, a longer life span, and lower health care costs.

> Good health practices have positive impacts on life span.

What is health promotion?

Health promotion is the process of enabling people to take control of and improve their health (World Health Organization, 2023). Simply stated, health promotion is teaching good health practices and finding ways to help people correct their poor health practices.

Healthy People 2030 sets forth comprehensive health goals for the nation with the aim of reducing mortality and morbidity for people of all ages. These objectives reflect priority public health issues and are associated with evidence-based interventions that can be used to guide teaching plans (Office of Disease Prevention and Health Promotion [ODPHP], n.d.).

Better late than never

Good health practices can benefit most people no matter when the practices begin. Of course, the earlier in life good practices are started, the fewer the poor habits that have to be overcome. Even so, later is better than never. For example, stopping cigarette smoking has immediate and long-term benefits. Immediately, the patient will experience improved circulation, pulse rate, and blood pressure. After 10 years, people who stop smoking can cut their risk of dying from cancer by 30% to 50% (National Cancer Institute, 2021).

Healthy People 2030: Vision

All people can achieve their full potential for health and wellness across the lifespan.

Healthy People 2030 has the following broad goals:

- achieve health and well-being free of preventable disease, disability, injury, and premature death
- eliminate health disparities, achieve health equity, improve health and well-being with health literacy
- create social and physical environments that promote wellness and the full potential of health for all
- promote well-being, healthy behaviors, and health development across all stages of life
- engage leadership and the public across multiple sectors to act and improve health and well-being of all

Healthy People 2030 objectives can be evaluated using the eight overall health and well-being measures (OHMs), which are organized into three tiers: well-being, healthy life expectancy, and summary mortality and health. Over the decade ending with 2030, the eight OHMs will be monitored and data will be used to determine the overall health and well-being of the population and improvements (U.S. Department of Health and Human Services, n.d.).

Health disparities

Health disparities are differences in any health-related factor that exists among population groups. Health disparities result from factors such as poverty, environment, socioeconomic status, educational inequalities, geographic location, ethnicity, age, health behaviors, access to health care, and more (Centers for Disease Control and Prevention, 2021; The National Institute on Aging [NIA], 2023).

Healthy aging

As people age, they are more likely to experience health issues and disorders. Some age-related variations in health are attributed to genetics, but most are due to physical, social, and environmental factors (NIA, 2023; World Health Organization, n.d.).

Challenges with aging

Society often sees older adults as frail and dependent. The World Health Organization (WHO) suggests society change our mindset about the aging process and focus on how we think, feel, and act, because this can promote health equity for all ages (World Health Organization, n.d.).

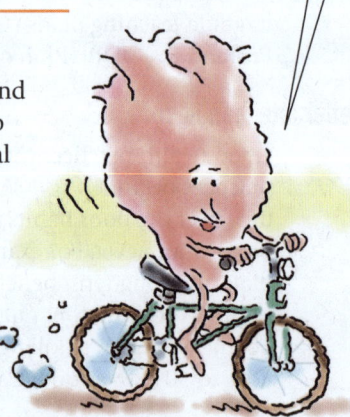

Maintaining healthy behaviors throughout life can contribute to improved physical and mental capacity.

Quick quiz

1. Which of the following is an example of health promotion?
    A. Administering antibiotics to a patient
    B. Splinting a patient's fractured bone
    C. Assisting a patient to stop smoking
    D. Inserting an IV catheter

Answer: C. Health promotion involves teaching good health practices as well as helping people correct poor health practices. Helping a patient to stop smoking helps them correct a poor health practice.

2. When describing disease development, which disease stage is described as producing generally mild, nonspecific signs and symptoms?
    A. Latent
    B. Acute
    C. Second latency
    D. Prodromal

Answer: D. The prodromal period is described as producing generally mild, nonspecific signs and symptoms.

3. The effect of illness on a family unit depends on several factors, including which of the following? (Select all that apply.)
    A. The seriousness and duration of the illness
    B. Which family member is impacted
    C. If the illness is due to poor health habits
    D. The family's social and cultural customs

Answer: A, B, and D. The effect of illness on a family unit depends on the seriousness and duration of the illness, which family member is impacted, and the family's social and cultural customs.

4. Health disparities result from multiple factors, including which of the following? (Select all that apply.)
    A. Access to health care
    B. Socioeconomic status
    C. Educational inequalities
    D. Geographic location

Answer: A, B, C, and D. Health disparities result from factors such as poverty, environment, socioeconomic status, educational inequalities, geographic location, ethnicity, age, health behaviors, and access to health care.

Scoring

☆☆☆ If you answered all four questions correctly, super! Your understanding of the spectrum of health and illness is spectacular.

☆☆ If you answered three questions correctly, great! You sure have been practicing your nursing practice.

☆ If you answered fewer than three questions correctly, don't despair! Keep "continuum" to review, and you'll soon have a healthy understanding of the chapter.

References

Agency for Healthcare Research and Quality AHRQ. (2020). *Health literacy universal precautions toolkit* (2nd ed.). https://www.ahrq.gov/health-literacy/improve/precautions/tool10.html

Centers for Disease Control and Prevention. (2021). *Health disparities.* https://www.cdc.gov/healthyyouth/disparities/index.htm

van Druten, V.P., Bartels, E.A., van de Mheen, D., de Vried, E., Kerckhotts, A.P., & Nahar-van Venrooij L.M. (2022). Concepts of health in different contexts: A scoping review. *BMC Health Services Research, 22*(1), 1–21. https://doi.org/10.1186/s121913-022-07702-2

National Cancer Institute. (2021). *Cigarette smoking: Health risks and how to quit.* https://www.cancer.gov/about-cancer/causes-prevention/risk/tobacco/quit-smoking-pdq

National Institute on Aging. (2023). *Strategic directions for research, 2020-2025 goal C.* https://www.nia.nih.gov/about/aging-strategic-directions-research/goal-health-interventions

National Institutes of Health. (2021). *Cultural respect.* https://www.nih.gov/institutes-nih/nih-office-director/office-communications-public-liaison/clear-communication/cultural-respect

Office of Disease Prevention and Health Promotion. (n.d.). *Healthy people 2030.* U.S. Department of Health and Human Services. https://health.gov/healthypeopleU.S

Parker, N., Schneegurt, M., Thi Tu, A.H., & Lister, P. (2021). *Characteristics and steps of Infectious diseases.* OpenStax. https:/bio.libretexts.org/@go/page/31850

U.S. Department of Health and Human Services. (n.d.). *Overall health and well-being measures.* https://health.gov/healthypeople/objectives-and-data/overall-health-and-well-being-measures

World Health Organization. (2023). *Health promotion.* https://www.who.int/westernpacific/about/how-we-work/programmes/health-promotion

World Health Organization. (n.d.). *Ageing and health.* https://www.who.int/news-room/fact-sheets/detail/ageing-and-health

Chapter 3

Ethical and legal considerations

Just the facts

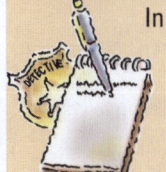

In this chapter, you'll learn:

♦ the significance of values and ethics in providing nursing care
♦ strategies to approach ethical dilemmas in patient care
♦ the nurse's roles and responsibilities to safeguard patients' rights
♦ the differences between intentional and unintentional torts.

Values

Values are attitudes, ideals, and beliefs an individual or group holds and uses to guide behaviors and decision-making (Poorchangizi et al., 2019). Values are sometimes expressed as what that individual or group considers right and what they consider wrong. Values are influenced by culture, family, environment, and religion (Habeeb, 2022). Professional values are standards for action that professional groups use to establish frameworks for evaluating behaviors. Some core nursing values are altruism, autonomy, integrity, and honesty (Poorchangizi et al., 2019). Values are crucial to developing ethical consciousness and guiding nurses in making important decisions. However, because values are highly individualized yet subject to influence from outside sources, it's not surprising that value conflicts are common among health care professionals.

Personal values

Clarifying personal values is an important part of developing professional ethics. A person may become more aware of their values by consciously reflecting on their behaviors (See *Developing values awareness*.)

Developing values awareness

Nurses, like all people, sometimes rely on hearsay, opinions, or prejudice instead of developing a strong sense of their own values. Sometimes, they don't stop to think about the values that are reflected in their conversation and behavior.

Consider the following dialogue in which three nurses express various value judgments. Think about the following questions:

What values does each nurse express? Do the values of the three conflict? Are individual nurses expressing consistent values? Do they show high regard for patient autonomy?

Shop talk

Kate: I can't believe it. I have to float to the ICU—and it's only my second week on the job. I hate floating, especially to intensive care.

Dean: So do I. The last time I floated to ICU, I was assigned to a 300-lb patient who had been driving drunk and wasn't wearing a seat belt. The guy was badly hurt, and I had to do all the positioning myself because the unit was so short-staffed. I just about killed my back. It isn't fair that they always assign male nurses to patients who are obese.

Pat: Floating is really a tough issue. I try to see it from the patient's side, though. I mean, maybe you were assigned to care for this patient because you're a good nurse and could give him the best care.

Kate: What bugs me is having to care for patients who obviously don't care about their own health. They don't watch their weight, they drive drunk, they don't use seat belts, and we get pulled from the work we're comfortable with to care for them. I can't even find time for a cigarette break.

Pat: Don't forget, Kate, we're supposed to take care of patients regardless of their health habits or lifestyle. No one's perfect, after all.

Kate: Yeah, I guess you're right, but floating makes me nervous anyway. I'm scared I'll really mess up because everything's so unfamiliar.

Dean: Let me give you some advice. No matter what you think about floating, don't say anything. If you're pegged as a complainer around here, your career is over.

Pat: You sound like you think nurses shouldn't ever speak out if something is wrong with the system. I think nurses do have the power to change things for the better, but that won't happen if we aren't willing to take some risks.

Dean: You're an idealist. I'm a realist. I ask, is it worth risking your job?

Pat: I think being a nurse means not being willing to compromise your standards of care just to keep a job.

Kate: What happened to the 300-lb patient? Is he still in ICU? Do you think I might get assigned to him?

Dean: Well, no. It's the craziest thing. We put all this time and effort into stabilizing his condition and keeping him infection-free, and one day, the health care provider decides to just turn everything off. Now I ask you, is that right?

Examining values

The nurses in this scenario make various moral judgments. By analyzing these types of conversations and attitudes, each nurse can better understand their own values:

- Kate criticizes the health habits of a trauma patient who is obese but insists on her own right to have time for a cigarette break. What values are guiding her opinions? Is her outlook consistent?

- Dean thinks that Kate should take an assignment for which she isn't prepared rather than risk losing favor with the administration. Is this attitude irresponsible or merely realistic?

- Pat is accused of being an idealist. Is that a fair judgment?

- What values are mirrored in each nurse's attitude about the practice of floating?

- At the end of the conversation, Dean mentions that the health care provider decided to withdraw treatment from the patient. If the three nurses were to discuss the ethical questions raised by the provider's decision, how do you think each nurse would respond?

- Would these three nurses have similar or conflicting views about what it means to be a patient advocate?

Values clarification

Each nurse and patient brings values to the health care system. These values include beliefs about such concepts as life, death, a higher power, organ transplantation, the right to die, and who should and shouldn't receive health care. The patient's values may change when faced with illness, injury, and possible death.

Values clarification refers to the process of raising consciousness so that value conflicts can be resolved (Witteman et al., 2021). You're likely to encounter many conflicting sets of values in the course of your professional career. To provide optimal support to the patient, you must undergo your own values clarification process.

First reflect…

Exercises, such as analyzing conversations between coworkers, offer one way to clarify values. Another approach is for the nurse to reflect on their own statements and actions.

…then choose…

You must choose among competing values to establish your own. Once your values are established, you can integrate them into your life and practice. This process prepares you to act on chosen values when confronted with difficult choices.

…and, finally, clarify

Making values decisions need not be haphazard. By clarifying your own values and checking to see if they're consistent with the established standards of the nursing profession, you can enhance your ability to make responsible judgments.

Ethics

Ethics is defined as conduct appropriate for all members of a group. It encompasses differentiating right conduct from wrong conduct (Haddad & Geiger, 2022). Health care workers today deal with many ethical issues. These issues involve protecting patient rights, balancing the demand to provide high-quality care, and managing costs with limited resources. There are six ethical principles in nursing. (See *Basic ethical principles*.)

OK, team, how would you handle a hypothetical situation like this…?

ETHICS DISCUSSION

PLATO   DESCARTES   HIPPOCRATES   ROUSSEAU

Codes of ethics

A code of ethics is a group of fundamental beliefs about what is morally right or wrong and reasons for maintaining those beliefs. It sets a central and necessary foundation for the profession's standards of behavior. A code of ethics includes main principles such as responsibility, accountability, advocacy, and confidentiality. Codes of ethics are revised periodically.

Two of the most important ethical codes for registered nurses are the ANA and Canadian Nurses Association codes (2017). The ANA *Code of Ethics for Nurses* (2015) guides the practicing nurse in using their professional skills to provide the most effective holistic care possible, such as serving as a patient advocate and striving to protect the health, safety, and rights of each patient. The International Council of Nurses (ICN, 2021), an organization based in Geneva, Switzerland, that seeks to improve the standards and status of nursing worldwide, has also published a code of ethics.

Basic ethical principles

Respect for human dignity is a primary ethical responsibility of nurses. It requires that each human be valued as a unique individual equal to all others and that all aspects of a person's life are appreciated. Respect for persons and dignity are the foundation of the six ethical principles in nursing.

Autonomy
Autonomy asserts that individuals have the right to determine their own actions and the freedom to make their own health care decisions. Respect for individuals is the core of the principle. Respect for autonomy refers to including patients in decisions about all aspects of their care.

Beneficence
Beneficence is the "doing of good," or taking positive actions toward others.

Nonmaleficence
Nonmaleficence is the duty to do no harm. The nurse must act with the intention of not causing intentional harm to a patient.

Justice
Justice refers to fairness. It implies that patients have a right to fair and impartial treatment. It means that no matter the characteristics of the patient (such as the patient's financial resources, age, ethnicity, or gender), they have the right to the same health care as any person with the same diagnosis.

Fidelity
Fidelity is the agreement to follow through with promises and commitments. For example, if the nurse tells a patient they will manage their pain, the nurse must follow through with actions to assess, intervene, and evaluate the pain management plan. When obtaining a nursing license, the nurse promises to remain qualified and competent to practice safely.

Veracity
Veracity is truth telling. Telling the truth is fundamental to developing and continuing trust among individuals (American Nurses Association [ANA], 2021).

Responsibility

Responsibility is respecting professional obligations. The nurse is responsible for their actions and those that they delegate. The nurse accepts responsibility for staying competent in practice.

Accountability

Accountability is the ability to answer for decisions, choices, and actions. It requires nurses to work within their scope of practice, comply with professional standards, use evidence to inform practice, and follow workplace policies.

Advocacy

Advocacy refers to supporting a particular cause. Causes can include the health, safety, and rights of patients, encompassing their right to privacy and their right to refuse treatment. Essentially, the nurse is championing the patient's voice. For example, although a nurse is not legally responsible for obtaining a patient's informed consent, the nurse is ethically responsible as the patient's advocate for reporting to the provider a patient's misunderstanding about treatment or withdrawal of consent. To be an effective advocate, a nurse must understand the ethical and legal principles of informed consent, including that the patient's consent is not valid unless they understand their condition, the proposed treatment, treatment alternatives, potential risks and benefits, and relative chances of success or failure.

Confidentiality

The Health Insurance Portability and Accountability Act (HIPAA) of 1996 was enacted in the spring of 2003 to strengthen and protect patient privacy. HIPAA mandates confidentiality and protects patients' personal health information, including information in the patient's medical record, conversations about the patient's care between health care providers, billing information, and the health insurer's computerized records (United States Department of Health and Human Services [USDHHS], 2021). In practice, information about a patient's medical condition can't be shared with those not involved in the patient's care.

Rights for All!

Under HIPAA, patients have the right to access their medical information, know when health information is shared, and make changes or corrections to their medical records. Patients also have the right to decide if they want to allow their information to be used for certain purposes, such as marketing or research (USDHHS, 2021). When patients receive health care, they must sign an authorization form before protected health information can be used for purposes other than routine treatment or billing. The form should be placed in the patient's medical record.

Privacy

Patient records with identifiable health information must be secured so that they aren't accessible to those who don't have a need for them. Identifiable health information may include the patient's name, Social Security number, medical record number, birth date, admission and discharge dates, and health history.

Social media

The advent of social networking has created many avenues to communicate both personally and professionally. However, the nature of social media poses some risks because it offers immediate sharing opportunities that allow little time for reflective thought. It also carries the added burden that items that are posted leave a digital footprint that can never truly be deleted. This can have both moral and ethical implications for all social media users. You can use social media in a positive way to share workplace experiences. Nevertheless, when interacting on social media as a nurse, you must remember patient privacy and consider the appropriateness of what is shared (National Council of State Boards of Nursing, 2018). Also, keep in mind that it is your responsibility to know your employer's policies regarding the use of social media in the workplace.

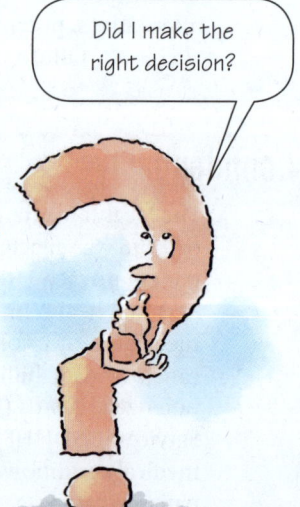

Did I make the right decision?

Ethical decisions

Every day, nurses make ethical decisions in their nursing practice. These decisions may involve patient care, actions related to coworkers, or nurse–provider relationships. At times, you may find yourself trapped in the middle of an ethical dilemma, pulled in every direction by your duties and responsibilities to your patient, your employer, and yourself. Even after you make a decision, you may ask yourself, "Did I make the right decision?"

It isn't automatic

There are no automatic solutions to all ethical conflicts. Although such conflicts may be painful and confusing, particularly in nursing, you don't have to have a philosophy degree to act ethically or to make decisions that fall within nursing's ethical codes. Nonetheless, you need to understand the principles of ethics that guide your nursing practice. Legally, nurses are responsible for using their knowledge and skills to protect the comfort and safety of their patients. Ethically, nurses, in their role as patient advocates, are responsible for safeguarding their patients' rights.

Ethical conflicts

Rapid advances in medical research have outpaced society's ability to solve the ethical problems associated with new health care technology. For nurses, ethical decision making in clinical practice is complicated by sociocultural factors, legal debates, growing professional autonomy, and consumer involvement in health care.

Decisions, decisions

Major areas of ethical conflict may include end-of-life decisions, determining medical futility, withholding or withdrawing treatment, advance directives, and organ donation. No matter what your nursing specialty, you'll probably encounter at least one of these conflicts during your nursing career.

Question of quality

It is sometimes difficult to determine what can be done to achieve a good quality of life and what can simply be achieved technologically speaking. Years ago, death was considered a natural part of life, and most people died at home, surrounded by their families. Today, most people die in hospitals, and death is commonly regarded as a medical failure rather than a natural event. Sometimes, it is hard for the nurse to know whether they are assisting in extending the patient's life or merely delaying the patient's death. To help with this issue, many inpatient facilities employ palliative care teams to assist with end-of-life decisions.

Consulting the committee

Most hospitals have ethics committees that review ethical dilemmas (see *The ethics committee*). The nurse may consider consulting the ethics committee if
- the health care provider disagrees with the patient or their family regarding treatment

The ethics committee

The ethics committee addresses ethical issues regarding the clinical aspects of patient care. It provides a forum for the patient, family, and health care providers to resolve conflicts.

The functions of an ethics committee include the following (Crico et al., 2020):
• policy development (such as developing policies to guide deliberations over individual cases)
• education (such as inviting guest speakers to visit and discuss ethical concerns)
• case consultation (such as debating the prognosis of a patient who's in a persistent vegetative state)
• addressing a single issue (such as reviewing all cases that involve a no-code or do-not-resuscitate [DNR] order)
• addressing problems of a specific population group (e.g., the American Academy of Pediatrics recommending that hospitals have a standing committee called the "infant bioethical review committee")
• addressing issues of organization ethics (such as business practice, marketing, admission, and reimbursement).

Pros and cons

If properly run, an ethics committee provides a safe outlet for voicing opposing views on emotionally charged ethical conflicts. The committee process can help lessen the bias that interferes with rational decision making. It enables members of disparate disciplines, including health care providers (doctors, nurse practitioners, physician assistants), nurses, clergy, social workers, hospital administrators, and ethicists, to express their views on treatment decisions.

Critics of the ethics committee think that committee decision making is too bureaucratic and slow to be useful in clinical crises and that one dominating committee member may intimidate others with opposing views. Furthermore, they contend that health care providers may view the committee as a threat to their autonomy in patient-care decisions. For these reasons, many ethics committees have a "rapid response team" of committee members who are on call to respond quickly in emergent ethical dilemmas. The rapid response team usually consists of three or four committee members who have had special training in negotiation and mediation. The entire committee will then review each case.

Selection of committee members

Ethics committees consist of members from various disciplines in the health care setting, including the patient's family, nurses, chaplains, physicians, social workers, and lawyers (Crico et al., 2020). The members should be diverse in their culture, skills, experiences, and knowledge. Committee members should be selected for their ability to work cooperatively in a group.

The nurse's role on a hospital ethics committee

Because of the nurse's close contact with the patient, their family, and other members of the health care team, the nurse is commonly in a position to identify ethical dilemmas, such as when a family is considering a DNR order for a relative. In many cases, the nurse is the first to recognize conflicts.

Before ethics committees were widely used, nurses had no official outlet for voicing their opinions in ethical debates. In many situations, health care providers made ethical decisions about patient care behind closed doors. Now, ethics committees provide nurses an avenue to express their views, hear the opinions of others, and understand more deeply the rationale behind ethical decisions.

• health care providers disagree among themselves about treatment options
• family members disagree about what should be done.

End-of-life decisions

End-of-life decisions are almost always difficult for patients, families, and health care professionals to make. Nurses are in a unique position as patient advocates assisting patients and their families through the process of death.

Your primary role as a patient advocate is to promote the patient's wishes. In many instances, however, the patient's wishes aren't known. That's when ethical decision making takes priority. Decisions aren't always easy to make, and the answers aren't usually clear-cut. At times, such ethical dilemmas may seem unsolvable.

Determining medical futility

Medical futility refers to treatment that isn't likely to benefit the patient, even though it may appear to be effective. For example, a patient with a terminal illness who's expected to die experiences cardiac arrest. Cardiopulmonary resuscitation (CPR) may be effective in restoring a heartbeat but may be deemed futile because it doesn't change the patient's outcome. CPR must be initiated unless written instruction otherwise was previously provided by the patient or if such information is included in the health care provider's order.

Withholding or withdrawing treatment

The issue of withholding or withdrawing treatment can certainly present some ethical dilemmas. When withdrawing treatment from a patient, even at the patient's request, controversy over the principle of *nonmaleficence* (to prevent harm) exists.

Harm alarm

Controversy can revolve around the definition of *harm*. Some feel that removing a patient from a ventilator and allowing death is an intentional infliction of harm. Others argue that keeping a person on a ventilator against the patient's will, thus prolonging death, is an intentional infliction of harm. (See *Approaching ethical decisions*.)

> Be advised . . . ethical dilemmas are chock-full of controversies.

Approaching ethical decisions

When you're faced with an ethical dilemma, consider these questions:
- What health issues are involved?
- What ethical issues are involved?
- What further information is necessary before a judgment can be made?
- Who will be affected by this decision? (Include the decision maker and other caregivers if they'll be affected emotionally or professionally.)
- What are the values and opinions of the people involved?
- What conflicts exist between the values and ethical standards of the people involved?
- Must a decision be made and, if so, who should make it?
- What alternatives are available?
- For each alternative, what are the ethical justifications?
- For each alternative, what are the possible outcomes?

Dealing with cardiac arrest

In cases of cardiac arrest (sudden stoppage of the heart), a critically ill patient may be described by a code status. Code status relates to the orders written by the health care provider describing what resuscitation measures should be carried out by the nurse. The orders are based on the patient's wishes regarding resuscitation measures. When cardiac arrest occurs, you must ensure that resuscitation efforts are initiated or that unwanted resuscitation doesn't occur.

Who decides?

The wishes of a competent, informed patient should always be honored. However, when a patient can't make decisions, the health care team—consisting of the patient's family, nursing staff, and health care providers—may have to make end-of-life decisions for the patient.

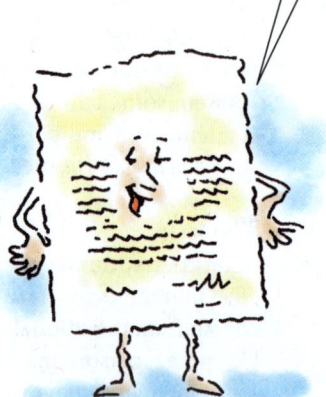

Remember, you're required by law to ask whether your patient has an advance directive or a durable power of attorney.

Advance directives

Most people prefer to make their own decisions regarding end-of-life care. It's important that patients discuss their wishes with their loved ones; however, many don't. Instead, total strangers may be asked to make important health care decisions when a patient can't do so. That's why it's important for people to make choices ahead of time and to make these choices known by completing an advance directive.

The Patient Self-Determination Act (1991) requires hospitals and other institutions to make information available to patients on advance directives. However, it isn't mandatory for patients to have an advance directive.

Where there's a will…

There are two types of advance directives:
- treatment directive, sometimes known as a *living will*
- appointment directive, sometimes known as a *durable power of attorney for health care.*

A living will identifies what treatments a patient will accept and refuse in case terminal illness renders the patient unable to make those decisions at the time. For example, a patient may be willing to accept artificial nutrition but not hemodialysis (House et al., 2022).

Durable power of attorney is the appointment of a person chosen by the patient to make decisions on the patient's behalf if the patient can no longer do so. A durable power of attorney for health care does not give the chosen individual authority to access business accounts; the power is strictly related to health care decisions.

After an advance directive is written, two witnesses must sign it. This document can be altered or canceled at any time. Laws can vary from state to state, so become familiar with procedures and laws in the state where you practice.

Organ donation

When asked, most people say they support organ donation. However, although tens of thousands of names are on waiting lists for organs in the United States alone, only a small percentage of qualified organs are ever donated. Organ transplantation is successful for many patients, giving them additional, high-quality years of life.

The National Organ Transplant Act (1984) governs the donation of organs and tissues. In addition, most states have legislation governing the procurement of organs and tissues. Some require medical staff to ask about organ donation on every death. Other states require the staff to notify a regional organ procurement agency that then approaches the family.

Medical criteria for organ donation vary from state to state. The following conditions usually preclude any organ or tissue donation:

- advanced age
- metastatic cancer
- history of hepatitis, HIV, or AIDS
- sepsis.

It is important for you to become familiar with the state laws and the policies where you practice. For example, many organ procurement agencies want to be notified of all deaths and imminent deaths so that they, not the medical staff, can determine whether the patient is a potential candidate for organ donation. Organ donation policies and laws may differ in each state.

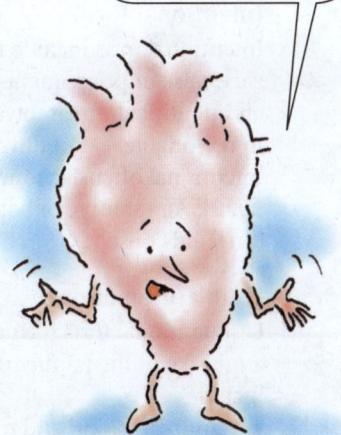

Learn about organ donation in your state. You're an important resource for patients and families making donation decisions.

Important discussions

When ethical problems arise, you need to discuss them candidly with all members of the health care team. Social workers, psychologists, clergy, and ethics committee members may also be involved to help resolve difficult ethical problems. A nurse who has a solid ethical understanding can be a resource to facilitate the decision-making process for the patient, family, and health care team.

Laws

Laws are binding rules of conduct enforced by authority. Ideally, laws are based on what's right and good. Realistically, though, the relationship between laws and ethics is complex. When a law is challenged as unjust or unfair, the challenge usually reflects some underlying clinical principle. Even so, there's a strong connection between ethics and laws regarding the nurse's role as a patient advocate.

Torts

A tort is an act or failure to act that is intentional, accidental, or negligent and causes harm to another person by violating a protected right (Ronquillo et al., 2022). Torts result in a civil trial to assess compensation for the plaintiff. Torts can be *intentional* or *unintentional*.

Intentional torts

Intentional torts include fraud, assault and battery, invasion of privacy, false imprisonment, and defamation of character. An assault is an intentional threat toward another person that places the person in reasonable fear of unwelcome contact. In contrast, battery is any intentional offensive touching without consent (Ronquillo et al., 2022). An example of battery would be performing a procedure without valid consent.

Unintentional torts

Unintentional torts include negligence and malpractice. *Negligence* is a mistake or the failure to be careful. Common sources of negligence include
- failure to assess and monitor a patient
- failure to notify the provider of significant changes in the patient's condition
- failure to give medications safely
- failure to properly delegate
- failure to follow policies.

Malpractice is defined as a professional person's wrongful conduct, improper discharge of professional duties, or failure to meet standards of care that results in harm to another person (Ronquillo et al., 2022). When nursing care falls below the standard of care, malpractice results. Several criteria are required to establish nursing malpractice, including a duty of care, a breach of the duty of care, failure of the nurse to meet the standard of care, and proven damage (Ronquillo et al., 2022).

Do no harm

Most malpractice suits result from a patient's dissatisfaction with care. When patients believe they haven't been treated with respect or dignity or that their needs and rights have been ignored or violated, they're more likely to initiate legal action. Keep in mind, however, that malpractice is more than an undesired outcome; for a patient to successfully file a malpractice lawsuit against a nurse, there must be evidence that some action or inaction that the nurse was obligated to perform resulted in harm to the patient (Ronquillo et al., 2022). Suppose the patient doesn't have compelling evidence; in that case, they may still file the suit, but the court may find it frivolous and it will generally be unsuccessful.

Regulation of nursing practice

The practice of nursing requires rules and regulations to ensure patient safety and a competent level of behavior in the professional role as a nurse. Nursing licensure allows practice as a professional nurse. Standards of nursing practice help ensure high-quality care and serve as criteria in legal questions of whether adequate care was rendered (ANA, 2021).

Licensure

Your nursing license entitles you to practice as a professionally qualified nurse. However, like most privileges, your nursing license imposes certain responsibilities. Registered nurses and licensed practical nurses are responsible for providing safe, quality care to patients. To meet this responsibility and protect the right to practice, nurses must understand the professional and legal significance of a nursing license.

Each nurse practice act contains licensing laws. They establish qualifications for obtaining and maintaining a nursing license. They also broadly define the legally permissible scope of nursing practice (ANA, 2021). Although they vary from state to state, most licensing laws specify:

- qualifications a nurse must have to be granted a license
- license application procedures for new licenses and reciprocal (state-to-state) licensing arrangements
- application fees
- authorization to use the title of Registered Nurse, Licensed Practical Nurse, or Vocational Nurse to applicants who receive their license
- grounds for license denial, revocation, or suspension
- license renewal procedures, including continuing education requirements.

Standards of nursing care

Standards of nursing care set minimum criteria for proficiency on the job, enabling each nurse to judge the quality of care provided (ANA, 2021). Standards of care reflect the knowledge and skills typically possessed and used by nurses actively practicing. States may refer to standards in their nurse practice act. Unless included in a nurse practice act, professional standards aren't laws but guidelines for sound nursing practice. You're expected to meet standards of nursing care for every nursing task you perform.

Legal issues affecting nursing

Nurses are faced with legal issues that may affect their nursing care. In the event of a malpractice lawsuit, a nurse's actual conduct is compared with nursing standards of care to determine whether the nurse acted in the same manner as a reasonably prudent nurse would act under the same circumstances. Common legal issues for nurses are related to patient rights, delegation, and documentation.

Patient rights

At one time, nurses were forbidden to give patients even the most basic information about their care or health, but in the 1960s, attitudes changed. Patients began demanding more information about their care and turned to nurses to assist them in getting the information.

Patient rights serve to protect patients when they seek health care. From the 1950s to the 1970s, the National League of Nursing and the American Hospital Association (AHA) conceptualized the Patient's Bill of Rights. Since that time, it has been modified and updated. The most recent version presented by the AHA, the Patient Care Partnership, defines a person's rights, such as respect for human dignity, privacy, confidentiality, and refusal of treatment (American Hospital Association, 2003).

Tell me all about it

The patient's bill of rights also ensures the patient's right to receive a full explanation of the cost of medical care, be fully informed, and be required to give consent before participating in experimental treatments because the patient exercises control over their own health care. These bills emphasize the patient's right to acquire information about all aspects of their care, including discharge education (American Hospital Association, 2003).

Informed consent

Being adequately informed about proposed treatment, procedures, surgery, or research in order to provide consent is a patient's legal right. The information included in the consent should be the risks, benefits, and alternatives of a procedure (Shah et al., 2022). So, it isn't surprising that the topic of informed consent appears in all current medical and nursing texts and that a signed informed consent form must be in the patient's records when invasive or experimental procedures, treatment, or surgery is anticipated.

You're free to provide patients with the information they need to give informed consent, but make sure it's within your scope of practice and nursing knowledge base to do so.

In the know

Informed consent means that the patient, or someone acting on their behalf, has enough information to know the risks related to undergoing the proposed treatment and the possible consequences if consent for the treatment is refused or withdrawn (Shah et al., 2022). Nurses may provide patients and their families with information that's within a nurse's scope of practice and knowledge base. However, a nurse shouldn't substitute their knowledge for a health care provider's knowledge and input.

Capacity to consent

Although the age of consent for medical care varies from state to state, typically, children under 16 years cannot provide informed consent; therefore, parents or legal guardians must consent to the treatment or interventions (Shah et al., 2022). Also, those with mental disorders may be held incompetent to consent. When there's a question about an individual's capacity to give consent, a legal determination may be sought from the appropriate court or an ethics committee. The bottom line in determining capacity is whether the person providing consent is impaired in their capacity or judgment to the extent that they do not understand the process and implications of treatment before it begins.

To assess the capacity to consent, a nurse may need to rely on their instincts as well as professional judgment. If the nurse believes the patient doesn't understand, they should reassess and discuss the consent issue with the patient, the guardian (if applicable), and the health care provider before the treatment begins.

Health Insurance Portability and Accountability Act

HIPAA protects the privacy, confidentiality, and security of all medical information. Patient information is available only to those who need it to provide care for the patient. Patients may also authorize others to have access to their information. These are the only groups who can lawfully receive oral, written, or electronic information. Failure to comply with HIPAA, intentionally or unintentionally, could result in criminal or civil penalties (USDHHS, 2021) (See *Patient rights under HIPAA*).

Patient rights under HIPAA

The goal of HIPAA is to provide safeguards against the inappropriate use and release of personal medical information, including all medical records and identifiable health information in any form (electronic, paper, and verbal). Patients are the beneficiaries of this privacy rule, which includes these rights:

1. The right to give consent before information is released for treatment, payment, or health care operations

2. The right to be educated about the provider's policy on privacy protection

3. The right to access their medical records

4. The right to request that their medical records be amended for accuracy

5. The right to access the history of nonroutine disclosures (disclosures that did not occur in the course of treatment, payment, or health care operations or those not specifically authorized by the patient)

6. The right to request that the provider restrict the use and routine disclosure of information. (Providers are not required to grant this request, especially if they think the information is important to the quality of patient care.)

Delegation

Delegation is giving another person the authority to act for another. It carries significant legal and safety issues in nursing practice. The nurse retains accountability and is legally liable for acts delegated to another person (ANA, 2015). The five delegation rights include the right *task*, the right *circumstance*, the right *person*, the right *direction/communication*, and the right *supervision/evaluation*.

Documentation

When a nurse accurately documents, it shows that the care provided meets the patient's needs and expressed wishes. It also supports that the nurse is following the accepted standards of nursing care mandated by the law, profession, and health care facility. Nurses should always document the nursing care provided, as well as the patient's response to that care.

Proper documentation communicates crucial information to caregivers, so they make fewer errors. The quality of documentation can determine whether the care provided will be communicated and understood in a court of law. Medical records are used as evidence in cases involving disability, personal injury, and mental competency. Poor documentation is the essential issue in many malpractice cases.

Quick quiz

1. Informed consent is an application of which ethical principle?
   A. Veracity
   B. Nonmaleficence
   C. Autonomy
   D. Beneficence

Answer: C. Autonomy involves including patients in all aspects of care, such as consenting to a procedure.

2. An example of an intentional tort would be:
   A. Failing to monitor a patient following surgery.
   B. Giving a medication without following the six rights of medication administration.
   C. Delegating medication administration to an unlicensed nursing assistant.
   D. Threatening to restrain a patient if they do not stop getting out of bed.

Answer: D. Threatening to restrain a patient is considered false imprisonment and is therefore an intentional tort. Other intentional torts include fraud, assault and battery, invasion of privacy, and defamation of character.

3. The Health Insurance Portability and Accountability Act (HIPAA) is responsible for which of the following?
   A. Mandating confidentiality about an individual's medical diagnosis.
   B. Ensuring hospitals make information about advance directives available to all patients.
   C. Developing rules and regulations for professional licensure.
   D. Identifying the rights of individuals to a clean and safe hospital room.

Answer: A. HIPAA mandates confidentiality about and protects patients' personal health information.

4. A nurse is caring for a patient with a terminal diagnosis who wants to stop treatment. However, the family requests every possible treatment to prolong life. The nurse contacts the health care provider to inform them of the patient's wishes. Which ethical code is the nurse utilizing?
   A. Advocacy
   B. Accountability
   C. Confidentiality
   D. Responsibility

Answer: A. Advocacy is standing up for the patient's desires.

Scoring

☆☆☆   If you answered all four questions correctly, bravo! Your understanding of ethical and legal issues is beyond reproach.

☆☆   If you answered three questions correctly, way to go! You've judged
correctly on most ethical and legal issues in this chapter.

☆   If you answered fewer than three questions correctly, don't fret! It
isn't grounds for malpractice. Review the chapter, and try again.

References

American Hospital Association (AHA). (2003). *The patient care partnership: Understanding expectations, rights, and responsibilities*. https://www.aha.org/system/files/2018-01/aha-patient-care-partnership.pdf

American Nurses Association (ANA). (2015). *Guide to the Code of Ethics for nurses with interpretive statements*. https://www.nursingworld.org

American Nurses Association (ANA). (2021). *Nursing scope and standards of practice* (4th ed.). https://www.nursingworld.org/practice-policy/scope-of-practice/

Canadian Nurses Association (CNA). (2017). *Code of ethics for registered nurses*. https://www.cna-aiic.ca/en/home

Crico C., Sanchini V., Casali P. G., & Pravettoni G. (2021). Evaluating the effectiveness of clinical ethics committees: A systematic review. *Med Health Care Philos, 24*(1), 135–151. https://link.springer.com/article/10.1007/s11019-020-09986-9

Habeeb S. (2022). Importance of professional values in nursing and healthcare. *Journal of Practical and Professional Nursing, 6*, 33. https//doi.org.10.24966/PPN-5681/100033

Haddad L. M., & Geiger R. A. (2022). *Nursing ethical considerations*. StatPearls. https://www.ncbi.nlm.nih.gov/books/NBK526054/

House S. A., Schoo C., & Ogilvie W. A. (2022). *Advance directives*. StatPearls. https://www.ncbi.nlm.nih.gov/books/NBK459133/

International Council of Nurses (ICN). (2021). *The ICN code of ethics for nurses*. https://www.icn.ch/system/files/2021-10/ICN_Code-of-Ethics_EN_Web_0.pdf

National Council of State Boards of Nursing (NCSBN). (2018). *A nurse's guide to the use of social media*. https://www.ncsbn.org/public-files/NCSBN_SocialMedia.pdf

National Organ Transplant Act, Public Law 98-507. (1984). https://www.govinfo.gov/content/pkg/STATUTE-98/pdf/STATUTE-98-Pg2339.pdf

Patient Self-Determination Act, 42, CFR 417. (1991). https://www.ecfr.gov/current/title-42/chapter-IV/subchapter-B/part-417

Poorchangizi B., Borhani F., Abbaszadeh A., Mirzaee M., & Farokhzadian J. (2019). The importance of professional values from nursing students' perspective. *BMC Nurs, 18*, 26, Article 26. https://doi.org/10.1186/s12912-019-0351-1

Ronquillo Y., Pesce M. B., & Varacallo M. (2022). *Tort*. StatPearls. https://www.ncbi.nlm.nih.gov/books/NBK441953/

Shah P., Thornton I., Turrin D., & Hipskind J. E. (2022). *Informed consent. StatPearls.* https://www.ncbi.nlm.nih.gov/books/NBK430827/

United States Department of Health and Human Services. (2021). *HIPPA for professionals.* Health Information Privacy. https://www.hhs.gov/hipaa/for-professionals/index.html

Witteman H. O., Ndjaboue R., Vaisson G., Dansokho S. C., Arnold B., Bridges J. F. P., Comeau S., Fagerlin A., Gavaruzzi T., Marcoux M., Pieterse A., Pignone M., Provencher T., Racine C., Regier D., Rochefort-Brihay C., Thokala P., Weernink M., White D. B., … Jansen J. (2021). Clarifying values: An updated and expanded systematic review and meta-analysis. *Med Decis Making,* 41(7), 801–820. https://doi.org/10.1177/0272989X211037946

Chapter 4

Nursing process

Just the facts

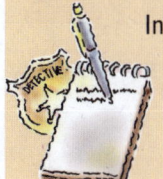

In this chapter, you'll learn:

◆ the five steps of the nursing process

◆ guidelines for performing an assessment based on the nursing process

◆ methods to prioritize patient problems and needs

◆ how to plan, implement, and evaluate nursing interventions.

A look at the nursing process

The nursing process is a systematic problem-solving approach to nursing care. Using the principles of critical thinking and clinical judgment, the nursing process determines the patient's priority problems, devises a plan to address them, implements the plan, and evaluates the effectiveness of the care provided (Toney-Butler & Thayer, 2023).

The nursing process emerged in the 1960s as team health care came into wider practice, and nurses were increasingly called upon to define their specific roles. However, the roots of the nursing process can be traced to World War II, when technology, medical advances, and a growing need for nurses began to transform the nursing profession (Taylor et al., 2023).

Step by step

The nursing process consists of five steps:
1. assessment
2. diagnosis/identification of patient needs
3. development of goals/plans
4. implementation
5. evaluation.

These five steps are dynamic and often overlap. Together, they resemble similar steps that many professions take to identify and correct problems.

Assessment

Assessment, the first step in the nursing process, begins when you first examine the patient. According to the American Nurses Association (n.d.) guidelines, the data collected should accurately reflect the patient's life experiences and patterns of living. Assessment continues throughout the nursing process as you obtain more information about the patient's evolving condition.

Getting the whole picture

During an assessment, you collect relevant information from various sources and use it to form a complete picture of your patient. As you collect the information, accurate documentation is imperative because:

- It guides you through the nursing process, helping you identify priority problems, set goals, plan, implement, and evaluate care.
- It serves as a vital communication tool for other team members, as a baseline for evaluating a patient's progress, and as legal documentation.

First impressions

During the initial assessment, consider the patient's immediate and emerging needs, including physical, psychological, spiritual, and social concerns. Gathering a patient's history is an essential first step in any assessment. Patient responses to questions asked about medications, health history, presentation, and reason for seeking care are extremely important.

After the history is established, you should complete a thorough physical assessment. The initial assessment helps you determine what care the patient needs and sets the stage for future assessments. The inferences you make from the data collected help to guide the plan of care. Remember that a patient's family, culture, and religion are important factors in the patient's response to illness and treatment.

Assessment types

There are four types of assessments. How they are used depends on the clinical situation, the time available, the purpose of the data collected, and the status of the patient.

Initial assessment

An initial, or admission, assessment occurs when the patient first comes to a health care setting. The initial assessment helps to determine what care the patient needs and sets the stage for further assessments. The most important item to determine is the reason the patient is seeking care. Gathering background information is crucial.

Focused assessment

A focused assessment is used to collect data about a specific problem that has been identified. The nurse must determine if the problem still exists and whether the status of the problem has improved, worsened, or resolved.

Time-lapsed reassessment

Time-lapsed reassessment takes place after the initial assessment and intervention to evaluate changes in the client's functional health. This type of assessment occurs on set intervals that can last a few hours up to a few months. Similar to a focused assessment, it is used to determine the status of already identified problems. Time-lapsed assessment may involve periodic outpatient clinic visits, health developmental screenings, or home care visits.

Emergency assessment

An emergency assessment occurs during a life-threatening situation. Rapid identification of and interventions for the patient's health problem is the primary goal. During an emergency assessment, the patient's priority problem usually centers on the patient's ABCDEs (airway, breathing, circulation, disability, and exposure/environmental control) (Peate & Brent, 2021). An emergency assessment is not a comprehensive assessment.

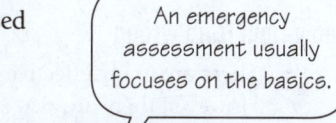

An emergency assessment usually focuses on the basics.

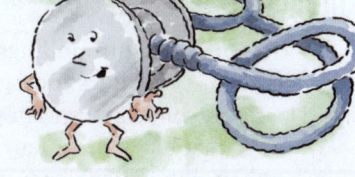

Health history

A health history includes physical, psychological, cultural, spiritual, and psychosocial data. It is the main source of information about the patient's health status and guides the physical examination that follows.

The history helps to:
- plan health care by anticipating needs
- assess the impact of illness on the patient and members of their family
- evaluate the patient's health education needs
- initiate discharge planning.

Effective techniques

Before collecting the health history, attempt to build rapport with the patient to ensure that they feel comfortable and respected. Use effective interview techniques to help the patient identify resources and improve problem-solving abilities. Remember, successful techniques for one situation may not be effective for another. Your approach and the patient's interpretation of your questions may vary. In general, you should:

- allow the patient time to think and reflect
- encourage the patient to talk
- encourage the patient to describe a particular experience
- indicate listening by paraphrasing the patient's response
- ask specific questions related to the patient's condition, history of present illness, and chief complaint.

Know right from wrong

There are many effective ways to communicate with a patient. However, there are also some approaches that can hinder the interview process. (See *Interview techniques to avoid*.)

Conducting an interview

The physical surroundings, psychological atmosphere, interview structure, and questioning style can all impact the interview flow and outcome, and so can your ability to adopt a communication style that fits your patient's needs and the situation at hand. To enhance the interview process, close the door to help prevent interruptions and face the patient to create an attentive and welcoming atmosphere.

Interview techniques to avoid

Some interview techniques cause problems between the nurse and patient. You should avoid:

- asking "why" or "how" questions
- asking probing or persistent questions
- using inappropriate language
- giving advice
- giving false reassurance
- changing the subject or interrupting
- using clichés or stereotypical responses
- giving excessive approval or agreement
- jumping to conclusions
- minimizing the patient's feelings
- using defensive responses.

Start by introducing yourself, then establish an interview time-frame and ask whether the patient has questions about the interview procedure. If time permits, spend a few minutes chatting informally before beginning the interview.

A note on notes

Lengthy note-taking may distract the patient. If you must take notes, tell the patient before the interview starts. Finish the interview by summarizing significant interview points, telling the patient the interview results, explaining how the physical assessment will be conducted, and discussing follow-up plans.

Be sure to be attentive while collecting information. Lengthy note-taking may distract the patient.

Short and sweet

A patient who is ill, experiencing pain, or sedated may have difficulty completing the health history. In such instances, obtain only the information pertaining to the immediate problem. To avoid tiring a seriously ill patient, obtain the history in several sessions or ask a close family relative or friend to supply essential information. However, because of Health Insurance Portability and Accountability Act (HIPAA) policies, personal information cannot be disclosed to family members or friends without consent of the patient (United States Department of Health and Human Services [USDHHS], 2021).

Open and closed

Typically, a health history includes two types of questions: open-ended, which encourage more subtle and flexible responses, and closed-ended, which require a yes-or-no response. Open-ended questions usually result in the most useful information and give patients the feeling that they're actively participating in and have some control over the interview. Closed-ended questions are useful when the interview requires brevity, for example, when a patient reports extreme pain or digresses frequently. No matter the type of questions you use, move logically from one history section to the next. Allow the patient to concentrate and give complete information on a subject before moving on.

Primary and secondary sources

There are two sources of data: primary and secondary. The patient is the primary source of data; data collected directly from the patient is considered the most reliable type of data. Unless circumstances prevent it, you should always collect information directly from the patient. Patients who have an altered level of consciousness, memory issues, or are in severe pain may be unreliable primary sources.

Secondary sources provide information that supports, validates, clarifies, and supplements the information gathered from the patient. These sources typically include family members, significant others, laboratory results, the health care record, diagnostic procedures, and health team members.

Biographic data

Begin obtaining the patient's health history by collecting personal information. This data section identifies the patient and provides important demographic information. The patient may fill out a form to gather information, including address, telephone number, age, gender, birth date, Social Security number, place of birth, ethnicity, marital status, occupation, education, religion, cultural background, and emergency contact person.

Health and illness patterns

Health and illness patterns include the patient's chief complaint; current, past, and family health history; status of physiologic systems; and developmental considerations.

Mind their P's and Q's

Determine why the patient is seeking health care by asking, "What brings you here today?" If the patient has specific symptoms, record that information in the patient's own words. Ask the patient with a specific symptom or health concern to describe the problem in detail, including the suspected cause. To ensure that you don't omit pertinent data, use the OPQRSTU mnemonic device, which provides a systematic approach to obtaining information. (See *OPQRSTU: What is the story?*)

Think back

Be sure to document the patient's whole history, including childhood and other illnesses, injuries, previous hospitalizations, surgical procedures, immunizations, allergies, and medications taken regularly. Information about the patient's past and current physiologic status (also called *review of systems*) is an essential health history component and helps identify potential or undetected physiologic disorders.

Tell me about your family

Information about the patient's relatives can reveal potential health problems. Some diseases, such as cardiovascular disease, alcoholism, depression, and cancer, may be genetically linked.

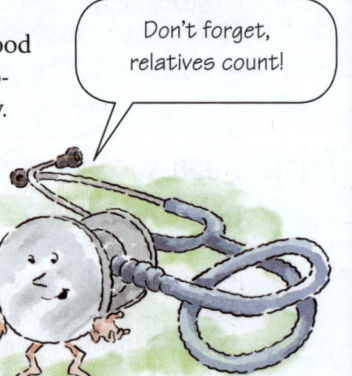

Don't forget, relatives count!

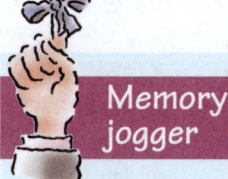

Memory jogger

What's the story?

Use the **OPQRSTU** mnemonic device to fully explore your patient's chief complaint. When you ask the questions below, you'll encourage the patient to describe their symptoms in greater detail.

	Questions for the patient
Onset	• When did the symptom start? • How long has it been going on?
Provocative or Palliative	• What provokes or relieves the symptom? • Does stress, anger, certain physical positions, or other things trigger the symptom? • What makes the symptom worsen or subside?
Quality or Quantity	• What does the symptom feel like, look like, or sound like? • Are you having the symptom right now? If so, is it more or less severe than usual? • To what degree does the symptom affect your normal activities?
Region or Radiation	• Where in the body does the symptom occur? • Does the symptom appear in other regions? If so, where?
Severity	• How severe is the symptom? How would you rate it on a scale of 1–10, with 10 being the most severe? • Does the symptom seem to be diminishing, intensifying, or staying the same?
Timing	• When did the symptom begin? • Was the onset sudden or gradual? • How often does the symptom occur? • How long does the symptom last?
Understanding	• What do you think caused the symptom? • How do you feel about the symptom? Do you have fears associated with it? • How is the symptom affecting your life? • What are your expectations from the health care team?

Others, such as hemophilia, cystic fibrosis, sickle cell anemia, and Tay–Sachs disease, are genetically transmitted.

Determine the general health status of the patient's immediate biological family members, including grandparents, siblings, aunts, uncles, and children. If any of them are deceased, record the year and cause of death. Use a genogram to record and organize family history data (see *Developing a genogram*).

Developing a genogram

A genogram provides a visual family health summary. It includes the patient and their spouse, children, and parents. To develop a genogram, first draw the relationships of family members to the patient, as shown, and then fill in the ages of living members and note deceased members and the ages at which they died. Additionally, record diseases that have a familial tendency (such as Huntington chorea) or an environmental cause (such as lung cancer from exposure to coal tar).

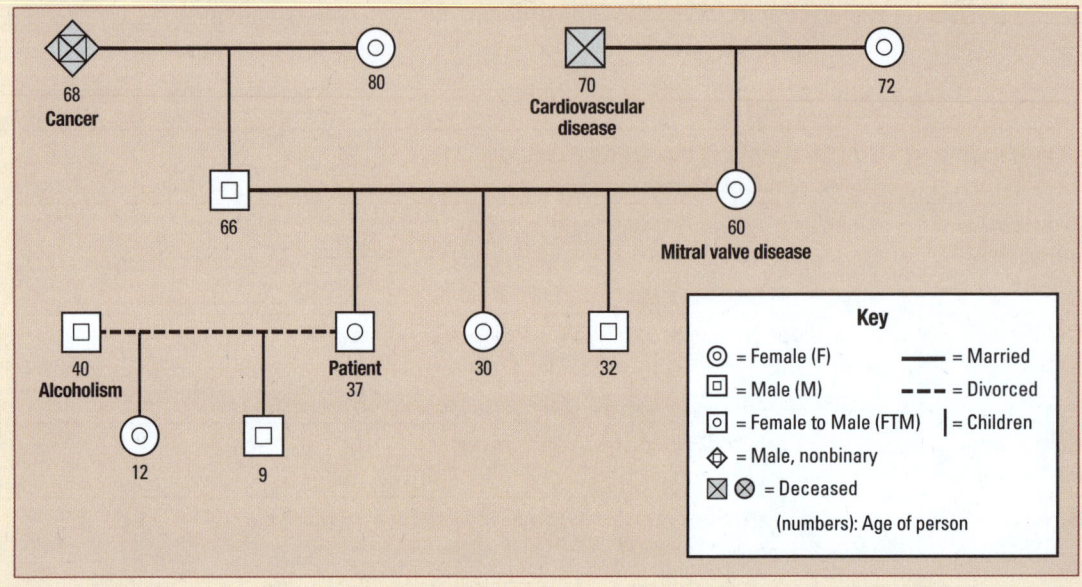

There are times and situations when there is not enough time for a genogram. If this is the case, the nurse must focus on questions about the family based on the patient's current health issue. For example, if a patient presents with cardiac chest pain as a 40-year-old, it would be pertinent to ask about any family member who may have a history of heart problems.

Physical examination

The second half of the assessment process involves performing a physical examination. Use the following techniques to conduct the examination:

- inspection
- palpation
- percussion
- auscultation.

There is one exception to this rule, the abdominal assessment. With this assessment, auscultation comes before palpation and percussion.

The objective data gathered during the physical examination may be used to confirm or rule out health problems that were suggested or suspected during the health history. You focus on these findings to plan and implement care and conduct patient teaching. For example, if the patient's blood pressure is high, they may need a low-sodium diet and instruction on how to regulate hypertension.

It's all in the details

The level of detail in the physical examination depends on the patient's condition, the clinical setting, and your facility's policies and procedures. The main components of the physical examination include:
- height and weight
- vital signs
- review of the major body systems. (See *Rapid review of the physical assessment.*)

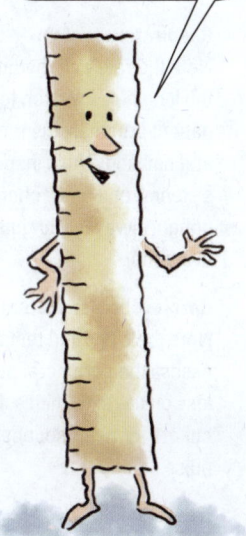

Besides measuring height and weight and taking vital signs, remember to review major body systems.

Problem–based care plans

The development of critical thinking skills and clinical judgment has become a major focus in the profession of nursing over the past decade (National Council of State Boards of Nursing [NCSBN], 2023). With this shift, the nursing process and nursing care have also evolved. The nursing process continues to be the framework for planning nursing care, with a shift to problem-based care plans. Similar to other methods of care planning, the steps for problem-based care plans include:
1. identifying patient problems/needs
2. prioritizing patient problems/needs
3. planning
4. implementation
5. evaluation.

Identifying and prioritizing

After you complete the patient assessment, it is important to analyze the collected data. The steps in this process, modeled to reflect critical thinking and clinical judgment, are as follows (NCSBN, 2023):

Rapid review of the physical assessment

During a physical examination, your main task is to record the patient's height, weight, and vital signs and review the major body systems. Here's a typical body system review for an adult patient.

Respiratory system

Note the rate and rhythm of respirations, and auscultate the lung fields. Watch for flaring or retractions as the patient breathes. Inspect the lips, mucous membranes, and nail beds. Also inspect the sputum, noting color, consistency, and other characteristics. If the patient has a cough, always distinguish whether the cough is productive or dry.

Cardiovascular system

Note the color and temperature of the extremities, and assess the peripheral pulses. Check for edema and hair loss on the extremities. Inspect the neck veins, and auscultate for heart sounds. Assess for regularity of apical pulse.

Neurologic system

Assess the patient's level of consciousness, noting their orientation to time, place, and person and their ability to follow commands. Assess pupillary reaction and accommodation (pupils equal, round, reactive to light, and accommodation [PERRLA]). Check the extremities for movement and sensation. Check grip strength bilaterally.

Eyes, ears, nose, and throat

Assess the patient's ability to see objects with and without corrective lenses. Assess their ability to hear spoken words clearly. Inspect the eyes and ears for discharge and the nasal mucous membranes for dryness, irritation, and blood. Inspect the teeth, gums, and condition of the oral mucous membranes, and palpate the lymph nodes in the neck.

Gastrointestinal system

Before starting the abdominal assessment, ask if the patient has any abdominal pain. If pain is present, assess that area last to avoid guarding through the assessment. Ask the patient to empty their bladder prior to the abdominal assessment. Auscultate for bowel sounds in all quadrants. Note abdominal distention or ascites. Gently palpate the abdomen for tenderness. Note whether the abdomen is soft, hard, or distended. Assess the condition of the mucous membranes around the anus.

Musculoskeletal system

Assess the range of motion of major joints. Look for swelling at the joints, contractures, muscle atrophy, or obvious deformity. Assess muscle strength of the trunk and extremities. Assess posture and gait.

Genitourinary and reproductive systems

Note any bladder distention or incontinence. If indicated, inspect the genitalia for rashes, edema, or deformity. (Inspection of the genitalia may be waived at the patient's request or if no dysfunction was reported during the interview.) If indicated, inspect the genitalia for sexual maturity. Also examine the breasts, noting any abnormalities. When taking a history, it is important to ask about the patient's sexual activity.

Integumentary system

Note any sores, lesions, scars, pressure ulcers, rashes, bruises, discoloration, or petechiae. Also note the patient's skin turgor.

Source: Jensen, S., & Servello, D. (2023). *Nursing health assessment: A clinical judgment approach* (4th ed.). Wolters Kluwer.

1. **Group significant data into logical clusters.** The patient's needs will not be based on a single sign or symptom but rather on a cluster of assessment findings.
2. **Identify data gaps or conflicting data.** Determine data and cues that do not fit into consistent patterns. Clarify information that conflicts with other assessment findings and determine what is causing the inconsistency.
3. **Recognize and analyze cues and trends in the assessment findings.** By analyzing and identifying patterns, the nurse can form a hypothesis about the patient's problems and needs and how to prioritize them.

Lippincott problem–based taxonomy

Once the patient's problems and needs have been identified and analyzed, the Lippincott Advisor Problem-Based Taxonomy can be used to classify patient problems and needs in a uniform and meaningful way (see the appendix, page 658). The problems found in the taxonomy are straightforward and translate readily into nursing care.

Validate

Once a problem is selected from the taxonomy, it is important to validate the choice. Review all clustered cues and data. Are they consistent? Do the patient findings confirm the choice? If not, it may be time to review the data and make a new choice.

Prioritize

After you've established the patient's problems and needs, several nursing diagnoses, categorize them in order of priority. Life-threatening problems must be addressed first, followed by health-threatening concerns. Also, consider how the patient perceives their health problems; their priorities may differ from yours. In addition, as the patient's condition changes, their priorities may change.

Maslow's hierarchy of needs

Maslow's hierarchy of needs (see box in Chapter 1 on page 19) classifies human needs based on the idea that lower-level, physiologic needs must be met before higher-level, abstract needs (Maslow, 1958). This framework can be useful when prioritizing nursing care. For example, if a patient has shortness of breath, they probably aren't interested in discussing family support systems. However, as the patient's breathing issues improve, their main concern may shift to who will provide support as they transition home.

Planning

After you've established and prioritized patient problems and needs, you'll develop a written plan of care. Putting the plan in writing enables it to serve as a communication tool among health care team members that helps ensure continuity of care. The plan consists of two parts:
1. Goals: Clearly defined goals describe results and behaviors to be accomplished within a specified timeframe.
2. Interventions: After you establish goals, you need to develop evidence-based nursing interventions to address patient needs and problems.

"SMART" measurement

Goals are required to develop the planning, implementation, and evaluation parts of a care plan. These goals should be specific, measurable, achievable, realistic, and time oriented (SMART). Defining goals that are SMART help to keep the entire care team on the same page (Doran, 1981). This process helps to streamline nursing care and gives the team a uniform method to evaluate the patient. (See *Make it SMART*.)

Make it SMART

The SMART acronym was created in the 1980s for use in corporate America. Since then, it has been adapted for use in the nursing profession. SMART goals help organize efforts and consequently improve chances of success. The letters in SMART stand for:

S: Specific—clearly state the desired result

M: Measurable—quantify observable markers of progress

A: Achievable—identify any barriers and a plan to address them

R: Realistic—determine if results can be achieved with resources available

T: Time oriented—specify when results should be achieved.

A SMART goal before and after:

BEFORE (not SMART): "The patient will stretch regularly."

AFTER (SMART): "The patient will attend a 30-minute yoga class 4 times a week for the next 2 months."

Source: Doran, G. T. (1981). There's a S.M.A.R.T. way to write management's goals and objectives. *Management Review, 70*(11), 35–36. https://community.mis.temple.edu/mis0855002fall2015/files/2015/10/S.M.A.R.T-Way-Management-Review.pdf

Intervention options

Before you implement a care plan explore evidence-based nursing interventions. Interventions based on the most recent evidence help to provide care that is uniform and improve safety, quality, and overall patient well-being (Adjoa-Kumah et al., 2022). Although nursing interventions should be based on evidence, within these parameters it is important to tailor them to fit each patient's specific needs. Additional considerations should include the patient's willingness to participate in the interventions, if the necessary equipment and resources are available, and preparations that would be needed to postpone or modify interventions, if required.

Implementation

The implementation phase is when you put your care plan into action. Implementation encompasses all nursing interventions directed at solving the patient's problems and meeting health care needs. Although as the nurse you coordinate implementation, you also seek help from the patient, the patient's family, and health care team members.

Monitor and gauge

After implementing the nursing process and plan of care, continue to monitor the patient to gauge the effectiveness of interventions and adjust as the patient's condition changes. Document each step of the process; this is essential because it serves as a record for all health care team members. Expect to review, revise, and update the entire plan of care regularly, according to facility policy. Remember that the plan is usually a permanent part of the patient's medical record.

Evaluation

Evaluation is a critical step in the process of nursing care. This step occurs after the nursing interventions have had time to impact the patient and their problems and needs. Evaluation is the process of deciding whether the selected interventions have enabled the patient to achieve the defined goals.

Start with the finish

Begin by reviewing patient goals for each patient problem or need. Observe and assess behavioral changes to judge how well the patient meets the related goals. Does the patient's behavior match these goals or fall short? Evaluation reveals patient progress and where alterations can be made. This step encourages you to reevaluate the plan and to use the nursing process to move forward with a new or different plan.

A successful resolution

The evaluation phase also allows you to judge the effectiveness of the nursing process as a whole. If the process has been applied successfully, the patient's health status will improve. Their health problems will have been addressed, and progress will have been made toward achieving optimum health. The patient will also be able to perform self-care measures with a sense of independence and confidence.

Concept mapping

Concept mapping is a way to show the flow of your critical thinking during patient care. Concept mapping allows students and nurses alike to see and understand the connections and thought processes of others. Concept maps show relationships between important concepts that are required to provide skillful and informed nursing care to patients (Schuster, 2020).

Unlike formal care planning, concept maps are developed using graphical or pictorial representations of concepts. After concepts are established, lines are used to identify relationships and links. The beauty of a concept map is that it allows the team to see the big picture when caring for patients (Schuster, 2020). See *Putting it together: Using a concept map* for an example concept map.

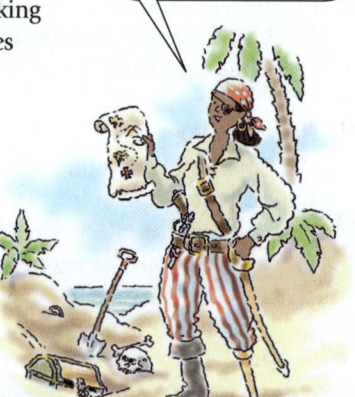

Concept mapping is a creative way to develop critical thinking skills.

Interdisciplinary team

Nurses aren't the only health care professionals involved in patient care. You'll need to collaborate with the interdisciplinary team to meet the diverse needs of your patient.

Share and share alike

The focus of an interdisciplinary team is on the patient and their goals. To provide more effective and comprehensive care, you need to understand each team member's role.

Putting it together: Using a concept map

A concept map can guide a nursing student's clinical day or help a nurse organize and conceptualize nursing care. For example, connections can be made between supplemental oxygen, vital signs, and activity intolerance in a patient with chronic obstructive pulmonary disease. Utilizing a concept map allows you to see relationships at a glance. After you plug in the basic information, you can add other elements such as laboratory values, medications, and assessment findings (Schuster, 2020).

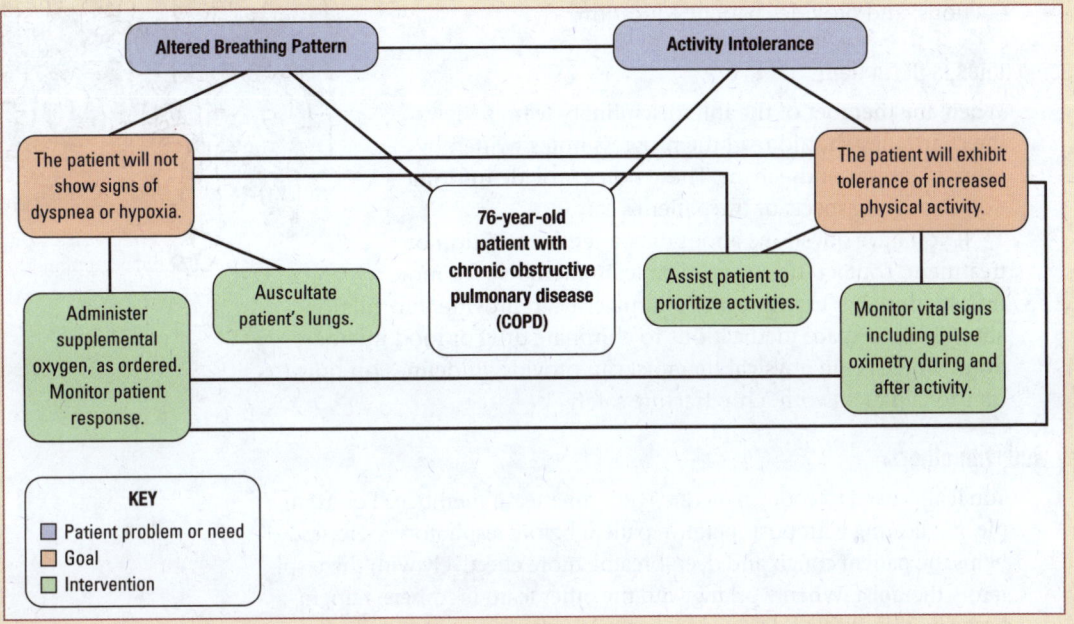

Members of the health care team include:

- **Health care provider:** can be a physician, nurse practitioner, or physician assistant. These professionals make decisions about the diagnosis and treatment of the patient
- **Registered dietitian:** assesses and monitors nutritional needs, makes nutritional recommendations, and provides patient education
- **Social worker:** provides support and counseling to patients and their families and helps with financial difficulties
- **Occupational therapist:** assists the patient in performing activities of daily living, participating in recreation, and working to their highest functional level

- **Physical therapist:** provides therapy to improve or restore physical functioning and prevent deconditioning
- **Respiratory therapist:** monitors and provides airway management
- **Pastoral care specialist:** provides spiritual and religious support to patients and their families
- **Pharmacist:** reviews, prepares, and dispenses the patient's medications; provides information and guidance in the preparation and administration of medications; and provides patient education.

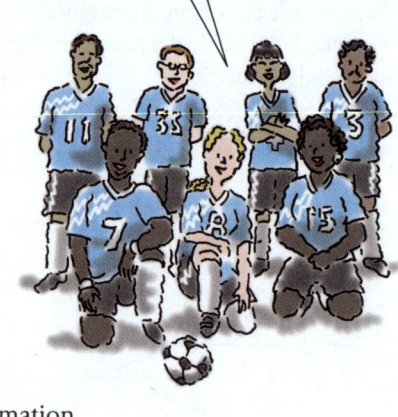

Interdisciplinary teamwork gets the job done!

Passing notes is permitted!

When any member of the interdisciplinary team reviews the chart, they should read the progress notes written by other members of the team. These notes provide information about all aspects of the patient's care.

If you have questions about the patient's condition or treatment, contact the appropriate team members for more information. For example, the pharmacist can provide information about how to space medications to eliminate drug or food interactions, whereas the physical therapist can provide guidelines on how to transfer a patient with a hip fracture safely.

Play well with others

You'll also need to coordinate care with other team members. For example, medicating your postoperative patient before respiratory exercises helps the patient cough and deep-breathe more effectively with the respiratory therapist. When working with the other team members, remember to be respectful and to use professional communication skills.

Quick quiz

1. The nurse is conducting an interview with a patient. What is one communication technique that should be used?
    A. giving advice
    B. asking persistent questions
    C. giving reassurance
    D. jumping to conclusions

Answer: C. Giving the patient reassurance helps to build rapport.

2. When exploring the patient's chief complaint, the nurse uses the OPQRSTU mnemonic. What does the "S" stand for?
    A. Significant
    B. Severity
    C. Systemic
    D. Strength

Answer: B. The "S" in the OPQRSTU mnemonic stands for severity.

3. The nurse is using SMART goals to build a patient's plan of care. The nurse knows that the "M" in SMART stands for:

    A. Measurable

    B. Meaningful

    C. Motivational

    D. Mindful

Answer: A. The "M" in SMART stands for Measurable.

4. After the patient's problems have been identified, the nurse then reviews all collected assessment data to see if it confirms the choice of patient problems. What is this process called?

    A. Intervention

    B. Evaluation

    C. Assessment

    D. Validation

Answer: D. Validation occurs when the nurse confirms that the data collected are consistent and confirm the choice of patient problems.

Scoring

☆☆☆ If you answered all four questions correctly, super! You're a nursing process pro.

☆☆ If you answered three questions correctly, great! You've got the nursing process pretty down pat.

☆ If you answered fewer than three questions correctly, chin up! Process this chapter one more time and try again.

References

American Nurses Association (ANA). (n.d.). *The nursing process.* https://www.nursingworld.org/practice-policy/workforce/what-is-nursing/the-nursing-process/

Doran, G. T. (1981). There's a S.M.A.R.T. way to write management's goals and objectives. *Management Review, 70*(11), 35–36. https://community.mis.temple.edu/mis0855002fall2015/files/2015/10/S.M.A.R.T-Way-Management-Review.pdf

Jensen, S., & Servello, D. (2023). *Nursing health assessment: A clinical judgment approach* (4th ed.). Wolters Kluwer.

Kumah, E. A., McSherry, R., Bettany-Saltikov, J., & van Schaik, P. (2022). Evidence-informed practice: Simplifying and applying the concept for nursing students and academics. *British Journal of Nursing, 31*(6), 322–330. https://www.britishjournalofnursing.com/content/professional/evidence-informed-practice-simplifying-and-applying-the-concept-for-nursing-students-and-academics/

Maslow, A. H. (1958). A dynamic theory of human motivation. In Stacey, C. L., & DeMartino, M. (Eds.), *Understanding human motivation* (pp. 26–47). Howard Allen Publishers. https://doi.org/10.1037/11305-004

National Council of State Boards of Nursing (NCSBN). (2023). *Clinical judgment measurement model: A framework to measure clinical judgment and decision making.* https://www.nclex.com/clinical-judgment-measurement-model.page

Peate, I., & Brent, D. (2021). Using the ABCDE approach for all critically unwell patients. *Healthcare Assistants, 15*(2):57–102. https://doi.org/10.12968/bjha.2021.15.2.84

Schuster, P. M. (2020). *Concept mapping: A clinical judgment approach to patient care* (5th ed.). F.A. Davis Company.

Taylor, C., Lynn, P., & Bartlett, J. (2023). *Fundamentals of nursing: The art and science of person-centered care* (10th ed.). Wolters Kluwer.

Toney-Butler, T., & Thayer, J. (2023). *Nursing process. StatPearls.* StatPearls Publishing. https://www.ncbi.nlm.nih.gov/books/NBK499937/

United States Department of Health and Human Services (USDHHS). (2021). *HIPAA for professionals.* https://www.hhs.gov/hipaa/for-professionals/index.html

Part II

General nursing skills

Chapter 5

Communication

Just the facts

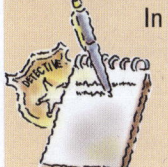

In this chapter, you'll learn:

◆ verbal and nonverbal methods of communication

◆ the phases of a therapeutic relationship

◆ how to incorporate therapeutic use of self

◆ how to identify and handle communication barriers

◆ the importance of communication in documenting patient care.

A look at communication

What is communication? Communication is a way to fulfill a person's basic need to relate to others. Communication is dynamic and ongoing and is a way to interact and develop relationships. It is also a way to effect change.

Nurses encounter many people during the course of their education and nursing career. They communicate with educators, patients, family members, and other members of the health care team. Learning to communicate effectively is a skill that sometimes takes time and effort (Taylor et al., 2023).

Verbal communication

Verbal communication is the transmission of messages through spoken or written language. For effective verbal communication, six criteria must be met:
- simplicity
- clarity
- timing and relevance
- adaptability
- credibility

Simplicity

In verbal communication, complex information should be stated in commonly understood terms, based on the level of comprehension. This is especially important when communicating with patients. For instance, when explaining a procedure to the patient, be careful to use terminology the patient will understand. Use short sentences that express the idea completely. Long explanations are sometimes difficult for people to understand because the context of the explanation gets lost.

Nix the jargon

Use terms appropriately to the patient's level of understanding; avoid using jargon and complex medical terms. Offer explanations in lay terms, and then use the related medical terms, if appropriate, so the patient can become familiar with them. For instance, if you ask a patient "Do you have to void?" they may not understand you're asking if they need to use the bathroom facilities. Instead, ask the patient if they have to urinate or go to the bathroom. Use words the patient is familiar with and that are appropriate to the level of comprehension.

Clarity

Verbal communication must be clear. Don't make the listener guess what you mean or make assumptions. For instance, if you're explaining a medication regimen to a patient who has never taken medicine before, don't tell them they must take the medication four times per day. Instead, be clear and tell the patient exactly how many hours should elapse before taking each dose of the medication.

Communicate in a respectful manner to maintain a hostile-free environment. Talk *to* the patient, not *at* them. Tell the patient how long the process will take. Always address an adult patient by their legal name, avoid using first names and nicknames. You may ask the patient their preferred name and how they would like to be addressed (Myrick & Karosas, 2021). Be patient, relaxed, and unhurried. If the patient has a visual or hearing impairment, make sure their glasses or hearing aid are accessible for them to use.

Early in the interview, try to evaluate the patient's ability to communicate and their reliability as a historian. If language poses a problem, enlist the aid of an interpreter. If you have doubts about what the patient is saying, before the interview proceeds further consider asking whether a family member or friend can be present or the patient might request that such a person assist them. Having another person present gives the nurse a chance to observe the patient's interaction with this person and provides more data for the history. However, the presence of another person may prevent the patient from speaking freely, so plan to talk with the patient privately at some time during the assessment.

Be concise and rephrase

Provide carefully structured questions to elicit significant information. Keep questions concise, rephrase those the patient doesn't understand, and use such nonverbal techniques as facial expressions, pointing, and touching to enhance meaning when appropriate.

To foster your patient's cooperation, take a little extra time to help them see the relevance of the questions. Repeating or explaining several times during the interview may be necessary. Give the patient plenty of time to respond to questions and directions (Taylor et al., 2023).

Timing and relevance

Make sure that the message is communicated at a time when the receiver is ready to receive it. If the patient is in pain, don't try to explain a procedure or provide teaching; the patient will be more receptive to communication when the pain subsides.

Score one for format!

Ensure the message is communicated in an appropriate format. If the patient has trouble visualizing what you're saying, try using written materials or diagrams to complement your verbal explanation; this will help them to understand better.

Adaptability

Communication that is effective is adaptable and states a message that reflects the situation. For instance, if you have a patient who speaks another language or who has a hearing or visual impairment, you should use interpreter services to communicate with them or employ other strategies. (See *Overcoming communication obstacles*.)

Overcoming communication obstacles

If a patient doesn't speak English or has difficulty understanding it, the facility/clinic likely has a group of interpreters and/or an interpretation service that can be called on for help. A trained medical interpreter—one who is familiar with medical terminology, knows interpreting techniques, and understands the patient's rights—would be ideal. Be sure to tell the interpreter to translate the patient's speech verbatim.

Avoid using one of the patient's family members or friends as an interpreter. Doing so violates the patient's right to confidentiality.

If your patient is hearing impaired, make sure the light is bright enough and that your mouth is not covered with an obstructive mask so the patient is able to see your lips move. Then face them and speak slowly and clearly. If necessary, have the patient use an assistive device, such as a hearing aid or an amplifier. If the patient uses sign language, locate a sign language interpreter.

Remember that communication may not necessarily be face-to-face; the nurse may have to communicate with patients over the phone or via electronic formats such as telehealth visits, emails, or patient portals. Adapt your communication based on the patient's needs.

Credibility

For communication to be credible, it must be stated in a trustworthy and believable manner.

Honestly now!

Communication must be accurate, consistent, and honest. Communication commonly spurs continued conversation, so be prepared and well versed in the subject and content area so you'll be able to answer any question that arises. If the patient asks questions or seeks information that is beyond the nurse's scope of practice, be honest, saying that you are unable to answer. However, explain that you'll convey their concerns to someone who will be able to provide an answer.

Verbal communication strategies

Verbal communication strategies range from alternating between open-ended and closed questions to employing such techniques as silence, facilitation, confirmation, reflection, clarification, summary, and conclusion.

An open…

Asking open-ended questions such as "How did you fall?" lets the patient respond more freely. The response may provide answers to many other questions. For instance, the patient might respond that they were unsteady on their feet just before eating, became dizzy, and fell. Based on the patient's answer, the nurse might deduce that the patient had a syncopal episode caused by hypoglycemia.

...and shut case

The use of closed questions may also be appropriate. Although closed questions are unlikely to provide extra information, they may encourage the patient to give clear, concise feedback. (See *Two ways to ask*.)

Silence is golden

Another technique is to allow moments of silence during the interview. Remain silent and allow the patient time to collect their thoughts and ideas before responding. In addition to encouraging the patient to continue talking, this technique also gives the nurse a chance to assess the patient's ability to organize thoughts.

Patience is the key to communicating with a patient who responds slowly to questions. However, make sure your patience can't be perceived as being patronizing. The patient will easily perceive patronization and may interpret it as a lack of genuine concern.

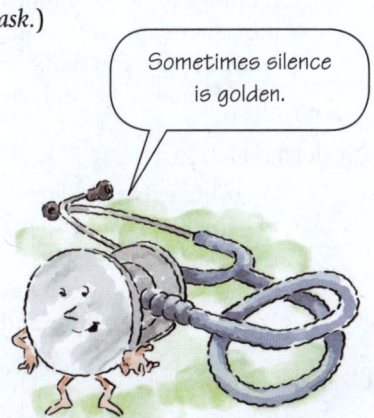

Sometimes silence is golden.

Two ways to ask

Questions can be characterized as *open-ended* or *closed*.

Open-ended questions

Open-ended questions require the patient to express feelings, opinions, and ideas. They also help the nurse collect more information than can be gathered with closed questions. Open-ended questions encourage a good nurse–patient relationship because they show interest in what the patient has to say. Examples of open-ended questions include:
- "Why did you come to the hospital tonight?"
- "How would you describe the problems you're having with your breathing?"
- "What lung problems, if any, do other members of your family have?"

Closed questions

Closed questions elicit "yes" or "no" answers or one- or two-word responses. Closed questions limit the development of the nurse–patient relationship. Although closed questions can help the nurse "zoom in" on specific points, they don't provide the patient with an opportunity to elaborate. Examples of closed questions include:
- "Do you ever get short of breath?"
- How long have you been experiencing breathing problems?
- "Are you the only one in your family with lung problems?"

Give them a boost

Using such phrases as "please continue," "go on," and even "uh-huh" encourages the patient to continue with their story. Known as *facilitation*, this feedback demonstrates interest in what is being said.

Confirmation conversation

Employing the technique of confirmation helps ensure that you and the patient are on the same track. For instance, ask "If I understand you correctly, you said," and then repeat the information the patient gave. Doing so helps to clear up any misconceptions.

Check and reflect

Try using reflection—repeating something the patient has just said—to help obtain more specific information. For example, a patient with a stomachache might say, "I know I have an ulcer." If so, you can repeat, "You know you have an ulcer?" Then the patient might say, "Yes. I had one before, and the pain is the same."

Clear skies

When information is vague or confusing, use the technique of clarification. For example, if the patient says, "I can't stand this," you might respond, "What can't you stand?" or "What do you mean by 'I can't stand this'?" Using this approach gives the patient an opportunity to explain their statement.

Put the landing gear down...

At the end of the patient interview, get in the habit of restating the information provided by the patient. Known as *summarization*, this technique ensures that the data you've collected are accurate and complete. Summarization also signals to the patient that the interview is about to end.

...and come in for a safe landing

Signal to the patient when you're ready to conclude the interview. This signal gives the patient an opportunity to gather thoughts and make any pertinent final comments. A statement such as "I think I have all the information I need now. Is there anything you would like to add?" can signal conclusion of the interview.

Nonverbal communication

Nonverbal communication transmits messages without using words and is commonly referred to as *body language*. Nonverbal communication includes facial expressions, posture, gait, hand gestures, tone of voice, positioning and space, touch, appearance, and level of alertness. Nonverbal communication can convey feelings of sadness, joy, and anxiety. It reflects self-concept, current mood, and health.

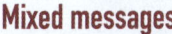

> Nonverbal communication transmits messages without using words.

Mixed messages

Nonverbal communication aids interpretation of verbal communication but requires acute observation by the receiver for accurate interpretation of the message. For instance, if a patient states that the pain has subsided but the nurse observes they are guarded and clenching the side rails on the bed, verbal communication is telling one thing but nonverbal actions are revealing something else.

Nonverbal communication strategies

To maintain a good relationship with the patient, remember that their cultural behaviors—including their nonverbal communication—may differ from your own. To make the most of nonverbal communication, do the following:

- Listen attentively and make eye contact frequently; however, be aware that people in some cultures may regard direct eye contact as disrespectful or aggressive.
- Use reassuring gestures, such as nodding your head, to encourage the patient to keep talking.
- Watch for nonverbal clues that indicate the patient is uncomfortable or unsure about how to answer a question. For example, they might lower their voice or glance around uneasily.
- Be aware of your own nonverbal behaviors that might cause the patient to stop talking or become defensive. For example, if you cross your arms, you might appear closed off from them. If you stand while they are sitting, you might appear superior. If you glance at your watch, you might appear to be bored or rushed, which could keep the patient from answering questions completely.
- Observe the patient closely to see whether they understand each question. If they don't appear to understand, repeat the question using different words or familiar examples. For instance, instead of asking, "Did you have respiratory difficulty after exercising?" ask, "Did you have to sit down after walking around the block?"

Therapeutic relationships

A therapeutic relationship occurs during nurse and patient interaction in a clinical setting. This interaction is the beginning of the nurse–patient relationship.

The building process

The nurse–patient relationship doesn't just happen; it is created with care and skill and built on the patient's trust of the nurse and on the nurse's respect of the patient. The building process follows a natural progression of four distinct phases:
1. preinteraction
2. orientation
3. working
4. termination.

Preinteraction phase

During the preinteraction phase, review the patient data that you might already have, such as the medical or surgical history and information gained from family members. If at all possible, after reviewing this information, try to anticipate any concerns or issues that might arise.

Orientation phase

During the orientation phase, you first meet the patient. More than likely, it will occur at the bedside when the patient is admitted. This time is the best time for you to talk to the patient and get to know them. However, the meeting isn't usually leisurely or controlled—especially if the patient is in the emergency department, in pain, or apprehensive. Even in difficult situations, though, you must use verbal and nonverbal communication skills to ease the patient's fears and begin to develop a relationship.

> Do your best to make a good first impression by remaining warm, open, and attentive to the patient's needs.

First impressions

During the orientation phase, the patient will be forming a first impression of the meeting. The patient will form an opinion about your interest in their health care by watching you closely. By acting in a warm, caring manner, you'll make this first impression, one that helps build a good nurse–patient relationship.

Trust building

Trust is a crucial part of the therapeutic relationship. If the patient doesn't trust you, they won't be open and answer your questions. Take time to close the curtain and sit down in a chair with the patient. These actions will convey that you are attentive and are not in a hurry to leave the room. Acting with integrity will also help the patient to develop confidence in you and your abilities.

Role clarification

Patients are becoming increasingly knowledgeable about their bodies. They have access to a wealth of information today via the Internet, newspapers, and magazines. As patients learn more about how to stay healthy, they're taking a more active role in their health care. You must recognize and respect this role. Patients' growing involvement in their own health care is helping to change the approach of many health care professionals from the authoritarian "Do as I say" mindset to the more cooperative "Here's why I recommend this" attitude. This shift in approach allows the patient to be a part of their own health care team.

Build rapport

As you begin to develop rapport with your patient, you develop a therapeutic relationship with them that is built on trust and a mutual desire to ensure that they receive the treatment they need.

Working phase

The working phase is a team-building stage that includes the nurse, the patient, and the entire health care team. During this phase, you use therapeutic communication to encourage the patient and help them to understand their condition and how to set goals.

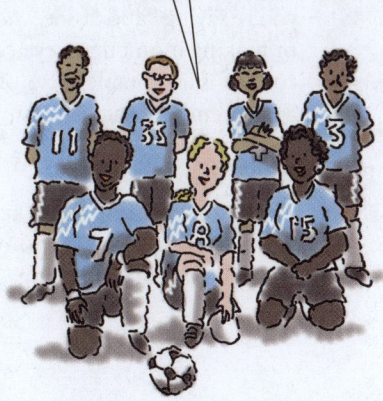

Let's remember … we're a team. By working together, we'll accomplish our goals.

Give and take

This phase is a give-and-take phase because you and the patient have specific roles to play and certain expectations of what will happen during the relationship. As the nurse, you expect the patient to be willing to participate in their health care by providing accurate information, asking questions about treatments, and participating in treatment procedures as appropriate. The patient, on the other hand, expects that their health care needs will be met by you and the other members of the health care team. They expect that in your role as the nurse you will act as their health care advocate, keeping them informed and providing them with appropriate treatments and procedures.

Termination phase

The termination phase is when the relationship is coming to an end. A simple way of ending the relationship is by saying good-bye at the end of your shift. However, termination can sometimes be more complex; it can include discharge planning and may also involve beginning to develop relationships with the patient's health care team as you make necessary referrals for home care nurse visits and rehabilitation.

Smooth sailing

When the termination phase is easy, the patient can have a smooth transition to other health care team members.

Therapeutic use of self

Using interpersonal skills in a healing way to help the patient is called *therapeutic use of self*. Three important techniques enhance therapeutic use of self:
- exhibiting empathy
- demonstrating acceptance
- giving recognition.

Path to empathy

To show empathy, use statements that acknowledge the patient's feelings, such as "That must have upset you."

Acceptance acts

To show acceptance, use neutral statements, such as "I hear what you're saying" and "I see." Nonverbal behaviors, such as nodding or making momentary eye contact (for those patients for whom eye contact is acceptable) also provide encouragement without indicating agreement or disagreement.

I recognize that

To give recognition, listen actively to what the patient says, occasionally providing verbal or nonverbal acknowledgment to encourage them to continue speaking.

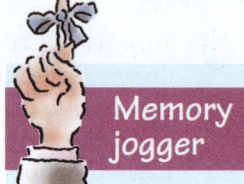

Memory jogger

When it comes to therapeutic interpersonal patient communication skills, lend an EAR! Make sure you show:

Empathy

Acceptance

Recognition.

Blocks to communication

Various factors contribute to the communication process and directly affect a person's ability to send and receive messages. If a patient has physical, behavioral, or learning impairments that can affect communication, the nurse needs to understand which factors influence communication so that any barriers can be cleared away. (See *Considering communication barriers*.)

Not so obvious

Although some communication barriers (including communicating with a patient who speaks another language or who has a hearing or visual impairment) are obvious, be sure to also consider the not-so-obvious barriers, such as those that could be encountered when dealing with a young child or an unconscious patient.

> Don't let communication barriers get in your way. There's always another route around a difficult situation.

Considering communication barriers

This diagram shows the components of nurse–patient communication. Note the factors that affect communication, such as orientation, preconceptions, and language. The nurse's sensitivity to these factors makes the difference between effective and ineffective communication.

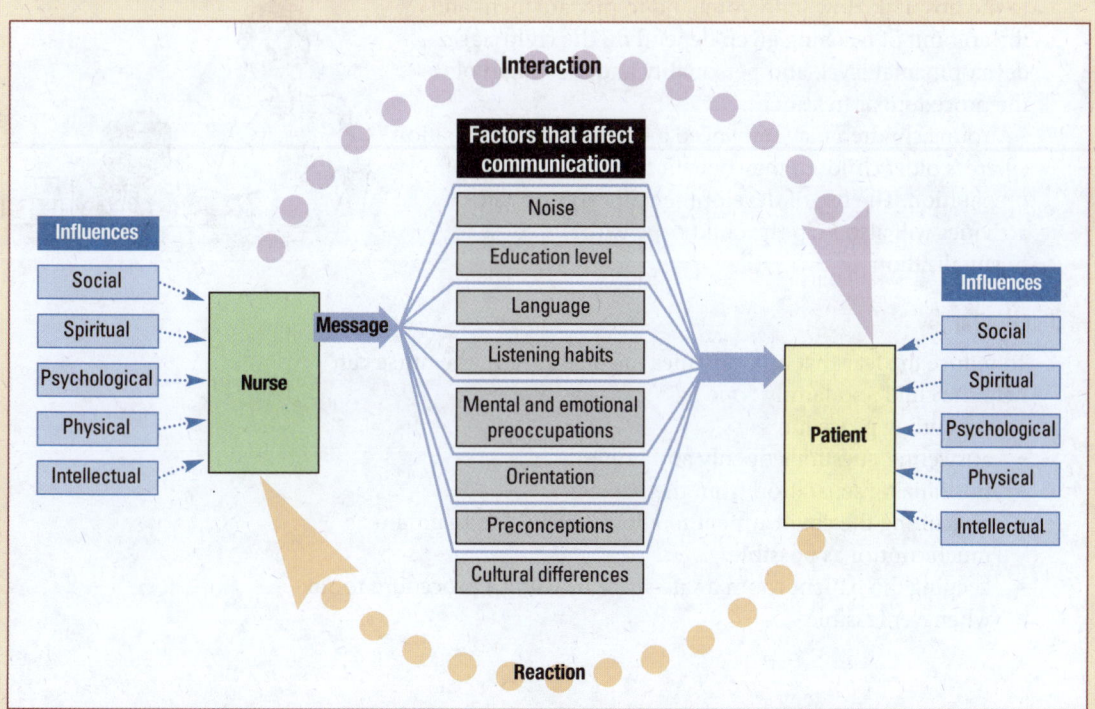

Interaction

Factors that affect communication
- Noise
- Education level
- Language
- Listening habits
- Mental and emotional preoccupations
- Orientation
- Preconceptions
- Cultural differences

Influences
- Social
- Spiritual
- Psychological
- Physical
- Intellectual

Nurse — Message

Patient

Influences
- Social
- Spiritual
- Psychological
- Physical
- Intellectual

Reaction

Pediatric patients

When dealing with a young patient, it is essential to keep in mind the child's developmental level. If your patient is a young child or an infant, you will need to communicate with the parents, caregivers, or guardian instead of or in addition to the child. When speaking with a child, get down at eye level with them and speak in terms they can understand. Make sure to take into consideration their developmental level.

In the case of a very young child, such as an infant, the nurse will need to communicate with the infant's parents, caregivers, or guardians. Always use a caring and compassionate tone with those caring for the infant because, more than likely, they're anxious about having their child hospitalized.

Let's pretend

Remember that children commonly regress to an earlier stage of development when they're ill. Role playing is one way to communicate with children to find out how they're feeling. Make sure to use language the child will understand.

Always be prepared

When possible, it is ideal to prepare the child for admission to the hospital. How far beforehand to prepare them and the amount of teaching given depend on the child's age, developmental level, and personality and the length of the procedure or treatment.

Young children may only need a few hours of preparation, whereas older children may benefit from several days of preparation. The use of developmentally appropriate activities will also help the child cope with the stress of hospitalization.

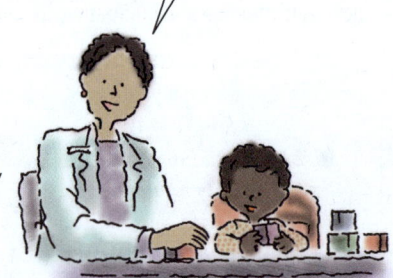

Having developmentally appropriate activities on hand can help a child cope with the stress of hospitalization.

Keep it in the family

To reduce the fear that accompanies hospitalization, the nurse can help the child and family cope by:
- explaining procedures
- answering questions openly and honestly
- minimizing separation from the parents
- structuring the environment to allow the child to maintain as much control as possible
- keeping the patient room a safe space by using a procedure room whenever feasible.

Unconscious patient

When caring for an unconscious patient, always try to communicate with them. Never assume that they can't hear you. Introduce yourself as you would to a conscious patient. Always explain every procedure the patient will undergo. Don't talk about the patient with other people in the room as if the patient isn't present. Always treat the unconscious patient with kindness, consideration, and respect, as you would a patient who is conscious.

Communicating by documentation

Patients are cared for by many health care professionals who work different shifts, so they may speak with one another infrequently. The medical record is the main source of information and communication among nurses, doctors, physical therapists, social workers, and other caregivers. Today, nurses are commonly considered managers of care as well as practitioners, and nurses usually document the most information. Everyone's notes are important because together they represent a complete picture of the patient's care.

> Everyone's notes are important because together they represent a complete picture of patient care.

Growing team

As health care facilities continue to streamline and redesign care delivery systems, tasks that were historically performed by nurses are now being assigned to multiskilled workers such as nursing assistants. To deliver highly specialized care, each caregiver must provide accurate, thorough information and be able to interpret what others have written about a patient. Then each can use this information to plan future patient care. Commonly, decisions, actions, and revisions related to the patient's care are based on documentation from various team members. A well-prepared medical record shows the high degree of collaboration among the entire health care team.

Quick quiz

1. When developing a therapeutic nurse–patient relationship, during what phase do you work with a patient to set goals?
    A. Orientation
    B. Working
    C. Preinteraction
    D. Termination

Answer: B. During the working phase, you will work with a patient to help them understand their condition and to set goals.

2. Which of the following factors influence nurse–patient communication? (Select all that apply.)
    A. Spiritual
    B. Physical
    C. Occupational
    D. Intellectual

Answer: A, B, and D. Social, spiritual, psychological, physical, and intellectual factors influence nurse–patient communication.

3. Which of the following would be considered an example of an encouraging phrase that would give the patient a boost to continue their story?
    A. "What can't you stand?"
    B. "Please continue."
    C. "If I understand you correctly, you said you've had a headache for three days?"
    D. "I think I have all the information that I need now."

Answer: B. the phrase "Please continue" is an example of an encouraging phrase that will facilitate the patient to continue their story.

4. What is the **BEST** way to communicate with an unconscious patient when performing procedures?
    A. Be as quiet as possible and don't speak to the patient.
    B. Show them pictures and videos of the procedure.
    C. Introduce yourself and explain every procedure to the patient.
    D. Explain everything to the family members while in the patient's room.

Answer: C. Introduce yourself and explain every procedure to the patient. Don't assume that they can't hear you. Don't talk about the patient with other people in the room as if the patient isn't present.

5. Health care providers can communicate verbally and nonverbally with their patients. Which of the following is an example of a positive nonverbal communication technique?

A. Crossing your arms across your chest to show you are comfortable
B. Standing over the patient to get a better viewpoint
C. Using facilitating gestures like smiling and nodding
D. Checking your watch to keep the interview on time

Answer: C. Utilizing facilitating and reassuring gestures like nodding your head and smiling encourages the patient to continue speaking and to answer your question.

Scoring

⭐⭐⭐ If you answered all four questions correctly, fantastic! You're a communication connoisseur.

⭐⭐ If you answered three questions correctly, super! You've got a handle on handling communication strategies.

⭐ If you answered fewer than three questions correctly, no worries! Reflect on the chapter and try again.

References

Myrick, K. M., & Karosas L. M. (2021). *Advanced health assessment and differential diagnosis: Essentials for clinical practice*. Springer Publishing Company.

Taylor, C., Lynn P., & Bartlett J. (2023). *Fundamentals of nursing: The art and science of person-centered care* (10th ed.). Wolters Kluwer.

Chapter 6

Health assessment

Just the facts

In this chapter, you'll learn:

- reasons to perform and complete a health history assessment
- techniques for effective communication during the health history assessment
- essential steps of a complete health history assessment
- pertinent questions specific to each step of a health history assessment.

A look at the health assessment

Assessments lay the foundation for health care. Knowing how to complete an accurate health assessment—from taking the health history to performing the physical examination—will help you recognize potential health problems, identify opportunities for patient education, and assist in developing an appropriate care plan. According to Jensen (2023), the health assessment "consists of taking a thorough health history and an extensive psychosocial and physical examination" (p. 230).

Any assessment involves collecting two kinds of data: objective and subjective. *Objective data* are obtained through clinical observation and physical assessment, and it is verifiable. For example, a red, swollen arm in a patient who is reporting arm pain is an example of data that can be seen and verified by someone other than the patient. *Subjective data* can't be verified by anyone other than the patient and are gathered solely from the patient's own account—for example, "My head hurts" or "I have trouble sleeping at night." Subjective and objective data collection is important to the nursing assessment (Toney-Butler & Unison-Pace, 2022). Thus, all data obtained by a medical professional during the health assessment interview must be documented appropriately. Furthermore, information gathered by any means can be crucial in guiding and directing patient care (Nichols Sundjaja & Nelson, 2022).

> The health history is an exploration of the patient's health—past and present.

Remember to examine both the past and the present

A health history is used to gather subjective data about the patient's past and present problems. A patient's past health history is as important as their current health problems because it can often indicate the status of the patient's current health. A health history can reveal data regarding chronic illnesses or prior disease that may not be related to current treatment but that may have lasting effects on the patient's health (Nichols et al., 2022).

Set yourself up for success

Discussing family and personal health history can be an intimidating and overwhelming activity for many people. It is important to keep in mind that the accuracy and completeness of the patient's answers largely depend on the nurse's skill as an interviewer. Therefore, it is crucial to establish a rapport with the patient to make them feel comfortable and safe. Before asking questions, take a moment to review the following communication guidelines to help successfully navigate the interview process.

Create the proper environment

To make the most of the patient interview, first create an environment in which the patient feels comfortable. If a patient does not feel at ease, the health care provider may not be able to extract all of the information needed to treat the patient appropriately. Some patients may feel anxious during the interview due to distractions of health concerns and stressors (Myrick & Karosas, 2021). So, before asking the first question, try to connect with the patient, calm their nerves, and explain the purpose of the interview. Consider the following guidelines:

- Choose a quiet, private, well-lit interview setting.
- Treat the patient with respect; this encourages trust, and the patient will likely provide more accurate and complete information.
- Make sure the patient is comfortable. Sit facing the patient; sitting with a patient indicates you have time to speak and listen to them. And, if possible, try to position yourself on the same eye level (Jensen, 2023).
- Address the patient by their legal name (for example, Jared Jones); avoid using first names or nicknames until you ask the patient their preferred name and/or the patient indicates how they prefer to be addressed (Myrick & Karosas, 2021). Don't utilize any terms of endearment such as "honey" or "sweetie."
- Introduce yourself, explain the purpose of the health history assessment, and reassure the patient that everything they say will be kept confidential.

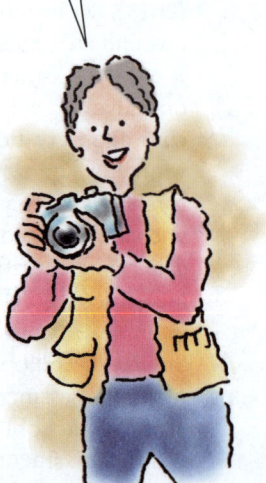

When interviewing a patient, remain focused on the task at hand.

- Describe what will happen during the health history interview and give the patient your best estimate on how long it will take.
- Use touch sparingly. Many people aren't comfortable with strangers hugging, patting, or touching them.
- Assess for language barriers. For example, does the patient speak and understand English? Can they hear you? (See *Overcoming communication obstacles* in Chapter 5, page 76).
- Taking your time, speak slowly and clearly, using easy-to-understand language. Avoid using medical terms.
- As discussed in Chapter 5, use both open-ended and close-ended questions. Start with open-ended questions to gather information (for example, tell me what brings you here today) followed by closed-ended questions (for example, questions that require yes or no or questions that require a one- or two-word response) to clarify (Myrick & Karosas, 2021). Open-ended questions allow the patient to express their thoughts/feelings, and closed or focused questions help the interviewer to obtain details in a time-efficient manner (Slade & Sergent, 2022).
- Communicate effectively. See Chapter 5 for tips on effective communication and how to overcome communication barriers.

Reviewing general health

Asking the right questions about the patient's general physical and emotional health is important to the interview process. Remember that as the health care professional, it is important for you to maintain a positive, professional attitude and to keep the interview flowing productively (Slade & Sergent, 2022).

Asking the right questions

A complete health history requires information from each of the following categories, obtained in this order:
1. biographic data
2. chief complaint
3. medical history
4. family history
5. psychosocial history
6. activities of daily living.

Biographic data

Start the health history by obtaining biographical information from the patient. Ask the patient for name, address, telephone number, emergency contact, birth date, age, birth place, ethnicity, race, employment, occupation, and relationship status (Jensen, 2023). It is also

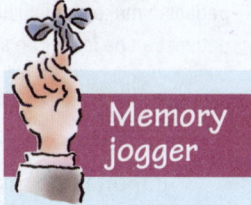

Memory jogger

To remember the categories you should cover in your health history and the order you should ask about them, remember that "**B**eing **C**omplete **M**akes **F**or **P**roper **A**ssessment":

Biographic data

Chief complaint

Medical history

Family history

Psychosocial history

Activities of daily living.

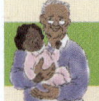

Advance directives

The Patient Self-Determination Act allows patients to prepare advance directives—written legal documents that specify their health care wishes in the event they become incapacitated or unable to make decisions (House et al., 2022).

Direction for directives

If a patient doesn't have an advance directive in place, the health care facility must provide them with information about how to establish one.

An advance directive may include:
• name of the person authorized by the patient to make medical decisions if the patient can no longer do so

• specific medical treatment the patient wants or doesn't want
• instructions regarding pain medication and comfort—specifically, whether the patient wishes to receive certain treatment even if the treatment may hasten their death
• information the patient wants to relay to their loved ones
• name of the patient's primary health care provider
• any other wishes.

important to ask what sex the patient was assigned at birth, as well as their current gender identity (Altarum Institute, 2022).

Also, ask the patient about health care, including who is their primary doctor and the date of their last health care visit. Investigate if they have ever been treated and/or if they are currently receiving treatment for the present problem. Finally, ask if they have an advance directive in place. (See *Advance directives*.)

Take a hint

The patient's answers to basic questions can provide important clues about their personality, medical problems, and reliability. Paying attention to these sometimes minor clues adds information to the overall assessment of the patient (Myrick & Karosas, 2021). If the information the patient provides isn't reliable (for example, if a patient can't furnish accurate information because of memory difficulties), this may be concerning (Jensen, 2023). If this is discovered during the heath assessment interview, ask the patient for the name of a friend or relative who could assist them and document the source of the information as well as whether an interpreter was necessary.

Chief complaint

Try to pinpoint why the patient is seeking health care or their *chief complaint.* In a nutshell, a chief complaint is a patient's list of symptoms and a description of what prompted the patient to seek care that is obtained at the beginning of a health care visit (National Quality Forum, 2019). Document this information in the patient's exact words to avoid misinterpretation. Ask how and when the symptoms developed, what led the patient to seek medical attention, and how the problem has affected their life and ability to function.

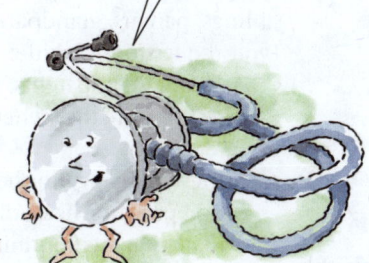

Identify the chief complaint. Remember, accuracy is key to a correct diagnosis.

Alphabet soup

To ensure that pertinent data are not omitted, use the PQRSTU mnemonic device (see *PQRSTU: What's the story?*), which provides a systematic approach to obtaining information.

Past medical history

A patient's past medical history involves any health issues that have occurred during their lifetime (Myrick & Karosas, 2021). Ask the patient about past and current medical problems, surgeries, hospitalizations, medications, pregnancy and childbirth (if applicable), etc. Typical questions include:

- What childhood illnesses did you have?
- Have you ever been hospitalized? If so, when and why?
- Have you ever had surgery? If so, when and why?
- Are you currently being treated for any problem? If so, for what reason, and who is your treating health care provider?
- Do you have any known environmental, food, or medication allergies? If so, what kind of allergic reaction do you have?
- Are you taking medications, including over-the-counter preparations, such as aspirin, vitamins, and cough syrup? If so, how much do you take, and how often do you take it? Do you use herbal preparations or take dietary supplements?
- Do you use any homemade remedies? If so, what remedy do you use, what are its ingredients, and how do you use it?
- Do you use other alternative or complementary therapies, such as acupuncture, therapeutic massage, or chiropractic care?
- When was your last physical examination? (Also inquire about their most recent screening assessments, such as their last dental, vision, and hearing examinations.) (Jensen, 2023)
- Have you received any immunizations? If so, which ones and when?

Family history

Questioning the patient about their family health history is a good way to uncover risks of having certain illness or disease. Family history is a useful tool for identifying common chronic disease (Filoche et al., 2021). Generally, family history questions apply only to first-degree relatives (for example, biological siblings, parents, grandparents) (Myrick & Karosas, 2021). Typical questions include:

- Are your grandparents, parents, and siblings living? If not, how old were they when they died? What were the causes of death?
- If they are living, do they have any history of diabetes, high blood pressure, heart disease, stroke, asthma, cancer, sickle cell anemia, hemophilia, cataracts, glaucoma, mental illness, alcohol use disorder, or other illnesses? (Jensen, 2023).

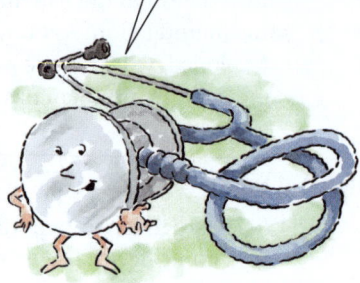

Risk for disease or illness can be identified from information about the health of a patient's family.

Psychosocial history

While obtaining the health history, you must assess both the physical and emotional needs of the patient (Toney-Butler & Unison-Pace, 2022). Find out how the patient feels about themselves, their place in society, and their relationships with others. Ask about occupation (past and present), education, economic status, and quality of life. Typical questions include:

- How have you coped with medical or emotional crises in the past? (See *Asking about abuse*, page 95.)
- Have you experienced any recent life changes that have impacted your behavior and/or personality?
- How would you describe your current quality of life?
- How adequate is the emotional support you receive from family and friends?
- How would you describe your current economic status?

Activities of daily living

Find out what is normal for the patient by asking them to describe a typical day. Make sure to include the following areas in your assessment.

Diet and elimination

Ask the patient about their appetite, special diets, and food allergies. Ask about the frequency of bowel movements and laxative use. Can they afford to buy enough food? Who cooks and shops at home?

Asking about abuse

Abuse is a sensitive subject. Anyone can be a victim of abuse: a significant other, a spouse, an older adult, a child, or a caregiver. Also, abuse can come in many forms: physical, psychological, emotional, or sexual. When taking a health history, ask two open-ended questions to explore abuse:

- Do you feel safe at home?
- When don't you feel safe?

Watch the reaction

Even if you don't immediately suspect an abusive situation, be aware of how your patient reacts to open-ended questions. Is the patient defensive, hostile, confused, or frightened? Assess how they interact with you and others. Do they seem withdrawn or fearful, or do they show other inappropriate behavior? Keep reactions in mind when you perform your physical assessment.

Must report

Health care providers have an ethical and legal role in reporting abuse (Thomas & Reeves, 2022). If any signs and/or suspicions of abuse arise during your assessment, follow your facility's and/or clinic's guidelines for mandated reporting.

Exercise and sleep

Ask the patient about their current exercise routine (for example, types of exercise, length of exercise, frequency). Inquire about their sleep habits (for example, ask them how many hours they sleep at night, ask them to describe their sleep patterns, ask if they feel rested after sleep, and ask if they experience any difficulties with sleep).

Work and leisure

Ask the patient what they do for a living and what they do during leisure time. Do they have hobbies?

Use of tobacco, alcohol, and other drugs

Ask the patient if they smoke cigarettes. If so, how many packs per day? Do they consume alcohol? If so, how much each day? Ask if the patient uses illicit drugs, and if so, what and how often. Also ask about past use of alcohol, smoking, or drug use. If ever used, ask how much and when they stopped.

Fudging the facts

Keep in mind that, because these topics are very personal, patients may understate the amount they use substances (including alcohol) because of embarrassment. The health care provider should always remain mindful of this fact but note that further clarifying questions may be warranted if there is a concern for health risks and/or if the

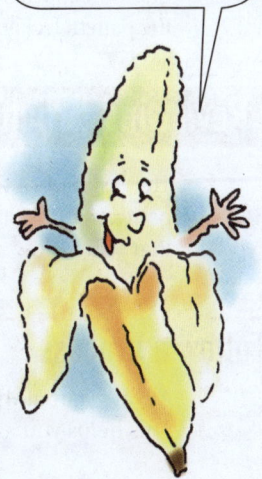

When asking about food and diet, be sure to ask if there are any food allergies.

patient's current lifestyle behaviors may be linked to their current disease state (Nichols et al., 2022). If you're concerned that answer responses are not accurate or truthful, you may want to overestimate the amount of substance use during questioning. For example, "You told me you drink beer. Do you drink about a six-pack per day?" The patient's response might be, "No, I drink about half that."

Religious observances

Ask the patient if they have religious beliefs that affect diet, dress, or health practices. Patients will feel reassured when you make it clear that you understand these points.

Maintaining a professional attitude

Assessment begins the moment you first greet your patient (Myrick & Karosas, 2021). Don't let your personal opinions interfere with your assessment. Always maintain a professional, neutral approach, and don't offer advice. For example, don't suggest that the patient enter a drug rehabilitation program. That type of response may make patients defensive, and they might not answer subsequent questions honestly. Also, avoid using leading questions such as "You don't do drugs, do you?" This type of question appears to be based on a personal value system, so it may make the patient feel guilty and might prevent them from responding honestly.

Reviewing structures and systems

The last part of the health history is a systematic assessment of the patient's body structures and systems. A thorough assessment requires that you follow a process while asking specific questions.

Follow a process

Always start at the top of the head and work your way down the body. This helps you avoid skipping an area accidentally.

Ask specific questions

Information gained from a health history forms the basis for the plan of care and enables you to distinguish physical changes and devise a holistic approach to treatment. As with other nursing skills, improvement comes with practice. Practicing the health history interview will improve your ability to reach patients and to demonstrate understanding and care (Slade & Sergent, 2022). (See *Evaluating a symptom*.)

Evaluating a symptom

Your patient is vague in describing the chief complaint. Using your interviewing skills, you discover the problem is related to abdominal distention. Now what? This flowchart will help you decide what to do next, using abdominal distention as the patient's chief complaint.

Question the patient to identify the symptom that's bothering them. They tell you, "My stomach gets bloated."

▼

Form a first impression.
Does the patient's condition alert you to an emergency? For example, do they say the bloating developed suddenly? Do they mention that other signs or symptoms occur with it, such as sweating and lightheadedness? (Both are indicators of hypovolemia.)

 YES   · **NO**

Take a brief history to gather more clues. For example, ask the patient if they have severe abdominal pain or difficulty breathing or if they ever had an abdominal injury.	Take a thorough history to get an overview of the patient's condition. Ask about associated signs or symptoms. Especially note gastrointestinal (GI) disorders that can lead to abdominal distention.
Perform a focused physical examination to determine the severity of the patient's condition quickly. Check for bruising, lacerations, changes in bowel sounds, or abdominal rigidity.	Thoroughly examine the patient to evaluate the chief sign or symptom and to detect additional signs and symptoms. Place the patient in a recumbent position and observe for abdominal asymmetry. Inspect the skin, auscultate for bowel sounds, percuss and palpate the abdomen, and measure abdominal girth.

Evaluate your findings. Are emergency signs or symptoms present, such as abdominal rigidity and abnormal bowel sounds?

Based on your findings, intervene appropriately to stabilize the patient. Notify the doctor immediately, place the patient in a supine position, administer oxygen, and start an IV line. GI or nasogastric tube insertion and emergency surgery may be needed.	Review your findings to consider possible causes, such as cancer, bladder distention, cirrhosis, heart failure, and gastric dilation.
After the patient's condition is stabilized, review your findings to consider possible causes, such as trauma, large-bowel obstruction, mesenteric artery occlusion, or peritonitis.	Evaluate your findings and devise an appropriate care plan. Position the patient comfortably, administer analgesics, and prepare the patient for diagnostic tests.

Let's start from the top and work our way down...

Here are some key questions to ask the patient about each body structure and system. (See also *Tips for assessing a severely ill patient*, at the end of this section on page 101.)

> Let's start at the top!

Skin, hair, and nails

Are you experiencing any current skin problems (for example, rashes, lesions, bruising, or swelling)? Any history of skin disease (for example, eczema, psoriasis, hyperpigmentation, mole changes, excessive dryness, or pruritus)? Have you had any recent hair loss or change in condition of your hair? Any change in nail shape, thickness, or color (Jensen, 2023)?

Head

Do you get headaches? If so, where are they located, how often do they occur, how long do they last, and how painful are they? Does anything trigger them, and how do you relieve them? Have you ever had a head injury? Do you have lumps or bumps on your head? Are you currently experiencing and/or have you ever experienced any head injuries, syncope, dizziness, or vertigo (Jensen, 2023)?

Eyes

Do you have any difficulty with your vision (for example, blurriness, double vision, blind spots, eye pain/discomfort, watering or discomfort, redness, swelling, discharge, glaucoma, and/or cataracts) (Jensen, 2023)? When was your last eye examination? Do you wear glasses? Does light bother your eyes? Do you have any known color blindness?

Ears

Do you have loss of balance, ringing in your ears, deafness, or poor hearing? Have you ever had ear surgery? If so, why and when? Do you wear a hearing aid? Are you having pain, swelling, or discharge from your ears? If so, has this problem occurred before, and how frequently?

Nose

Do you have nasal problems that impair your ability to smell or that cause breathing difficulties, snoring at night, frequent sneezing, sinus pain, or discharge? Have you ever had sinusitis or nosebleeds? Have you ever had nasal surgery? If so, why and when?

Mouth and throat

Do you have any current or past issues with mouth sores, dryness, hoarseness, change in voice, loss of taste, dental pain, or bleeding gums? Do you wear dentures and, if so, do they fit? Do you have a sore throat, fever, or chills? Do you have difficulty swallowing? If so, is the problem with solids or liquids? Is it a constant problem or does it accompany a sore throat or another problem? What, if anything, makes it go away?

Neck

Do you have swelling, soreness, lack of movement, stiffness, or pain in your neck? If so, did something specific cause it to happen such as too much exercise? How long have you had this symptom? Does anything relieve it or aggravate it?

Breast

Have you noticed any pain, lumps, a change in breast contour, or discharge from your nipples (Jensen, 2023)? Have you ever had breast cancer? If no, has anyone in your family had it? Do you perform monthly breast self-examinations? Have you ever had a mammogram? When, and what were the results?

Respiratory

Do you have any history of wheezing, chest pain while breathing, any lung diseases (for example, asthma, tuberculosis, emphysema, pneumonia, or bronchitis), or shortness of breath on exertion or while lying in bed? Do you have a productive cough? If so, do you cough up blood-tinged sputum? Do you have night sweats? Have you ever had a chest x-ray or tuberculin skin test? If so, when, and what were the results?

Cardiovascular

Do you have any current and/or history of chest pain, palpitations, irregular heartbeat, fast heartbeat, shortness of breath, a persistent cough, or swelling? Do you have high blood pressure, coronary artery disease, or heart murmurs? Have you ever had an electrocardiogram? If so, when, and what were the results?

Peripheral Vascular

Do you have any current and/or history of cold extremities, varicose veins, or intermittent pain in your legs, extremity swelling, skin discoloration, or ulcers (Jensen, 2023)? Have you ever been diagnosed with anemia or blood abnormalities? Do you bruise easily or become fatigued quickly? Have you ever had a blood transfusion? If so, did you have any type of adverse reaction?

Gastrointestinal

Have you had nausea, vomiting, loss of appetite, heartburn, abdominal pain, frequent belching, or passing of gas? Have you lost or gained weight recently? How often do you have a bowel movement, and what color, odor, and consistency are your stools? Have you noticed a change in your regular elimination pattern? Do you use laxatives frequently?

Have you had hemorrhoids, rectal bleeding, hernias, gallbladder disease, or liver disease?

Genitourinary

Do you have urinary problems, such as burning during urination, incontinence, urgency, retention, reduced urinary flow, and dribbling? Do you get up during the night to urinate? If so, how many times? What color is your urine? Have you ever noticed blood in it? Have you ever been treated for kidney stones?

Reproductive

Questions for people assigned female at birth

Assess menstrual history (for example, How old were you when you started menstruating? When was your last menstrual cycle? How often do you get your period, and how long does it usually last? Do you have pain or pass clots?). If you're postmenopausal, at what age did you stop menstruating? If you're in the perimenopausal stage, what perimenopausal symptoms are you experiencing? Have you ever been pregnant? If so, how many times? How many pregnancies resulted in live births? How many resulted in miscarriage or still birth?

Do you have any history of vaginal itching, discharge, frequent vaginal infections, or a sexually transmitted infection (STI)? When was your last gynecologic examination and Papanicolaou (Pap) test? What were the results? Are you sexually active? If yes, do you use birth control, and if so, what method do you currently use?

Questions for people assigned male at birth

Have you noticed penile pain, sores, discharge, lesions, or testicular lumps? Do you perform monthly testicular self-examinations? Have you ever had a prostate examination and, if so, when? Have you had a vasectomy? If yes, do you use birth control, and if so, what method do you currently use? Have you ever had a sexually transmitted infection (STI)?

Musculoskeletal

Do you have difficulty walking, sitting, or standing? Are you steady on your feet, or do you lose your balance easily? Do you have arthritis, gout, a back injury, muscle weakness, or paralysis?

Neurologic

Do you ever experience tremors, twitching, numbness, tingling, or loss of sensation in a part of your body? Have you ever had seizures? Are you less able to get around than you think you should be?

Endocrine

Do you have any history of diabetes or thyroid disease? Have you been unusually tired lately? Do you feel hungry or thirsty more often than usual? Have you lost weight for unexplained reasons? How well can you tolerate heat or cold? Have you noticed changes in your hair distribution? Do you take hormone medications?

Psychosocial

Do you ever experience mood swings or memory loss? Do you ever feel anxious, depressed, or unable to concentrate? Are you feeling unusually stressed? Do you ever feel unable to cope?

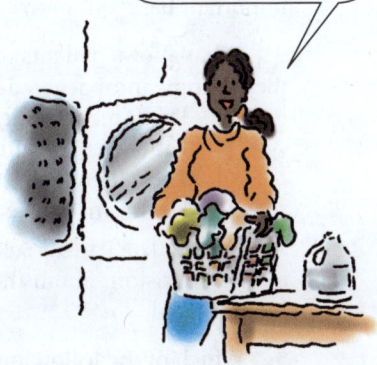

It may read like a long laundry list, but all these questions are crucial to a thorough assessment.

Tips for assessing a severely ill patient

When the patient's condition doesn't allow a full assessment—for example, if the patient is in severe pain—get as much information as possible from other sources. With a severely ill patient, keep these key points in mind:

• Identify yourself to the patient and the family.

• Stay calm to gain the patient's confidence and to allay anxiety.

• Stay on the lookout for important information. For example, if a patient is seeking help for ringing in their ears, don't overlook a casual mention by the patient of a periodic "racing heartbeat."

• Avoid jumping to conclusions. Don't assume that the patient's complaint is related to the admitting diagnosis. Use a systematic approach and collect the appropriate information; then, draw conclusions.

Quick quiz

1. When obtaining a health history from a patient, the nurse should first ask about:
   A. Chief complaint.
   B. Family history.
   C. Name of primary health care provider.
   D. Biographic data.

Answer: D. Take care of the biographic data first; otherwise, you might get involved in the patient history and forget to ask the very important basic questions.

2. What allows patients to state their wishes regarding health care if they become incapacitated?
   A. First Amendment.
   B. Patient's Bill of Rights.
   C. The Patient Self-Determination Act.
   D. Health Insurance Portability and Accountability Act.

Answer: C. The Patient Self-Determination Act allows patients to make decisions about their health care when they become incapacitated.

3. Which of the following is an appropriate setting in which to obtain a health history?
   A. A quiet, well-lit area of a clinic's lobby.
   B. A quiet, well-lit office or examination room.
   C. A noisy, well-lit area of a clinic's hallway.
   D. An open bay emergency room with curtain closed.

Answer: B. A health history should be obtained in a quiet, private, well-lit interview setting (for example, an office or examination room with a door).

4. When reviewing the body systems, the interview should always start with what area?
   A. Any system; the order does not matter
   B. Skin, hair, nails
   C. Musculoskeletal
   D. Cardiovascular

Answer: B. Remember, start at the top (scalp and hair) and work your way down. This makes it less likely to forget a body system.

Scoring

⭐⭐⭐ If you answered all four questions correctly, bravo! You're our intrepid interviewer.

⭐⭐ If you answered three questions correctly, that's cool! You're our hip historian.

⭐ If you answered fewer than three questions correctly, that's OK! Review the chapter and you'll know all the questions—and answers.

References

Altarum Institute. (2022). *Sexual health and your patients: A provider's guide*. Retrieved from https://nationalcoalitionforsexualhealth.org/tools/for-healthcare-providers/asset/Provider-Guide_May-2022.pdf

Filoche, S., Stubbe, M. H., Grainger, R., Robson, B., Paringatai, K., Wilcox, P., Jefferies, R., & Dowell, A. (2021). How is family health history discussed in routine primary healthcare? A qualitative study of archived family doctor consultations. *BMJ Open*, *11*(10), e049058. https://doi.org/10.1136/bmjopen-2021-049058

House, S. A., Schoo, C., Ogilvie, W. A. (2022). *Advance directives*. StatPearls. Retrieved from https://www.ncbi.nlm.nih.gov/books/NBK459133/

Jensen, S. (2023). *Nursing health assessment: A clinical judgment approach* (4th ed.). Wolters Kluwer.

Myrick, K. M., & Karosas, L. M. (2021). *Advanced health assessment and differential diagnosis: Essentials for clinical practice*. Springer Publishing Company.

National Quality Forum. (2019). *Advancing chief complaint-based quality measurement*. Retrieved from https://www.qualityforum.org/Projects/c-d/Chief_Complaint-Based_Quality_of_Emergency_Care/Final_Report.aspx

Nichols, J. R., Sundjaja, J. H., & Nelson, G. (2022, September 5). *Medical history—statpearls - NCBI bookshelf*. StatPearls. Retrieved February 24, 2023, from https://www.ncbi.nlm.nih.gov/books/NBK534249/

Slade, S., & Sergent, S. R. (2022, April 28). *Interview techniques*. In *StatPearls*. StatPearls Publishing. Retrieved from https://www.ncbi.nlm.nih.gov/books/NBK526083/

Thomas, R., & Reeves, M. (2022). *Mandatory reporting laws*. In: *StatPearls*. StatPearls Publishing. Retrieved from https://www.ncbi.nlm.nih.gov/books/NBK560690/

Toney-Butler, T. J., & Unison-Pace, W. J. (2022, August 29). *Nursing admission assessment and examination*. StatPearls. Retrieved February 24, 2023, from https://www.ncbi.nlm.nih.gov/books/NBK493211/

Taking vital signs

A look at vital signs assessment

Accurate measurements of a patient's height, weight, and vital signs provide critical information about body functions. It is essential to record baseline vital signs and statistics during a patient's initial assessment. After that, measurements should be recorded at regular intervals, depending on the patient's condition, the health care provider's orders, and the facility's policy. A series of vital signs readings usually provides more valuable information than a single set.

Vital tips

It is best to assess vital signs simultaneously because two or more abnormal values provide important clues about potential patient problems. For example, a rapid, thready pulse along with low blood pressure may signal shock.

If vital signs are abnormal, wait a minute or two after the initial readings and then reassess to ensure they are accurate. Remember that normal assessments vary with the patient's age. For example, temperature decreases with age, and respiratory rate may increase with age or the underlying disease. Also, remember that an abnormal value for one patient may be a normal value for another. Each patient has their own baseline values, making recording accurate vital signs during the initial assessment essential.

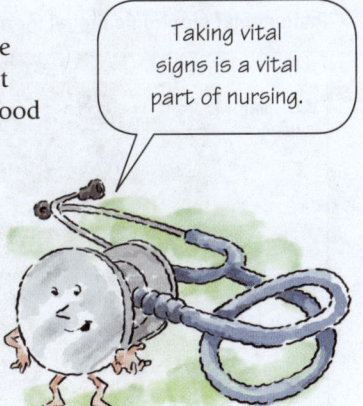

Taking vital signs is a vital part of nursing.

Body temperature

Body temperature represents the balance between heat produced by metabolism and heat produced by muscular activity. Some heat is lost through the skin, lungs, and body waste. A stable temperature pattern promotes the proper function of cells, tissues, and organs; a change in this pattern usually signals the onset of illness.

Types of thermometers

A patient's temperature can be taken with an oral, rectal, or axillary electronic digital thermometer. A tympanic temperature can only be taken with a tympanic thermometer.

Tympanic thermometer

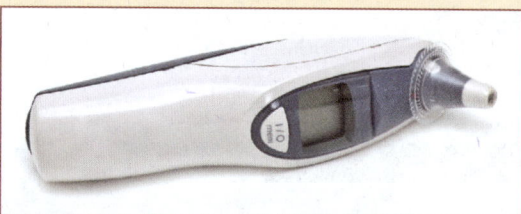

(Image from Shutterstock/Anna Stasevska)

Individual electronic digital thermometer

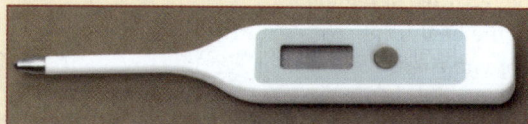

Institutional electronic digital thermometer

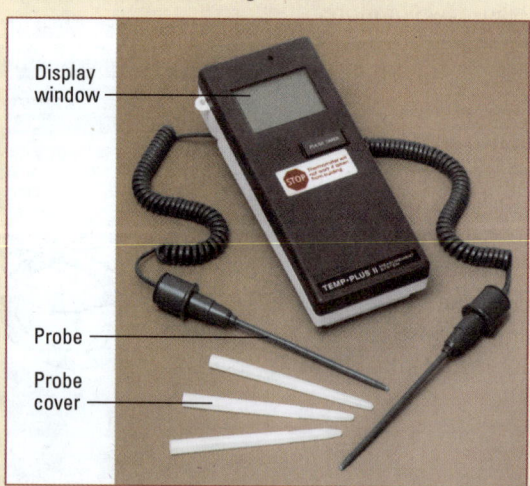

Display window

Probe

Probe cover

Infrared thermometer

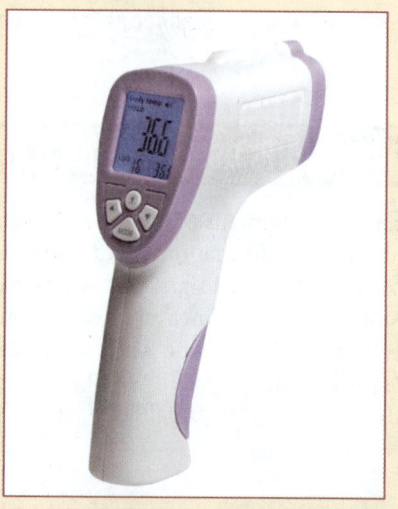

(Image from Shutterstock/VladyslaV Travel photo)

How temperature readings compare

A person's body temperature can be taken in any of the following ways:

Method	Normal temperature	Nursing care
Oral	97.7°–99.5° F (36.5°–37.5° C)	Adults and older children who are awake, alert, oriented, and cooperative
Axillary (armpit)	96.7°–98.5° F (35.9°–3.6.9° C)	Infants, young children, and patients with impaired immune systems when infection is a concern
Rectal	98.7°–100.5° F (37.1°–38.1° C)	Infants, young children, and confused or unconscious patients
Temporal artery	97.4°–100.1° F (36.3°–37.8° C)	Adults, children, infants, and conscious and cooperative patients
Tympanic (ear)	98.2°–100° F (36.8°–37.8° C)	Adults and children, conscious and cooperative patients, and confused or unconscious patients

Choose one

Oral temperature in adults normally ranges from 97.7° to 99.5° F (36.5° to 37.5° C). Rectal temperatures are the most accurate type of reading and are usually 1° F (0.6° C) higher. Axillary (armpit) temperature, which is the least accurate type of temperature reading, is usually 1° to 2° F (0.6° to 1.1° C) lower. Tympanic (in the ear) temperature reads 0.5° to 1° F (0.3° to 0.6° C) higher. (See *Types of thermometers*, page 106 and *How Temperature Readings Compare*.)

Normal ups and downs

Body temperatures can fluctuate with rest and activity. The lowest readings typically occur between 4 and 5 a.m.; the highest readings, between 4 and 8 p.m. Other factors also influence temperature. (See *Differences in temperature*.)

From F to C and back again

To convert a Celsius measurement to a Fahrenheit measurement, multiply the Celsius temperature by 1.8 and add 32. To convert Fahrenheit to Celsius, subtract 32 from the Fahrenheit temperature and divide by 1.8.

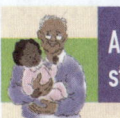

Ages and stages

Differences in temperature

Besides activity level, other factors that influence temperature include sex assigned at birth, age, emotional conditions, and environment. Keep these principles in mind:

• People assigned female at birth normally have higher temperatures than people assigned male at birth do, especially during ovulation.

• Normal temperature is highest in neonates and lowest in older adults.

• A hot external environment can raise temperature; a cold environment can lower it.

Supplies

Necessary supplies for taking a patient's temperature include an electronic or tympanic thermometer, facial tissue, disposable thermometer sheath or probe cover, and gloves. If a rectal temperature is being taken, you will need a water-based lubricant and a rectal thermometer.

How it's done

- Introduce yourself and explain the procedure to the patient.
- If you're taking an oral temperature, ask the patient if they have had hot or cold liquids, have been chewing gum, or have smoked within the past hour. If the patient answers "yes" to any of these questions, wait 20 to 30 minutes to take a measurement, or switch to another route with the appropriate thermometer in order to get an accurate temperature reading.

Taking an oral temperature

- Put on gloves.
- Insert the probe into a disposable probe cover.
- Position the probe tip under the patient's tongue on either side of the frenulum as far back as possible. Placing the tip in this area promotes contact with superficial blood vessels and ensures a more accurate reading.
- Instruct the patient to close their lips while instructing them to not bite down with their teeth to avoid breaking the thermometer.
- Leave the probe in place until the maximum temperature appears on the digital display. Then remove the probe, dispose of the probe cover, note the temperature, and document it in the patient's record.

Taking a rectal temperature

- Before beginning, check with the health care provider to make sure that a rectal temperature is necessary. Taking a temperature rectally can cause rectal perforation, so if there is doubt, choose another route.
- Put on gloves.
- Insert the probe into a disposable probe cover and apply lubricant to the probe cover.
- Position the patient on their side with the top leg flexed, and drape the patient to provide privacy. Then fold back the bed linens to expose the anus.
- Lift the patient's upper buttock and insert the thermometer about ½" (1 cm) for an infant and 1½" (3.8 cm) for an adult.
- Gently direct the thermometer along the rectal wall toward the umbilicus to avoid perforating the anus or rectum and to help ensure an accurate reading. (The thermometer will register hemorrhoidal artery temperature instead of fecal temperature.)
- Hold the thermometer in place until it beeps to prevent damage to rectal tissues caused by displacement.

- Carefully remove the thermometer, wiping it if necessary. Then wipe the anal area to remove any feces.
- Remove gloves, wash hands, and document the results.

Taking an axillary temperature

- Position the patient with the axilla exposed.
- Put on gloves, and gently pat the axilla dry with a facial tissue because moisture conducts heat. Avoid harsh rubbing, which generates heat.
- Ask the patient to reach across their chest and grasp the opposite shoulder, lifting the elbow.
- Position the thermometer in the center of the axilla, with the tip pointing toward the patient's head.
- Tell the patient to keep grasping their shoulder, lower the elbow, and hold it against their chest to promote skin contact with the thermometer.
    - Leave the thermometer in place for the appropriate length of time. Axillary temperatures take longer to register than oral or rectal temperatures because the thermometer *isn't enclosed in a body cavity*.
    - Grasp the end of the thermometer, and remove it from the axilla. Remove gloves, wash hands, and document the results.

With a tympanic thermometer

- Make sure the lens under the probe is clean and shiny. Attach a disposable probe cover.
- Stabilize the patient's head, and gently pull their ear down and back (for children up to age 3) or up and back (for adults and children older than age 3). (See *Taking an infant's temperature.*)
- Insert the thermometer until the entire ear canal is sealed. The thermometer should be inserted toward the tympanic membrane in the same way an otoscope is inserted.
- Press the activation button, and hold for 1 second. The temperature will appear on the display. (See *Tips about temperature,* page 110.)

With a noncontact infrared thermometer

- Noncontact infrared thermometers (NCITs) may be used to reduce cross-contamination risk and to minimize the risk of spreading disease.
- The person using the device should follow the manufacturer's guidelines and instructions for the use of the specific NCIT being used.
- Use in a draft-free space, out of direct sun and away from radiant heat sources.
- Place the NCIT in the testing environment or room for 10 to 30 minutes prior to use to allow the NCIT to adjust to the environment.

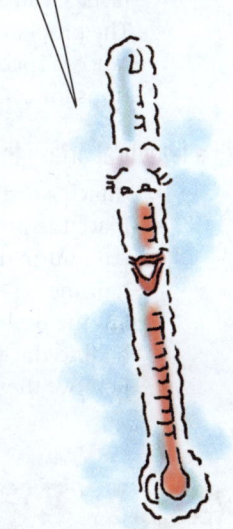

Remember, an armpit isn't an enclosed body cavity, so I'll need to be kept in place a little longer for an accurate reading.

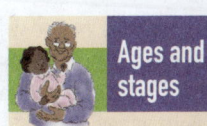

Ages and stages

Taking an infant's temperature

Due to the seriousness of febrile illness for infants under 3 months of age, accuracy of the temperature reading is essential. For these patients, take three temperature readings and use the highest one.

In preparation for taking a temperature measurement with an NCIT, the nurse should ensure the following (U.S. Food and Drug Administration, 2023):

- The test area of the forehead is clean, dry, and not blocked during measurement.
- The person's body temperature or temperature at the forehead test area has not been increased or decreased by wearing excessive clothing or head covers (headbands, bandanas, etc.), or by using facial cleansing products.
- The proper distance between the NCIT and the forehead. This distance is specific to each NCIT. Consult the manufacturer's instructions for correct measurement distances.

With a temporal artery thermometer

- Attach a disposable probe cover.
- Place the probe in the middle of the forehead. While keeping the red button depressed, slide the probe across the forehead to the hairline.
- Lift the probe from the forehead and touch the patient's neck just behind the earlobe. Release the button and record temperature.
- Remove the plastic disposable cover and dispose of the cover.

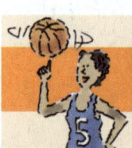

Stay on the ball

Tips about temperature

Keep these tips in mind when taking a patient's temperature:

- Oral measurement is contraindicated in young children and infants and in patients who are unconscious, disoriented, or prone to seizures or those who must breathe through their mouth.
- Always ask the health care provider before performing a rectal temperature. Rectal measurement is contraindicated in patients with diarrhea, recent rectal or prostatic surgery or injury (because it may injure inflamed tissue), or recent myocardial infarction (because anal manipulation may stimulate the vagus nerve, causing bradycardia or another rhythm disturbance).
- Use the same thermometer for repeat temperature taking to ensure consistent results.
- If a patient is receiving nasal oxygen, an oral temperature is still possible because oxygen administration raises oral temperature by only 0.37° F (0.21° C).

Source: Cleveland Clinic. (2023). *What is normal body temperature?* https://health.cleveland-clinic.org/body-temperature-what-is-and-isnt-normal/.

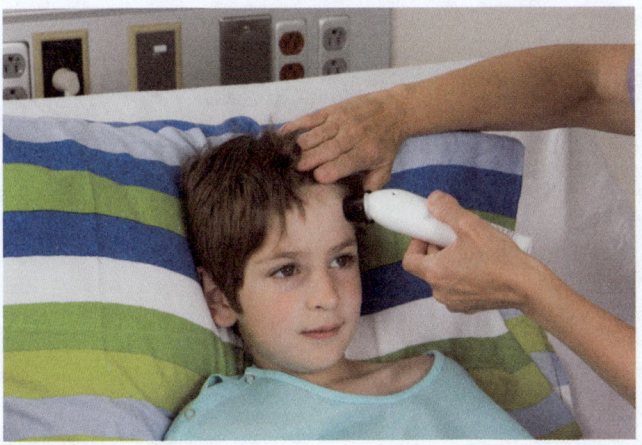

(Image reprinted with permission from Lynn, P. (2015). *Taylor's clinical nursing skills* (4th ed., Skill 2-1, Figure 1D). Wolters Kluwer.)

Pulse

The patient's pulse reflects the amount of blood ejected with each heartbeat. The recurring wave—called a *pulse*—can be palpated at locations on the body where an artery crosses over bone or firm tissue. To assess the pulse, palpate one of the patient's arterial pulse points and note the rate, rhythm, and amplitude of the pulse. A normal pulse for an adult is between 60 and 100 beats/minute.

The radial pulse

The radial pulse is the most accessible. During cardiovascular emergencies, the femoral or carotid pulses may be palpated. These vessels are larger and more accurately reflect the heart's activity. (See *Pinpointing pulse sites*.)

Rate, rhythm, and volume

Taking a patient's pulse involves determining the number of beats per minute (the pulse rate), the pattern or irregularity of the beats (the rhythm), and the volume of blood pumped with each beat. (See *Alternate site for taking a pulse*.) If the pulse is faint or weak, consider using a Doppler ultrasound blood flow detector. (See *Using a Doppler device*, page 112.)

Supplies

A watch with a second hand, a stethoscope (for auscultating apical pulse), and, if necessary, a Doppler ultrasound blood flow detector.

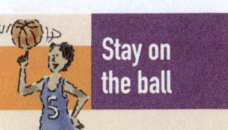

Stay on the ball

Pinpointing pulse sites

Pulses can be assessed at several sites, including those shown in this illustration.

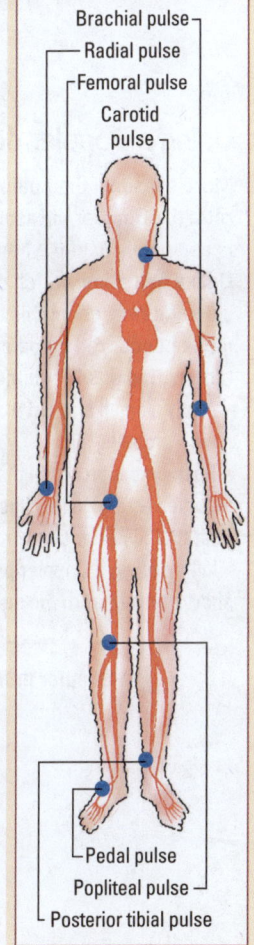

Brachial pulse
Radial pulse
Femoral pulse
Carotid pulse
Pedal pulse
Popliteal pulse
Posterior tibial pulse

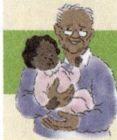

Alternate site for taking a pulse

The most common site for taking a pulse is the radial artery in the wrist. This holds true for adults and children older than age 3.

For infants and children younger than age 3, however, it is better to listen to the heart with a stethoscope rather than palpate a pulse. Because auscultation is done at the apex of the heart, the pulse measurement is the *apical pulse*.

Using a Doppler device

More sensitive than palpation for determining pulse rate, the Doppler ultrasound blood flow detector is especially useful when a pulse is faint or weak. Unlike palpation, which detects arterial wall expansion and retraction, this instrument detects the movement of red blood cells. Here is how to use it (Johns Hopkins Medicine, 2023):

• Apply a small amount of transmission gel to the ultrasound probe.

• Position the probe on the skin directly over the selected artery. In the illustration below, the probe is over the posterior tibial artery.

• When using a Doppler probe with an amplifier (as shown below), turn the instrument on, and moving counterclockwise, set the volume control to the lowest setting. If the model used doesn't have a speaker, plug in the earphones and slowly raise the volume.

• To obtain the best signals, put gel between the skin and the probe and tilt the probe 45° from the artery. Slowly move the probe in a circular motion to locate the center of the artery and the Doppler signal—a hissing noise at the heartbeat. Avoid moving the probe rapidly because this distorts the signal.

• Count the signals for 60 seconds to determine the pulse rate.

• After you've measured the pulse rate, clean the probe with a soft cloth soaked in antiseptic solution or soapy water. Don't immerse the probe.

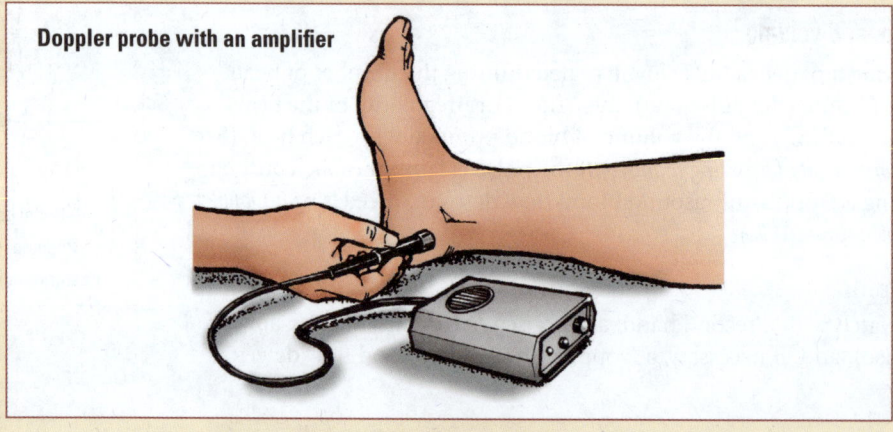

Doppler probe with an amplifier

How it's done

- Introduce yourself and explain the procedure to the patient.
- Make sure the patient is comfortable and relaxed because an awkward, uncomfortable position may affect their heart rate.

Taking a radial pulse

- Place the patient in a sitting or supine position, with their arms at the side or across the chest.

Keep the thumb out of it

- To feel the pulse, press your index and middle fingers on the radial artery inside the patient's wrist. Only moderate pressure should be used; excessive pressure may occlude blood flow distal to the pulse site. The thumb shouldn't be used to take the patient's pulse; the thumb has a strong pulse of its own and may be easily confused with the patient's pulse.

1, 2, 3 … 60

- After locating the pulse, count the beats for 60 seconds to get the number of beats per minute. Counting for a full minute provides a more accurate picture of irregularities.
- While counting the rate, assess pulse rhythm and volume by noting the pattern and strength of the beats. If an abnormality is detected, repeat the count and note whether the irregularity occurs in a pattern or randomly. If there is still doubt, take an apical pulse. (See *Identifying pulse patterns*, page 114.)

Taking an apical pulse

- Help the patient to a supine position.

Warm the scope first, please

- The diaphragm or bell of the stethoscope can be warmed on the palm of the hand. Placing a cold stethoscope against the patient's skin may startle them and momentarily increase their heart rate.
- Place the bell or diaphragm of the stethoscope over the apex of the heart (typically located at the fifth intercostal space, left of the midclavicular line).
- Count the beats for 60 seconds, and note their rate, rhythm, volume, and intensity.

Taking an apical-radial pulse

- When taking an apical-radial pulse, you may need to find another nurse to assist you. One nurse can auscultate the apical pulse while the other palpates the radial pulse.
- Help the patient to the supine position.
- Locate the apical and radial pulses, and then determine a time to begin counting. Each nurse should count beats for 60 seconds.

Identifying pulse patterns

This chart lists different types of pulse patterns along with their rates, rhythms, and causes and incidence.

Type	Rate	Rhythm	Causes and incidence
Normal	60 – 80 beats/min; in neonates, 120–140 beats/min	● ● ● ●	• Varies with such factors as physical activity, sex assigned at birth, and age (infants and children have higher pulse rates than adults; older adults have lower pulse rates)
Tachycardia	More than 100 beats/min	●●●●●●●	• Accompanies stimulation of the sympathetic nervous system resulting from emotional stress (such as anger, fear, or anxiety) or the use of certain drugs (such as caffeine) • May result from exercise or such health conditions as heart failure, anemia, and fever, which increase oxygen requirements, and thus, pulse rate
Bradycardia	Less than 60 beats/min	● ● ●	• Accompanies stimulation of the parasympathetic nervous system resulting from drug use, especially cardiac glycosides, and such conditions as cerebral hemorrhage and heart block • May also be present in very fit athletes and persons with hypothyroidism
Irregular	Uneven time intervals between beats (e.g., periods of regular rhythm interrupted by pauses or premature beats)	●●●● ●●	• May indicate cardiac irritability, hypoxia, digoxin toxicity, potassium imbalance, or a more serious arrhythmia if premature beats occur frequently (occasional premature beats are normal)

Source: Johns Hopkins Medicine. (2022). *Vital signs (body temperature, pulse rate, respiration rate, blood pressure)*. https://www.hopkinsmedicine.org/health/conditions-and-diseases/vital-signs-body-temperature-pulse-rate-respiration-rate-blood-pressure

Working alone

- First, auscultate the apex of the heart, holding the stethoscope in place with the hand wearing the watch. Next, palpate the radial artery with the other hand. This process helps you feel any discrepancies between the apical and radial pulses.
- Note that some of the heartbeats detected at the apex can't be detected at peripheral sites. When this occurs, the apical pulse rate is higher than the radial pulse rate; the difference is documented as a pulse deficit.

Leaps and bounds

Pulse amplitude should also be assessed. To do so, use a numerical scale or descriptive term to rate or characterize the strength. Numerical scales differ slightly among facilities, but the following scale is commonly used:

Type of pulse	Description	Measured as:
absent pulse	not palpable	0
weak or thready pulse	hard to feel, easily obliterated by slight finger pressure	+1
normal pulse	easily palpable, obliterated by strong finger pressure	+2
bounding pulse	readily palpable, forceful, not easily obliterated by pressure from the fingers	+3

ABSENT

weak

NORMAL

BOUNDING

(See *Documenting pulse*.)

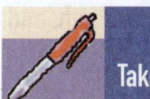

Take note!

Documenting pulse

- When documenting a pulse, be sure to record pulse rate, rhythm, and volume as well as the time of measurement.
- "Full" or "bounding" describes a pulse of increased volume; "weak" or "thready," a pulse of decreased volume.
- When recording an apical pulse, include the intensity of heart sounds.
- When recording an apical-radial pulse, chart the rate according to the pulse site—for example, A/R pulse = 80/76.

Respiration

Respiration is the exchange of oxygen and carbon dioxide between the atmosphere and the body. External respiration, or breathing, occurs through the work of the diaphragm and chest muscles and delivers oxygen to the lower respiratory tract and alveoli.

Rate, rhythm, depth, and sound

Respiration is measured according to rate, rhythm, depth, and sound. For an adult, a respiratory rate of 12 to 20 breaths per minute is considered normal (Sapra et al., 2022). These measurements reflect the body's metabolic state, diaphragm and chest muscle condition, and airway patency. The number of breaths per minute is highly regulated to enable cells to produce the optimum amount of energy at any given time (Chourpiliadis & Bhardwaj, 2022).

The respiratory rate is documented as the number of cycles per minute, with inspiration and expiration making up one cycle; rhythm is the regularity of these cycles. Depth is the volume of air inhaled and exhaled with each respiration; the sound is the audible digression from normal, effortless breathing.

Supplies

A watch with a second hand and a stethoscope.

How it's done

- Introduce yourself and explain the procedure to the patient.
- The best time to assess a patient's respirations is immediately after taking their pulse rate. Keep your fingertips over their radial artery and count respirations without telling the patient. Otherwise, the patient will become conscious of the rate, and it may change.

Watch the movement

- Count respirations by observing the rise and fall of the chest as the patient breathes. Alternatively, position the patient's opposite arm across the chest, and count respirations by feeling its rise and fall. Consider one rise and one fall as one respiration.
- Count respirations for 30 seconds and multiply by two, or count for 60 seconds if respirations are irregular to account for variations in respiratory rate and pattern.
- Observe chest movements for depth of respirations. If the patient inhales a small volume of air, record the depth as shallow; if the patient inhales a large volume, record the depth as deep.
- Observe the patient for use of such accessory muscles as the scalene, sternocleidomastoid, trapezius, and latissimus dorsi. Such use indicates weakness of the diaphragm and the external intercostal muscles, the major muscles of respiration.

Listen to the sounds

- As respirations are observed, watch for and record such breath sounds as stertor, stridor, wheezing, and expiratory grunting.

- ○ *Stertor* is a snoring sound resulting from secretions in the trachea and large bronchi. Listen for it in comatose patients and in patients with a neurologic disorder.
  - ○ *Stridor* is an inspiratory crowing sound that occurs in patients with laryngitis, croup, or upper respiratory tract obstruction with a foreign body. (See *How age impacts respiration*.)
  - ○ *Wheezing* is caused by a partial obstruction in the smaller bronchi and bronchioles. This high-pitched, musical sound is common in patients with emphysema or asthma.
  - ○ To detect other breath sounds, such as crackles and rhonchi, you must use a stethoscope.
- Watch the patient's chest movements and listen to their breathing to determine the rhythm and sound of respirations. (See *Identifying respiratory patterns*, page 118.)
  - ○ Respiratory rates of less than 8 breaths/minute or more than 40 breaths/minute are usually considered abnormal and should be reported promptly.
- Observe the patient for signs of dyspnea, such as an anxious facial expression, flaring nostrils, a heaving chest wall, and cyanosis. To detect cyanosis, look for the characteristic bluish discoloration of the nail beds and lips, under the tongue, in the buccal mucosa, and in the conjunctiva.
  - ○ When assessing a patient's respiratory status, consider personal and family history. Ask if they have ever smoked and, if so, the number of years and the number of packs per day. (See *Documenting respirations*.)

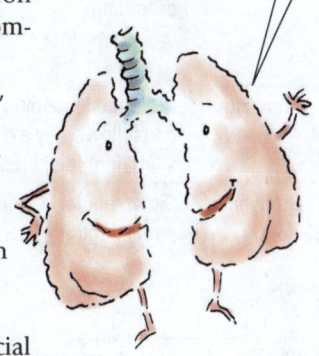

Observing, counting, and listening . . . assessing respirations is an exercise in multitasking!

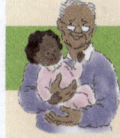

Ages and stages

How age impacts respiration

When assessing respirations in pediatric and older patients, keep these points in mind (Sapra et al., 2022):

- When listening for stridor in infants and children with croup, check for sternal, substernal, and intercostal retractions.
- In infants, an expiratory grunt indicates imminent respiratory distress.
- In patients over the age of 65, an expiratory grunt indicates partial airway obstruction.
- A child's respiratory rate may double in response to exercise, illness, or emotion.
- Normally, the rate for neonates is 30 to 80 breaths/minute; for toddlers, 20 to 40 breaths/minute; and for children of school age and older, 15 to 25 breaths/minute.
- Children usually reach the adult rate (12 to 20 breaths/minute) at about age 15.

Identifying respiratory patterns

This chart presents different types of respirations along with their characteristics, patterns, and possible causes.

Type	Characteristics	Pattern	Possible causes
Apnea	Periodic absence of breathing	———————	• Mechanical airway obstruction • Conditions affecting the brain's respiratory center in the lateral medulla oblongata
Apneustic	Prolonged, gasping inspiration followed by extremely short, inefficient expiration	∿∿∿∿∿	• Lesions of the respiratory center
Bradypnea	Slow, regular respirations of equal depth	∿∿∿	• Normal pattern during sleep • Conditions affecting the respiratory center, such as tumors, metabolic disorders, respiratory decompensation, and the use of opiates or alcohol
Cheyne-Stokes	Fast, deep respirations for 30–170 seconds punctuated by periods of apnea lasting 20–60 seconds	∿∿∿	• Increased intracranial pressure, severe heart failure, renal failure, meningitis, drug overdose, and cerebral anoxia
Eupnea	Normal rate and rhythm	∿∿∿	• Normal respiration
Kussmaul	Fast (more than 20 breaths/min), deep (resembling sighs), labored respirations without pause	∿∿∿∿	• Renal failure and metabolic acidosis, particularly diabetic ketoacidosis
Tachypnea	Rapid respirations, rate rises with body temperature at about 4 breaths/min for each degree Fahrenheit above normal	∿∿∿∿	• Pneumonia, compensatory respiratory alkalosis, respiratory insufficiency, lesions of the respiratory center, and salicylate poisoning

Source: Sapra, A., Malik, A., & Bhandari, P. (2022). Vital sign assessment. *StatPearls*. Treasure Island (FL): StatPearls Publishing. https://www.ncbi.nlm.nih.gov/books/NBK553213/

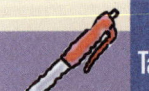

Take note!

Documenting respirations

Record the rate, depth, rhythm, and sound of the patient's respirations.

Accessory to the act . . . of breathing

The use of accessory muscles can enhance lung expansion when oxygenation drops. Patients with chronic obstructive pulmonary disease (COPD) or respiratory distress may use neck muscles, including the sternocleidomastoid muscles, and abdominal muscles for breathing. Posture changes during normal breathing may also suggest such problems as COPD. Normal respirations should be quiet and easy, so it is important to note any abnormalities.

Oxygen saturation

Measurement of oxygen saturation determines the percentage of oxygen that is bound to hemoglobin. This measurement can be completed noninvasively using a pulse oximeter. A pulse oximeter measures the oxygen saturation of a patient's arterial blood using a LED light and receiver that are typically placed on a patient's finger. Normal pulse oximetry readings range between 92% and 100%. When a patient's pulse oximetry reading falls below 92%, additional assessments may be necessary to determine the next steps or the need for intervention (Jensen, 2023).

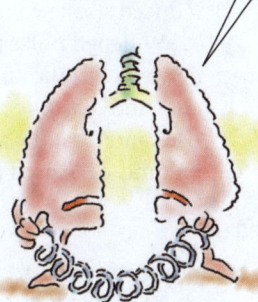

In respiratory disorders, such as COPD, I have to rely on accessory muscles to help me expand.

Blood pressure

Blood pressure, which is the force that blood exerts on arterial walls, is affected by the force of ventricular contractions, arterial wall elasticity, peripheral vascular resistance, and blood volume and viscosity (Ismail et al., 2022). Blood pressure measurements consist of systolic pressure and diastolic pressure readings.

Systolic (contract) vs. diastolic (relax)

Systolic pressure occurs when the left ventricle contracts. It reflects the integrity of the heart, arteries, and arterioles. A normal systolic pressure ranges from 100 to 119 mm Hg. *Diastolic pressure* occurs when the left ventricle relaxes. It indicates blood vessel resistance. Normal diastolic pressure ranges from 60 to 79 mm Hg (American Heart Association (AHA), 2023). In principle, the systolic blood pressure corresponds to the increase in oscillation when blood flows through the cuff, and the diastolic pressure corresponds to the disappearance of the oscillation. The diastolic pressure is generally more significant as it measures the heart at rest. Both pressures are measured in millimeters of mercury (mm Hg) with a sphygmomanometer and a stethoscope, usually at the brachial artery.

Systolic pressure – diastolic pressure = pulse pressure

Pulse pressure, or the difference between systolic and diastolic pressures, varies inversely with arterial elasticity. Normally, systolic pressure exceeds diastolic pressure by about 40 mm Hg. Narrowed pulse pressure, or a difference of less than 30 mm Hg, occurs when systolic pressure falls and diastolic pressure rises. These changes reflect reduced stroke volume, increased peripheral resistance, or both.

Widened pulse pressure, a difference of more than 50 mm Hg between systolic and diastolic pressures, occurs when systolic pressure rises and diastolic pressure remains constant or when systolic pressure rises and diastolic pressure falls. These changes reflect increased stroke volume, decreased peripheral resistance, or both.

Going up?

Blood pressure rises with age, weight gain, prolonged stress, and anxiety. (See *Effects of age on blood pressure.*)

Supplies

Sphygmomanometer (blood pressure cuff with gauge), stethoscope, and automated vital signs monitor (if available). Blood pressure cuffs come in six standard sizes, ranging from neonate to extra-large adult. Disposable cuffs are available.

An automated vital signs monitor is a noninvasive device that measures pulse rate, systolic and diastolic pressures, and mean arterial pressure at preset intervals. (See *Using an electronic vital signs monitor,* page 120.)

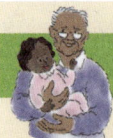

Ages and stages

Effects of age on blood pressure

Neonate – 17 years of age
- At birth, systolic and diastolic blood pressure readings are significantly lower than in adults (systolic 50–70 and diastolic 30–50) (Flynn et al., 2017).
- As the child grows, blood pressure readings increase each year until readings stabilize and meet adult measurements.
- In 2017, the American Academy of Pediatrics (AAP) (Flynn et al., 2017) presented new clinical practice guidelines to screen and manage high blood pressure in children and adolescents. This guidance presents a sex-, age-, and height-based chart to determine normal blood pressure readings for each age group. This chart can be found here: https://www.nhlbi.nih.gov/files/docs/guidelines/child_tbl.pdf

Adult—18 and older
Normal blood pressure reading for adults (AHA, 2023):
- Systolic: 90 to 120
- Diastolic: 60 to 80

Using an electronic vital signs monitor

An electronic vital signs monitor allows the nurse to continually track a patient's vital signs without having to reapply a blood pressure cuff each time. The steps below can be followed with most monitors.

Some automated vital signs monitors are lightweight and battery-operated and can be attached to an IV pole for continual monitoring. It is important to note the capacity of the monitor's battery and plug in the machine whenever possible to keep it charged.

Before using any monitor, check its accuracy. Determine the patient's pulse rate and blood pressure manually, using the same arm for the monitor cuff. When both readings are complete, compare the results. If the results differ, contact the supply department or the manufacturer's representative for monitor calibration.

Preparing the device

• Collect the monitor, dual air hose, and pressure cuff. Then make sure the monitor unit is firmly positioned near the patient's bed.
• Explain the procedure to the patient. Describe the alarm system so that the patient won't be frightened if the alarm is triggered.
• Make sure the power switch is off. Then plug the monitor into a properly grounded wall outlet. Secure the dual air hose to the front of the monitor.
• Connect the pressure cuff's tubing to the other ends of the dual air hose and tighten the connections to prevent air leaks. Keep the air hose away from the patient so that it isn't accidentally dislodged.
• Wrap the cuff loosely around the patient's arm or leg, allowing two fingerbreadths between the cuff and the arm or leg. Position the cuff's "artery" arrow over the palpated brachial artery. Then secure the cuff for a snug fit.
• Never apply the cuff to a limb that has an IV line in place or to an individual who has had breast or lymph node excision on that side or has an arteriovenous graft, shunt, or fistula.

Monitor Settings

• When ready, turn on the monitor and select parameters for measurement. Some monitors have special settings for cuff size and location. Be sure to follow all necessary guidelines for the monitor being used.

Collecting data

• Once the monitor is configured, push the appropriate button to start the machine blood pressure measurement.
  – If measurements are to be repeated at set intervals, you'll need to tell the monitor how often to obtain data. Automatic readings can be set at necessary time intervals.
  – After the measurements are collected the monitor will display the last data obtained along with the time elapsed. Newer monitors will also display the last several measurements if automatic readings were employed.

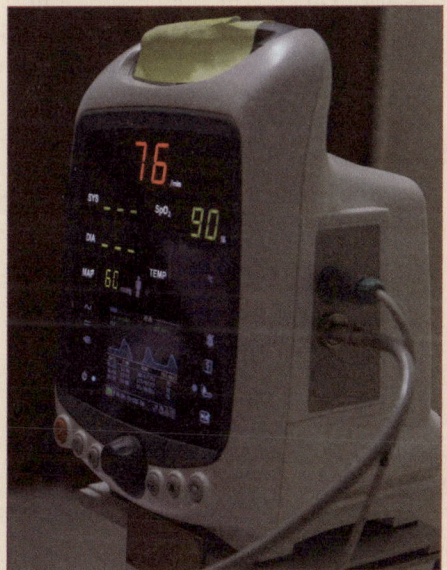

(Image from Shutterstock/bochimsang12.)

Source: Ismail, S., Nayan, N., Jaafar, R., & May, Z. (2022). Recent advances in non-invasive blood pressure monitoring and prediction using a machine learning approach. *Sensors, 22*(16), 6195. https://doi.org/10.3390/s22166195

Getting ready

- Carefully choose a cuff of appropriate size for the patient. An extremely narrow cuff may cause a false-high reading; an extremely wide one, a false-low reading.

How it's done

- Introduce yourself and explain the procedure to the patient.
- The patient can lie in a supine position or sit upright while the blood pressure measurement is taken. The patient's arm should be extended at heart level and be well supported. If the artery is below heart level, the reading may be artificially increased. Make sure the patient is relaxed and comfortable when measuring the blood pressure so it stays at a normal level.

Don't compromise

- Don't take a blood pressure measurement on the same arm of an arteriovenous fistula or hemodialysis shunt because blood flow through the device may be compromised. In addition, don't take a blood pressure measurement on the affected side of a mastectomy because it may compromise lymphatic circulation, worsen edema, and damage the arm. Finally, don't take blood pressure on the same arm as a peripherally inserted central catheter because it may damage the device.
- Wrap the deflated cuff snugly around the patient's upper arm.

Go with the bell

- Palpate the brachial artery. Center the bell of the stethoscope over the part of the artery where you detect the strongest beats and hold it in place with one hand. The bell of the stethoscope transmits low-pitched arterial blood sounds more effectively than the diaphragm. (See *Using a sphygmomanometer.*)
- Using the thumb and index finger of your other hand, turn the thumbscrew on the rubber bulb of the air pump clockwise to close the valve.
- Pump air into the cuff while auscultating for the sound over the brachial artery to compress and, eventually, occlude arterial blood flow. Continue pumping air until the mercury column or aneroid gauge registers 160 mm Hg or at least 30 mm Hg above the level of the last audible sound.
- Carefully open the valve of the air pump. Then deflate the cuff no faster than 5 mm Hg/s while watching the mercury column or aneroid gauge and auscultating for the sound over the artery.

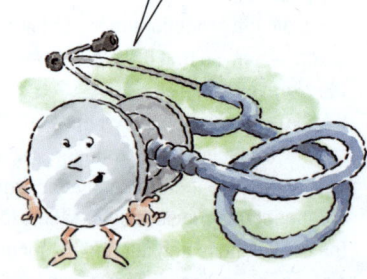

Be aware of preexisting conditions or problems that can compromise the blood pressure reading or your patient's health.

Using a sphygmomanometer

Here is how to use a sphygmomanometer properly:
- For accuracy and consistency, position the patient with their upper arm at heart level and their palm turned up.
- Apply the cuff snugly, 1″ (2.5 cm) above the brachial pulse, as shown in the top photo.
- Position the manometer at eye level.
- Palpate the brachial or radial pulse with your fingertips while inflating the cuff.
- Inflate the cuff to 30 mm Hg above the point where the pulse disappears.
- Place the bell of the stethoscope over the point where you felt the pulse was felt, as shown in the bottom photo. Using the bell helps you hear more clearly Korotkoff sounds, which indicate the pulse.
- Release the valve slowly and note the point when the Korotkoff sounds reappear. The start of the pulse sound indicates the systolic pressure.
- The sounds will become muffled and then disappear. The last Korotkoff sound heard indicates the diastolic pressure.

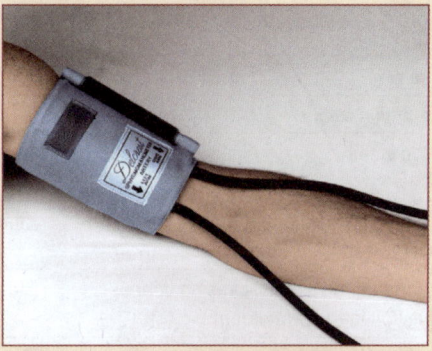

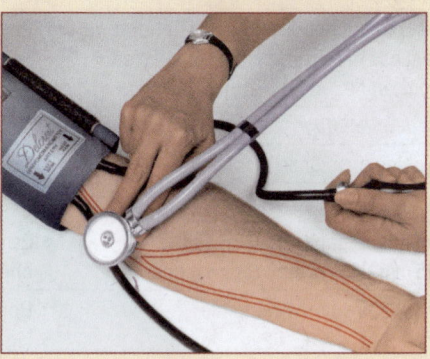

Tune in to the five sounds

- When you hear the first beat or clear tapping sound, note the pressure on the column or gauge, that is, the systolic pressure. (The beat or tapping sound is the first of five Korotkoff sounds. The second sound resembles a murmur or swish; the third, crisp tapping; the fourth, a soft, muffled tone; and the fifth, the last sound heard.)
- Continue to release air gradually while auscultating for the sound over the artery.
- Note the diastolic pressure, the fourth Korotkoff sound. If you continue to hear sounds as the column or gauge falls to zero (common in children), record the pressure at the beginning of the fourth sound. This step is important because, in some patients, a distinct fifth sound is absent. (For information on situations that can cause false-high or false-low readings, see *Correcting problems of blood pressure measurement.*)

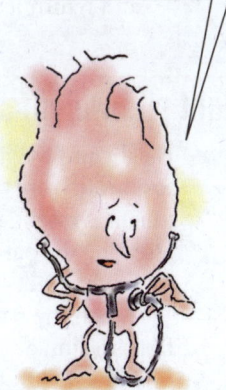

> That's one (tap) . . . two (swish) . . . three (tap) . . . four (muffle) . . . five . . .

Correcting problems of blood pressure measurement

This chart lists blood pressure measurement problems along with their causes and appropriate nursing actions.

Causes	Nursing actions
False-high reading	
Cuff too small	Make sure the cuff bladder is 20% wider than the circumference of the arm or leg being used for measurement.
Cuff wrapped too loosely, reducing its effective width	Tighten the cuff.
Cuff deflated too slowly, causing venous congestion in the arm or leg	Never deflate the cuff more slowly than 2 mm Hg per heartbeat.
Mercury column tilted	Read pressures with the mercury column vertical.
Measurement poorly timed (e.g., after the patient has eaten, ambulated, appeared anxious, or flexed their arm muscles)	Postpone the blood pressure measurement or help the patient relax before measuring the blood pressure.
False-low reading	
Arm or leg positioned incorrectly	Make sure the patient's arm or leg is level with the heart.
Mercury column below eye level	Read the mercury column at eye level.
Auscultatory gap (sound fades out for 10–15 mm Hg and then returns) unnoticed	Estimate systolic pressure by palpation before measuring it. Then check this pressure against measured pressure.
Low-volume sounds inaudible	Before reinflating the cuff, instruct the patient to raise their arm or leg to decrease venous pressure and amplify low-volume sounds. After inflating the cuff, tell the patient to lower their arm or leg. Then deflate the cuff and listen. If still unable to detect low volume sounds, chart palpated systolic pressure.

One more time

- To confirm blood pressure findings, rapidly deflate the cuff. Record the pressure, wait 1 to 2 minutes, and then repeat the procedure and record the pressures. After doing so, remove and fold the cuff, and return it to storage.

Height and weight

Height and weight are routinely measured when a patient is admitted to a health care facility. An accurate record of the patient's height and weight is essential for calculating dosages of drugs and contrast agents, assessing the patient's nutritional status, and determining the height-to-weight ratio.

Weigh the patient at the same time each day (usually before breakfast), in similar clothing, and using the same scale. If the patient uses crutches, weigh the patient with the crutches. Then weigh the crutches and any heavy clothing and subtract their weight from the total to determine the most accurate record of the patient's weight.

Weight and fluid status

Because body weight is the best overall indicator of fluid status, daily monitoring is important for patients receiving a diuretic or a medication that causes sodium retention. Rapid weight gain may signal fluid retention, and rapid weight loss may indicate diuresis.

Scales for every position

Weight can be measured with a standing scale, a chair scale, or a bed scale. Height can be measured with the measuring bar on a standing scale. If a patient is unable to stand, height can be measured in bed in a supine position using a measuring tape.

Supplies

Standing scale with measuring bar. A chair scale for patients in a wheelchair (if needed for patient transport) or a bed scale. A patient can be measured for height using a tape measure if the patient is lying in bed and unable to stand.

Getting ready

Be sure to select the appropriate scale. Typically, a standing scale is used for an ambulatory patient, and a chair or bed scale is used for an acutely ill or debilitated patient. Make sure the scale is balanced. Standing scales and, to a lesser extent, bed scales may become unbalanced when transported.

How it's done

- Introduce yourself and explain the procedure to the patient.
- The explanation may differ based on the type of measurement devices used.

Using a standing scale

- If indicated, place a protective cover on the scale's platform.
- Tell the patient to remove their robe and slippers or shoes. If the scale has wheels, lock them before the patient steps on. Assist the patient onto the scale and remain close to them to prevent falls.

Upright balance scale

- If an upright balance scale is being used, slide the lower rider to the groove representing the largest increment below the patient's estimated weight. Grooves represent 50, 100, 150, and 200 lb.
- Slide the small upper rider until the beam balances. Add the upper and lower rider figures to determine the weight.

Multiple weight scale

- If using a multiple-weight scale, move the appropriate ratio weights onto the weight holder to balance the scale; ratio weights are labeled 50, 100, and 200 lb.
- Add ratio weights until the next weight causes the main beam to fall.
- Adjust the main beam poise until the scale balances.
- To obtain the weight, add the sum of the ratio weights to the figure on the main beam.
- Return ratio weights to their rack and the weight holder to its proper place.

Digital scale

- If a digital scale is being used, make sure the display reads 0 before use.
- Read the display with the patient standing as still as possible.

Raising the bar

- To measure height, tell the patient to stand erect on the scale's platform. Raise the measuring bar above the patient's head, extend the horizontal arm, and lower the bar until it touches the top of the patient's head. Then read the patient's height.
- Help the patient off the scale and give the patient their robe and slippers or shoes. Then return the measuring bar to its initial position.

Using a chair scale

- Transport the patient to the weighing area or the scale to the patient's bedside.
- Lock the scale in place to prevent it from moving accidentally.
- If a scale with a swing-away chair arm is being used, unlock the arm. When unlocked, the arm swings back 180° to permit easy access.
- Position the scale beside the patient's bed or wheelchair with the chair arm open. Transfer the patient onto the scale, swing the chair arm to the front of the scale, and lock it in place.
- Weigh the patient by adding ratio weights and adjusting the main beam poise. Then unlock the swing-away chair arm as before, and transfer the patient back to their bed or wheelchair.
- Lock the main beam to avoid damaging the scale during transport. Then unlock the wheels and remove the scale from the patient's room.

Using a bed scale

- Cover the bed scale stretcher with a protective cover. Balance the scale with the drawsheet in place to ensure an accurate measurement.
- Provide privacy, and tell the patient about the procedure of being weighed on a special bed scale.
- When rolling the patient onto the stretcher, be careful not to dislodge IV lines, indwelling catheters, and other supportive equipment.
- Position the scale next to the patient's bed, and lock the scale's wheels. Then turn the patient onto their side, facing away from the scale.
- Release the stretcher frame to the horizontal position, and pump the hand lever until the stretcher is positioned over the mattress. Lower the stretcher onto the mattress, and roll the patient onto the stretcher.
- Raise the stretcher 2″ (5 cm) above the mattress. Then add ratio weights, and adjust the main beam poise as for the standing and chair scales.
- After weighing the patient, lower the stretcher onto the mattress, turn the patient onto their side, and remove the stretcher. Be sure to leave the patient in a comfortable position.

Using a digital bed scale

- Release the stretcher to the horizontal position; then lock it in place. Turn the patient onto their side, facing away from the scale.
- Roll the base of the scale under the patient's bed. Adjust the lever to widen the base of the scale, providing stability. Then lock the scale's wheels.
- Center the stretcher above the bed, lower it onto the mattress and roll the patient onto the stretcher. Then position the circular weighing arms of the scale over the patient, and attach them securely to the stretcher bars.
- Pump the handle with long, slow strokes to raise the patient a few inches off the bed. Make sure the patient doesn't lean on or touch the headboard, side rails, or other bed equipment because doing so will affect weight measurement.
- Depress the OPERATE button, and read the patient's weight on the digital display panel. Then press in the scale's handle to lower the patient.
- Detach the circular weighing arms from the stretcher bars, roll the patient off the stretcher and remove it, and position comfortably in bed.
- Release the wheel lock and withdraw the scale. Return the stretcher to its vertical position.

Quick quiz

1. The nurse is preparing to take a patient's oral temperature with an electronic thermometer. When asking the patient temperature pre-assessment questions, which answer would allow the nurse to continue the assessment immediately?
    A. I just smoked a cigarette.
    B. I just had a cup of hot coffee.
    C. I just had a sip of room-temperature water.
    D. Do I need to spit my gum out?

Answer: C. Patients should not have hot or cold liquids, smoke cigarettes, or chew gum prior to having their temperature taken orally.

2. The health care provider has asked a patient to monitor their temperature four times a day for a week. The patient has noted that their temperature is always lowest during what time period?
    A. Between 4 and 5 a.m.
    B. Between 8 and 9 a.m.
    C. Between 4 and 8 p.m.
    D. Between 9 and 11 p.m.

Answer: A. Temperature normally fluctuates with rest and activity. The lowest readings typically occur between 4 and 5 a.m.; the highest readings, between 4 and 8 p.m.

3. The nurse is concerned because a patient is making a snoring sound while sleeping. What respiratory sound does the nurse suspect?
    A. Stertor
    B. Stridor
    C. Wheezing
    D. Expiratory grunting

Answer: A. Stertor is a snoring sound that results from secretions in the trachea and large bronchi.

4. A nurse is preparing to take a patient's blood pressure. Which of the following patient assessments would indicate that the nurse could not use the patient's arm for a blood pressure measurement? (Select all that apply.)
    A. Mastectomy
    B. Hemodialysis shunt
    C. Peripherally inserted central catheter (PICC)
    D. Immunization injection 1 week prior

Answer: A, B, and C. Previous mastectomy, hemodialysis shunt, and a peripherally inserted central catheter would indicate the need to take blood pressure in the other arm. Immunization injections are not a contraindication for the application of a blood pressure cuff.

Scoring

⭐⭐⭐ If you answered all four questions correctly, congratulations! You're a vital signs expert.

⭐⭐ If you answered three questions correctly, great! You've got the pulse on vital signs assessment skills.

⭐ If you answered fewer than three questions correctly, don't despair. Take a deep breath, listen to your heart, and know that you still measure up to a good nurse!

References

American Heart Association (AHA). (2023). *High blood pressure.* https://www.heart.org/en/health-topics/high-blood-pressure

Chourpiliadis, C., & Bhardwaj, A. (2022). *Physiology, respiratory rate. StatPearls.* StatPearls Publishing. https://www.ncbi.nlm.nih.gov/books/NBK537306/

Cleveland Clinic. (2023). *What is normal body temperature?* https://health.cleveland-clinic.org/body-temperature-what-is-and-isnt-normal/

Flynn, J., Kaelber, D., Baker-Smith, C., Blowey, D., Carroll, A., Daniels, S., de Ferranti, S., Dionne, J., Falkner, B., Flinn, S., Gidding, S., Goodwin, C., Leu, M., Powers, M., Rea, C., Samuels, J., Simasek, M., Thaker, V., & Urbina, E. (2017). Clinical practice guideline for screening and management of high blood pressure in children and adolescents. *Pediatrics, 140*(3), 320171904. https://doi.org/10.1542/peds.2017-1904

Ismail, S., Nayan, N., Jaafar, R., & May, Z. (2022). Recent advances in non-invasive blood pressure monitoring and prediction using a machine learning approach. *Sensors, 22*(16), 6195. https://doi.org/10.3390/s22166195

Jensen, S. (2023). *Nursing health assessment: A clinical judgment approach.* (4th ed.). Wolters Kluwer.

Johns Hopkins Medicine. (2022). *Vital signs (body temperature, pulse rate, respiration rate, blood pressure).* https://www.hopkinsmedicine.org/health/conditions-and-diseases/vital-signs-body-temperature-pulse-rate-respiration-rate-blood-pressure

Johns Hopkins Medicine. (2023). *Vascular studies.* https://www.hopkinsmedicine.org/health/treatment-tests-and-therapies/vascular-studies

Sapra, A., Malik, A., & Bhandari, P (2022). *Vital sign assessment. StatPearls.* StatPearls Publishing. https://www.ncbi.nlm.nih.gov/books/NBK553213/

U.S. Food and Drug Administration. (2023). *Non-contact infrared thermometers.* https://www.fda.gov/medical-devices/general-hospital-devices-and-supplies/non-contact-infrared-thermometers

Chapter 8

Asepsis and infection control

Just the facts

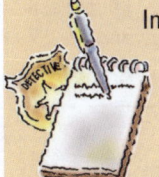

In this chapter, you'll learn:

♦ types of infections and microorganisms

♦ how microorganisms cause infections

♦ proper hand hygiene

♦ why personal protective equipment is important and how it is used.

A look at infection

Infection is the invasion and multiplication of microorganisms in or on body tissues. These microorganisms have evaded the first line of host defenses that normally produce an immune response, resulting in localized or generalized signs and symptoms. This reproduction injures the host by causing cellular damage from microorganism-produced toxins, intracellular multiplication, or competing with host metabolism (Bennett et al., 2020).

The host's own immune response may worsen the tissue damage. The damage may be localized (an infected wound) or systemic (fever or septic shock). The infection's severity depends on three main components: the pathogenicity of invading microorganisms, the quantity of invading microorganisms, and the strength of host defenses (Block et al., 2022). The very young and the very old are especially susceptible to infections. In addition, individuals who are hospitalized are also at risk for contracting a hospital-acquired infection (CDC, 2021a).

Severity of infection depends on invading organisms and the strength of host defenses.

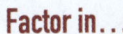

Factor in…

Certain factors contribute to an increased risk of infection. For example, travel can expose people to diseases for which they have little natural immunity. Additionally, certain underlying illnesses, expanded use of immunosuppressants, surgery, and other invasive procedures increase the risk of infection by opportunistic microorganisms.

Types of human–microbe interactions

- **Transient microorganisms:** microorganisms encountered as they "pass through" the body, for example, in consumed food or water; these are usually harmless but can lead to infection.
- **Commensal microorganisms:** "commensal" literally means "eating at the same table." Microorganisms that are present normally on or in the human body from which the host or organism may or may not derive benefit. Usually, this is a mutually beneficial relationship and does not cause harm or disease.
- **Pathogens:** microorganisms that cause disease. Pathogenic microorganisms can also be transient or commensal and can develop into infections after evading the immune system.
- **Opportunistic pathogens:** microorganisms that cause disease in persons with defense mechanisms that are compromised in some way.
- **Accidental pathogens:** microorganisms that cause disease by accidental introduction into the body through animal, insect, or environmental contact. Examples include rabies from a dog bite or Lyme disease from a tick bite (Bennett et al., 2020).

> The average human has about 4 to 5 pounds of microorganisms living on and inside them! Most are bacterial species and are normally protective.

Types of infection

There are four major types of infection:

- *Subclinical*, also called *silent* or *asymptomatic*, is a laboratory-verified infection or presence of a microorganism that causes no signs and symptoms or damage to the host.
- *Colonized* is a multiplication of microbes that produces no signs, symptoms, or immune responses. Colonization by a microorganism can also be defined as "critically colonized," which means the colonization has a high risk of developing into an active infection due to the high quantity or high virulence (pathogenicity) of the microorganism and host factors. Because a person with a subclinical infection or colonization may not have symptoms, this person can be a carrier and transmit the infection to others (Edwards-Jones, 2020).
- *Dormant*, also called *latent*, occurs after a microorganism has been dormant in the host, sometimes for years. An exogenous infection results from environmental pathogens; an endogenous infection, from the host's normal flora (e.g., *Escherichia coli* displaced from the colon, which may cause urinary tract infection).
- *Active infection*, also known as *infectious disease*, is when the interaction between the host and the microorganism causes physiological damage from the microorganism's toxins or from the host's own immune response, resulting in signs and symptoms of infection (Bennett et al., 2020).

Types of infecting organisms

The forms of microorganisms responsible for infectious diseases include bacteria, viruses, fungi, and protozoa. Larger organisms, such as helminths (worms), may also cause disease.

Bacteria

Bacteria are single-cell microorganisms with well-defined cell walls that can multiply independently on artificial media without the need for other cells (Bennett et al., 2020). In some areas of the world, poor sanitation heightens the risk of infection and bacterial diseases commonly cause death and disability. Even in industrialized countries, they are still the most common fatal infectious diseases. (See *Bacteria: Oh, the damage they can do!*, page 134.)

Shaping up

Bacteria can be classified by shape:

- *spherical*—cocci
- *rod shaped*—bacilli
- *spiral shaped*—spirilla.

Response, motility, capsulation, spores, and O$_2$

Bacteria also can be classified by:

- *response to staining*—gram positive, gram negative, or acid fast
- *motility*—motile or nonmotile
- *tendency toward capsulation*—encapsulated or nonencapsulated
- *capacity to form spores*—sporulating or nonsporulating
- *oxygen requirements*—aerobic (need oxygen to grow) or anaerobic (don't need oxygen to grow).

Spirochetes

Spirochetes, a type of bacteria, is flexible, slender, undulating spiral rods that have cell walls. Most are anaerobic. The three pathogenic forms in humans include *Treponema*, *Leptospira*, and *Borrelia*.

Viruses

Viruses are subcellular organisms made up of only an RNA or a DNA nucleus covered with proteins. They're the smallest known organism so tiny that they're visible only through an electron microscope.

An invasion occasion

Viruses can't replicate independent of host cells. Rather, they invade a host cell and stimulate it to participate in the formation of additional virus particles. The estimated 400 viruses that infect humans are classified according to their size, shape (spherical, rod shaped, or cubic), or means of transmission (respiratory, fecal, oral, or sexual) (Bennett et al., 2020).

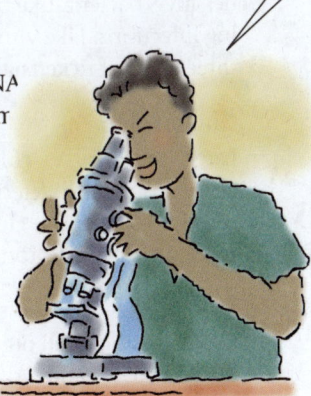

How can such a tiny thing cause so much trouble?

Bacteria: Oh, the damage they can do!

Bacteria and other infectious organisms are constantly present in and on the human body and can cause infections. Some are beneficial, such as the intestinal bacteria that produce vitamins and are protective. Others are harmful, causing illnesses ranging from acute otitis media to life-threatening septic shock.

To infect a host, bacteria must first enter it. They do this by adhering to the mucosal surface and directly invading the host cell or attaching to epithelial cells and producing toxins that invade host cells. To survive and multiply within a host, bacteria or their toxins adversely affect biochemical reactions in cells. The result is a disruption of normal cell functions or cell death (as shown below).

For example, the diphtheria toxin damages heart muscle by inhibiting protein synthesis. In addition, as some organisms multiply, they extend into deeper tissue and eventually enter the bloodstream.

Some toxins cause blood to clot in small blood vessels. The tissues supplied by these vessels may be deprived of blood and damaged (as shown below).

Other toxins can damage the cell walls of small blood vessels, causing leakage. This fluid loss results in decreased blood pressure, which in turn impairs the heart's ability to pump enough blood to vital organs (as shown below).

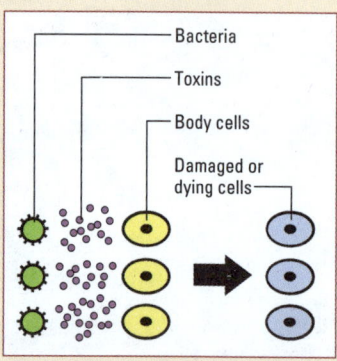

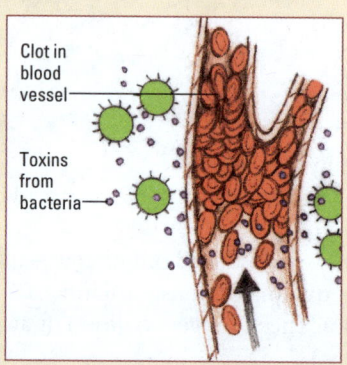

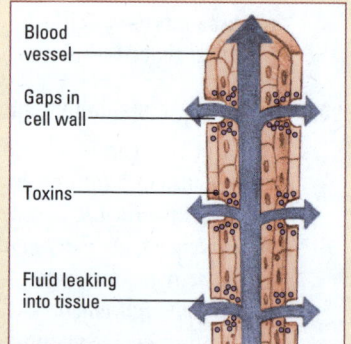

Rickettsiae

Relatively uncommon in the United States, rickettsiae are small, gram-negative, bacteria-like organisms that commonly induce life-threatening infections. Like viruses, these require a host cell for replication. The three types of rickettsiae are *Rickettsia*, *Coxiella*, and *Rochalimaea*.

Chlamydiae

Larger than viruses, chlamydiae have recently been found to be intracellular obligate bacteria. Unlike other bacteria, they depend on host cells for replication. However, unlike viruses, chlamydiae are susceptible to antibiotics.

Fungi

Fungi are single-cell organisms that have nuclei enveloped by nuclear membranes. Although these organisms have rigid cell walls like plant cells, they lack chlorophyll, the green matter

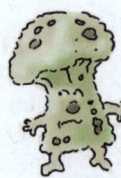

I think there may be a fungus among us.

necessary for photosynthesis. They also show relatively little cellular specialization. Fungi occur as yeasts (single-cell, oval-shaped organisms) or molds (organisms with hyphae or branching filaments). Depending on the environment, some fungi may occur in both forms. Fungal diseases in humans are called *mycoses*.

Protozoa

Protozoa are the simplest single-cell organisms of the animal kingdom but show a high level of cellular specialization. Like other animal cells, they have cell membranes rather than cell walls, and their nuclei are surrounded by nuclear membranes.

Helminths

The three groups of helminths that invade humans include nematodes, cestodes, and trematodes. Nematodes are cylindrical, unsegmented, elongated helminths that taper at each end. Their shape has earned them the designation *roundworm*. Cestodes, better known as *tapeworms*, have bodies that are flattened front to back with distinct, regular segments. Tapeworms also have heads with suckers or sucking grooves. Trematodes have flattened, unsegmented bodies and are called *blood, intestinal, lung,* or *liver flukes*, depending on their infection site (Bennett et al., 2020).

Lines of defense

The human body has a powerful defense system against invading organisms that want to:

- establish a habitat
- evade body defenses
- replicate
- spread (usually to a preferred site)
- ultimately, transmit to another host to do it all over again.

Humans have three main lines of defense to protect against these mechanisms: physical barriers, the innate (instinctive) immune response, and the adaptive (or learned) immune response (Netea et al., 2020).

First line of defense: Physical barriers

- **Skin:** Acts as a protective wall against invading organisms. When this seal is broken, colonized bacteria that are naturally present on the skin, such as *Streptococcus, Fusobacterium,* and many others, can invade and cause disease.
- **Mucous membranes:** These moist walls are rich with microorganisms and cover every inner body surface that has contact with the outside environment. Mucous membranes are present in the respiratory, intestinal, and genitourinary tracts and provide protection through bumpy paths, sticky mucosal secretions, and emission of inflammatory cells.

Second line of defense: Innate immunity and the inflammatory response

When the first line of defense is breached, the innate immune system is mobilized. The rapid increase of response proteins and chemokines stimulates the movement of white blood cells and other phagocytic cells to the site of invasion. This migration of cells results in the generalized signs and symptoms of infection, such as fever and body aches, and is the preceptor for the specific adaptive immune response (Netea et al., 2020).

The smart defense system: The adaptive immune response

If the patient is immunocompetent, after their first encounter with a pathogen, antibodies—also known as immunoglobulins—produced in the lymphatic system are able to identify, neutralize, and clear specific pathogens using a "memory" function. There are two types of immunity (Bennett et al., 2020):

- *Active acquired immunity:* developed after natural exposure or immunization
- *Passive acquired immunity:* gained from donor to recipient (i.e., birthing parent to baby via the placenta), through immunotherapy, or even convalescent plasma (plasma from donors who have recovered from the disease).

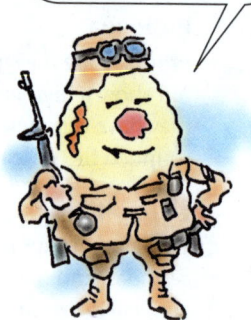

My army will mount a robust immune response against the invasion!

Modes of transmission

Infectious diseases are transmitted directly (by contact) or indirectly. Indirect transmission may occur via droplet transmission, airborne transmission, vector-borne transmission, or vehicle-borne transmission.

Close contact

In contact transmission, the susceptible host comes into direct contact (as in sexually transmitted diseases) or indirect contact (contaminated inanimate objects) with the source. Direct transmission may also occur via droplet spread, the close-range spray of contaminated droplets into the conjunctiva or mucous membranes.

How is the air?

Airborne transmission results from inhalation of contaminated evaporated saliva droplets (as in pulmonary tuberculosis or bacterial meningitis), which sometimes are suspended in airborne dust particles or vapors. These particles are airborne because they are small and light. (Think droplet = larger particles that drop to the ground vs. airborne = lighter particles that float in the air.)

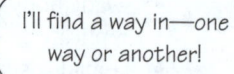

I'll find a way in—one way or another!

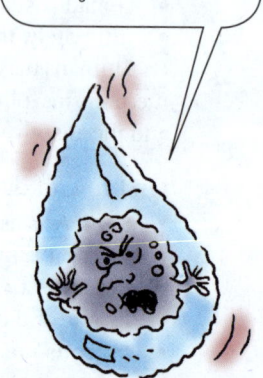

Hector vector

Vector-borne transmission occurs when an intermediate carrier (vector), such as a flea or a mosquito, transfers an organism. Vehicle-borne transmission occurs when water, food, or blood products introduce organisms into a susceptible host via ingestion or inoculation.

Preventing health care–associated infections (HAIs)

Here are some tips to help prevent HAIs (Haque et al., 2020):
- Follow good hand-washing techniques and encourage other staff members to do the same.
- Follow strict infection control procedures.
- Document hospital infections as they occur.
- Identify outbreaks early and take steps to prevent their spread.
- Eliminate unnecessary procedures or devices that contribute to infection.
- Strictly follow necessary isolation techniques.
- Observe all patients for signs of infection, especially patients who are at high risk for infection.
- Keep staff members and visitors with obvious infection as well as known carriers away from susceptible patients.

Health care–associated infections

Formerly known as *nosocomial infections*, health care–associated infections (HAIs) develop while a patient is in a health care facility or another facility. According to the Centers for Disease Control and Prevention (CDC), every day, about 1 in every 31 hospitalized patients has an infection caused by receiving medical care. Annually, in the United States, almost 3 million people will become infected with bacteria that are resistant to antibiotics. In addition, over 35,000 patients will die each year as a direct result of these infections (Centers for Disease Control and Prevention (CDC), 2019). Most HAIs result from group A *Streptococcus pyogenes*, *Staphylococcus*, *Escherichia coli*, *Klebsiella*, *Proteus*, *Pseudomonas*, *Clostridium difficile*, and *Candida albicans*, among others.

Most HAIs are transmitted by direct contact and are usually associated with an invasive device or procedure. They can be categorized into site-specific infections: catheter-associated urinary tract infections, central line–associated bloodstream infections, surgical-site infections, and ventilator-associated pneumonia (CDC, 2021).

Many risks for many reasons

HAIs continue to pose a problem because most facility patients are older and more debilitated than in the past. The advances in treatment that increase longevity in patients with diseases that alter immune defenses also create a population at high risk for infection. Moreover, the growing use of invasive and surgical procedures, immunosuppressants, and antibiotics predisposes patients to infection and helps create new strains of antibiotic-resistant bacteria. The growing number of facility personnel that come in contact with each patient increases the risk of exposure. (See *CDC isolation precautions*, pages 138–139.)

CDC isolation precautions

The CDC's *Guidelines for Isolation Precautions in Hospitals,* developed by the CDC (2022) and the Hospital Infection Control Practices Advisory Committee, help facilities maintain up-to-date isolation practices.

Standard precautions

The guidelines contain two tiers of precautions. The first, called *standard precautions,* are those designated for the care of all facility patients regardless of their diagnosis or presumed infection. Standard precautions are the primary strategy for preventing HAI. These precautions apply to:
- blood
- all body fluids, secretions, and excretions, except sweat, regardless of whether they contain visible blood
- skin that is not intact
- mucous membranes.

Transmission-based precautions

The second tier of precautions, *transmission-based precautions*, are instituted for patients who are known to be or suspected of being infected with a highly transmissible infection—that is, one that needs precautions beyond those defined in standard precautions. There are three types of transmission-based precautions: airborne precautions, droplet precautions, and contact precautions.

Airborne precautions

Airborne precautions apply to patients known or suspected to be infected with microorganisms transmitted by airborne droplet nuclei. These precautions are designed to reduce the risk of airborne transmission of infectious agents. Microorganisms carried through the air can be dispersed widely by air currents, making them available for inhalation or deposit on a susceptible host in the same room or a longer distance away from the infected patient. Airborne precautions include special air handling and ventilation procedures to prevent the spread of infection. They require the use of respiratory protection such as a mask, in addition to standard precautions, when entering an infected patient's room. The mask should be either N95 or a powered air purifying respirator. A patient under airborne precautions must be placed in a special room known as an *airborne infection isolation room.*

Airborne infection isolation room

At a minimum, airborne infection isolation rooms must:

- Provide negative pressure with a minimum of 12 air exchanges per hour
- Exhaust directly to the outside or through HEPA (high efficiency particulate air) filtration.

Droplet precautions

These precautions are designed to reduce the risk of transmitting infectious agents through large-particle (exceeding 5 µm) droplets. Such transmission involves contact of infectious agents with the conjunctivae or the nasal or oral mucous membranes of a susceptible person. Large-particle droplets don't remain in the air and generally travel short distances of 3 feet (1 m) or less. They require the use of a mask, in addition to standard precautions, to protect the mucous membranes.

Contact precautions

These precautions are designed to reduce the risk of transmitting infectious agents by direct or indirect contact. Direct-contact transmission can occur through patient care activities that require physical contact. Indirect-contact transmission involves a susceptible host coming in contact with a contaminated object, usually inanimate, in the patient's environment. Contact precautions require the use of gloves, a mask, and a gown—in addition to standard precautions—to avoid contact with the infectious agent. Stringent hand washing is also necessary after removal of the protective items.

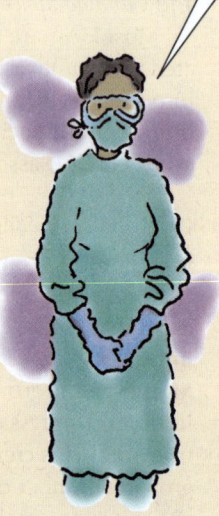

Always take precautions and wear personal protective gear when warranted!

CDC isolation precautions *(continued)*

Always take the right precautions! This chart shows the different types of precautions and provides examples of infections for which specific precautions would be used.

Precautions	Indications
Standard precautions	Designated for all patients regardless of diagnosis or presumed infection
Airborne precautions (used in addition to standard precautions)	Patients known to have or suspected of having a serious illness transmitted by airborne droplet nuclei, such as: • measles • tuberculosis • varicella • COVID-19
Droplet precautions (used in addition to standard precautions)	Patients known to have or suspected of having a serious illness transmitted by large-particle droplets, such as: • invasive *Haemophilus influenzae* type b disease, including meningitis, pneumonia, epiglottitis, and sepsis • invasive *Neisseria meningitides* disease, including meningitis, pneumonia, and sepsis • other serious bacterial respiratory infections spread by droplets, such as diphtheria; *Mycoplasma* pneumonia; pertussis; pneumonic plague; and streptococcal (Group A) pharyngitis, pneumonia, or scarlet fever in infants and young children • other serious viral infections spread by droplets, including adenovirus, influenza, mumps, parvovirus B19 (with most serious risk to fetuses), and rubella.
Contact precautions (used in addition to standard precautions)	Patients known to have or suspected of having a serious illness that can be transmitted by direct patient contact or by contact with items in the patient's environment. Examples of such illnesses include: • Gastrointestinal, respiratory, skin, or wound infections or colonization with multidrug-resistant bacteria judged by the infection control program (based on current state, regional, or national recommendations) to be of special clinical and epidemiologic significance • enteric infections with a low infectious dose or prolonged environmental survival, including *Clostridium difficile* or, for diapered or incontinent patients, enterohemorrhagic *Escherichia coli* O157:H7, *Shigella*, hepatitis A, or rotavirus • respiratory syncytial virus, parainfluenza virus, or enteroviral infections in infants and young children • skin infections that are highly contagious or that may occur on dry skin, including diphtheria (cutaneous); herpes simplex virus (neonatal or mucocutaneous); impetigo; major (noncontained) abscesses, cellulitis, or decubiti; pediculosis; scabies; staphylococcal furunculosis in infants and young children; zoster (disseminated or in an immunocompromised host) • viral or hemorrhagic conjunctivitis • viral hemorrhagic infections (Ebola, Lassa, or Marburg).

(Continued)

CDC isolation precautions *(continued)*

Precautions	Indications
Special contact precautions for neutropenic patients (used in addition to standard precautions)	Neutrophils are immature white blood cells and are the important warrior cells that our body uses to fight infection. In certain patients, especially those receiving chemotherapy, these neutrophils are extremely lowered. In these patients, they can become infected from their environment. Precautions include: • No live flowers, fruits, or vegetables. All food must be well cooked. • Private room • Patient must wear a mask when out of the room. Health care providers should wear a mask if any illness persists • Strict handwashing.

Source: Centers for Disease Control and Prevention (CDC). (2022). Guidelines for isolation precautions: Preventing transmission of infectious agents in healthcare settings. https://www.cdc.gov/infectioncontrol/guidelines/isolation/index.html

Need for accurate assessment

Accurate assessment helps identify infectious diseases and prevents avoidable complications. Complete assessment consists of a patient history, a physical examination, and diagnostic tests.

All the details

The history should include the patient's gender, age, address, occupation, and place of work; known exposure to infection; and date of disease onset. It should also detail information about recent hospitalization, blood transfusions, sexual history, vaccination, travel or camping trips, and exposure to animals. If a patient has contracted an HAI in the recent past, depending on the policy of the institution, the patient may be put in isolation precautions.

Diseases, drugs, diet...

If applicable, ask the patient about illicit drug use and possible exposure to sexually transmitted diseases. Also, ask about usual dietary patterns, unusual fatigue, and factors that may predispose the patient to infection, such as neoplastic disease and alcohol use. Notice if the patient is listless or uneasy, lacks concentration, or has any obvious abnormality of mood or affect.

Suspicious? Assess the skin

In suspected infection, a physical examination includes an assessment of the skin, mucous membranes, liver, spleen, and lymph nodes. Check for and note the location and type of drainage from skin lesions. Record skin color, temperature, and turgor; ask if the patient has pruritus or itching. Skin with a warm or red appearance is always considered suspect.

Follow the fever

Monitor the patient's temperature, using the same route consistently, and watch for a fever, the best indicator of many infections. Note and record the pattern of temperature change and the effect of antipyretics. Typically, antipyretics are used sparingly. Be aware that certain analgesics may contain antipyretics, which will mask a fever (Ludwig & McWhinnie, 2019). Watch for seizures in cases of high fever, above 105° F, especially in children.

Mostly up, sometimes down

Check the patient's pulse rate. Infection commonly increases the pulse rate, but some infections such as typhoid fever may decrease it. In severe infection or when complications are possible, monitor the patient for hypotension, hematuria, oliguria, hepatomegaly, jaundice, palpable and painful lymph nodes, bleeding from gums or into joints, and altered level of consciousness. Obtain diagnostic tests and appropriate cultures, as ordered.

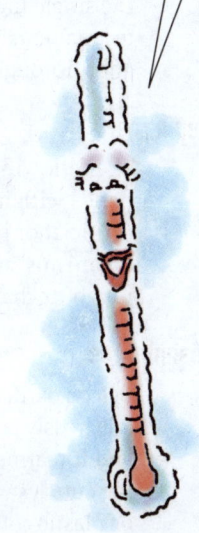

Always remember that a fever is often the best sign of infection.

Preventing infection

Comprehensive immunization (including immunization of travelers to and persons from endemic areas); improved nutrition, living conditions, and sanitation; and correction of other environmental factors are some broad steps the healthcare community can take to prevent infection.

Individual action

Individual health care professionals can also prevent infection by:
- employing drug prophylaxis when necessary
- using strict hand-hygiene techniques
- following standard precautions
- using correct isolation garb.

Drug prophylaxis

Although prophylactic antibiotic therapy may prevent certain diseases, the risk of superinfection and the emergence of drug-resistant strains may outweigh the benefits. So prophylactic antibiotics are usually reserved for patients at high risk for exposure to dangerous infection.

Hand hygiene

The hands are the conduits for almost every transfer of potential pathogens from one patient to another, from a contaminated object to the patient, or from a staff member to the patient. Hand hygiene is the single most important procedure in preventing infection. To protect patients from HAIs, hand hygiene must be performed routinely and thoroughly.

Keep it real

The following minimize the risk of contamination: clean and healthy hands with intact skin; short, natural fingernails; and no rings. Artificial or painted fingernails may serve as a reservoir for microorganisms, and microorganisms are more difficult to remove from rough or chapped hands.

Present arms

Before participating in any sterile procedure or when hands are grossly contaminated, it is important to wash both hands and forearms and clean under fingernails and in and around the cuticles with a fingernail brush, disposable sponge brush, or plastic cuticle stick. Use these softer implements because brushes, metal files, or other hard objects may injure the skin and, if reused, may be a source of contamination.

Your hands are healing tools, so always keep them clean, healthy, and ready to assist.

Soap for most

Follow your facility's policy concerning when to wash with soap and when to use an antiseptic cleaning agent. Nurses should wash their hands:
- before starting a shift
- before and after patient contact
- before and after performing any bodily functions, such as using the bathroom
- before preparing or serving food
- before preparing or administering medications
- after contact with a patient's excretions, secretions, or blood
- after completing their shift.

Antiseptic when susceptible

Use an antiseptic cleaning agent before performing invasive procedures, wound care, and dressing changes and after contamination. Antiseptics are also recommended for hand washing in isolation rooms, newborn nurseries, and before caring for any highly susceptible patient.

Hold the alcohol

If hands aren't visibly soiled, an alcohol-based hand rub is preferred for routine decontamination. An alcohol-based hand sanitizer should not be used if contact with items contaminated with *Clostridium difficile* or *Bacillus anthracis* (Anthrax) is anticipated. These organisms can form spores, and alcohol does not kill spores. Wash hands with soap and water or antiseptic soap and water if either of these organisms is known or suspected to be present.

Home sweet home

If a nurse is providing care in the patient's home, they may need to bring their own supply of soap and disposable paper towels. If there is no running water, alcohol-based hand sanitizer can be used to disinfect hands.

Supplies
Hand washing
- Hand-washing soap or detergent
- Warm running water
- Paper towels
- Optional: antiseptic cleaning agent, fingernail brush, disposable sponge, or plastic cuticle stick.

Hand sanitizing
Hand sanitizing alcohol-based hand rub.

How it's done
Hand washing
- Remove rings or artificial fingernails as facility policy dictates because they harbor dirt and skin microorganisms.
- Remove watch or wear it well above the wrist.
- Keep nails short, no more than ¼″ beyond the end of the finger. Nails grown longer than that may harbor more microorganisms.
- Get hands and wrists wet with warm water and apply soap from a dispenser. Don't use bar soap because it allows cross-contamination.
- Hands should be held below elbow level to prevent water from running up arms and back down, thus contaminating clean areas.
- Work up a generous lather by rubbing both hands together vigorously for about 10 seconds. Soap and warm water reduce surface tension, and this reduced tension, aided by friction, loosens surface microorganisms, which wash away in the lather.
- Pay special attention to the areas under fingernails and around cuticles, and to the thumbs, knuckles, and sides of the fingers and

hands, because microorganisms thrive in these protected or over-looked areas.

- Avoid splashing water because microorganisms spread more easily on wet surfaces and because slippery floors are dangerous. Avoid touching the sink or faucets because they are considered contaminated.
- Rinse hands and wrists well because running water flushes suds, soil, and microorganisms away.
- Pat hands and wrists dry with a paper towel. Avoid rubbing, which can cause abrasion and chapping.
- If the sink isn't equipped with knee or foot controls, turn off the faucets by gripping them with a dry paper towel to avoid recontamination.
- Because frequent hand washing strips the skin of natural oils, this simple procedure can result in dryness, cracking, and irritation. However, these effects are probably more common after repeated use of antiseptic cleaning agents, especially in people with sensitive skin. To help minimize irritation, rinse hands thoroughly, making sure they're free from residue.
- To prevent dry or chapped hands, apply an emollient hand cream after each washing or switch to a different cleaning agent. Avoid creams and lotions with strong perfumes because they may irritate a patient with asthma or cause nausea in some patients.
- Some nurses may develop dermatitis from hand washing. If this occurs, they may need to be evaluated by an employee or an occupational health care provider to determine the next steps.

Use hand cream to avoid dry, chapped hands caused by frequent hand washing. Be sure to always use the lotion provided by the facility.

Hand sanitizing

- Apply a small amount of the alcohol-based hand rub to all surfaces of the hands.
- Rub hands together until all the product has dried (usually about 20 to 30 seconds).

Standard precautions

The CDC recommends that the following standard blood and body fluid precautions be used for *all* patients. These standard precautions are especially important in emergency care settings where the risk of blood exposure is increased and the patient's infection status is usually unknown. Implementing standard precautions doesn't eliminate the need for other transmission-based precautions, such as airborne, droplet, and contact precautions.

Sources of potential exposure

Standard precautions apply to blood, semen, vaginal secretions, cerebrospinal fluid, synovial fluid, pleural fluid, peritoneal fluid, pericardial fluid, and amniotic fluid. These fluids are most likely to transmit bloodborne pathogens (for example, hepatitis and HIV). Standard precautions also apply to other body fluids, including stool, nasal secretions, saliva, sputum, tears, vomitus, and breast milk.

Barrier precautions

- Wear gloves when touching blood and body fluids, mucous membranes, or broken skin of all patients; when handling items or touching surfaces soiled with blood or body fluids; and when performing venipuncture and other vascular access procedures.
- Change gloves when they become soiled and wash hands before and after contact with each patient.
- Wear a mask and protective eyewear or a face shield to protect mucous membranes of the mouth, nose, and eyes during procedures that may generate drops of blood or other body fluids.
- In addition to a mask and protective eyewear or a face shield, wear a gown or an apron during procedures that are likely to generate splashing of blood or other body fluids.
- After removing gloves, thoroughly wash hands and other skin surfaces that may be contaminated with blood or other body fluids.

To learn more about the use of personal protective equipment, see *Donning and removing personal protective equipment (PPE)* at the end of this chapter.

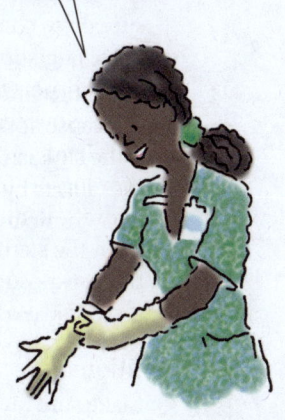

Gloves—the perfect accessory for those infectious nursing occasions.

Precautions for invasive procedures

- During all invasive procedures, wear gloves. Also wear a surgical mask and goggles or a face shield.
- During procedures that commonly generate droplets or splashes of blood or other body fluids or bone chips, wear protective eyewear and a mask or face shield.
- During invasive procedures that are likely to cause splashing or splattering of blood or other body fluids, wear a gown or an impervious apron.
- If a nurse assists in vaginal or cesarean deliveries, they should wear gloves and a gown when handling the placenta or the infant and during umbilical cord care.

Work practice precautions

- Prevent injuries caused by needles, scalpels, and other sharp instruments or devices when cleaning used instruments, disposing of used needles, and handling sharp instruments after procedures.

- To prevent needle-stick injuries, DO NOT recap used needles, bend or break needles, remove them from disposable syringes, or manipulate them. Use safety-protected needles and needleless IV systems whenever possible.
- Place disposable syringes and needles, scalpel blades, and other sharp items in puncture-resistant containers for disposal, making sure these containers are located near the area of use.
- Place large-bore reusable needles in a puncture-resistant container for transport to the reprocessing area.
- If the glove tears or a needle stick or other injury occurs, remove the gloves, wash hands, and wash the site of the needle stick thoroughly; then put on new gloves as quickly as patient safety permits. Remove the needle or instrument involved in the incident from the sterile field. Promptly report injuries and mucous membrane exposure to the appropriate infection control officer.
- Never reuse a one-time use needle or vial.

Additional precautions

- Make sure mouthpieces, one-way valve masks, resuscitation bags, or other ventilation devices are available in areas where the need for resuscitation is likely.
- If a nurse is experiencing exudative lesions or weeping dermatitis, they must refrain from direct patient care and handling patient care equipment until the condition resolves.

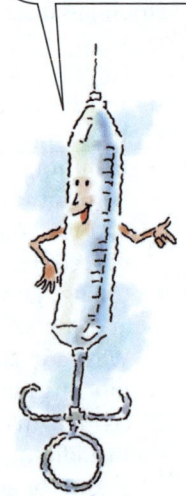

Handling syringes is sticky business. Take all necessary precautions to avoid injury and infection.

Using isolation equipment

Isolation procedures may be implemented to prevent the spread of infection from patient to patient, from the patient to health care workers, or from health care workers to the patient. They may also be used to reduce the risk of infection in immuno-compromised patients. Selection of proper equipment and adequate training of those who use it is central to the success of these procedures.

Once is enough

Use gowns, gloves, goggles, and masks only once, and discard them in the appropriate container before leaving a contaminated area. If a mask designated by its manufacturer as reusable is being used, save it for further use unless it is damaged or damp. Be aware that isolation garb loses its effectiveness when wet because moisture permits organisms to seep through the material. Change masks and gowns as soon as moisture is noticeable or according to the manufacturer's recommendations or facility policy.

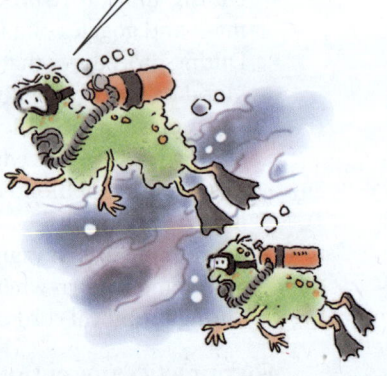

I wouldn't have guessed in a million years it would be so easy breaking in through all those barriers. . .

Supplies

Materials required for isolation typically include barrier clothing, an isolation cart or anteroom for storing equipment, and a door card stating that isolation precautions are in effect.

Barrier clothing:

- gowns
- gloves
- goggles
- masks (Each staff member must be trained in their proper use.)

Isolation supplies:

- specially marked laundry bags
- plastic trash bags
- an isolation cart may be used when the patient's room has no anteroom. It should include a work area (such as a pull-out shelf) and drawers or a cabinet area for holding isolation supplies.

Getting ready

To prepare for nursing care in an isolation area, remove the cover from the isolation cart, if necessary, and set up the work area. Check the cart or anteroom to ensure that correct and sufficient supplies are in place for the designated isolation category.

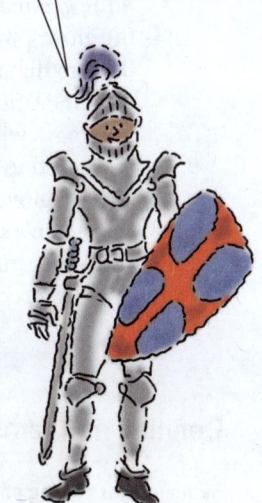

Barrier clothing isn't what it used to be, thank goodness! Now we use gowns, gloves, goggles, and masks—a bit more comfortable if you ask me!

Recommended standard precautions

Component	Recommendations
Hand hygiene	After touching blood, body fluids, secretions, excretions, contaminated items; immediately after removing gloves; between patient contacts.
Personal protective equipment (PPE)	
Gloves	For touching blood, body fluids, secretions, excretions, contaminated items; for touching mucous membranes and nonintact skin
Gown	During procedures and patient-care activities when contact of clothing/exposed skin with blood/body fluids, secretions, and excretions is anticipated
Mask, eye protection (goggles), face shield	During procedures and patient-care activities likely to generate splashes or sprays of blood, body fluids, secretions, especially suctioning, endotracheal intubation
Patient placement	Prioritize for single-patient room if patient is at increased risk of transmission, is likely to contaminate the environment, does not maintain appropriate hygiene, or is at increased risk of acquiring infection or developing adverse outcome following infection.

Adapted from Centers for Disease Control and Prevention (CDC). (2016). Standard precautions for all patient care. https://www.cdc.gov/infectioncontrol/basics/standard-precautions.html

How it's done

- Remove all jewelry and watches on hands and wrists. These actions help prevent the spread of microorganisms hidden under these items.
- Wash hands with an antiseptic cleaning agent to prevent the growth of microorganisms under gloves.

Putting on isolation garb

- Put the gown on, ensuring that it covers all clothing. Tie the strings or fasten the snaps or pressure-sensitive tabs at the neck.
- All masks should be placed snuggly over the nose and mouth. Ensure that the mask ear loops are secure around the ears or that the strings are tied tightly behind the head high enough so the mask will not slip off. The adjustable nose bridge should be squeezed to fit the nurse's nose firmly but comfortably.
- Put on gloves. Pull the gloves over the cuffs to cover the edges of the gown's sleeves.
- For more information regarding this process see the *Donning and removing personal protective equipment (PPE)* box below.

Donning and removing personal protective equipment (PPE)

Sequence for putting on PPE

The type of PPE used will vary based on the level of precautions required, such as standard and contact, droplet, or airborne infection isolation precautions. The procedure for putting on and removing PPE should be tailored to the specific type of PPE.

1. Gown
- Fully cover torso from neck to knees, arms to end of wrists, and wrap around the back.
- Fasten in back of neck and waist.

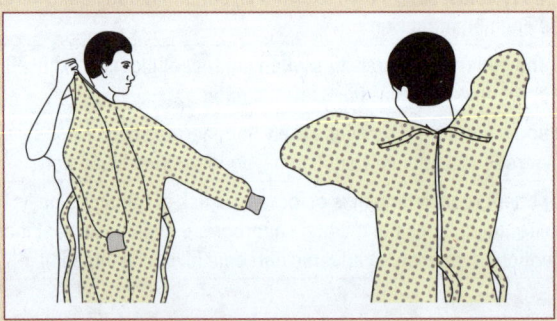

Donning and removing personal protective equipment (PPE) *(continued)*

2. Mask or respirator
- Secure ties or elastic bands at middle of head and neck.
- Fit flexible band to nose bridge.
- Fit snug to face and below chin.
- Fit-check respirator.

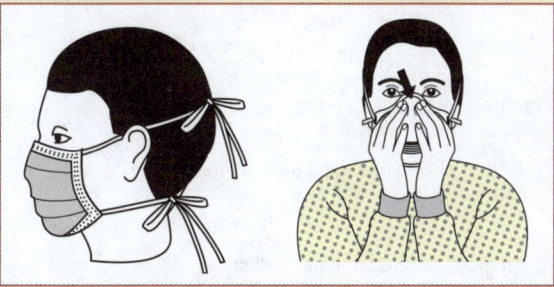

3. Goggles or face shield
- Place over face and eyes and adjust to fit.

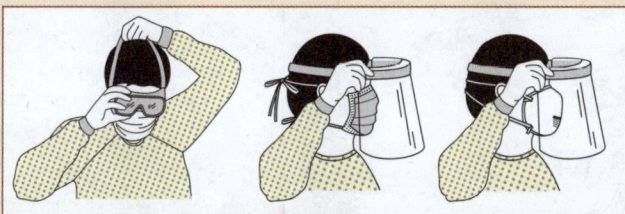

4. Gloves
- Extend to cover wrist of isolation gown.
- Use safe work practices to protect yourself and limit the spread of contamination.
- Keep hands away from face.
- Limit surfaces touched.
- Change gloves when torn or heavily contaminated.
- Perform hand hygiene.

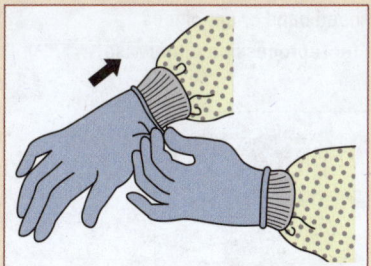

(Continued)

Donning and removing personal protective equipment (PPE) *(continued)*

How to safely remove personal PPE, Example 1
There are a variety of ways to safely remove PPE without contaminating your clothing, skin, or mucous membranes with potentially infectious materials. Here is one example. **Remove all PPE before exiting the patient room** except a respirator, if worn. Remove the respirator **after** leaving the patient room and closing the door. Remove PPE in the following sequence:

1. Gloves
• Outside of gloves is contaminated!
• If your hands get contaminated during glove removal, immediately wash your hands or use an alcohol-based hand sanitizer.
• Using a gloved hand, grasp the palm area of the other gloved hand and peel off first glove.
• Hold removed glove in gloved hand.
• Slide fingers of ungloved hand under remaining glove at wrist and peel off second glove over first glove.
• Discard gloves in a waste container.

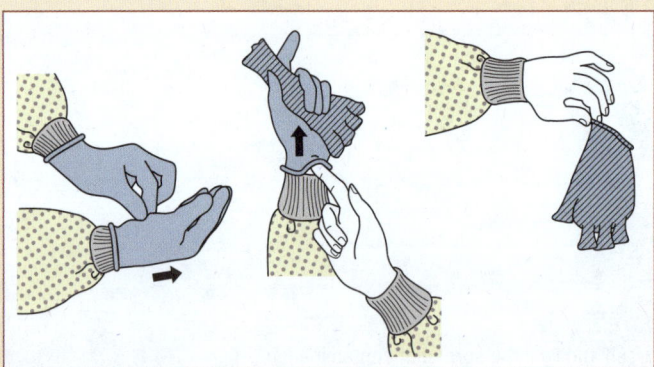

2. Goggles or face shield
• Outside of goggles or face shield is contaminated!
• If your hands get contaminated during goggle or face shield removal, immediately wash your hands or use an alcohol-based hand sanitizer.
• Remove goggles or face shield from the back by lifting head band or ear pieces.
• If the item is reusable, place in designated receptacle for reprocessing. Otherwise, discard in a waste container.

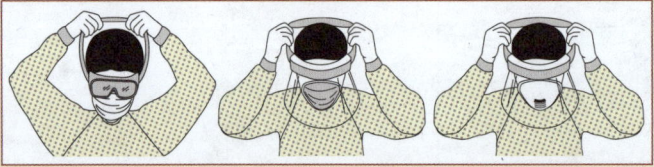

Donning and removing personal protective equipment (PPE) *(continued)*

3. Gown

• Gown front and sleeves are contaminated!
• If your hands get contaminated during gown removal, immediately wash your hands or use an alcohol-based hand sanitizer.
• Unfasten gown ties, taking care that sleeves don't contact your body when reaching for ties.
• Pull gown away from neck and shoulders, touching inside of gown only.
• Turn gown inside out.
• Fold or roll into a bundle and discard in a waste container.

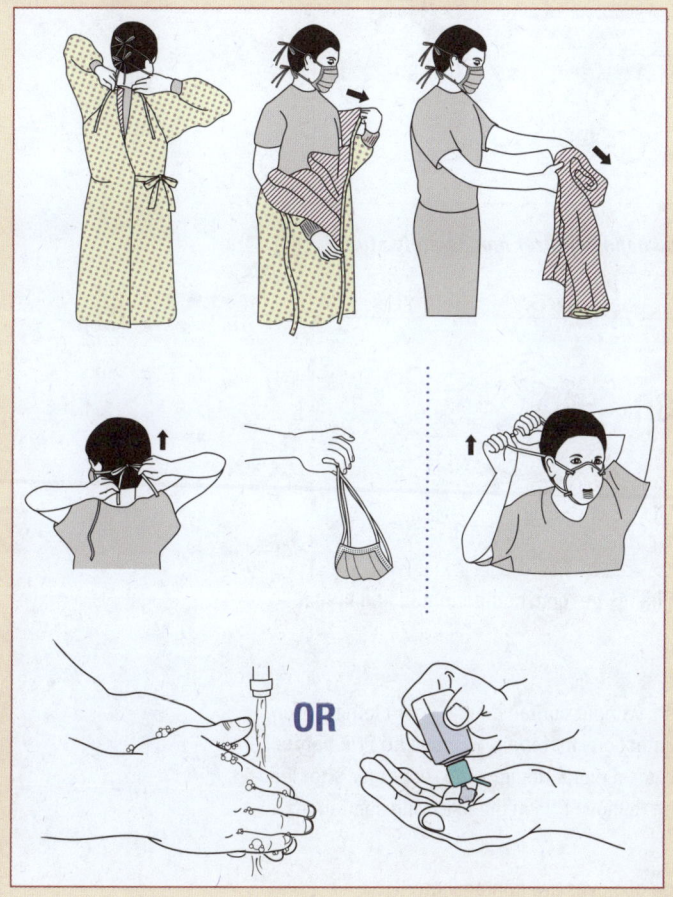

OR

(Continued)

Donning and removing personal protective equipment (PPE) *(continued)*

4. Mask or respirator
- Front of mask/respirator is contaminated—DO NOT TOUCH!
- If your hands get contaminated during mask/respirator removal, immediately wash your hands or use an alcohol-based hand sanitizer.
- Grasp bottom ties or elastics of the mask/respirator, then the ones at the top, and remove without touching the front.
- Discard in a waste container.

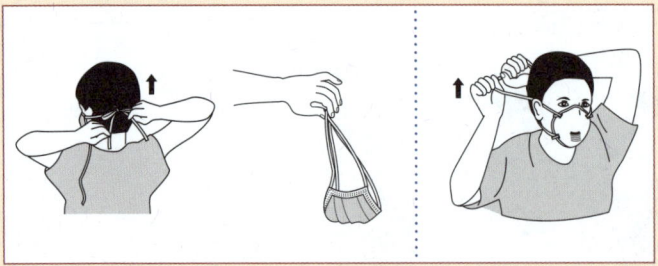

5. Wash hands or use an alcohol-based hand sanitizer immediately after removing all PPE.

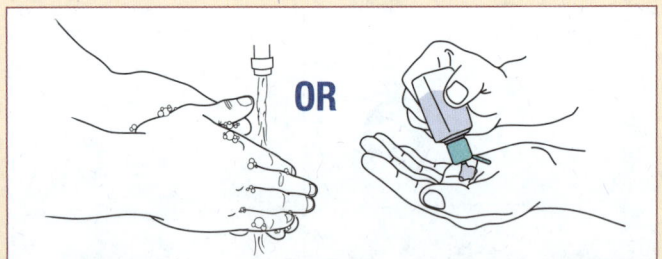

Perform hand hygiene between steps if hands become contaminated and immediately after removing all PPE.

How to safely remove PPE, Example 2
Here is another way to safely remove PPE without contaminating your clothing, skin, or mucous membranes with potentially infectious materials. **Remove all PPE before exiting the patient room** except a respirator, if worn. Remove the respirator **after** leaving the patient room and closing the door. Remove PPE in the following sequence:

1. Gown and gloves
- Gown front and sleeves and the outside of gloves are contaminated!
- If your hands get contaminated during gown or glove removal, immediately wash your hands or use an alcohol-based hand sanitizer.
- Grasp the gown in the front and pull away from your body so that the ties break, touching outside of gown only with gloved hands.

Donning and removing personal protective equipment (PPE) *(continued)*

• While removing the gown, fold or roll the gown inside-out into a bundle.
• As you are removing the gown, peel off your gloves at the same time, only touching the inside of the gloves and gown with your bare hands. Place the gown and gloves into a waste container.

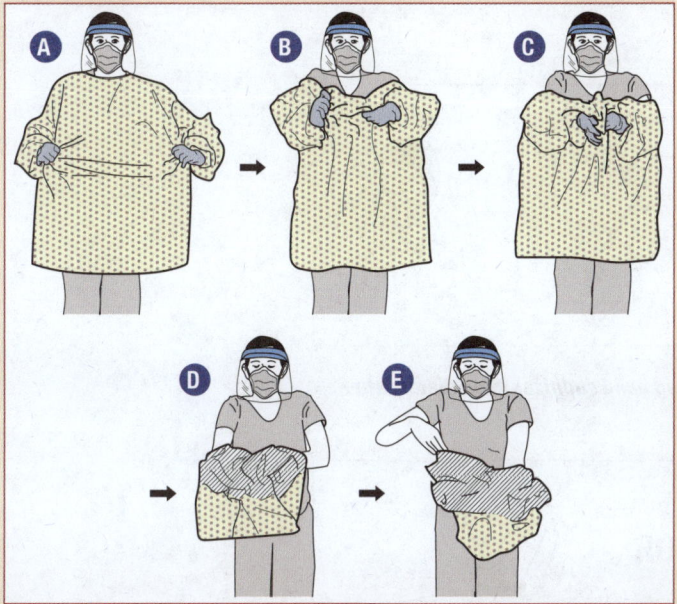

2. Goggles or face shield

• Outside of goggles or face shield is contaminated!
• If your hands get contaminated during goggle or face shield removal, immediately wash your hands or use an alcohol-based hand sanitizer.
• Remove goggles or face shield from the back by lifting head band and without touching the front of the goggles or face shield.
• If the item is reusable, place in designated receptacle for reprocessing. Otherwise, discard in a waste container.

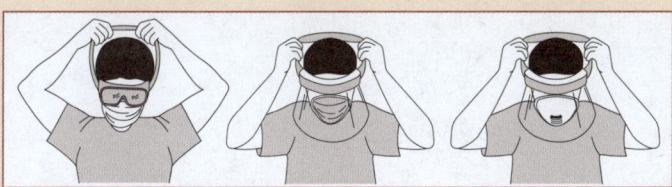

(Continued)

Donning and removing personal protective equipment (PPE) *(continued)*

3. Mask or respirator
- Front of mask/respirator is contaminated—DO NOT TOUCH!
- If your hands get contaminated during mask/respirator removal, immediately wash your hands or use an alcohol-based hand sanitizer.
- Grasp bottom ties or elastics of the mask/respirator, then the ones at the top, and remove without touching the front.
- Discard in a waste container.

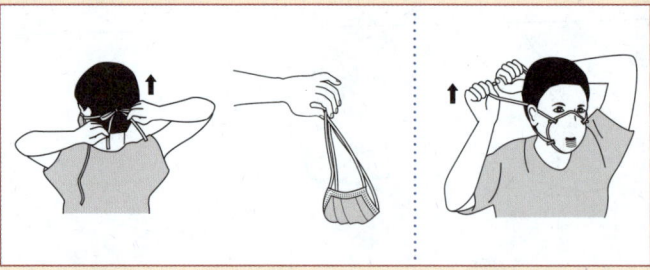

4. Wash hands or use an alcohol-based hand sanitizer immediately after removing all PPE.

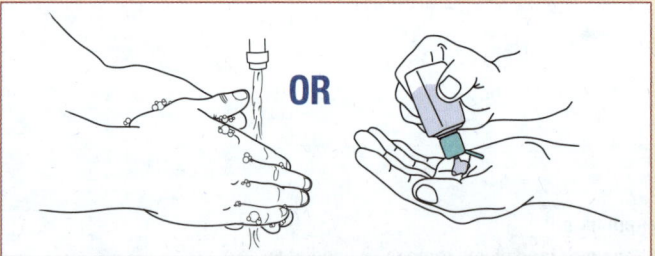

Perform hand hygiene between steps if hands become contaminated and immediately after removing all PPE.

Quick quiz

1. What type of microorganisms cause infections in persons with defense mechanisms that are compromised in some way?
    A. Transient
    B. Opportunistic
    C. Communal
    D. Colonized

Answer: B. Opportunistic pathogens take advantage of persons with compromised immune systems that are caused by disease, immuno-suppressive drugs, or procedures.

2. Which immune response can be described as follows? The rapid increase of response proteins and chemokines stimulates the move-ment of white blood cells and other phagocytic cells to the site of invasion.
    A. Adaptive immune response
    B. Passive immunity
    C. Innate immune response
    D. Physical barriers

Answer: C. The following describes the innate immune response, which is the second line of defense for invading organisms: The rapid increase of response proteins and chemokines stimulates the move-ment of white blood cells and other phagocytic cells to the site of invasion.

3. A nurse is teaching a patient about methods of infection control. Which of the following methods is most effective?
    A. Isolation precautions
    B. Wearing sterile gloves
    C. Neutropenic precautions
    D. Hand washing

Answer: D. Hand washing with soap and water or an alcohol-based hand sanitizer is the most effective infection control method.

4. A nurse is caring for a patient who has measles. Which type of equipment will the nurse use?
    A. N95 mask
    B. Face shield
    C. Standard surgical mask
    D. None is needed.

Answer: A. N95 mask. Measles is an airborne pathogen; therefore, airborne precautions are used.

Scoring

 If you answered all four questions correctly, bravo! You're super at preventing superinfection.

 If you answered three questions correctly, great! There are no spirochetes on you.

If you answered fewer than three questions correctly, chin up! Review the chapter and you'll be discarding this quiz properly in no time.

References

Bennett, J., Dolin, R., & Blaser, M. (2020). *Principles and practice of infectious diseases.* Elsevier.

Block, H., Rossaint, J., & Zarbock, A. (2022). The fatal circle of NETs and NET-associated DAMPs contributing to organ dysfunction. *Cells, 11*(12), 1919. https://doi.org/10.3390/cells11121919

Centers for Disease Control and Prevention (CDC). (2016). Standard precautions for all patient care. https://www.cdc.gov/infectioncontrol/basics/standard-precautions.html

Centers for Disease Control and Prevention (CDC). (2019). *Antibiotic resistance threats in the United States.* US Dept of Health and Human Services. https://www.cdc.gov/drugresistance/biggest-threats.html

Centers for Disease Control and Prevention (CDC). (2021a). Healthcare-associated infections (HAIs). https://www.cdc.gov/hai/index.html

Centers for Disease Control and Prevention (CDC). (2021b). Sequence for donning and removing personal protective equipment PPE. https://www.cdc.gov/HAI/prevent/ppe.html#anchor_1634672522151

Centers for Disease Control and Prevention (CDC). (2022). Guidelines for isolation precautions: Preventing transmission of infectious agents in healthcare settings. https://www.cdc.gov/infectioncontrol/guidelines/isolation/index.html

Edwards-Jones, V. (2020). Antimicrobial stewardship in wound care. *British Journal of Nursing, 29*(15), S10–S16. https://doi.org/10.12968/bjon.2020.29.15.S10

Haque, M., McKimm, J., Sartelli, M., Dhingra, S., Labricciosa, F. M., Islam, S., Jahan, D., Nusrat, T., Chowdhury, T. S., Coccolini, F., Iskandar, K., Catena, F., & Charan, J. (2020). Strategies to prevent healthcare-associated infections: A narrative overview. *Risk Management and Healthcare Policy, 13*, 1765–1780. https://doi.org/10.2147/RMHP.S269315

Ludwig, J., & McWhinnie, H. (2019). Antipyretic drugs in patients with fever and infection: Literature review. *British Journal of Nursing, 28*(10), 610–618. doi: https://doi.org/10.12968/bjon.2019.28.10.610

Netea, M., Domínguez-Andrés, J., Barreiro, L., Chavakis, T., Divangahi, M., Fuchs, E., Joosten, L., van der Meer, J., Mhlanga, M., Mulder, W., Riksen, N., Schlitzer, A., Schultze, J., Stabell Benn, C., Sun, J., Xavier, R., & Latz, E. (2020). Defining trained immunity and its role in health and disease. *Nature Reviews Immunology, 20*(6), 375–388. https://doi.org/10.1038/s41577-020-0285-6

Chapter 9

Medication basics

Just the facts

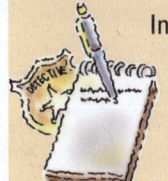

In this chapter, you'll learn:

- basics of medication administration
- drug administration routes
- key concepts of pharmacokinetics and pharmacodynamics
- dosage and administration considerations
- various drug delivery systems
- common medication errors.

Administering medication safely

Safe medication administration is one of the most crucial skills when providing care for patients in day-to-day nursing practice. From legal, ethical, and practical standpoints, medication administration is much more than simply a delivery service. Medication administration is a highly technical skill that requires you to exercise wide-ranging knowledge, analytical skill, professional judgment, and clinical expertise.

To deliver medications safely and accurately, you must have a sound working knowledge of:

- drug terminology
- routes of delivery
- effects of drugs once inside the body.

Pharmacology is the scientific study of the origin, nature, chemistry, effects, and uses of drugs. This chapter reviews some concepts basic to pharmacology—and essential to the safe administration of medication—starting with the most basic of all: drug names.

The name game

The typical drug has three or more names (see *What's in a name?*):

- The *chemical name* describes the drug's atomic and molecular structure.

What's in a name?

Most drugs have three names—chemical, generic, and trade/brand—as this example demonstrates. Some drugs may have more than one trade name. The best way to avoid confusion is to use the generic name when speaking or writing about a drug.

Chemical name

> 7-chloro-1,3-dihydro-1-methyl-5-phenyl-2H-1,4-benzodiazepin-2-one

Generic name

> diazepam

Trade name or brand name

> Valium

- The *generic name* is a shorter, simpler version of the drug's chemical name.
- The *trade name* (also known as the *brand name* or *propriety name*) is the name selected by the drug company that sells it. Trade names are protected by copyright laws.

A class act

Drugs that share similar characteristics are grouped together into pharmacologic classes or families. For example, the class known as *beta-adrenergic blockers* contains several drugs with similar properties.

Drugs can also be grouped according to their therapeutic class, which classifies drugs according to their use. For example, thiazide diuretics and beta-adrenergic blockers are both antihypertensives, but they belong to different pharmacologic classes because they share few characteristics.

Routes of administration

A drug's administration route influences the quantity given and the rate at which the drug is absorbed and distributed. These variables in turn affect the drug's action and the patient's response. Routes of administration that involve the gastrointestinal (GI) tract are known as *enteral routes*, which are from the mouth to the rectum. Enteral routes include oral, sublingual, translingual, buccal, tube feedings, and rectal. Routes that don't involve the GI tract are known as *parenteral routes*. Parenteral routes can be useful for treating a patient who can't take a drug orally. The sections that follow compare the advantages and disadvantages of various drug administration routes.

Topical route

The topical route is used to deliver a drug via the skin or a mucous membrane. The advantages of delivering drugs by this route include:
- easy administration
- few allergic reactions
- fewer adverse reactions than drugs administered by systemic routes.

Avoid a mess with topical meds

Delivering precise doses of medications can be difficult with the topical route because some medications can be messy to apply—and even messier for the patient to wear! Keep in mind that topical medications may stain the patient's clothing and bed linens. When applying topical medications, follow proper application techniques, and wear gloves.

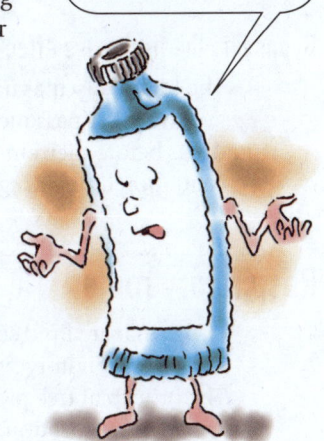

Besides being messy, some topical medications have a very distinctive smell.

Ophthalmic administration

Ophthalmic administration involves drugs such as creams, ointments, and liquid drops that are placed in the conjunctival sac or directly onto the surface of the eye. Intraocular inserts and collagen shields can be used to deliver drugs to the eye as well. For all types of ophthalmic administration, take care to avoid contaminating the medication container or transferring organisms to the patient's eye.

Convenience at a price

Ocusert Pilo, one type of intraocular insert, supplies pilocarpine to the ciliary muscles to treat glaucoma. Because this eye medication disk releases the drug for an entire week, it's more convenient than eyedrops. However, intraocular inserts cost much more than eyedrops, may be uncomfortable, and may produce adverse effects. The patient should be encouraged to speak with the health care provider regarding the pros and cons of intraocular inserts before deciding to use this type of ophthalmic.

Wielding the shield

Collagen shields that have been soaked in a drug solution can be applied to the eye to treat corneal ulcers and severe iridocyclitis (inflammation of the iris and ciliary body). Collagen shields may prove more effective than injections of collagen beneath the conjunctiva, where the substance is poorly absorbed.

Make sure that eardrops are at room temperature before administration. Otherwise, they can cause pain or vertigo.

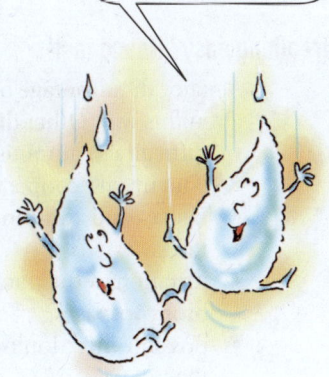

Otic administration

Otic administration involves drugs that are placed directly into the ear. Solutions placed into the ear can be used to treat infection or inflammation of the external ear canal, produce local anesthesia, or soften built-up cerumen (earwax) for easier removal.

Bring otic solutions to room temperature before administering them because cold solutions can cause pain or vertigo.

Nasal administration

Nasal administration involves drugs that are placed directly into the patient's nostrils (transnasal). Medicated solutions can be placed into the patient's nostrils from a dropper or as an atomized spray from a squeeze bottle or pump device.

Bypassing the first-pass effect

The highly vascular nasal mucosa allows systemic absorption while avoiding first-pass metabolism by the liver (the liver breaks down drugs before they enter circulation, resulting in a reduction of the concentration of the drug).

Respiratory route

Drugs that are lipid soluble and available as gases can be administered into the respiratory system by way of the bronchi and bronchial tree. The bronchial tree provides an extensive, highly perfused region for enhanced absorption. Smaller doses of potent drugs can be given by this route to minimize their adverse effects. Because this route is easily accessible, it provides a convenient alternative when other routes are unavailable.

Emergency!

In emergencies, some injectable drugs (such as atropine, lidocaine, and epinephrine) can be given directly into the lungs via an endotracheal tube. A drug administered into the trachea is absorbed into the bloodstream from the alveolar sacs. Surfactant, for example, is administered to premature neonates via the trachea to improve their respiratory function. Also, atropine can be administered to patients with symptomatic bradycardia and no vascular access to increase their heart rate.

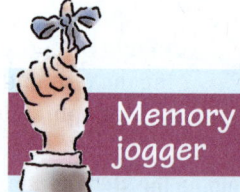

Memory jogger

Remember ALE to recall the emergency medications that can be administered through an endotracheal:

Atropine

Lidocaine

Epinephrine

Breathing easy? Not so fast!

A major disadvantage of the respiratory route is that few drugs can be given this way. Other disadvantages include:
- difficulty in administering accurate doses—or full doses, if the patient isn't cooperative
- nausea and vomiting when certain drugs are delivered into the lungs
- irritation of the tracheal or bronchial mucosa, causing coughing or bronchospasm
- possible infection from the equipment used to deliver drugs into the lungs.

Buccal, sublingual, and translingual routes

Certain drugs are given via routes that prevent destruction or trans-formation of the drug in the stomach or small intestine. These routes include buccal (in the pouch between the cheek and teeth), sublingual (under the tongue), and translingual (on the tongue). Drugs given by these routes act quickly because the oral mucosa's thin epithelium and abundant vasculature allow direct absorption into the bloodstream.

Cheeky checklist

These routes can be used if the patient can take nothing by mouth, can't swallow, or is intubated. In addition, because drugs given via these routes are absorbed in the bloodstream, they don't cause GI irritation. However, only drugs that are highly lipid soluble may be given by these routes and they may irritate the oral mucosa.

Oral route

Oral administration is usually the safest, most convenient, and least expensive method. For that reason, most drugs are administered by this route to patients who are conscious and able to swallow.

Down in the mouth

The oral route does have some disadvantages, which include:
- first-pass metabolism may take place because the drug moves through the intestine or liver, resulting in decreased concentration of the drug.
- slow and unpredictable absorption rates make oral drugs unreliable in emergencies. (See *Enteral administration: Why absorption varies.*)

Enteral administration: Why absorption varies

A drug that's administered enterally—orally or by gastric tube—can undergo variable rates of absorption due to:
- changes in the pH of the GI tract
- changes in intestinal membrane permeability
- fluctuations in GI motility
- fluctuations in GI blood flow
- food in the GI tract
- other drugs in the GI tract.

- oral drugs may irritate the GI tract, stain the patient's teeth, or taste unpleasant.
- oral drugs can be accidentally aspirated if the patient has trouble swallowing or is combative.

Gastric route

The gastric route allows direct instillation of medication into the GI system of patients who can't ingest the drug orally. A variety of tubes can be placed for instillation. Medications in oil, as well as enteric-coated or sustained-release tablets or capsules, can't be administered by this route.

Rectal and vaginal routes

Suppositories, ointments, creams, or gels may be inserted into the rectum or vagina to treat local irritation or infection. Some drugs applied to the mucosa of the rectum or vagina can be absorbed systemically. Drugs may also be delivered to the rectum in a medicated enema or to the vagina in a medicated douche.

> Some drugs can be administered by the rectal or vaginal route to treat local irritation or infection.

The up side

Drugs administered by the rectal or vaginal route don't irritate the upper GI tract, as some oral medications do. Also, these routes avoid destruction by digestive enzymes in the stomach and small intestine.

The down side

However, there are some disadvantages to the rectal and vaginal routes:

- The rectal route is usually contraindicated when the patient has a disorder affecting the lower GI tract, such as rectal bleeding or diarrhea.
- Drug absorption may be irregular or incomplete with these routes.
- The rectal route usually can't be used in an emergency.
- Because rectal administration typically stimulates the vagus nerve, this route may pose a risk for cardiac patients.
- Drugs given rectally may irritate the rectal mucosa.
- Administering a drug by the rectal or vaginal route may cause discomfort and embarrassment for the patient.

Intradermal route

Intradermal drug administration is used mainly for diagnostic purposes when testing for allergies or tuberculosis. To administer drugs intradermally, inject a small amount of serum or vaccine between the skin layers just below the stratum corneum. Because this route results in little systemic absorption, it produces mainly local effects.

Don't get too deep

When using the intradermal route, be sure not to inject the substance too deeply. If this occurs, the drug will have to be reinjected, which may cause additional stress to the patient, increase cost, and delay treatment.

Subcutaneous route

When using the subcutaneous route, small amounts of a drug are injected beneath the dermis and into the subcutaneous tissue, usually in the patient's upper arm, thigh, or abdomen. Patients with diabetes use this technique to give themselves insulin. The drug is absorbed slowly from the subcutaneous tissue, thus prolonging its effects.

Tissue issues

Disadvantages to the subcutaneous route include the following:
- Subcutaneous injection may damage tissue.
- The subcutaneous route can't be used when the patient has occlusive vascular disease and poor perfusion because decreased peripheral circulation delays absorption. Exceptions to this are heparin (enoxaparin) and insulin.
- The subcutaneous route can't be used when the patient's skin or underlying tissue is grossly adipose, edematous, burned, hardened, swollen at the common injection sites, damaged by previous injections, or diseased.

Implants eliminate nonadherence

Besides injection, another method of subcutaneous administration is to implant beneath the skin pellets or capsules that contain small amounts of a drug. From the dermis, the medication seeps slowly into the tissues. One example of an implant drug is goserelin acetate, which is used to manage prostate and breast cancer; it's inserted into the upper abdominal wall.

Because subcutaneous implants require no patient action after they're in place, they eliminate the problem of patients not adhering to a treatment regimen. Their major drawback is the need for minor surgery to insert or remove them.

Intramuscular route

The intramuscular (IM) route allows you to inject drugs directly into various muscle groups at varying tissue depths. This route is used to give aqueous suspensions and solutions in oil and to give medications that are not available in oral form. Drugs administered by the IM route take effect relatively quickly, and aqueous IM medications can be given to adults in doses of up to 5 mL in some sites. Another benefit of the IM route is that it may eliminate the need for an intravenous (IV) site.

Intramuscular miscues

Despite the advantages, there are many disadvantages to the IM route

- A drug delivered via the IM route may precipitate in the muscle, thereby reducing absorption.
- The drug may not absorb properly if the patient is hypotensive or has a poor blood supply to the muscle.
- Improper technique can cause accidental injection of the drug into the patient's bloodstream, possibly causing an overdose or an adverse reaction.
- The IM route may cause pain and local tissue irritation, damage bone, puncture blood vessels, injure nerves, or break down muscle tissue.
- Medications delivered via the IM route are not well absorbed in patients with severe muscle wasting.

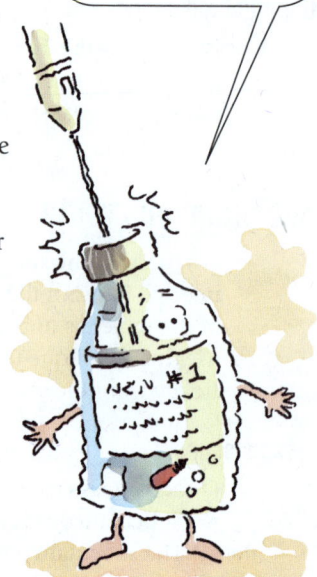

IM injections are helpful in a lot of situations, but they require proper technique to prevent pain, tissue breakdown, nerve injury, and even accidental overdose.

Intravenous route

The IV route allows injection of substances directly into the bloodstream through a vein. Appropriate substances include drugs, fluids, diagnostic contrast agents, and blood or blood products. Administration can range from a single dose to an ongoing infusion delivered with great precision.

In the IV league

Because the drug or solution is absorbed immediately and completely, the patient's response is rapid. Instant bioavailability (the drug's availability for target tissues) makes the IV route the first choice for giving drugs during an emergency. Unlike the enteral route, the IV route has no first-pass effect in the liver; in addition, unlike the IM route, it avoids damage to muscle tissue caused by irritating drugs. Because absorption into the bloodstream is complete and reliable, large drug doses can be delivered at a continuous rate.

This road can be bumpy

Life-threatening adverse reactions may arise if IV drugs are administered too quickly, if the flow rate isn't carefully monitored, or if incompatible drugs are mixed together. Also, the IV route increases the risk of complications, such as extravasation, vein irritation, systemic infection, and air embolism. Follow the IV administration guidelines in Chapter 11 Intravenous therapy to help pave the way to success.

Specialized infusions

Under certain circumstances, drug infusion may take place directly at the site of intended activity. Using specialized catheters and devices, drugs and solutions can be delivered to an organ or its blood vessels to manage emergencies, treat disease, infuse tumors, or relieve pain. These infusions may be given by the epidural, intrapleural, intraperitoneal, intra-articular, or intraosseous routes. (See *Reviewing specialized infusions*.)

Reviewing specialized infusions

Sometimes drug therapy needs to be administered directly to a specific site in the patient's body. Specialized routes of drug administration are shown in the chart.

Route	Characteristics
Epidural infusion	• The drug is injected into the epidural space, outside or above the dura mater. • The drug is absorbed into cerebrospinal fluid and works directly on the central nervous system. • Epidural anesthesia or analgesia is given through a special catheter and is considered safe and versatile. It may be tailored to affect a specific area of the body from the legs up to the upper abdomen. • The drug infused through an epidural catheter must be preservative-free to prevent serious neurotoxicity or spinal cord injury. • Epidural catheters should be labeled "for epidural use only" to prevent the accidental injection of other drugs into the epidural space.
Intrapleural infusion	• The drug is injected into the pleural cavity. • The drug crosses the pleural membrane and enters the pleural space, where it works locally at the disease site. • Chemotherapy is an example of a drug given by this type of infusion to minimize systemic effects and increase drug effects on the tumor.
Intraperitoneal infusion	• The drug is injected into the peritoneal cavity. • The drug or solution crosses the peritoneal membrane and enters the peritoneal space where it works locally. • This administration route is used for peritoneal dialysis in which the peritoneum functions as a semipermeable membrane. • Fluid or electrolyte imbalances can be corrected, toxins removed, and normal renal excretion facilitated using this route.

(Continued)

Reviewing specialized infusions *(continued)*

Route	Characteristics
Intra-articular infusion	• The drug is injected into the synovial cavity of a joint to suppress inflammation, prevent contractures, and delay muscle atrophy. • This route is most often used to treat rheumatoid arthritis, gout, systemic lupus erythematosus, osteoarthritis, and other joint disorders. • Corticosteroids, anesthetics, and lubricants are most commonly administered into the shoulder, elbow, wrist, finger, knee, ankle, or toe joints. • This route is used sparingly because of the risk of infection.
Intraosseous infusion	• The drug is injected into the rich vascular network of a long bone for rapid absorption. • Drugs and solutions administered through bone marrow are absorbed as rapidly as those administered by IV. • With a special intraosseous access needle, this route has been used successfully in children and adults for emergency infusions when normal vascular access isn't possible.

Pharmacokinetics

A solid understanding of pharmacokinetics—the movement of a drug through the body—can help you predict your patient's response to a prescribed drug regimen and anticipate potential problems. Any time you give a drug, a series of physiochemical events takes place in the patient's body and includes four basic processes:

- Absorption
- Distribution
- Metabolism
- Excretion.

(See *What happens after drug administration.*)

Absorption

Before a drug can act on the body, it must be absorbed into the bloodstream. How well a patient's body absorbs a drug depends on several factors. These include:

- the drug's physiochemical properties
- the drug's form
- the route of administration
- the drug's interactions with other substances in the GI tract
- various patient characteristics, especially the site and the condition of the absorbing surface.

These factors can also determine the speed and amount of drug absorption.

What happens after drug administration

Drug disposition begins as soon as a drug is administered. The drug proceeds through pharmacokinetic, pharmacodynamic, and pharmacotherapeutic phases. This chart shows the various phases, the activities that occur during them, and the factors that influence those activities.

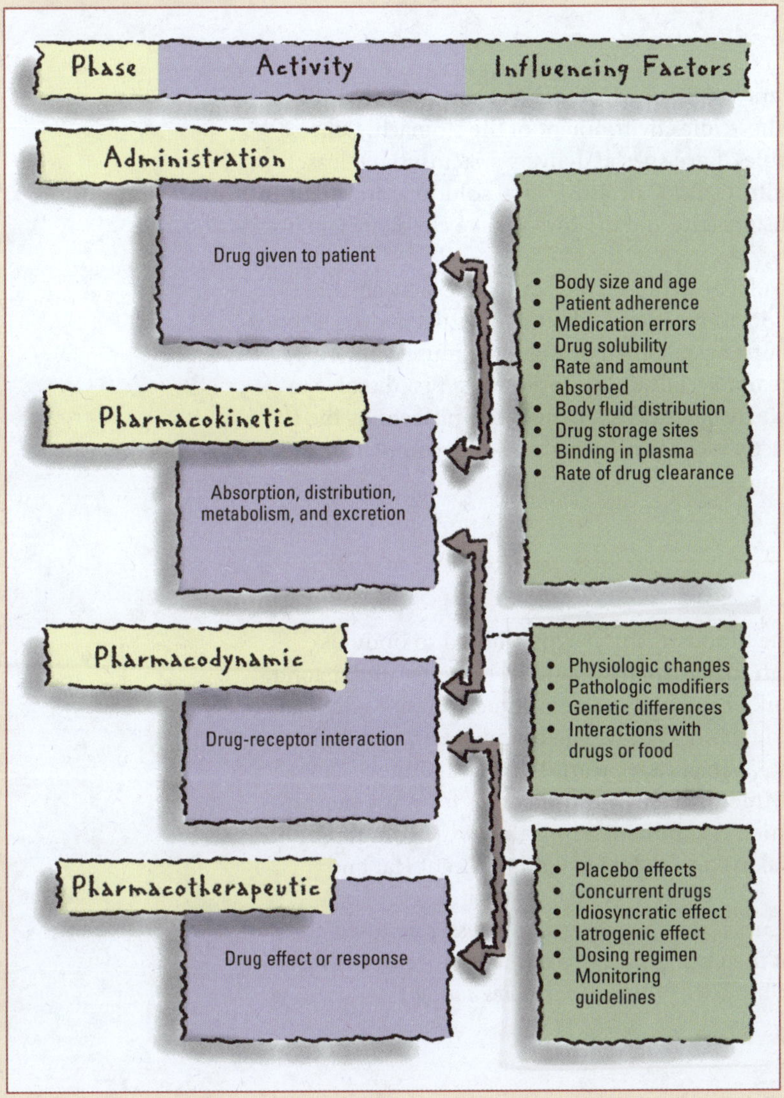

Phase	Activity	Influencing Factors
Administration	Drug given to patient	• Body size and age • Patient adherence • Medication errors • Drug solubility • Rate and amount absorbed • Body fluid distribution • Drug storage sites • Binding in plasma • Rate of drug clearance
Pharmacokinetic	Absorption, distribution, metabolism, and excretion	
Pharmacodynamic	Drug-receptor interaction	• Physiologic changes • Pathologic modifiers • Genetic differences • Interactions with drugs or food
Pharmacotherapeutic	Drug effect or response	• Placebo effects • Concurrent drugs • Idiosyncratic effect • Iatrogenic effect • Dosing regimen • Monitoring guidelines

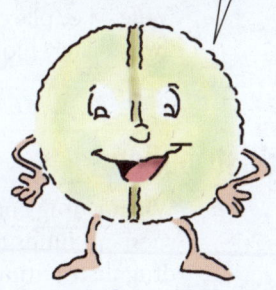

Here's an easy way to see what happens to a drug after it has been administered.

Becoming bioavailable

When taken orally, some drug forms, such as tablets and capsules, may have to disintegrate before free particles are available to dissolve in the gastric juices. Only after dissolving in these juices can the drug be absorbed, circulate in the bloodstream, and thus become bioavailable. A bioavailable drug is one that's ready to produce a physiologic effect.

Timing is everything

Some tablets have enteric coatings, which delay disintegration until after the tablets leave the acidic environment of the stomach. Others, such as liposome capsules, have special delivery systems that release the drug only at a specific osmotic pressure. Oral solutions and elixirs, which don't have to disintegrate and dissolve to take effect, are usually absorbed more rapidly.

If the patient has had a bowel resection, anticipate slow absorption of any oral drug you administer. And remember that a drug given via the IM route must first be absorbed through the muscle before it can enter the bloodstream. Rectal suppositories must first dissolve to be absorbed through the rectal mucosa. Drugs administered by the IV route—i.e., placed directly into the bloodstream—are completely and immediately bioavailable.

Distribution

When a drug enters the bloodstream, it's distributed to body tissues and fluids through the circulatory system. To better understand drug distribution, think of the body as a system of physiologic compartments defined by blood flow. The bloodstream and highly perfused organs—such as the brain, heart, liver, and kidneys—make up the central compartment. Lesser perfused areas form the peripheral compartment, which is subdivided into the tissue compartment (viscera, muscle, and skin) and the deep compartment (fat and bone).

Highly perfused tissues receive the drug before lesser perfused areas do. Each compartment then stores portions of the drug, releasing it as plasma drug levels decline. (See *How the body stores a drug.*)

Leaping lipid barriers

Distribution also depends partly on a drug's ability to cross lipid membranes. Some drugs can't cross certain cell membranes and thus have limited distribution. For example, antibiotics have trouble permeating the prostate gland, abscesses, and exudates.

How the body stores a drug

The body can store a drug in fat, bone, or skin. Knowing the characteristics of each drug storage compartment will help you understand how distribution can affect a drug's duration of action.

Fat storage

A drug that dissolves easily in lipids migrates to adipose tissue (what we commonly think of as fatty tissue). Because this tissue lacks receptors for drug action, the drug remains inactive there. Eventually, it's released by fat cells to exert its pharmacologic effect. With some drugs, this slow, prolonged action is an advantage. For example, slow release of anesthetic barbiturates provides effective anesthesia during surgery. With other drugs, such prolonged action can be dangerous.

Bone storage

Bone acts as a storage compartment for certain drugs. Lead and some chemicals can also accumulate in bone, resulting in prolonged exposure to toxins.

Skin storage

Storage of drugs in the skin typically causes photosensitivity. Tetracycline and amiodarone are examples of drugs that are stored in the skin.

It has to be free

Distribution can also be affected if the drug binds to plasma proteins, especially albumin. Only a free, unbound drug can produce an effect at the drug receptor site, so such binding greatly influences the drug's effectiveness and duration of action.

Disease disrupts distribution

Certain diseases impede drug distribution by altering the volume of distribution—the total amount of drug in the body in relation to the amount in plasma. Heart failure, dehydration, and burns are examples of such disorders. If the patient has heart failure, expect to increase the dosage because the drug must be distributed to a larger fluid volume. On the other hand, if the patient is dehydrated, expect to decrease the dosage because the drug will be distributed to a much smaller fluid volume. (See *Dosing dilemma*.)

Metabolism and excretion

Most drugs are metabolized in the liver and excreted by the kidneys. The rate at which a drug is metabolized varies with the individual. Some patients metabolize drugs so quickly that their blood and

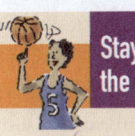

Stay on the ball

Dosing dilemma

Some drugs—such as digoxin, gentamicin, and tobramycin—are poorly distributed to fatty tissue. Therefore, dosing based on actual body weight in a highly obese patient may lead to overdose and serious toxicity.

Go lean

When administering such drugs, calculate the dose based on lean body weight, which you can estimate from actuarial tables that give average weight ranges for various heights.

tissue levels prove therapeutically inadequate. Others metabolize drugs so slowly that even ordinary doses can produce toxic results. Metabolism of medications in the older adult can be slow, resulting in increased plasma concentrations related to decreased muscle, increased body fat, and aging of the kidneys or liver (Rochon, 2023).

Slow or fast? Here's some help...

Drug metabolism may be faster in people who smoke than in people who don't smoke because cigarette smoke contains substances that induce production of hepatic enzymes. Also, a diet high in fat or carbohydrates may slow the metabolism of certain drugs, whereas a diet high in protein may speed metabolism.

Hepatic diseases, or diseases that interfere with hepatic blood flow or transport of drugs to the liver, may affect one or more of the liver's metabolic functions. Thus, in patients with hepatic disease, drug metabolism may be increased or decreased. All patients with hepatic disease must be monitored closely for drug effects and toxic reactions.

The kidneys can be key

Some drugs, such as digoxin and gentamicin, are eliminated almost unchanged by the kidneys. Thus, inadequate renal function causes the drug to accumulate, producing toxic effects. Some drugs can block renal excretion of other drugs, thereby allowing them to accumulate and enhancing their effects. In contrast, some drugs can promote renal excretion of other drugs, thus diminishing their effects.

Different escape routes

Although most drugs are excreted by the kidneys, some are excreted hepatically, via the bile and into stool. A few drugs leave the body in sweat, saliva, and breast milk. Certain volatile anesthetics—for example, halothane—are eliminated primarily by exhalation. When natural excretion mechanisms fail, as in drug overdose or renal dysfunction, many drugs can be removed through dialysis.

Underlying disease

Underlying disease can have a marked influence on drug action and effect. For example, acidosis may cause insulin resistance. Genetic diseases, such as glucose-6-phosphate dehydrogenase (G6PD) deficiency and hepatic porphyria, may turn drugs into toxins. As a result, patients with G6PD deficiency may develop hemolytic anemia when given sulfonamides or certain other drugs.

It's in your genes

Genetics may affect how medication is absorbed or metabolized (Pharmacogenomics, 2023).

Toxic conditions

The liver works to help break down some medications in the blood. If a drug is toxic or there is too much of a drug for the liver to break down, the liver can become damaged, resulting in drug-induced hepatitis (inflammation of the liver) (Drug-Induced Hepatitis, 2023).

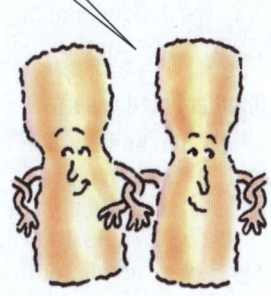

So many conditions and factors can influence a person's response to drug therapy, even genes.

Sphere of influence

Other conditions that may influence a patient's response to drug therapy include infection; fever; stress; starvation; hypersensitivity; sunlight; exercise; variations in circadian rhythm; alcohol intake; pregnancy; lactation; immunization; barometric pressure; and GI, renal, hepatic, cardiovascular, and immunologic function. (See *Age-old influence*.)

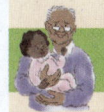

Ages and stages

Age-old influence

The patient's age has an important influence on a drug's overall action and effect. Older adults usually have decreased hepatic function, less muscle mass, and diminished renal function. Consequently, to avoid toxicity they need lower doses and, sometimes, longer dosage intervals.

Neonates have underdeveloped metabolic enzyme systems and inadequate renal function, which can also lead to toxicity. They need highly individualized dosages and careful monitoring.

Types of medication orders

In an outpatient setting, the process of ordering a medication is rather simple. Most often, a prescriber transmits an electronic digital prescription to a community or mail-order pharmacy (known as e-prescribing). Or, a prescriber may write an order on a prescription pad and give that piece of paper to the patient. The patient then takes the written prescription to the pharmacy to have it filled (Prescribing, 2023).

Inpatient med orders

In an inpatient setting, the process may be somewhat more complex. Several types of medication orders can be used in the inpatient setting, including:
- standard orders
- single (or one-time) orders
- stat orders
- p.r.n. orders
- standing orders
- verbal orders
- telephone orders.

Standard orders

A *standard order* is a prescription that remains in effect indefinitely or for a specified period. The prescriber either writes the order—along with instructions, such as for diet, radiographs, and laboratory work—on the order sheet in the patient's chart or enters the order into a computer, and then the order is printed out on a computer-generated patient record.

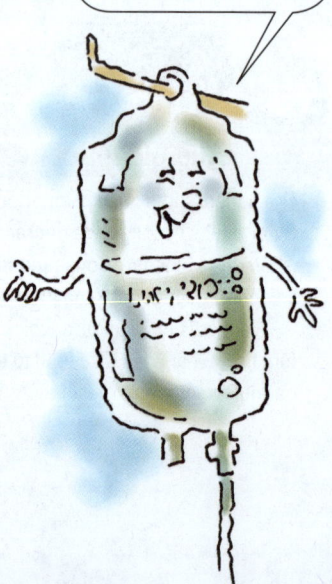

Be sure to check your facility's policies on certain drugs and doses when following standard orders.

Following orders

The order must specify the name of the medication, dosage, route of administration, frequency, duration (if time limited), and indication (if p.r.n.). (See *Components of a medication order*.) For example, the order might be written this way: *Amoxil 500 mg P.O. q 8 hr × 10 days.*

Administration times of the medication are scheduled based on the order, the facility's policies, and pertinent characteristics of the medication itself, such as onset and duration of action and whether it's to be given with or without food.

Wait for further orders

If a standard order doesn't specify a termination time, the order usually remains in effect until the prescriber writes another order to replace or discontinue it. For some types of drugs, however, the

Components of a medication order

For a hospitalized patient, a prescriber writes a medication order on an order sheet in the patient's chart or enters the order into the computer system. An example of a written order is shown here.

Component list

Whether written or entered into the computer, all drug orders must contain:

- patient's full name
- date and time of the order
- name of the drug being ordered
- dosage form
- dose amount
- administration route
- time schedule for administration
- prescriber's signature or computer code.

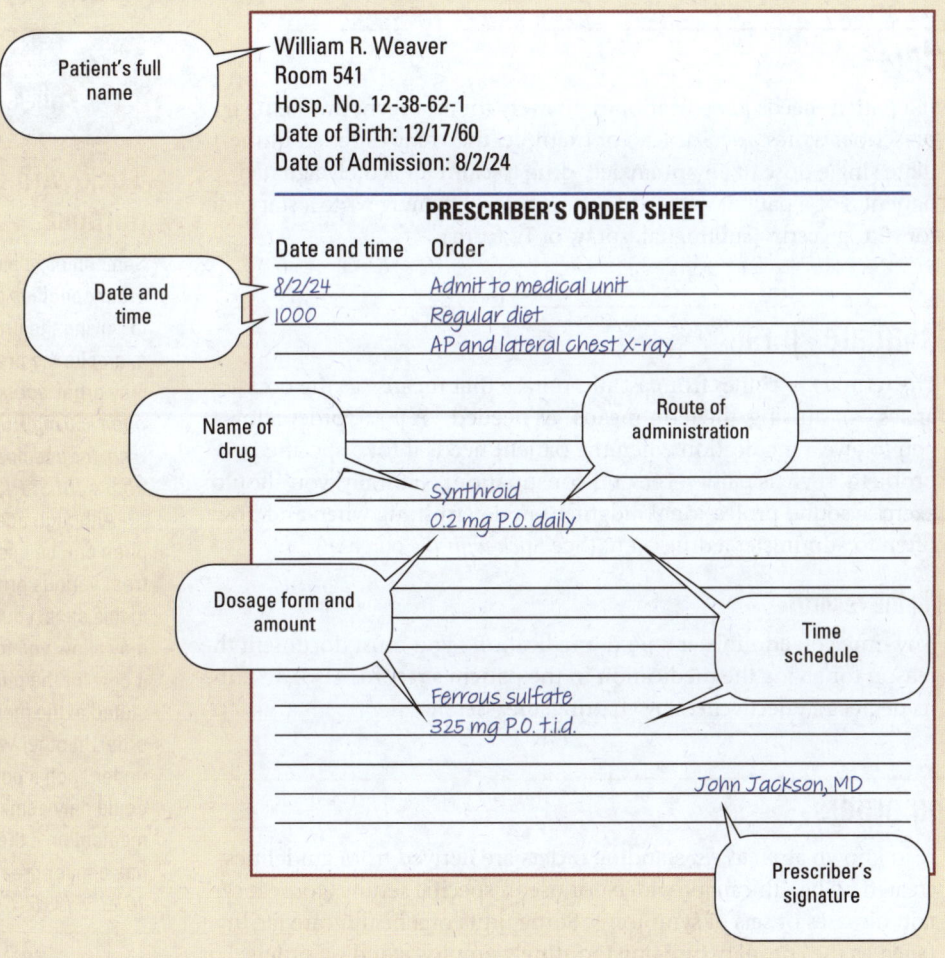

Patient's full name

William R. Weaver
Room 541
Hosp. No. 12-38-62-1
Date of Birth: 12/17/60
Date of Admission: 8/2/24

PRESCRIBER'S ORDER SHEET

Date and time	Order
8/2/24	Admit to medical unit
1000	Regular diet
	AP and lateral chest X-ray

Date and time

Name of drug

Route of administration

Synthroid
0.2 mg P.O. daily

Dosage form and amount

Time schedule

Ferrous sulfate
325 mg P.O. t.i.d.

John Jackson, MD

Prescriber's signature

amount of time covered by the order may be limited by facility policy. For example, opioid orders may have a controlled delivery time of 3 days. Some antibiotics may have a controlled delivery time of 7 days. If the patient still needs the drug after the termination date has passed, the prescriber must write another order. The same is true for postoperative medications; the prescriber must rewrite standard orders for all medications that are to continue after surgery.

Single (one-time) orders

When a medication is to be given only once, a prescriber writes what's called a *single order*. For example, they may order one injection of tetanus toxoid for a patient with a puncture wound who received a primary tetanus toxoid series more than 5 years earlier.

Stat orders

If a patient needs a medication right away for an urgent problem, a prescriber writes a stat order. For example, they may order an immediate single dose of an antianxiety drug to calm an acutely agitated patient. For a patient with acute chest pain, they may write a stat order for nitroglycerin (sublingual, spray, or IV form).

Orders that are "p.r.n."

The term *p.r.n.* comes from a Latin phrase that means "as the occasion arises." In nursing, the term means "as needed." A p.r.n. order allows you to give a medication when the patient needs it for a specified problem, such as pain, fever, and constipation. Naturally, you should exercise sound professional judgment in determining when and how often to administer a drug p.r.n. (See *Stick with the purpose.*)

Record it in the record

Any time you administer a p.r.n. medication , you must document the reason for giving the medication in the patient's record. Also, describe its degree of effectiveness by charting a reassessment.

Standing orders

Also known as *protocols*, standing orders are derived from guidelines created by health care providers for use in specific settings to treat certain diseases or sets of symptoms. Some units of a health care facility (such as the coronary care unit) routinely employ standing orders. For

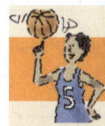

Stay on the ball

Stick with the purpose

Sometimes, a p.r.n. order specifies a reason for giving the drug. For example, the prescriber may order *acetaminophen 650 mg P.O. q 4 hr, p.r.n. for a temperature above 101.3° F (38.5° C)*.

Although acetaminophen can be used to treat various problems, in this case, your facility may allow you to give it only for the purpose stated in the medication order. In other words, under such a policy, you could only administer the medication if the patient has a fever greater than *101.3° F (38.5° C)*.

example, the unit may have standing orders for morphine sulfate to treat chest pain, for lidocaine to treat ventricular tachycardia, and for furosemide to treat pulmonary congestion.

Does a standing order need an order? Yes!

Standing orders specify which drugs you're permitted to administer and under which circumstances. The health care provider must still review each individually ordered medication for each patient. That is, there must be an order to enact the standing orders. Standing orders may also provide guidelines or algorithms for making dosage adjustments. For example, you may need to change the dosage of a heparin infusion based on your patient's anticoagulation studies.

A test of skills

Standing orders require the nurse to use considerable judgment and expertise in assessing a patient's need for a drug and detecting any dose-related adverse reactions that could occur. No standing order should be automatically implemented without a careful review regarding its appropriateness for a given patient at a given time.

> It may sound like double-talk, but make sure the patient's chart includes an order to give a standing order before administering a protocol drug.

Verbal and telephone orders

Medication orders given orally rather than in writing are known as *verbal orders*. Whenever possible, avoid them, because miscommunications can happen when verbal orders are exchanged. (See *Telephone order accuracy*.)

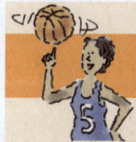

Stay on the ball

Telephone order accuracy

If you must take a medication order over the telephone, follow these steps to help ensure its accuracy:

• Have another nurse listen in on the call to confirm that they heard the same order as you.

• Repeat the name of the ordered drug to the prescriber to verify that you heard it correctly. Have the prescriber spell the drug name, if necessary.

• Repeat the individual digits of the dose ordered—for example, "You ordered fifteen, one-five, milligrams

of meperidine; is that right?" The prescriber can then confirm the amount or correct it with something like, "No, I ordered fifty, five-zero, milligrams of meperidine."

• Write out the order, noting that it was a verified telephone order, then sign and date it.

• Administer the medication as ordered.

• The prescriber must cosign the written order within the time allotted by your facility.

In an emergency, repeat, repeat

In urgent situations a verbal order sometimes can't be avoided. Repeat the order aloud to verify with the prescriber the order was understood. For example, let's say the patient goes into hypoglycemic or insulin shock and the health care provider tells you to immediately prepare 50 mL of 50% glucose for IV administration. To verify the order, show the provider the label on the empty glucose vial and say the drug's name out loud. Doing this allows the provider the opportunity to confirm the accuracy of the drug and its dose.

Signature required!

Anytime you accept a verbal order, it's your responsibility to ensure the accuracy of the communication. This holds true even in an emergency. During an emergency, if communication is unclear, ask the prescriber to spell the drug's name. Afterward, write and sign the order that was verbally given by the prescriber, then have the prescriber sign the order as soon as possible. The facility often has a policy that indicates the time frame the prescriber has to sign the verbal order.

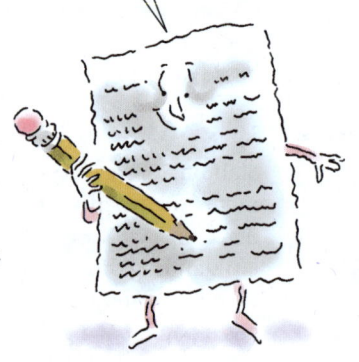

Getting a signature after a verbal order is just as important as getting it right!

Administration procedures

When it comes to administering medications correctly, you must understand the medication order and apply judgment and knowledge about the correctness of the order of the medication in light of your understanding of the patient's condition.

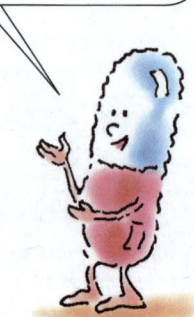

Use your good judgment before administering a medication.

The order is verified

Research the drug in the drug guide, and verify that a medication order is appropriate for the patient involved. After that, the next step is to prepare the drug correctly for administration. (See *Orders into action*.)

After you transcribe the medication order, go to a quiet area to prepare the medication for delivery, following the 6 rights of medication administration.

Orders into action

After you receive a written medication order, transcribe it into the electronic medication record or a working document approved by your health care facility. For example, your facility may require you to use a medication administration record (MAR), a medication Kardex, medication cards or tickets, or a computer printout.

Stepping away from errors

To reduce the risk of overlooking a medication order, your facility may require the nurses to periodically check all MARs against the original order sheets.

The 6 rights

Following a tried-and-true set of safeguards known as the *6 rights* can quickly and easily help you avoid the most basic and common sources of medication error. Each time you administer a medication, confirm that you have the:

- right drug
- right dose
- right patient
- right time
- right route
- right documentation.

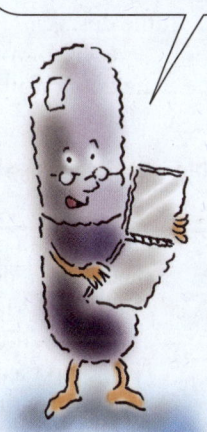

Before giving a drug, make sure you confirm the 6 rights of medication administration. Read the patient their rights!

Right drug

Always compare the name of an ordered drug with the name printed on the container label. Take your time and do it carefully; drugs with similar-sounding and similar-looking names may have very different indications and effects.

Sounds like…

For example, Celexa (citalopram hydrobromide) and Celebrex (celecoxib) sound quite similar. But Celexa is a selective serotonin reuptake inhibitor used to treat depression. Celebrex is a nonsteroidal anti-inflammatory drug used to treat osteoarthritis and rheumatoid arthritis. Other similar-sounding drugs may raise a similar risk of mix-ups.

Verify the name

When a medication is individually wrapped in single doses, check the name when removing it from the drawer and again when unwrapping and giving the drug to the patient. Before actually administering the drug, always explain to the patient the drug name and the reason the medication was prescribed.

From the mouth of the patient

Besides carefully checking the ordered drug name against the container label, also check the patient's reaction to the drug as you try to administer it. If they say, "I usually take one pink pill, but you've given me two yellow pills," stop and recheck the order. Perhaps there is a simple explanation for the difference, such as the pink pill contains 10 mg of the drug and the yellow ones contain 5 mg each. Or perhaps you'll discover that you're giving the patient the wrong medication. Either way, you must carefully follow up on any comment a patient makes about changes in a medication before you continue to administer it.

Right dose

The growing use of unit-dose medications (in which a single dose of medication is wrapped and labeled for individual use) has greatly reduced the risk of giving a patient the wrong drug dose. Also, many commercially prepared medications are available in various tablet sizes, decreasing the number of calculations you must do to determine the dosage.

Even so, you must know how and when to perform the appropriate dose calculations.

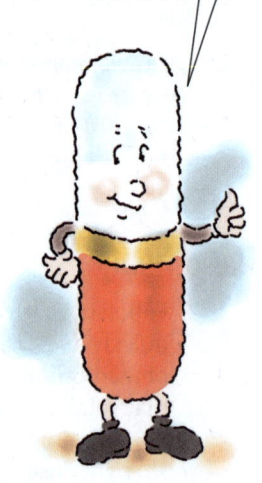

Before giving me to the patient, always mention my name and explain why I'm prescribed.

Double-check the dose

Whenever possible, double-check all your calculations with another nurse or with a pharmacist. Many hospitals require these double checks when dosage calculations involve children's medications. Additionally, for high-alert medications, many have policies requiring a witness verification to ensure the correct dose will be administered. High-alert medications include those with narrow safety margins, such as heparin and insulin.

Know your scope

You must stay within your scope of practice when administering medications. You may never alter the drug dosage or route specified in a prescriber's order. If the route is no longer appropriate, or the dose is not effective, you should communicate your concerns with the prescriber.

Sometimes a prescriber's original medication order specifies a range of dosages. If this is the case, you must determine the appropriate dose for the patient—within that range.

Right patient

To reduce the risk of medication errors, never assume that the patient in the bed is indeed the patient named on the medication label. To verify the right patient, always use two patient identifiers (neither of which should be the patient's room number) before giving any medication. Many hospitals use the bar code medication administration method, which requires the nurse to scan their identification badge, the patient's bracelet, and the medication bar code on the drug that is to be administered to the patient. (Follow your facility's policy for patient identification.)

Roll call

As an additional check, the patient's name and date of birth should also be checked each and every time before administering medication. Ask the patient their name by saying, "Please state your name; it's best not to say something like, "You're John, right?" because the patient could misunderstand you, they could be confused, or they could be a different John than the one scheduled for a medication.

Right time

The considerations that make an administration time the "right" time may be therapeutic, practical, or both. For therapeutic purposes, the right time is one that appropriately maintains the level of drug in the patient's bloodstream. For practical purposes, the right time is one that's convenient for the staff and the patient. Therapeutic goals take precedence over practical ones.

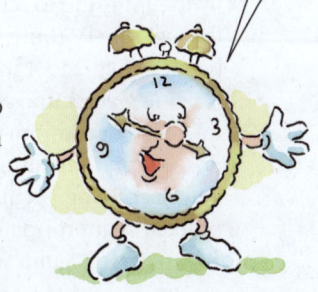

The right time to give a drug depends on the patient's individual circumstances.

Working around the clock

Some medications may need to be timed to allow the medication to be evenly spaced around the clock. This approach helps to maintain a consistent level of the drug in the patient's bloodstream.

For some drugs, you may need to collect assessment data to help determine whether it's the right time to give another dose. For example, before giving digoxin, you should assess the patient's apical pulse rate, determined by cardiac auscultation for 1 minute (because digoxin increases myocardial contraction and may lower the heart rate; it should be used cautiously in patients with bradycardia or avoided if the apical pulse is less than 60 beats per minute); before giving morphine, you should assess the patient's respiratory rate (because morphine is a central nervous system depressant and can reduce respiratory rate, it should be avoided in patients with bradypnea [less than 12 breaths per minute]).

The perfect plan

Besides maximizing the therapeutic effect, giving medications at specified, evenly spaced intervals provides some practical benefits. For one thing, it allows administration times to be planned around meals or for medications to be given during less busy times on the nursing unit. For example, instead of scheduling a once-daily medication at 8 a.m., which is commonly close to the time nurses change shifts, schedule it at 9 a.m..

Another practical benefit of a standardized administration time is that it can establish a habit for the patient. This may make it easier for the patient to keep taking the medication appropriately when they get home.

Administer on time

Regardless of the reasons behind the administration times established for the patient, those times need to be followed carefully. In fact, many facilities consider it a medication error if the nurse fails to give a medication within 30 minutes before or after its scheduled administration time.

Right route

Always pay careful attention to the administration route specified in the medication order, on the product's label, and in the drug guide. Also, make sure the ordered form of the drug is appropriate for the intended route. Only drugs labeled "for injection" should be used for injections of any kind.

Before giving the drug, consider whether the amount ordered is appropriate for the route by which it is being prepared. For example, 10 mg is an appropriate amount of morphine sulfate to be given by the IM route to relieve pain in an adult. However, administered through the IV route, the equivalent dose of morphine sulfate would be more like 2 to 4 mg (a much smaller dose because the medication is being given intravenously). If the patient is taking the drug orally, they may need more than 10 mg to achieve the same effect (a larger dose because the drug will be broken down by the liver or intestines before entering circulation). To determine whether the amount ordered is appropriate for the route of administration, always refer to a current drug guide.

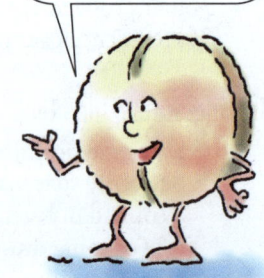

The rate of absorption of a drug varies depending on the route.

Different routes, different speeds

Remember that the route by which a drug is given affects the rate at which it gets absorbed into the patient's bloodstream. Because certain forms of a drug may be intended for specific routes, be careful not to interfere with a drug's action by changing routes or circumventing the chemical preparation. For example, an enteric-coated tablet or sustained-release capsule should not be crushed. (See *Working with sustained-release drugs*, page 181.)

Working with sustained-release drugs

A growing number of drugs are being formulated to exert an effect over many hours. The components of each drug dose dissolve at different rates, thus releasing the drug gradually but continuously into the patient's bloodstream. Convenient for staff and patients, sustained-release drugs require fewer doses per day and provide steadier control over symptoms.

Easy identification

Sustained-release drugs are supplied as plain tablets, coated tablets, and capsules filled with tiny granules. They may be identified by an *SR* (for sustained release) after the drug name, or they may have one of several prefixes attached to the name that suggests an extended effect. Some common examples include *Quinaglute Dura-Tabs*, *Dimetapp Extentabs*, *Chlor-Trimeton Repetabs*, and *Desoxyn Gradumets*. Other names include *Spansules and Gyrocaps*.

Don't split, crush, or chew

Never split or crush a sustained-release drug. Warn the patient not to chew the drug and to never open a sustained-release capsule to mix the granules into foods or beverages. These actions could alter the drug's absorption rate, put too much drug into the patient's bloodstream too quickly, or reduce the drug's overall effect.

Rate of absorption can be altered. For example, the speed at which topical nitroglycerin enters a patient's bloodstream can be increased by spreading it over a larger area of skin and covering it with plastic wrap. Or, if a patient chews or swallows a sublingual drug, such as sublingual nitroglycerin, the rate of absorption and effectiveness will be decreased.

Right documentation

After administering the medication following the first 5 rights, the 6th right is to document the administration correctly on the right patient, while following your facility's policy on documenting medications. Ways of documenting include computerized charting, paper charts, and barcode scanning (barcode scanning is discussed in Chapters 10 and 11).

Procedural safeguards

The 6 rights of medication administration afford a basic level of protection against medication errors. However, most experts consider them the minimum requirement. Here are some additional measures you should take to help avoid medication errors.

Storage and preparation

Follow these guidelines when storing and preparing drugs:

- Store and handle drugs carefully to maintain their stability and potency. Remember that some drugs can be altered by temperature, air, light, and moisture; make sure to follow all drug-specific precautions. Some drugs may need to be kept in brown bottles. Some IV bags may need to be covered with foil or dark plastic to block the light during infusion.
- Always keep drugs in the containers in which the pharmacy dispensed them. Cap all containers tightly. Many pill bottles have small cylinders inside the container that serve to absorb moisture and keep the product fresh; these cylinders should not be removed.
- Store drugs at room temperature unless instructed to refrigerate them. Refrigeration causes moisture to form and could alter some drugs through condensation.
- As required by law, keep opioids and controlled substances under double lock.

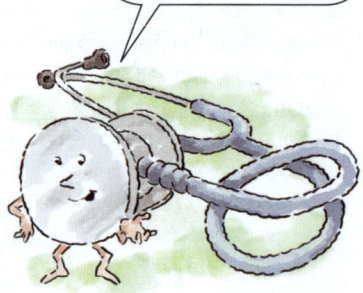

Always follow the manufacturer's recommendations and your facility's guidelines for storing and handling all medications.

Out of date? Out of the question!

- Always note a drug's expiration date—the date after which it loses some amount of potency. Never administer an outdated drug or one that looks or smells unusual.
- If the original package looks like someone may have tampered with it, don't give the drug; instead, return it in its package to the pharmacy for an investigation.
- Check the medication label three times—when you take it from the shelf, drawer, or dispensing unit; before putting it into the medication cup; and before administration—to make sure you are giving the prescribed medication. For a unit-dose medication, check the label just after obtaining the medication and again before discarding the wrapper.
- You may need to reconstitute a drug dispensed as a powder just before you administer it. If medication is left over after you remove your dose, label the container with the date, time, strength, and your initials or signature.
- Never administer a drug that wasn't labeled properly after reconstitution.
- Discard any drug that will reach its expiration date before another dose is scheduled.
- If you find an unlabeled syringe with medication inside, discard it.
- Let a refrigerated drug reach room temperature before administering it, unless instructed otherwise.

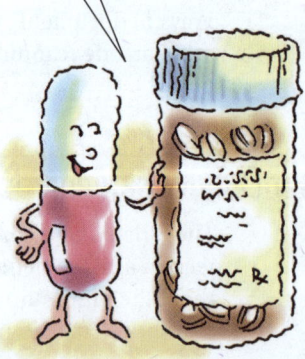

Check all medication labels and packaging carefully. Note the expiration date, too.

Handling orders for bedside medications

If a medication order specifies that you should leave a drug at the patient's bedside for self-administration, label the drug with:
- patient's name
- drug name
- dosage
- instructions the patient needs.

   Drugs commonly left at the patient's bedside include antacids and nitroglycerin tablets.

Supervision requires a super nurse

In most health care facilities, you're responsible for supervising a patient whose drugs are left at the bedside. For example, you must know how many nitroglycerin tablets the patient took, the exact times of self-administration, the degree of relief obtained, and any unusual reactions they had to the drug. Record this information in the patient's chart and report it to the prescriber.

Administration

Follow these guidelines when administering drugs:
- Before administering a medication based on new orders, review the patient's medication history for known allergies or other problems. Always ask the patient if they have any allergies to medications including over-the-counter medications.
- If the patient has a known drug allergy, make sure the chart clearly displays the allergy.
- Never administer a drug that you are unfamiliar with. Review the medication in the drug guide before administering it.
- Never leave a drug unattended. Always stay with the medication, or return it to a locked storage place.
- Assess the patient's physiologic and psychological condition before administering any medication.
- Stay with the patient until they take the medication to verify that they took it as directed.
- Never leave medication doses at a patient's bedside unless you have a specific order to do so. (See *Handling orders for bedside medications.*)
- Administer only medications that you have personally prepared or verified that the pharmacist prepared.
- Never administer a drug that another nurse asks you to give to their patient.
- Don't open individually prepared doses (unit-dose medications) until you're at the bedside and have confirmed the patient's identity.
- When administering an oral drug, urge the patient to drink a full glass of water, if appropriate. Doing so helps move the medication out of the esophagus and into the stomach. It also dilutes the drug, thus reducing the chance of gastric irritation.

Write it down!

- Document drugs immediately after you administer them. Delayed charting, especially of p.r.n. medications, can result in repeated doses. Documenting before giving a medication can lead to missed doses.
- Record your observations of the patient's positive and negative responses to the medication. For example, if you give an antibiotic to a patient with pneumonia, chart positive responses such as decreased sputum, reduced fever, and easier breathing to confirm the drug's effectiveness. Also, chart adverse reactions such as skin eruptions or gastric upset. Severe adverse reactions may prompt the prescriber to substitute another drug.

Drug delivery systems

The drug delivery system is yet another area of medication administration that you'll need to master. Your facility may use one of several systems by which drugs can be obtained from the pharmacy. In each one, the nurse serves a vital coordinating function between the prescriber and the pharmacist.

Systems analysis

Regardless of the delivery system used by your facility, the health care provider, nurses, and pharmacists must collaborate to make it work effectively. Common drug delivery systems include:
- unit-dose system
- automated systems
- individual prescriptions.

Unit-dose system

In a unit-dose system, the pharmacist dispenses a supply of wrapped, labeled individual doses of all forms of drugs: oral, injectable, and IV solutions with additives. The pharmacist usually dispenses sufficient drugs and IV solutions to last 24 hours; they may also prepare trays of medications for you to administer at specified hours.

Keep it under wraps

The pharmacist may prepare unit doses or purchase them commercially. You should keep the drugs in the labeled wrappers until you administer them. The unit-dose system reduces the likelihood of drug administration errors.

Automated systems

In essence, an automated drug delivery system is a computerized version of the unit-dose system. A pharmacist fills an electronic drug-dispensing unit and keeps it locked. The unit then delivers individually wrapped and labeled medications when they are requested. A computer records all drug transactions on electronic tape and furnishes requested printouts.

To avoid the possibly disastrous effects from computer downtime, facilities that use automated dispensing systems must have a backup plan for dispensing medications and documenting their delivery.

Freeing time for patients

An automated system greatly simplifies record keeping because the computer can monitor and track drugs from the original inventory to patient billing. This can save nurses time and allow you to spend more time teaching and consulting with patients.

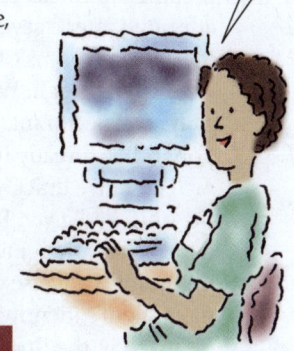

Automated systems simplify record keeping and possibly free up time to spend with the patient.

Common medication errors

In addition to following your facility's policies faithfully, you can help prevent medication errors by studying common errors and determining how to prevent them from happening. Some interventions that have helped decrease medication errors include the use of automated dispensing cabinets with labels for high-risk medications such as anticoagulants, insulins, and opioids. Another method used in automated dispensing cabinets is tall man lettering to help avoid confusion with similar-sounding drug names (e.g., HYDROcodone and oxyCODONE) (Workman & LaCharity, 2023). (See *Avoiding med mix-ups*.)

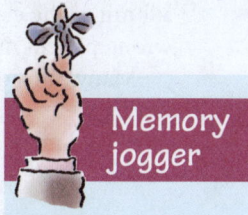

Memory jogger

A method helpful to remember high-risk medications is the acronym PINCH:

Potassium

Insulin

Narcotics

Chemotherapy

Heparin or any other strong antiplatelet medication

Source: Workman, M.L., & LaCharity, L.A. (2023). *Evolve resources for understanding pharmacology.* Elsevier Publishing.

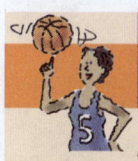

Stay on the ball

Avoiding med mix-ups

Many nurses have confused an order for morphine with one for hydromorphone. Both drugs come in 4-mg prefilled syringes. If morphine is given when the health care provider really ordered hydromorphone, the patient could develop respiratory depression or even arrest.

Consider posting a prominent notice in the medication room that warns the staff about this common mix-up. Or try attaching a fluorescent sticker printed with "not morphine" to each hydromorphone syringe and a sticker of a different color printed with "not hydromorphone" to each morphine syringe.

A case of mistaken identity

Drug names aren't the only kinds of words that can be confused. Patient names can cause trouble as well if the nurse fails to verify each person's identity. This problem can be especially troublesome if two patients have the same first name.

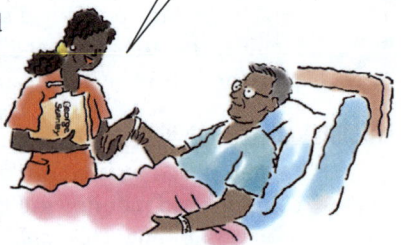

> Always check the patient's identity by verifying their name with their printed armband.

Consider this clinical scenario: Robert Brewer, age 5 years, was hospitalized for measles. Robert Brinson, also age 5 years, was admitted after a severe asthma attack. The boys were assigned to adjacent rooms on a small pediatric unit. Each had a nonproductive cough. When Robert Brewer's nurse came to give him an expectorant, the child's mother told the nurse that Robert had already inhaled a medication through a mask.

The nurse quickly figured out that another nurse, new to the unit, had given Robert Brinson's medication (acetylcysteine, a mucolytic) to Robert Brewer in error. Fortunately, no harmful adverse effects ensued. Had the nurse checked the patient's identity more carefully, however, no error would have occurred in the first place.

When consistently used, barcode scanners to confirm patient identification at the bedside and the ability to scan the medications and submit to the electronic medical record can also decrease the risk of wrong patient medication errors.

Many infusion pumps today can be programmed using a drug library so that the correct drug is infused with safe, programmed volumes and rates. Keep in mind that for best benefit of these time-saving devices, the settings must be programmed (MacDowell et al., 2021).

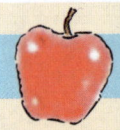

Education corner

Reducing medication errors through patient teaching

The nurse isn't the only one who's at risk for making medication errors. Patients are at an even greater risk because they may have a lack of knowledge about the medications.

Clearly, patient teaching is a crucial aspect of your responsibility in minimizing medication errors and their consequences—especially as more patients receive outpatient rather than inpatient care.

Teaching tips

Help minimize medication errors by:
- teaching the patient about their diagnosis and the purpose of their drug therapy
- providing the patient with their drug information in writing
- asking if they take over-the-counter medications at home in addition to prescribed drugs
- asking about herbal remedies and other nutritional supplements
- telling the patient what kinds of drug-related problems warrant a call to the health care provider
- urging the patient to report anything about their drug therapy that concerns or worries them.

Checking ID

Always check each patient's full name and birthdate. Also, teach each patient (or parent/caregiver) to offer an identification bracelet for inspection and to state a full name and birthdate when anyone enters the room with the intention of giving a medication. In addition, urge patients to speak up if an identification bracelet falls off, is removed, or gets lost so it can be replaced right away. (See *Reducing medication errors through patient teaching*.)

Allergy alert

After you've verified your patient's full name, take time to check whether they have any drug allergies—even if they are in distress. If the patient has an allergy, immediately document the allergy in the appropriate places such as the chart, MAR, wristband, and the pharmacy and report that information to the health care provider.

A re-enaction of an allergic reaction

Consider this real-life example: A health care provider issued a stat order for chlorpromazine for a distressed patient. By the time the nurse arrived with it, the patient had grown more distressed and was demanding relief. Unnerved by the patient's demeanor, the nurse gave the drug without checking the patient's MAR or documenting the order—and the patient had an allergic reaction to it.

Even in an urgent situation, you should always resist the temptation to act first and assess or document later. Skipping that crucial assessment step could easily lead to a medication error. (See *Safe alternative*.)

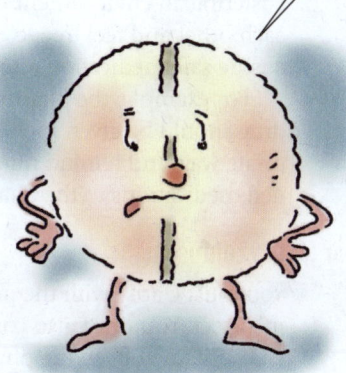

An allergic reaction is nothing to sneeze at. Take the time to check for drug allergies before giving any medication.

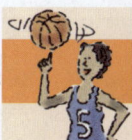

Stay on the ball

Safe alternative

A patient who's severely allergic to peanuts could have an anaphylactic reaction to ipratropium aerosol given by metered-dose inhaler. Ask the patient or the parents/caregivers whether they are allergic to peanuts before administering this drug.

If you find that they have such an allergy, the nasal spray and inhalation solution form of ipratropium should be ordered; because it doesn't contain soy lecithin, this form of the drug is safe for patients who are allergic to peanuts.

Order errors

Each year in the United States, 7,000 to 9,000 people die as a result of a medication error (Tariq et al., 2023). Many medication errors stem from a combination of mistakes that could have been caught at any of several steps along the way. For a medication to be administered correctly, each member of the health care team must fulfill the appropriate role. The health care provider must write the order correctly, and legibly. The pharmacist must evaluate whether the order is appropriate and then fill it correctly. In addition, the nurse must evaluate whether the order is appropriate and then administer it correctly.

Chain reaction

A breakdown anywhere along this chain of events can lead to a medication error. That is why it's so important for members of the health care team to act as a real team, checking each other and catching any problems that arise before those problems affect the patient's health. Fostering an environment in which professionals can double-check each other and feel free to communicate concerns or issues helps ensure safe medication administration.

For example, the pharmacist can help clarify the number of times a drug should be given each day, help to label drugs in the most appropriate way, and remind nurses to always return unused or discontinued medications to the pharmacy.

Clear up the confusion

You must clarify with the prescriber any orders that seem unclear or incorrect. You must also correctly handle and store any multidose vials obtained from the pharmacist. Following facility policies regarding medication storage and storing drugs in their original containers can help avoid errors. (See *Container confusion*.)

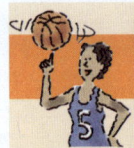

Stay on the ball

Container confusion

Even a confusing container can cause a medication error. For example, it's easy to mistake eyedrops for the developers used for the fecal occult blood test (Hemoccult test). Some patients have sustained permanent eye damage as a result. The best way to avoid this mistake is to keep Hemoccult developers in an appropriate room (such as the utility room). Never keep them in a patient's room. Follow the facility policy regarding storage of Hemoccult developers (many allow storage only in the laboratory).

Label liability

Only administer drugs that you've prepared personally. Never give a drug that has an ambiguous label or no label at all. Here's an actual example of an error that could happen: A nurse placed an unlabeled cup of phenol (used in neurolytic procedures) next to a cup of guanethidine (a postganglionic-blocking agent). The health care provider accidentally injected the phenol instead of the guanethidine, causing severe tissue damage to a patient's arm. The patient needed emergency surgery and developed neurologic complications.

Obviously, this was a compound problem. The nurse should have labeled each cup clearly, and the health care provider shouldn't have given an unlabeled substance to a patient.

Route trouble

Many medication errors stem at least in part from problems related to the route of administration. The risk of error increases when a patient has several lines running for different purposes.

Caught in a tangle of lines

Consider this example: A nurse prepared a dose of digoxin elixir for a patient who had a central IV line and a jejunostomy tube—and she mistakenly administered the drug into the central IV line. Fortunately, the patient had no adverse reaction. To help prevent such mix-ups in administration route, prepare all oral medications in a syringe that has a tip that is small enough to fit an abdominal tube but too big to fit a central line.

Bubble trouble

Here's another error that could have been avoided: To clear air bubbles from a 9-year-old patient's insulin drip, a nurse disconnected the tubing and raised the pump rate to 200 mL/hour to flush the bubbles through quickly. The nurse then reconnected the tubing and restarted the drip, but they forgot to reset the rate back to 2 U/hour. The child received 50 units of insulin before the error was detected. To prevent this kind of error, never increase a drip rate to clear bubbles from a line. Instead, remove the tubing from the pump, disconnect it from the patient, and use the flow-control clamp to establish gravity flow.

Nurses carry a great deal of responsibility for making sure that patients get the right drugs in the right concentrations at the right times and by the right routes. By diligently applying the guidelines offered here, you can minimize the risk of medication errors and maximize the therapeutic effects of your patients' drug regimens.

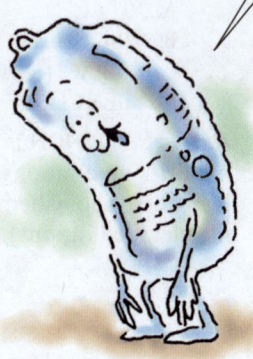

Bubbles can be trouble. Never adjust flow rate to clear bubbles from tubing.

Quick quiz

1. Which term is used to describe the state of a medication being ready to produce a physiologic effect?

    A. Pharmacokinetics.

    B. Biomechanics.

    C. Pharmacology.

    D. Bioavailability.

Answer: D. A bioavailable drug is one that's ready to produce a physiologic effect.

2. How do changes to the body associated with aging affect the half-life of medications?

    A. The half-life will be shorter.

    B. The half-life will increase each year of life after age 50 years.

    C. The half-life will be longer.

    D. The half-life will be unchanged.

Answer: C. The half-life of medications in older adults is longer because of the decreased muscle, increased body fat, and decreased function of the kidneys and liver in that population.

3. A group of nursing students is discussing the differences between enteral and parenteral routes. Which statement is accurate?

    A. "The parenteral route administers the drug into the GI tract."

    B. "The enteral route includes subcutaneous or IM injections."

    C. "IV medications are neither parenteral nor enteral routes."

    D. "Enteral routes include sublingual, buccal, and rectal."

Answer: D. Enteral routes include oral, sublingual, translingual, buccal, tube feedings, and rectal. Routes that don't involve the GI tract are known as *parenteral routes*. Parenteral routes can be useful for treating a patient who can't take a drug orally; parenteral medications include subcutaneous, IM, and IV.

4. What acronym can nurses use to identify high-risk medications?

    A. TEACH.

    B. PINCH.

    C. COACH.

    D. BENCH.

Answer: B. PINCH is the acronym that nurses can use to identify high-risk medications. P stands for Potassium, I for Insulin, N for Narcotics, C for Chemotherapy, and H for Heparin (or other antiplatelet medications).

Scoring

⭐⭐⭐ If you answered all four questions correctly, excellent! You're on the route to greatness.

⭐⭐ If you answered three questions correctly, you're getting the essentials! You used the key concepts to unlock the door to understanding.

⭐ If you answered fewer than two questions correctly, don't worry! Go back and review this chapter, and soon you'll be pharmaco-dynamite.

References

Drug-Induced Hepatitis. (2023). Johns Hopkins Medicine. https://www.hopkinsmedicine.org/health/conditions-and-diseases/hepatitis/druginduced-hepatitis

MacDowell, P., Cabri, A., & Davis, M. (2021). *Medication administration errors*. Agency for Healthcare Research and Quality. https://psnet.ahrq.gov/primer/medication-error-and-adverse-drug-events

Pharmacogenomics. (2023, October 04). *Cleveland clinic*. Retrieved October 25, 2023, from https://my.clevelandclinic.org/health/diagnostics/21093-pharmacogenomics#:~:text=Individuals%20who%20do%20not%20respond,someone%20responds%20to%20a%20medication

Prescribing. (2023). Texas Medical Association. https://www.texmed.org/erx/#:~:text=Physicians%20and%20other%20prescribers%20in,grants%20a%20one%2Dyear%20delay

Rochon, P. (2023). *Drug prescribing for older adults. UptoDate*. https://uptodate.com/contents/drug-prescribing-for-older-adults

Tariq, R., Vashisht, R., Sinha, A., & Scherbak, Y. (2023). *Medication dispensing errors and prevention*. NCBI bookshelf. https://ncbi.nlm.nih.govNBK19065

Workman, M.L., & LaCharity, L.A. (2023). *Evolve resources for understanding pharmacology*. Elsevier Publishing.

Chapter 10

Medication administration

Just the facts

In this chapter, you'll learn:

◆ how to administer drugs by the oral route, nasogastric tube, and gastric route

◆ the correct procedures for administering topical, ophthalmic, otic, and nasal drugs

◆ advantages and disadvantages of rectal and vaginal administration methods

◆ how to administer drugs via the respiratory route

◆ principles of injecting drugs

◆ methods for preparing an injection

◆ proper techniques for administering drugs intradermally, subcutaneously, and intramuscularly.

Administering oral drugs

Oral drug administration offers the safest, most convenient, and least costly way to administer a host of drugs. Usually, the nurse gives tablets, capsules, or liquid drugs (such as an elixir, syrup, or suspension) by the oral route. However, oral drugs are also available as powders, granules, and oils.

Taste test

Some drugs need to be mixed with flavoring, juice, or applesauce before delivery to make them more palatable.

Giving a tablet or capsule

Tablets or capsules may be given whole. However, some scored tablets may need to be split for dosing purposes. Crushing a tablet may also be necessary to ease administration. (See *Crushing a tablet* and *Splitting a scored tablet*, page 194.)

Splitting a scored tablet

To split a scored tablet, follow these steps:
- Wash your hands.
- If you're using your fingers to split a scored tablet, first don gloves.
- Notice the location of the score mark.
- Use both hands to grip the tablet on either side of the score mark, and then push down on the edges to break the tablet along the score line.
- If splitting the tablet using a cutting device, place the tablet into the device so the score mark lines up with the blade.
- Close the lid of the cutting device to force the blade through the tablet.
- Place the correct dose in a medication cup.
- Administer the prescribed dose with sufficient liquid in a separate cup for the patient to swallow it comfortably.

Crushing a tablet

To crush a tablet, follow these steps:
- Check in a drug reference book or drug reference program to see if the medication can be crushed. **Never crush an enteric-coated tablet or timed-release capsule.**
- Wash your hands.
- Remove the unit-dose tablet from the patient's medication drawer or pour the tablet from its container.
- To crush the tablet, utilize the work area's crushing device or a mortar and pestle.
- Place the tablet in the chosen device and crush it completely.
- To save time and to keep the device clean, crush a unit-dose tablet in its unopened wrapper. Then make sure to empty the wrapper completely.
- Place the crushed tablet into the fluid or food for administration, and mix it thoroughly.

Supplies
- prescribed medication in tablet or capsule form
- medication cup
- glass of water or other liquid to help the patient swallow the drug
- crushing device or mortar and pestle (if crushing a tablet)
- gloves or cutting device (if splitting a scored tablet)

Getting ready
- Verify the order for a tablet or capsule in the patient's chart.
- Wash your hands.

Practice pointers
- If a drug needs to be poured from its container, open the container and pour the required number of tablets or capsules into the lid of the container. Then put them in the medication cup.
- Assess the patient's ability to swallow before giving them an oral drug. Impaired swallowing can lead to aspiration.

How it's done
- If a unit-dose tablet or capsule is being given, remove it from the patient's medication drawer. Then place the unwrapped medication into the cup.
- Confirm the patient's identity using at least two patient identifiers (not including the patient's room number).
- If an electronic bar code scanning system is used, the nurse should log in or scan their identification badge, the patient's bracelet, and the medication bar code.
- Help the patient to a sitting position.

One at a time, please

- Offer the tablets or capsules one at a time. Have the patient place it in their mouth and take enough liquid to swallow it comfortably.
- If the drug is chewable, make sure the patient chews it thoroughly before swallowing it.

Look for the designer label

- Don't give tablets or capsules from a poorly labeled bottle or unlabeled bottle.
- Never give a tablet or capsule that has been poured by someone else.

No returns, no surprises

- Never return an opened or unwrapped drug to the patient's medication drawer. Instead, properly dispose of it and notify the pharmacy.

Can I get a witness?

- Remember that another nurse must witness and cosign the disposal of an opioid. (See *Documenting oral drug administration.*)
- If the patient questions the drug or the amount being given, double-check their medication record. If the drug and dose are correct, reassure and inform the patient about the drug and any changes in dosage. (See *Teaching about giving a tablet or capsule.*)

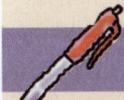

Take note!

Documenting oral drug administration

After administering a tablet or capsule, be sure to record:

- drug given
- dose given
- date and time of administration
- signing out of the drug on the patient's medication record
- patient's ability to swallow the drug administered (if the patient has had problems swallowing oral drugs)
- patient's vital signs (if the drug could impact their vital signs)
- any adverse reactions that arise
- patient's refusal and notification of a doctor, if needed (if a patient refuses a tablet or capsule)
- omission or withholding of a drug for any reason.

Administering a liquid drug

For an infant, child, or patient who has trouble swallowing pills, a liquid drug may be given. If the patient has a nasogastric (NG), gastrostomy, or jejunostomy tube, the drug may be given through the tube rather than orally.

Supplies
- measuring cup
- damp paper washcloth or towel
- prescribed medication

Getting ready
- Verify the order in the patient's chart.
- Consult the drug guide if you haven't given the drug previously or if you're unfamiliar with the purpose, dosage, contraindications, possible side effects, or nursing considerations.
- Wash your hands.
- Take the bottle from the patient's medication drawer or from the shelf.

How it's done
- Shake the bottle well and then uncap it. Place the cap upside down on a clean surface to avoid contaminating the inside surface.

Graduate to the next level
- While holding a graduated medicine cup at eye level, use your thumb to mark the correct level on the cup.
- Hold the bottle so the liquid flows from the side opposite the label so that the liquid won't stain or obscure the label if it runs down the bottle.
- Pour the drug into the cup until the bottom of the meniscus reaches the correct dose mark.
- Set down the cup and read the bottom of the meniscus again, still at eye level, to double-check for accuracy. If you've poured too much, discard the excess rather than pour it back into the bottle.

Give lip service
- Remove drips from the lip of the bottle using a clean damp washcloth or towel. Then clean the sides of the bottle with the washcloth, if necessary.

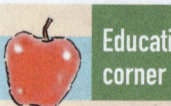

Education corner

Teaching about giving a tablet or capsule
- Caution the patient not to chew tablets that aren't supposed to be chewed, especially enteric-coated ones.
- Teach the patient about the drug being administered, including its name, purpose, and possible adverse effects.
- If the patient will be taking the tablets or capsules independently at home, make sure the patient thoroughly understands and plans to follow the regimen.
- Be sure to tell the patient to report anything that could be an adverse reaction to the drug.

- Confirm the patient's identity using at least two patient identifiers (not including the patient's room number).
- If an electronic bar code scanning system is used, the nurse should log in or scan their identification badge, the patient's bracelet, and the medication bar code.
- To administer a liquid drug to an infant, follow the steps outlined in *Administering a liquid drug to an infant*.

Practice pointers

- Don't give medication from a poorly labeled or unlabeled container.
- Never give a medication that has been poured by someone else.

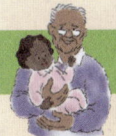

Ages and stages

Administering a liquid drug to an infant

To administer a liquid drug to an infant, follow these steps:

- Verify the infant's identity using at least two patient identifiers (not including the patient's room number).
- Wash your hands.
- Place a bib or towel under the infant's chin.
- Withdraw the correct amount of liquid drug from the medication bottle using an oral syringe.
- Hold the syringe in a vertical position at eye level to check the dose amount.
- Check the syringe for any excess air or bubbles and remove them before confirming the dose.
- Hold the infant securely, and raise the infant's head to about a 45° angle.
- Place the dropper at the corner of the infant's mouth so the drug will run into the pocket between the cheek and gum. This action keeps the infant from spitting out the drug and reduces the risk of aspiration.
- If necessary to facilitate swallowing, you may place the drug in a nipple and allow the

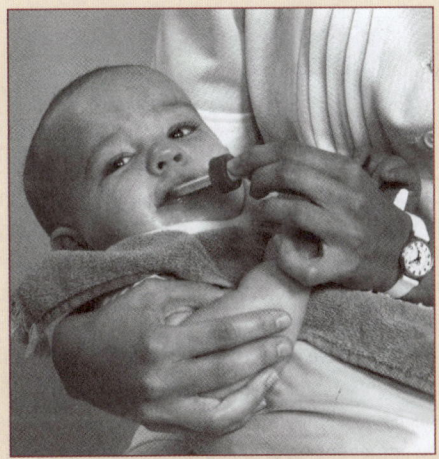

infant to suck the contents. Lift the infant's head and give the drug slowly to prevent aspiration. Don't mix a medication in a bottle, because if the infant does not drink all the contents of the bottle, they may not receive the full drug dosage.

Source: Smith, L., Leggett, C., & Borg, C. (2022). Administration of medicines to children: A practical guide. *Australian Prescriber, 45*(6), 188–192. https://doi.org/10.18773/austprescr.2022.067

- Assess the patient's ability to swallow before administering a liquid drug.
- If the patient questions the drug or the amount being given, double-check their medication record. If the drug and dose are correct, reassure and inform the patient about the drug and any changes in dosage.

Sip tips

- To avoid damaging or staining the patient's teeth, give acidic drugs or iron preparations through a straw.
- Liquid drugs that have an unpleasant taste are usually more palatable when taken through a straw because the liquid contacts fewer taste buds.
- When administering oral medications to pediatric patients, remember the helpful hints listed in *Administering oral medications to pediatric patients.*

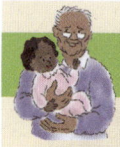

Ages and stages

Administering oral medications to pediatric patients

The oral route of drug administration is the preferred route in children due to comfort and safety. When administering oral medications to pediatric patients, use these guidelines:

- An effective liquid medication administration technique for young children involves administering the medication into the corner pocket of the patient's cheek to prevent the medication from running back out.
- If the patient is a toddler, to promote honesty and trust, don't mix a drug with food or call it "candy," even if it has a pleasant taste.

- Have the child drink a liquid drug from an oral syringe or calibrated medication cup, rather than from a spoon, because it's easier and more accurate.
- If the drug is available only in tablet form, crush it and mix it with compatible syrup after consulting the pharmacist.
- If the patient is an older child who can swallow a tablet or a capsule, have them place the pill on the back of the tongue and swallow it with water. Remember, milk or milk products, as well as specific juices, may interfere with drug absorption.

Source: Smith, L., Leggett, C., & Borg, C. (2022). Administration of medicines to children: A practical guide. *Australian Prescriber, 45*(6), 188–192. https://doi.org/10.18773/austprescr.2022.067

Gastric administration

If a patient has an NG or a gastrostomy tube, drugs can be delivered directly to the gastric mucosa through the tube. If they have a jejunostomy tube, drugs can be delivered to the intestinal lumen.

Going down the tubes

An NG tube extends from the patient's nose into the stomach. Patients may have an NG tube in place if they have trouble swallowing or an altered level of consciousness. In either case, it may be necessary to administer oral drugs through the tube rather than by the oral route.

Crossing over

Unlike an NG tube, a gastrostomy tube crosses the abdominal wall to enter the stomach. It may be surgically inserted, or it may be placed during an endoscopic, a laparoscopic, or a radiologic procedure.

A gastrostomy tube reduces the risk of aspiration, and it's more comfortable for the patient than an NG tube. The nurse uses the tube to deliver feeding solutions and drugs directly into the patient's stomach.

Supplies
- prescribed medication
- towel or linen-saver pad
- gloves
- facial tissues
- container of water
- 50- or 60-mL piston-type, catheter-tipped syringe (also known as an enteral syringe)
- pH test strip (to confirm tube placement)
- bulb syringe
- crushing device or mortar and pestle for crushing drug
- liquid in which to dissolve the drug just before instilling it (if giving a crushed tablet)

Getting ready
- All drugs delivered through an NG or a gastrostomy tube must be in liquid form so they can pass easily through the tube. If the patient's drug comes in tablet form, it will need to be crushed and dissolved in water. If the drug comes in capsule form, the contents will need to be emptied into water.
- Consult the pharmacist before crushing a pill or emptying the contents of a capsule to verify acceptable practice for the drug and its intended action.
- Verify the order in the patient's chart.
- Consult the drug guide if you haven't given the drug previously or if you're unfamiliar with the purpose, dosage, contraindications, possible side effects, or nursing considerations.

- Check the medication administration record (MAR) and drug allergies.
- Confirm the patient's identity using at least two patient identifiers (not including the patient's room number).
- Check the label on the medication before preparing to make sure the medication is being given correctly.
- If an electronic bar code scanning system is used, the nurse should log in or scan their identification badge, the patient's bracelet, and the medication bar code.
- Explain the procedure to the patient.
- Wash your hands and put on gloves.

How it's done

- Prepare the drug for delivery by crushing a tablet and mixing it in water or by opening a capsule and mixing the contents in water. The exact amount of water may vary by drug but generally will not exceed 30 mL. Consult the pharmacist for specific water amount recommendations.
- Help the patient into a semi-Fowler position.
- Always verify the placement of an NG tube before administering any medication. Unclamp the NG tube, attach a bulb syringe to the end of the tubing, and aspirate a small amount of stomach contents from the NG tube.

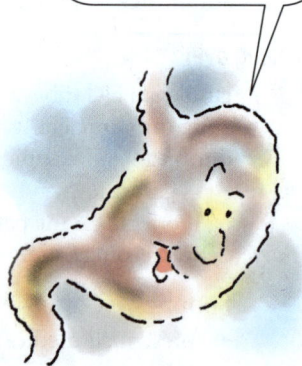

> Always aspirate a small amount of stomach contents and check the pH to verify correct tube placement before administering drugs through a gastric tube.

Grassy green

- Examine the aspirate and place a small amount on a pH test strip. Indications of correct gastric placement are (1) if the aspirate has a typical gastric fluid appearance (grassy-green, brown, or clear and colorless with mucous shreds) and (2) the pH is less than or equal to 5.0. An ongoing tube feeding may buffer the gastric pH.
- If no gastric contents appear when the syringe is drawn back, the tube may have risen into the esophagus and will need to be advanced before proceeding.
- If resistance is met when aspirating gastric contents, stop the procedure. Resistance may indicate a nonpatent tube or improper tube placement. (Keep in mind that some smaller tubes may collapse when aspiration is attempted.)
- If examination of the aspirate confirms tube placement in the stomach, resistance probably means that the tube is lying against the stomach wall. To relieve resistance, withdraw the tube slightly or turn the patient.
- After tube placement is confirmed, remove the syringe from the end of the tube.
- Draw water into the piston-type syringe, and use it to irrigate the tube with about 30 mL of water. Then reclamp the tube, remove the syringe from the tube, and remove the piston from the syringe.

- Reinsert the syringe tip into the distal end of the NG tube, making sure it fits snugly.
- With the syringe attached to the opening of the tube, hold the syringe upright and slightly above the level of the patient's nose.
- Unclamp the tube and slowly pour the drug into the syringe, using it as a funnel.

Slow flow

- Allow the drug to flow slowly through the tube. If it flows too quickly, lower the syringe. If it flows too slowly, raise the syringe slightly.
- As the syringe empties, add more of the drug. To prevent air from entering the patient's stomach, don't let the syringe drain completely before adding more of the drug to it.
- After the full dose has been given, pour 30 to 50 mL of water into the syringe.

Getting carried away

- Let the water flow through the tube to rinse it and to carry the drug into the patient's stomach.
- Next, clamp the tube and remove the syringe.
- If the tube is attached to suction, depending on the patient's ability to tolerate it and if the doctor writes an order, clamp the tube for 30 minutes after the drug is given. This will allow time for the drug to be absorbed and not lost to suction.
- Have the patient remain in a semi-Fowler position for at least 30 minutes after administration *to prevent esophageal reflux* (backward or return flow of stomach contents into the esophagus).
- Clean and store the equipment or dispose of it as appropriate.

Practice pointers

- Remember that all drugs instilled through the tube must be in liquid form. Check with a pharmacist if unsure whether a tablet can be safely crushed or a capsule safely opened.
- Never crush an enteric-coated or sustained-release drug.

Full follow-through

- Because capsules tend not to dissolve completely, always follow them with water to flush the tube and prevent occlusion.
- Dilute liquid drugs with water to decrease their osmolality (Pereira et al., 2020).
- If more than one drug must be given through an NG tube, give each one separately, flushing the tube with 10 to 15 mL of water between doses to avoid drug interactions.
- Irrigate the tube with 30 mL of irrigant before and after drug instillation.

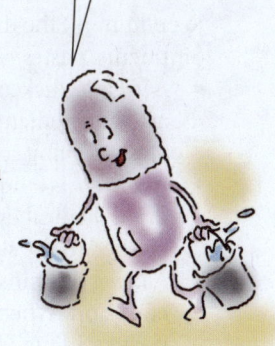

Water flushes between doses are a must to prevent drug interactions and clogging the tube.

Check the vent

- If the patient has a Salem sump tube, watch for fluid reflux in the vent lumen. Reflux means that pressure in the patient's stomach exceeds atmospheric pressure, possibly because the primary lumen is clogged or the suction system was set up incorrectly. Don't clamp the vent tube to stop the reflux.
- Some drugs, such as phenytoin, are altered by the presence of feeding solutions in the patient's stomach. Enteral tube feedings may need to be paused 2 hours before and/or after giving phenytoin; check with the health care provider (Vallerand & Sanoski, 2021).

Administering topical drugs

Topical drugs exert their effects after being applied to a patient's skin or the mucous membrane in the patient's mouth or throat.

Most forms are local

Topical drugs may take the form of a lotion, cream, ointment, paste, powder, or spray that is applied to an affected skin area. Other topical drug forms include a spray, mouthwash, gargle, and lozenge to treat a problem in the patient's mouth or throat.

Usually, these topical administration methods are used to obtain local, rather than systemic, drug effects. The drug moves through the epidermis and into the dermis, based in part on the vascularity of the region to which it's applied.

Transdermal transport

Certain types of topical drugs, known as transdermal drugs, are meant to enter the patient's bloodstream and exert a systemic effect after applying a paste or patch to the patient's skin.

Know the difference

Keep in mind the differences between gels, tinctures, lotions, creams, ointments, pastes, and powders:

- A *gel* is a thickened, water-based emulsion containing dissolved active ingredients. As a gel dries, leaving a film on the skin, it creates a cooling sensation due to water evaporation.
- A *tincture* is a liquid topical medication that is usually made of dried medical extracts dissolved in alcohol. When a tincture is applied to the skin, it absorbs quickly due to the alcohol conduit.
- A *lotion* contains an insoluble powder suspended in water or an emulsion. When a lotion is applied, it leaves a uniform layer of powder in the film on the patient's skin.

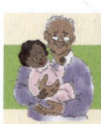

Ages and stages

Topical tips for tots

Remember these tips when giving topical drugs to pediatric patients:

- When applying powder, shake it into your gloved hand, and then apply it; this avoids creating puffs of powder that you or the child could accidentally inhale.
- Use topical corticosteroids cautiously and sparingly on diaper-covered body areas. Disposable diapers or rubber pants act like an occlusive dressing, possibly increasing systemic absorption of the drug.

- A *cream* is an oil-in-water emulsion in semisolid form. It lubricates the skin and acts as a barrier.
- An *ointment* is a semisolid substance that, when applied to the skin, helps to retain body heat and provides prolonged contact between the skin and the drug.
- A *paste* is a stiff mixture of powder and ointment. It provides a uniform coat to reduce and repel moisture.
- A *powder* is an inert chemical that may contain medication. It helps dry the skin and reduces friction and maceration. (See *Topical tips for tots.*)

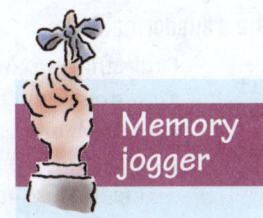

Memory jogger

Trans means "across" or "through"; *dermal* means "related to the skin." A transdermal drug moves *through the skin* and into the bloodstream.

Administering a transdermal drug

Transdermal drugs deliver a constant, controlled amount of medication through the skin and into the bloodstream, thereby achieving a steady, prolonged systemic effect.

Patch it up!

To give a transdermal drug, either apply a measured amount of ointment to a selected area of the patient's skin or apply a transdermal patch that contains medication. (See *Understanding a transdermal patch.*)

Understanding a transdermal patch

A transdermal patch is made up of several layers. The outermost layer is an aluminized polyester barrier that holds the drug in the patch. The next layer is the drug reservoir, which contains the main dose of the drug. The next layer, a membrane, controls the release of the drug from the reservoir.

Stick with it

The innermost adhesive layer keeps the patch on the patient's skin and holds a small amount of the drug as it moves from the patch into the skin. The dots in this illustration show the drug moving through the skin and into the bloodstream.

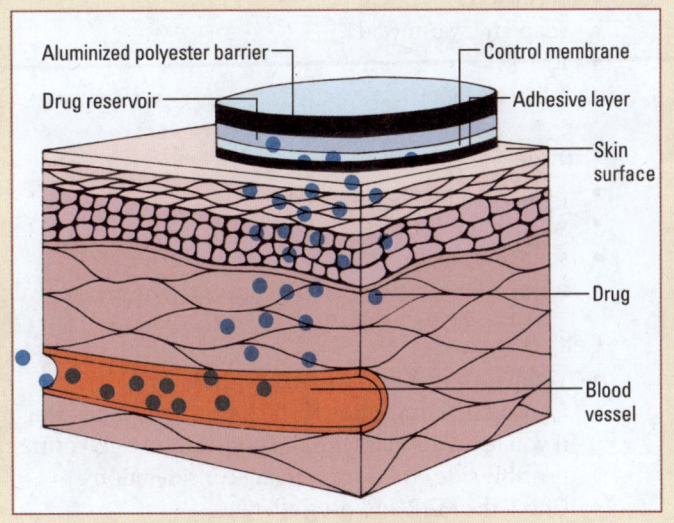

The transdermal team

Drugs that are commonly given via the transdermal route include:
- nitroglycerin to control angina
- scopolamine to treat motion sickness
- estradiol to provide hormone replacement during and after menopause
- clonidine to treat hypertension
- fentanyl to control chronic pain.

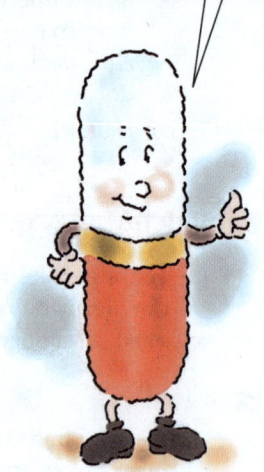

Generally, patches deliver drugs for longer periods of time than ointments do.

A matter of time

Choosing the most appropriate form of the drug (ointment or patch) depends largely on the desired delivery time. Typically, a patch delivers the drug for a longer period. For example, transdermal nitroglycerin ointment dilates coronary vessels for 4 to 8 hours, whereas a nitroglycerin patch lasts 8 to 24 hours. Other examples of duration of drug delivery in patch form include scopolamine, which lasts up to 72 hours; estradiol, which lasts up to a week; clonidine, which lasts up to 24 hours; and fentanyl, which lasts up to 72 hours (Vallerand & Sanoski, 2021).

Supplies

Transdermal ointment
- prescribed medicated ointment
- application strip or measuring paper
- semipermeable dressing or plastic wrap
- gloves
- washcloth
- soap and warm water
- towel
- adhesive tape

Transdermal patch
- prescribed medicated patch
- washcloth
- soap and water
- towel

Getting ready
- Verify the order in the patient's chart.
- Consult the drug guide if you haven't given the drug previously or if you're unfamiliar with the purpose, dosage, contraindications, possible side effects, or nursing considerations.
- Check the MAR and drug allergies.
- Confirm the patient's identity using at least two patient identifiers (not including the patient's room number).
- Wash your hands and put on gloves.

How it's done

To apply a transdermal ointment or a transdermal patch, follow these steps.

Applying a transdermal ointment

- Choose the application site, which is usually a dry, hairless spot on the patient's chest or arm.
- To promote absorption, wash the site with soap and warm water. Dry it thoroughly.
- If the patient has a previously applied medication strip at another site, remove it and wash this area to clear away drug residue.

Splitting hairs

- If the application site is hairy, clip excess hair rather than shaving it; shaving causes irritation, which may be exacerbated by the drug.
- Squeeze the prescribed amount of ointment on the application strip or measuring paper as shown. Don't touch the drug with your bare skin.
- Apply the strip, drug side down, directly to the patient's skin.
- Maneuver the strip slightly to spread a thin layer of the ointment to the skin under the strip, but don't rub the ointment into the skin (Vallerand & Sanoski, 2021).
- Secure the application strip to the patient's skin by covering it with a semipermeable dressing.

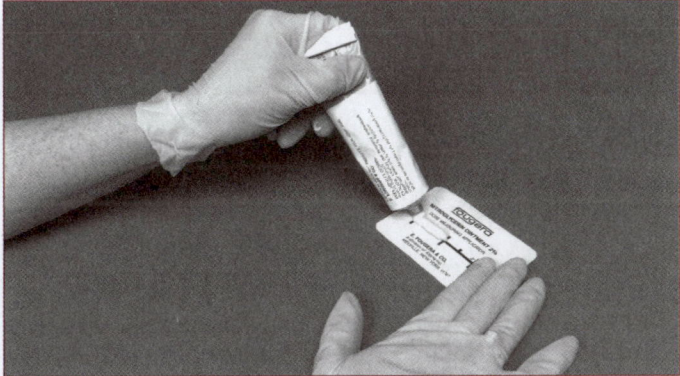

Skintight

- Press firmly with the palm of one hand to ensure that the dressing adheres well, especially around the edges.
- Label the strip with the date, time, and your initials.
- Remove gloves and wash your hands.

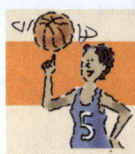

Stay on the ball

Discarding a patch

There is still a substantial amount of drug remaining in a used patch. To avoid possible harm to children or animals, fold the patch in half with the adhesive layer inside and discard into a closed container that is not accessible to children or pets (Vallerand & Sanoski, 2021).

Applying a transdermal patch

- Remove the old patch. (See *Discarding a patch*, page 206.)
- Choose a dry, hairless application site. Be sure to rotate application sites. Don't attempt to apply the patch to an area with alterations in skin integrity.
- If necessary, clip any hair from the site, but don't shave the area. The most commonly used sites are the upper arm, the chest, the back, and behind the ear (Vallerand & Sanoski, 2021).
- Clean the application site with soap and warm water. Dry it thoroughly.
- Open the drug package and remove the patch.
- Without touching the adhesive surface, remove the clear plastic backing.
- Apply the patch to the application site without touching the adhesive.

Practice pointers

- Apply any transdermal drug at the prescribed intervals to ensure a continuous effect.
- Don't apply the drug if the patient has skin allergies or has experienced skin reactions to the drug.
- Always make sure to remove the old patch, keeping in mind that some patches are clear and therefore hard to see. Not removing the old patch may cause an adverse reaction.
- Avoid areas of broken or irritated skin; the drug could increase the irritation.
- Don't apply a transdermal drug to scarred or callused skin because either condition may impair absorption.
- When a patient with a transdermal patch in place requires defibrillation, special care must be taken. For more information, see *A shocking experience.*
- Teach the patient about taking transdermal drugs. (See *Teaching about transdermal medications*, page 207.)

Something new

Transdermal drug delivery systems can be made even more effective by using enhancers.

Physical and chemical enhancers can be used to boost the movement of a transdermal drug into the skin. Some examples of enhancers are sonophoresis, microneedles, and nanoemulsions (Jeong et al., 2021).

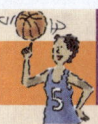

Stay on the ball

A shocking experience

Don't place a defibrillator paddle on a transdermal patch. The aluminum on the patch can cause electrical arcing during defibrillation, resulting in smoke, thermal burns, and ineffective electrical cardioversion. If a patient's patch is on a standard paddle site, remove the patch before applying the paddle.

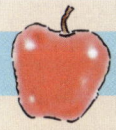

Education corner

Teaching about transdermal medications

• Review drug-specific precautions the patient must know. For example, make sure the patient knows to thoroughly wipe off an old application of nitroglycerin ointment before applying a new dose.

• Ensure the patient knows how to choose an appropriate application site. Tell the patient to avoid scarred or callused areas, bony prominences, and hairy surfaces.

• Warn the patient not to get transdermal ointment on their hands and to wash them thoroughly after applying a transdermal drug.

• Make the patient aware they need to keep the area around the application site as dry as possible.

• If the patient will be applying scopolamine, tell them not to drive or operate machinery until the patient knows how the drug impacts their body.

• If the patient will be using clonidine patches, tell the patient to check with their primary health care provider before using nonprescription cough preparations. Over-the-counter preparations may counteract the effects of the drug.

• Warn the patient about the possible adverse reactions that can occur with transdermal drug delivery, such as skin irritation, itching, and rashes.

• Be sure to alert the patient to potential adverse reactions to the drug being delivered. For example:

– Nitroglycerin may cause headaches and, in older adults, postural hypotension.

– Scopolamine commonly causes a dry mouth and drowsiness.

– Estradiol may cause nausea, fluid retention, thromboembolic disorders, mental depression, or hepatic dysfunction. It can also increase the risk of endometrial cancer, thromboembolic disease, and birth defects.

– Clonidine frequently causes drowsiness and dry mouth and may also cause severe rebound hypertension, especially if withdrawn suddenly. (See *Documenting transdermal drug administration*.)

Take note!

Documenting transdermal drug administration

Be sure to record:
• date and time of a transdermal application
• medication used
• location of the ointment or patch on the patient's body
• effects of the medication
• patient teaching that was provided.

Administering ophthalmic drugs

Typically, ophthalmic drugs (diagnostic and therapeutic) are given in the form of drops or ointment. When administering some types of drugs, a medicated disk is inserted into a patient's eye. Other times, a patch is applied over a patient's eye after instilling an ophthalmic drug.

Instilling eye drops

Eye drops can be used for many diagnostic and therapeutic purposes, including:
- dilating the pupil
- staining the cornea to detect abrasions or scars
- anesthetizing the eye
- lubricating the eye
- protecting the vision of a neonate
- treating certain eye disorders, such as infections or glaucoma.

Supplies
- prescribed eye drops
- sterile cotton balls
- gloves
- warm water or normal saline solution
- sterile gauze pads
- facial tissues
- eye dressing (if necessary)

Getting ready
- Verify the order in the patient's chart.
- Consult the drug guide if you haven't given the drug previously or if you're unfamiliar with the purpose, dosage, contraindications, possible side effects, or nursing considerations.
- Check the MAR and drug allergies.
- Read the label to make sure the drug is intended for ophthalmic use.

Seeing is believing
- Check the expiration date on the eye drop container, and inspect the drops for cloudiness, discoloration, and precipitates. If the solution appears abnormal in any way, don't use it.

- Keep in mind that some ophthalmic drugs are in suspension form and normally appear cloudy. When in doubt, check with a pharmacist.
- Take extra care when verifying an order for eye drops because different drugs or dosages may be ordered for each eye.
- Confirm the patient's identity using at least two patient identifiers (not including the patient's room number).
- Explain the procedure to the patient.
- Wash your hands and put on gloves.

How it's done
- If the patient has an eye dressing in place, remove it by gently pulling it down and away from the patient's forehead.

Careful cleanup
- If the patient has discharge around the eye, moisten sterile cotton balls or sterile gauze pads with warm water or normal saline solution.
- Wipe the eye gently to clean away debris, moving from the inner canthus to the outer canthus, as shown. Use a fresh sterile cotton ball or sterile gauze pad for each stroke.
- If the patient has crusted secretions around their eye, moisten a sterile gauze pad with warm water or normal saline solution. Then have the patient close their eye, and place the moist pad over the closed eye for 1 to 2 minutes.
- Remove the pad and reapply new moist sterile gauze pads, as needed, until the secretions become soft enough that you can remove them without injuring the tender ocular tissues.

Full tilt
- To help minimize systemic reactions to eye drops, see *Minimizing systemic reactions to eye drops*, page 210. In addition, take care to avoid dropper contamination during administration.
- Remove the dropper cap from the bottle (unless the bottle has a built-in dropper) and draw the eye drops into the dropper, taking care not to contaminate the dropper.
- Ask the patient to look up and away to move the cornea away from the lower lid, which minimizes the risk of touching the cornea with the dropper if the patient blinks.
- Steady the hand holding the dropper or eye drop bottle by resting it against the patient's forehead. Gently pull down the patient's lower eyelid as shown.

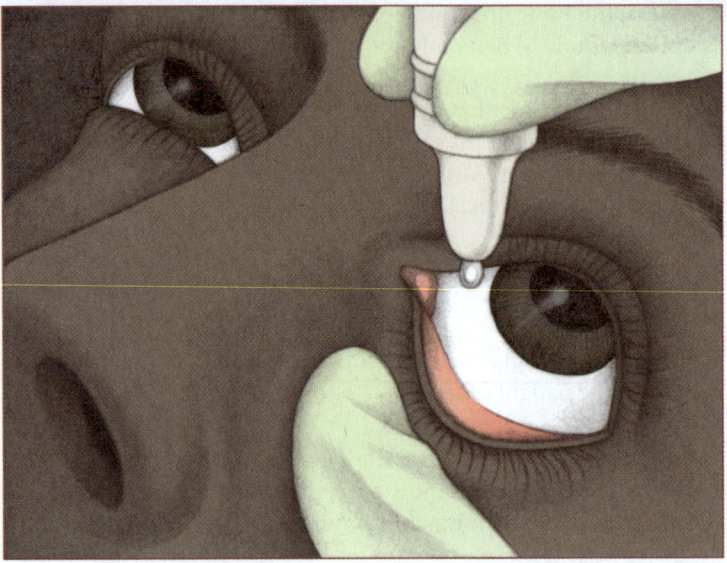

- Instill the prescribed number of drops into the conjunctival sac, not onto the patient's eyeball. Then release the patient's eyelid and have the patient blink to distribute the drops throughout their eye.

Practice pointers

- If the guidelines for using and storing the multidose medication are followed, the medication can be used until the manufacturer's expiration date (American Society of Ophthalmic Registered Nurses [ASORN], 2022).

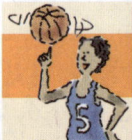

Stay on the ball

Minimizing systemic reactions to eye drops

Systemic reactions to eye drops—such as tachycardia, palpitations, flushing, dry skin, ataxia, and confusion—can be minimized by having the patient press a finger over the tear duct at the inner canthus as the drops are administered. This action compresses the nasolacrimal tear ducts, thus preventing the drops from draining out of the eye (Usgaonkar et al., 2021).

In addition, have the patient tilt their head back and toward the side of the affected eye. If drops will be placed in the left eye, ask the patient to tilt to the left, or to the right if drops will be placed in the right eye. By tilting their head, the patient reduces the chance that the drops will drain into the tear duct at the inner canthus and cause systemic effects.

- To prevent contamination, never use the same eyedrop container for more than one patient.

Worth the wait

- If the patient needs more than one type of eye medication, wait about 5 minutes between administering different doses (Gudgel, 2021).
- Teach the patient the correct procedure for instilling eye drops at home, if prescribed. (See *Teaching about eye drops.*)
- For tips on teaching an older patient, see *All about sensation.*

Administering ophthalmic ointment

An ointment formulation helps keep an ophthalmic drug in contact with the treatment area for as long as possible, which is an especially useful tactic for pediatric patients. Usually, an antibiotic ointment is used to treat eye infections.

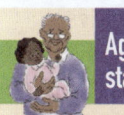

Ages and stages

All about sensation

If the patient is an older adult, they may have trouble sensing whether a drop has gone into their eye. If so, suggest that the patient chill the eye drops before using them. Most people find it easier to feel a drop entering the eye when the drop is cold.

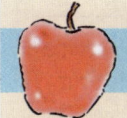

Education corner

Teaching about eye drops

- Explain why the doctor prescribed the eye drops.
- Stress the importance of proper handwashing before self-administering eye drops.
- Teach the patient to make sure they know it is the right medication, how many drops to administer, and into which eye.
- For patient comfort, tell the patient to warm the drops to room temperature by holding the bottle between their hands for about 2 minutes. However, if the patient has trouble getting the drop into the eye, chilling the eye drop first helps the patient know if the drop gets into their eye.
- If the patient is using more than one kind of eye drop, tell the patient to wait 5 minutes between administering the different types.

- Teach the patient to protect the container from light and heat.
- Teach the patient the potential adverse effects of the medication and when the patient should notify the doctor.
- Stress to the patient the importance of never placing any medication in their eyes unless the label reads "for ophthalmic use" or "for use in eyes."
- If the patient can see through the eyedrop container, teach the patient to hold it up to the light and look at it. If the liquid is discolored or if it contains sediment, tell the patient not to use it but to take the container back to the pharmacy and have it checked.
- Provide written instructions so the patient can review the proper administration steps after they get home.

Supplies

- prescribed eye ointment
- sterile cotton balls
- gloves
- warm water or normal saline solution
- sterile gauze pads
- facial tissues
- eye dressing (if necessary)

Getting ready

- Verify the order in the patient's chart.
- Consult the drug guide if you haven't given the drug previously or if you're unfamiliar with the purpose, dosage, contraindications, possible side effects, or nursing considerations.
- Check the MAR and drug allergies.
- Read the label to make sure the drug is intended for ophthalmic use.
- Double-check the medication order when administering ophthalmic ointment because different drugs or dosages may be ordered for each eye.
- Confirm the patient's identity using at least two patient identifiers (not including the patient's room number).
- Explain the procedure to the patient.
- Wash your hands and put on gloves.

How it's done

- If the patient has an eye dressing in place, remove it by gently pulling it down and away from the forehead.
- If the patient has discharge around the eye, moisten sterile cotton balls or sterile gauze pads with warm water or normal saline solution.
- Gently wipe the eye to clean away debris, moving from the inner canthus to the outer canthus. Use a fresh sterile cotton ball or sterile gauze pad for each stroke.
- If the patient has crusted secretions around their eye, moisten a sterile gauze pad with warm water or normal saline solution. Have the patient close their eye, then place the moist pad over it for 1 to 2 minutes.
- Remove the pad and reapply new moist sterile gauze pads, as needed, until the secretions are soft enough for you to remove without injuring the tissue.

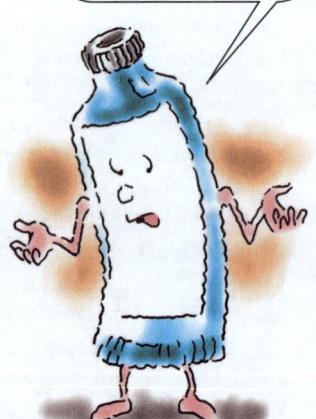

Remember, a little dab will do...but avoid touching the tube against the patient's eye.

Conquering crust

- If the tip of the ointment tube has crusted, wipe it with a sterile gauze pad to remove the crust.

- Ask the patient to look up and away to move the cornea away from the lower lid, which minimizes the risk of touching the cornea with the tip of the ointment tube if the patient blinks.
- Steady the hand holding the ointment tube against the patient's forehead. Use the other hand to gently pull down their lower eyelid.

Avoiding eye contact

- Squeeze a small ribbon of ointment along the edge of the conjunctival sac from the inner to the outer canthus, as shown. Don't let the tip of the tube touch the patient's eye. (If it does, discard the tube.)

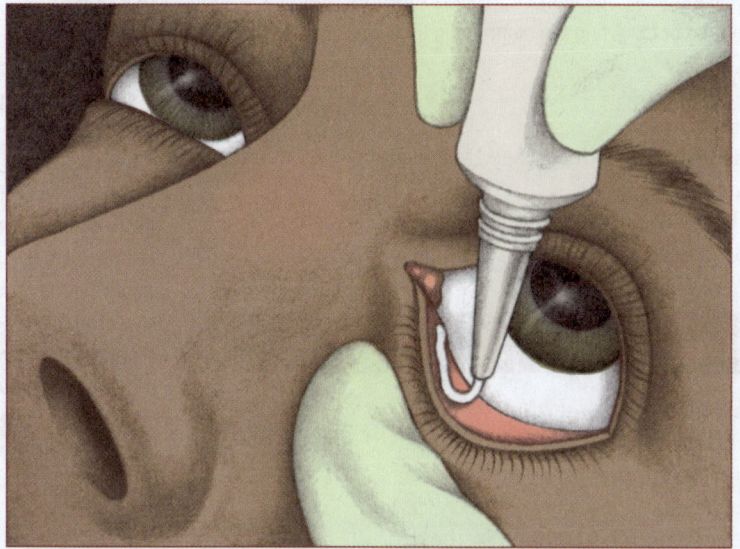

- Cut off the ribbon of ointment by turning the tube. Then release the patient's eyelid and have the patient roll their eyes behind closed lids to help distribute the drug.
- Use a clean tissue to remove excess ointment that leaks from the patient's eye. Use a fresh tissue for each eye to prevent cross-contamination.
- Lastly, apply a new eye dressing, if indicated.

Practice pointers

- If the guidelines for using and storing the medication are followed, the multidose medication can be used until the manufacturer's expiration date (ASORN, 2022).

An ounce of prevention

- Systemic reactions are unlikely with ophthalmic ointments because they don't empty quickly into the lacrimal duct, as eye drops do.

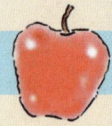

Take note!

Education corner

Teaching about ophthalmic ointment

- Explain why the doctor prescribed the ointment, and review the proper steps for using the ointment at home.
- Tell the patient to wash their hands before and after applying eye ointment. Be sure to warn the patient not to contaminate the lid of the ointment tube or to touch the tip of the tube to the eye or to the skin around the eye.
- Tell the patient to apply ointment from the inner to the outer corner of the eye. Let the patient know that their vision may be blurry for several minutes after putting the ointment in their eye.

- Carefully document the procedure. (See *Documenting ophthalmic drug administration.*)
- Teach the patient how to apply ophthalmic ointment for home use, if prescribed. (See *Teaching about ophthalmic ointment.*)

Administering otic drugs

Otic drugs may be instilled to:
- treat infections and inflammation
- soften cerumen for later removal
- produce local anesthesia
- aid removal of a foreign object trapped in the ear.

Instilling ear drops

Otic drugs are not typically given to a patient with a perforated eardrum (although it may be permitted with certain medications and with sterile technique). Certain otic drugs may be prohibited in other conditions as well. For example, hydrocortisone is contraindicated if the patient has a viral or fungal infection.

Supplies
- prescribed ear drops
- penlight
- facial tissues (or cotton-tipped applicators)
- cotton balls
- emesis basin for warm water
- gloves

Documenting ophthalmic drug administration

After administering an ophthalmic drug, be sure to record:
- eye treated
- date and time
- prescribed drug
- dose administered
- patient's response to the instillation procedure (note the appearance of the patient's eye before and after they receive eye drops.)
- patient or family teaching that was provided.

Getting ready

- Verify the order in the patient's chart.
- Consult the drug guide if you haven't given the drug previously or if you're unfamiliar with the purpose, dosage, contraindications, possible side effects, or nursing considerations.
- Check the MAR and drug allergies.
- To avoid adverse reactions caused by the instillation of cold ear drops (such as vertigo, nausea, and pain), warm the drops to body temperature by placing the container in a basin of warm water.

Now hear this

- Don't make the drops too hot.
- Confirm the patient's identity using at least two patient identifiers (not including the patient's room number).
- Wash your hands.
- Explain the procedure to the patient.

How it's done

- Have the patient lie on their side, with the affected ear facing up.
- Straighten the patient's ear canal. (See *Positioning a patient for ear drops*, page 215.)

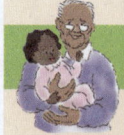

Ages and stages

Positioning a patient for ear drops

Before instilling ear drops, have the patient lie on their side. Then straighten the patient's ear canal to help the drops reach the eardrum. In an adult, gently pull the auricle up and back; in an infant or young child, gently pull it down and back as shown.

Adult

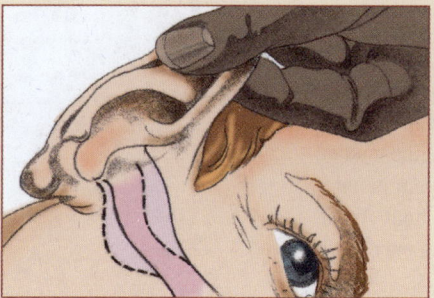

Child

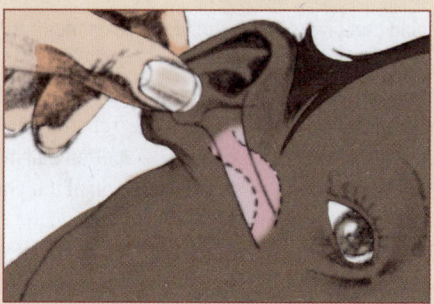

Light the way

- Using a penlight, examine the ear canal for drainage. If drainage is present, clean the canal with a tissue or cotton ball because drainage can reduce the effectiveness of the drug.
- Straighten the patient's ear canal once again and instill the ordered number of drops. To avoid patient discomfort, aim the dropper so the drops fall against the side of the ear canal, not on the eardrum.

Disappearing act

- Hold the ear canal in position until the drug disappears down the canal. Then release the ear.
- Tell the patient to remain on their side for 5 to 10 minutes to allow the drug to travel down the ear canal.
- If included in the provider's orders, tuck a cotton ball loosely into the opening of the ear canal. Don't push it too far into the ear, however, because this can keep secretions from draining and increase pressure on the eardrum.
- Clean and dry the outer ear.
- Help the patient into a comfortable position.
- Remove gloves, wash hands, and document.

Practice pointers

- Some conditions make the normally sensitive ear canal quite tender, so be especially gentle when instilling ear drops. (See *Otic tips for tots.*)
- Take special care not to injure the eardrum. Never insert any object, even a cotton-tipped applicator, so far into the ear canal that its tip can't be seen.

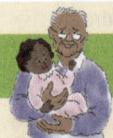

Ages and stages

Otic tips for tots

When teaching caregivers how to administer ear drops to their child, include this helpful information:
• Warm the drops for their child's comfort by holding the bottle in their hands for about 2 minutes.
• For children under age 3 years, gently pull the earlobe down and back to straighten the child's ear canal; up and back for children over age 3 years

(American Academy of Pediatrics [AAP], 2022).
• If necessary to keep the medication from running out of the ear, place a cotton ball moistened with the medication at the entrance to the ear canal. Remove the cotton after 1 hour. Avoid using dry cotton because it may absorb the medication.

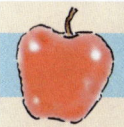

Teaching about ear drops

• Remind the patient never to insert any object into their ear.
• Review the importance of washing hands thoroughly before self-administering ear drops.
• Make sure the patient knows how many drops to give and into which ear.

• Teach the patient to call the pharmacist or doctor, and not to use the medication, if the liquid looks discolored or contains sediment.
• Provide written guidelines to caregivers who will be administering ear drops to a child at home.

Documenting otic drug administration

After administering an otic drug, be sure to record:
• ear treated
• name of the drug instilled
• date and time instilled
• dose given, and the patient's response to the instillation procedure
• appearance of the patient's ears before and after instilling ear drops
• teaching aids given to the patient or family.

• If the patient has vertigo, keep the bedside rails up and assist as necessary. Also, move slowly to avoid aggravating any vertigo.
• Carefully document the procedure. (See *Documenting otic drug administration.*)
• Teach the patient how to instill ear drops if they have been prescribed for home use. (See *Teaching about ear drops.*)

Administering nasal drugs

For the most part, nasal drugs produce local effects.

Instilling nose drops

Nasal drops are used to treat a specific nasal area, and sprays and aerosols disperse the drug through the nasal passages.

The nose knows

The most commonly administered nasal drugs are:
• vasoconstrictors, which coat and shrink swollen mucous membranes
• local anesthetics, which promote patient comfort during such procedures as bronchoscopy
• corticosteroids, which reduce inflammation caused by allergies or nasal polyps.

Supplies
- prescribed nasal medication
- gloves

Getting ready
- Verify the order on the patient's chart.
- Consult the drug guide if you haven't given the drug previously or if you're unfamiliar with the purpose, dosage, contraindications, possible side effects, or nursing considerations.
- Check the MAR and drug allergies.
- Confirm the patient's identity using at least two patient identifiers (not including the patient's room number).
- Explain the procedure to the patient and position them as needed to make sure the drops reach the intended site.

How it's done
- Shake the medication vial.
- Instruct the patient to blow their nose.
- Nasal medications can be in the form of drops or sprays.
- To administer drops:
- Instruct the patient to tilt their head back.
- Place the dropper about ⅓ inch (1 cm) inside the nostril. Angle the tip slightly toward the inner corner of the patient's eye. Squeeze the dropper bulb to dispense the correct number of drops into each nostril.
- After instilling the prescribed number of drops, instruct the patient to keep their head tilted back for about 5 minutes. Encourage the patient to expectorate any medication that runs into the throat. If the patient coughs, help the patient to sit up.
- To administer spray:
- Instruct the patient to sit upright, with their head tilted slightly forward.
- Place the spray nozzle about ⅓ inch (1 cm) inside the nostril. Angle the tip slightly toward the inner corner of the patient's eye. Squeeze the vial to administer the correct number of sprays into one nostril.
- After administering the prescribed number of sprays, instruct the patient to sniff slowly in, then bend the head forward and breathe through the mouth. Then repeat the administration steps for the other nostril (Kc et al., 2020).

Practice pointers
- Stay with the patient after administering nasal medications. Urge the patient to breathe through their mouth for several minutes. Observe the patient closely for possible respiratory problems.

Administering rectal drugs

Rectal drugs may be administered to a patient who's unconscious, vomiting, or unable to swallow or take anything by mouth. Rectally administered drugs can produce either local or systemic effects. The most common forms of rectal drugs include:
- suppositories
- medicated enemas.

Dodging digestion and bypassing biotransformation

Because rectal administration bypasses the upper gastrointestinal (GI) tract, drugs given by this method aren't destroyed by digestive enzymes in the stomach or small intestine. Also, these drugs don't irritate the upper GI tract, as some oral drugs can. In addition, rectal drugs bypass the portal system, thus avoiding biotransformation in the liver. Biotransformation, or drug metabolism, refers to the body's ability to change a drug from its dosage form to a more water-soluble form that can be excreted. Once in the liver, drugs are metabolized by enzymes.

Rectal drug downsides

Rectal drugs also have some disadvantages. The administration procedure may cause discomfort or embarrassment to the patient. Also, the drug may be incompletely absorbed, especially if the patient is unable to retain it or if the rectum contains feces. As a result, the patient may need a higher dose than if taken in oral form.

Administering rectal suppositories

A suppository is a firm, bullet-shaped object made from a substance that melts at body temperature (such as cocoa butter). As the suppository melts, it releases the drug into the patient's rectum, where it can be absorbed across the rectal mucosa. Most suppositories are about 1½ inches (4 cm) long (or smaller for infants and children). Rectal suppositories commonly contain drugs that reduce fever; induce relaxation; stimulate peristalsis and defecation; or relieve pain, vomiting, and local irritation.

Supplies
- prescribed rectal drug
- several 4 × 4-inch gauze pads
- gloves
- linen-saver pad
- water-soluble lubricant
- bedpan (if necessary)

Getting ready

- Verify the order on the patient's chart.
- Consult the drug guide if you haven't given the drug previously or if you're unfamiliar with the purpose, dosage, contraindications, possible side effects, or nursing considerations.
- Check the MAR and drug allergies.
- Confirm the patient's identity using at least two patient identifiers (not including the patient's room number).
- Provide privacy.

How it's done

- Place the patient on their left side in Sims position (semiprone with the right knee and thigh drawn up and the left arm along the patient's back). Cover the patient with the bedcovers, exposing only the buttocks.
- Place a linen-saver pad under the buttocks to protect the bedding.
- Wash hands and put on gloves.
- Remove the suppository from its wrapper and apply a water-soluble lubricant to it.
- Lift the patient's upper buttock to expose the anus.
- Tell the patient to take several deep breaths through their mouth to relax the anal sphincter and reduce anxiety and discomfort during insertion.

Tapered end first

- With your dominant hand, insert the tapered end of the suppository into the patient's rectum. (See *Inserting a rectal suppository in an adult.*)
- Ensure the patient's comfort. Ask the patient to lie quietly and, if applicable, to retain the suppository for an appropriate time. A suppository given to relieve constipation should be retained as long as possible (at least 20 minutes) for it to be effective. If necessary, press on the patient's anus with a gauze pad until the urge to defecate passes.
- If the patient can't retain the suppository and pressing on the anus with a gauze pad doesn't relieve the urge to defecate, place the patient on a bedpan.
- For information on administering a rectal suppository to a child, see *Using rectal suppositories in pediatric patients.*

Practice pointers

- Some rectal suppositories must be stored in the refrigerator to keep them firm and to maintain the drug's effectiveness.
- Before administering rectal medication, inspect the patient's anus. If the tissues are inflamed or if hemorrhoids are present, withhold

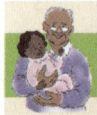

Ages and stages

Using rectal suppositories in pediatric patients

Rectal administration via suppository may be a good alternative when the oral route cannot be used, but it is important to understand it is a less reliable method in children than in adults. Remember to insert the suppository only up to the first knuckle joint of your finger. If the patient is an infant, use the smallest finger to insert the drug.

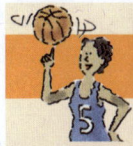

Inserting a rectal suppository in an adult

When inserting a rectal suppository in an adult, use your index finger to direct the suppository along the rectal wall toward the patient's umbilicus, so the membrane can absorb the drug. Continue to advance the suppository until it passes the internal anal sphincter.

the suppository and notify the health care provider. The drug could aggravate the condition.

- To minimize the risk of local trauma, this route may need to be avoided if the patient has had recent rectal, colon, or prostate surgery.
- Rectal suppositories are contraindicated in certain patients. (See *Contraindications for rectal suppositories.*)

Administering medicated enemas

When an enema is given, fluid is instilled into a patient's rectum for a variable amount of time. If the patient is being prepared for a diagnostic or surgical procedure or if the enema is being given to relieve constipation, a cleansing enema may be performed.

Cleaning crew

A cleansing enema is a procedure that involves instilling unmedicated fluid into a patient's rectum simply to clean the patient's rectum and colon. The patient expels the irrigant almost completely within about 15 minutes.

Pay attention… the topic is retention

Enemas can also be used to deliver such drugs as lactulose, which acidifies the colon contents and lowers blood ammonia levels. To deliver a drug, a retention enema is typically given. A retention enema is a type of enema that requires the patient to retain the fluid in their rectum and colon for 30 to 60 minutes, if possible, before expelling it. A retention enema can also be used as an emollient to soothe irritated colon tissues.

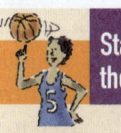

Contraindications for rectal suppositories

Avoid giving rectal suppositories to a patient who has:

- cardiac arrhythmias or has had a myocardial infarction, because inserting a rectal suppository typically stimulates the vagus nerve
- undiagnosed abdominal pain, because if the pain stems from appendicitis, the peristalsis caused by rectal administration could rupture the appendix
- recently undergone colon, rectal, or prostate surgery, because rectal suppositories increase the risk of local trauma.

Enema enemies

Enemas stimulate peristalsis by distending the colon and by stimulating nerves in the rectal walls. Consequently, an enema should not be given to a patient who has had:

- recent colon or rectal surgery
- myocardial infarction
- undiagnosed abdominal pain, which could be caused by appendicitis (giving an enema to a patient with appendicitis can irritate the inflamed area of the appendix and precipitate perforation).

Most importantly, give an enema cautiously to any patient who has cardiac arrhythmias, because inserting anything into the rectum stimulates the vagus nerve and could cause an increase in cardiac arrhythmias.

Supplies

- prescribed solution (usually in a premixed, commercially prepared container)
- disposable enema kit
- gloves, 4 × 4-inch gauze pads
- bedpan
- toilet paper
- emesis basin
- linen-saver pad
- water-soluble lubricant (see *Choosing enema supplies.*)

Grab bag

If a large volume of solution is needed for a patient's enema, an enema bag will be needed to perform the procedure instead of a commercially prepared solution and a disposable enema kit. You may also need an IV pole to hang the enema bag and a bath thermometer to test the temperature of the solution.

Choosing enema supplies

When choosing supplies for an enema, consider the drug prescribed as well as the patient's age, size, and condition. Remember that physical size is always more important than age. For example, if the patient is a small 9-year-old, use the smallest tube possible for that age group.

Remember to use smaller tubing and a smaller volume of fluid when giving a retention enema, to create less pressure in the patient's rectum to make it easier to retain the fluid.

Getting ready

- Verify the order on the patient's chart.
- Confirm the patient's identity using at least two patient identifiers (not including the patient's room number).
- Explain the procedure to the patient.
- To minimize peristalsis, have the patient empty their bladder and rectum before beginning.

Explain the need to retain

- Once the enema is instilled, explain to the patient they need to retain it in the rectum for a prescribed length of time until the drug is absorbed.
- Have the patient wear a gown, and provide privacy.

How it's done

- Help the patient onto the left side in Sims position. If the patient is uncomfortable in that position, reposition onto the right side or, if necessary, onto the back. Place a linen-saver pad under the patient to protect the bedding.

For disposable enemas

- Put on gloves, and remove the cap from the rectal tube.
- Check the amount of lubricant that's already on the tube. If needed, squeeze water-soluble lubricant onto a 4 × 4-inch gauze pad, and dip the tip of the rectal tube into the lubricant.
- Gently squeeze the enema container to expel air.
- Lift the patient's upper buttock to expose the anus.

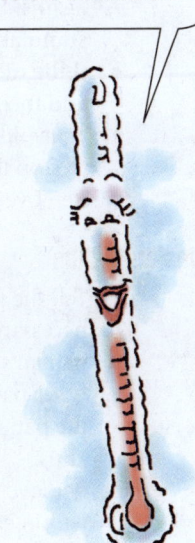

It's important to test the temperature of enema solution before instillation.

Waiting to inhale

- Tell the patient to take a deep breath. As the patient inhales, insert the rectal tube into the rectum, pointing the tube toward the umbilicus.
- If the patient is an adult, advance the tube about 4 inches (10 cm). Pediatric patients require different guidelines. (See *Administering enemas to children*.)

Squeeze until empty

- Squeeze the solution container until it's empty. Then remove the rectal tube and discard the used enema container, the packaging it came in, and the used gloves.

For enema bags

- Prepare the prescribed solution and warm it to body temperature or slightly higher. Test the temperature using a bath thermometer.

- Put on gloves, close the clamp on the enema tubing, and fill the enema bag with the solution.
- Hang the enema bag on an IV pole and adjust the bag so it's slightly above bed level.

Tip of the day

- Remove the protective cap from the end of the enema tubing. The tip of the tubing should be prelubricated. If it isn't, lubricate it with a small amount of water-soluble lubricant.
- Unclamp the tubing, flush the solution through it, then reclamp the tubing.
- Lift the patient's upper buttock. While holding the tube in your other hand, touch the patient's anal sphincter with the tip of the tube to stimulate contraction. Then insert the tube into the patient's anus.
- As the sphincter relaxes, tell the patient to breathe deeply through the mouth as the tube is gently advanced.

Hold on

- Release the clamp on the tubing. Make sure to continue holding the tube in the patient's rectum, because bowel contractions and pressure from the anal sphincter can expel the tube.
- Regulate the flow rate by lowering or raising the bag according to the patient's retention ability and level of comfort. Don't raise it higher than 18 inches (45.7 cm) for an adult (Taylor et al., 2023).
- If the flow stops, the tubing may be blocked with feces or wedged against the rectal wall. Gently turn the tubing to free it without stimulating defecation.
- If the tubing becomes clogged, withdraw it, flush it with solution, and then reinsert it.
- To avoid inserting air into the patient's rectum, clamp the tubing to stop the flow just before the enema bag empties.
- Remove the tubing, and dispose of the setup.

A matter of time

- Tell the patient to retain the solution for the prescribed time. If necessary, hold a 4 × 4-inch gauze pad against the anus until the patient's urge to defecate passes.
- If the patient is apprehensive, place them on a bedpan and have the patient hold toilet tissue or a rolled washcloth against their anus.
- Remove and dispose of your gloves, and place the call button within easy reach. Tell the patient to call for help to get out of bed, especially if the patient feels weak or faint.

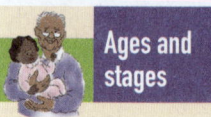

Ages and stages

Administering enemas to children

Advance the tube to just past the anal sphincter into the rectum. For an older child, this may be 3 or 4 inches (7.5 to 10 cm); for a young child, up to 2 inches (5 cm); and for an infant, 1 inch (2.5 cm).

Flow rate

Regulate the flow rate by lowering or raising the bag according to the patient's retention ability and level of comfort. Don't raise it higher than 12 inches (30.5 cm) for a child or 6 to 8 inches (15 to 20 cm) for an infant. Assess the patient for signs of cramping and discomfort, and adjust the flow rate accordingly.

Practice pointers

- Before giving a retention enema, check the patient's elimination pattern. A constipated patient may need a cleansing enema to keep feces from interfering with drug absorption. A patient with a fecal impaction may need to have the drug delivered by another route.
- Keep in mind that a patient with diarrhea may not be able to retain the enema solution for the prescribed time.
- Before administering a rectal medication, inspect the patient's anus for hemorrhoids, which could make insertion more difficult and painful for the patient.

Administering vaginal drugs

Vaginal drugs are available in many forms, including:
- suppositories
- creams
- gels
- ointments
- solutions.

These medicated preparations can be inserted to treat infection (particularly *Trichomonas vaginalis* and candidiasis), treat inflammation, or prevent conception. Vaginal administration is most effective when the patient can remain lying down afterward to retain the drug.

Giving a vaginal drug

Most vaginal drugs come packaged in or with an applicator that the nurse or patient can use to insert the drug into the anterior and posterior fornices. When in contact with the vaginal mucosa, suppositories melt, diffusing the drug as effectively as creams, gels, and ointments.

Supplies

- prescribed vaginal drug (with an applicator, if necessary)
- gloves
- water-soluble lubricant
- small sanitary pad
- absorbent towel
- linen-saver pad
- small drape
- cotton balls
- 4 × 4-inch gauze pad
- paper towel
- soap and water (if necessary)

Getting ready

- Verify the order on the patient's chart.
- Consult the drug guide if you haven't given the drug previously or if you're unfamiliar with the purpose, dosage, contraindications, possible side effects, or nursing considerations.
- Check the MAR and drug allergies.
- If possible, plan to give the drug at bedtime, when the patient is recumbent.
- Confirm the patient's identity using at least two patient identifiers (not including the patient's room number).
- Explain the procedure to the patient and provide privacy.
- Ask the patient to empty their bladder.

Self–administration is an option

- Ask the patient whether they would rather insert the medication themselves. If so, provide appropriate instructions.

How it's done

- If the patient decides not to self-administer, help the patient into the lithotomy position.
- Place a linen-saver pad under the patient's buttocks and a small drape over their legs. Expose only the perineum.
- Wash your hands and put on gloves.
- Squeeze a small portion of water-soluble lubricant onto a 4 × 4-inch gauze pad.

Package deal

- Unwrap the suppository, and coat it with the lubricant. If the drug is a small suppository in a prepackaged applicator, lubricate the tip of the suppository with water-soluble lubricant. If the drug is a foam or gel, fill the applicator as prescribed, and lubricate the tip of the applicator with the water-soluble lubricant.
- Separate the patient's labia.

Examination before administration

- Examine the patient's perineum. If it's excoriated, withhold the drug and notify the health care provider. The patient may need a different type of drug.
- If discharge is present, wash the area.
- To wash the area, soak several cotton balls in warm, soapy water.
- While holding the labia open with one hand, wipe once down the left side of the patient's perineum with a cotton ball.
- Discard the cotton ball, pick up another one, and use the new cotton ball to wipe once down the right side of the perineum.
- Discard the cotton ball, pick up another one, and use it to wipe once down the middle of the patient's perineum.

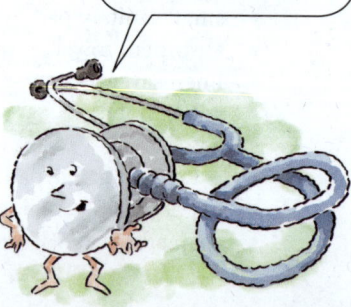

You'll need at least three cotton balls to clean the patient's perineum, so have a supply on hand.

Rounded tip first

- With the patient's labia still separated, insert the rounded tip of a suppository into the patient's vagina, advancing it along the posterior wall of the vagina or as far as it will go (Taylor et al., 2023).
- If you're using an applicator, insert it into the patient's vagina. (See *How to administer a vaginal drug using an applicator*, page 227.)

Time to lie down

- Tell the patient to lie down on their back for 5 to 10 minutes with their knees flexed to help promote absorption and allow the medication to flow into the posterior fornix. If a suppository has been inserted, tell the patient to remain recumbent for at least 30 minutes to allow time for it to melt.
- Place a small sanitary pad in the patient's underwear to keep clothes or bedding from becoming soiled.

Practice pointers

- Refrigerate vaginal gels, foams, and suppositories that melt at room temperature.

How to administer a vaginal drug using an applicator

If an applicator is used to administer a vaginal drug to a patient, follow these steps:

• Use your dominant hand to insert the applicator for its full length into the patient's vagina. Direct the applicator down initially, toward the patient's spine, and then back up toward the cervix, as shown.

• Press the plunger until all the medication is ejected from the applicator.

• Discard the applicator, or if the applicator is reusable according to the manufacturer, wash it with soap and warm water before storing it.

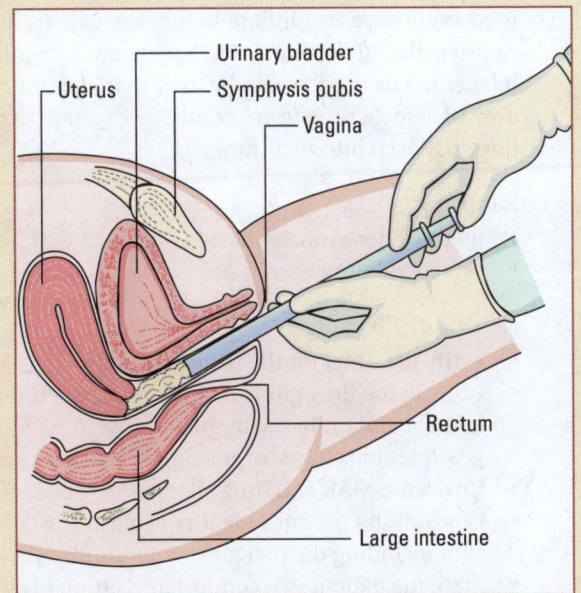

Figure reprinted with permission from Lippincott Williams and Wilkins. (2008). *Lippincott's visual encyclopedia of clinical skills* (figure on p. 595). Wolters Kluwer.

Administering respiratory medication

Several devices and procedures can be used to produce a fine, drug-carrying mist that a patient can inhale deep into their lungs.

Quick route to the capillaries

When the drug enters the lungs, it moves almost immediately into the lining of the patient's bronchi or alveoli and then into the adjacent capillaries. Drugs are administered in this way because the inhaled route is the most effective method to get the medicine where it's supposed to go—directly to the airways. In addition, the total dose is low and decreases the chance of systemic effect.

A breath of fresh air

To deliver drugs to the respiratory tract, some type of handheld inhaler (sometimes including special attachments with holding chambers called *spacers*) or a nebulizer is usually used.

Using a metered-dose inhaler

Many inhalant drugs, such as bronchodilators (which help to open the bronchial airways of the lungs) and corticosteroids (which are used as effective anti-inflammatory agents), are available in small canisters that are inserted into a metered-dose inhaler. A metered-dose inhaler is a device that can be used to trigger the release of a measured dose of aerosol drug from a canister. The patient can then inhale the fine mist deep into their lungs.

Supplies
- metered-dose inhaler device
- prescribed drug

Getting ready
- Verify the order on the patient's chart.
- Consult the drug guide if you haven't given the drug previously or if you're unfamiliar with the purpose, dosage, contraindications, possible side effects, or nursing considerations.
- Check the MAR and drug allergies.
- Confirm the patient's identity using at least two patient identifiers (not including the patient's room number).
- Place the patient in a comfortable sitting position.

How it's done
- Shake the inhaler canister well.

- Remove the cap from the canister, turn the canister upside down, and insert the stem of the canister into the small hole in the flattened portion of the mouthpiece as shown.
- If the inhaler has not been used before or has not been used within the last week, it should be primed by holding it at arm's length and compressing the canister.

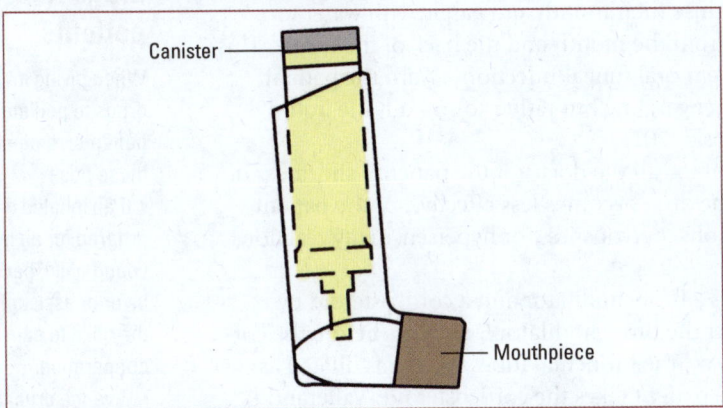

Canister

Mouthpiece

- Ask the patient to exhale and then to seal their lips around the mouthpiece of the inhaler. If using a spacer, the patient should seal their lips around the mouthpiece of the spacer (American Lung Association [ALA], 2022).
- Tell the patient to inhale slowly through the mouth and to continue inhaling until the lungs feel full.

Once is enough

- As the patient begins to inhale, compress the drug canister into the plastic housing of the inhaler to release a metered dose of the drug. Do this only once.
- Tell the patient to hold their breath for 10 seconds or as long as possible. Then instruct the patient to exhale slowly through pursed lips, as though whistling. Doing so produces back pressure, which helps to keep the bronchioles open, thus increasing the absorption and diffusion of the drug (ALA, 2022).

Practice pointers

- If the patient can't coordinate well enough to inhale the drug as soon as it is discharged, a spacer device may be added to the inhaler.
- Some inhaled bronchodilators may cause restlessness, palpitations, nervousness, and hypersensitivity reactions such as rash, urticaria, and bronchospasm.

Horse sense

- If the patient takes an inhaled corticosteroid, watch for hoarseness or fungal infection in the mouth or throat (Vallerand & Sanoski, 2021).
- To give inhaled drugs to pediatric patients, see *Giving inhaled drugs to pediatric patients.*
- Have the patient rinse their mouth and gargle with water to remove the drug from the mouth and the back of the throat. This step helps to prevent oral fungal infections. Warn the patient not to swallow after gargling but rather to spit out the liquid (Vallerand & Sanoski, 2021).
- Instruct the patient to call the doctor if the patient's shortness of breath worsens, the drug becomes less effective, or the patient develops palpitations, nervousness, or hypersensitivity reactions such as a rash.
- If the patient takes a bronchodilator and a corticosteroid by inhaler, administer the bronchodilator 5 minutes before the corticosteroid. That way, the bronchial tubes will be as dilated as possible when the patient takes the corticosteroid (Vallerand & Sanoski, 2021).
- Have the patient wait at least 1 minute between doses of a single inhaled drug.

Identification, please!

- If the patient takes an inhaled corticosteroid, urge the patient to carry medical identification announcing the possibility of needing supplemental corticosteroids during stress or a severe asthma attack.

Preparing an injection

The ability to inject drugs into a patient's skin, subcutaneous tissue, or muscle is a key nursing skill that must be exercised with great accuracy and care.

Quick and potent

Injecting medications promotes a rapid onset of drug action and high drug levels in a patient's blood, in part, because this route of administration sidesteps the breakdown that can take place in the GI tract and liver.

Proper prior preparation

To prepare for an injection, you need to know how to correctly choose a needle and how to withdraw a liquid drug from a vial or ampule.

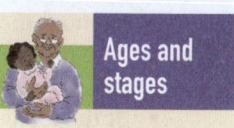

Ages and stages

Giving inhaled drugs to pediatric patients

When giving inhaled drugs to pediatric patients, remember these tips:

- If an inhaled drug is ordered for an infant or young child, have a caregiver or assistant hold the child to gain their cooperation.
- Give the drug through an aerosol nebulizer so the child doesn't have to hold their breath to retain the drug.
- For an older child, consider using a metered-dose inhaler, but only after proper patient education and return demonstration. Also, consider adding a spacer to the inhaler.
- Don't use this type of inhaler if you think the patient won't be able to get an appropriate dose into the lungs (rather than into the mouth and throat).

You may need to reconstitute the drug or combine drugs in a single syringe. After the drug is properly prepared, you must have the knowledge and skills to administer the injection to the appropriate site using the correct techniques. Once the injection is complete, the nurse must carefully dispose of needles and sharps in the nearest container, making sure to never recap a needle.

Start at the very beginning

Typically (unless a special needleless injection system is being used), the first step in preparing for injection is to choose the proper syringe and needle. When doing so, consider the route of administration, the size of the patient, and the most likely injection site. (See *Selecting syringes and needles*, pages 232 and 233.) The next step requires withdrawing the drug from its vial or ampule into a syringe, possibly together with another drug.

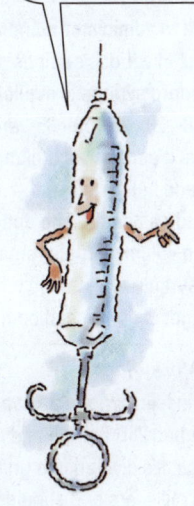

Injecting a drug into a patient tests a nurse's skills. It requires a great deal of accuracy and care. Get my point?

Withdrawing a drug from a vial

Withdrawing a drug from a vial may require the following two steps:
1. reconstitution
2. withdrawal.

Supplies
- medication vial
- vial or ampule of an appropriate diluent
- alcohol pads
- syringe
- two needles of appropriate size
- filter needle (if indicated, to screen particles that may be created during reconstitution)

Getting ready
- Verify the order on the patient's chart.
- Consult the drug guide if you haven't given the drug previously or if you're unfamiliar with the purpose, dosage, contraindications, possible side effects, or nursing considerations.
- Check the MAR and drug allergies.
- Wash your hands.

How it's done
- Place the vial on a countertop.
- Wipe the rubber diaphragm on top of the vial with an alcohol pad.

Selecting syringes and needles

When giving injections, success often depends on the ability to choose the proper syringe and needle for the task.

Syringes

Illustrated here are four types of commonly used syringes, shown without the protection devices that prevent needle-stick injuries.

Standard syringe

Used to administer numerous drugs in various settings, the standard syringe is available in 3-, 5-, 10-, 20-, 25-, 30-, 35-, and 50-mL sizes. It consists of a plunger, barrel, and hub. The syringe may also include a needle. The dead space is the volume of fluid remaining in the syringe and needle when the plunger is depressed completely.

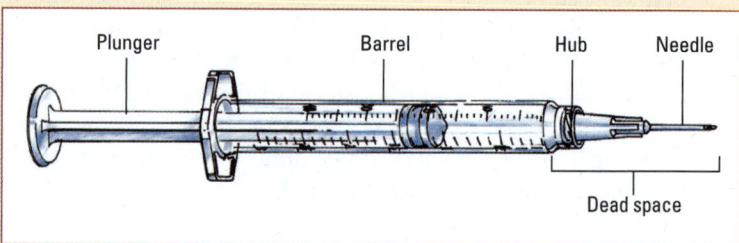

Plunger Barrel Hub Needle

Dead space

Insulin syringe

The insulin syringe has an attached 25G needle and no dead space. It's divided into units rather than milliliters and should be used ONLY for insulin administration.

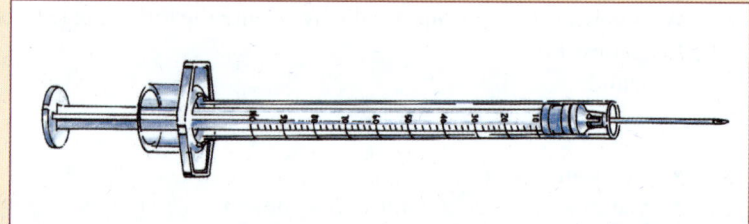

Tuberculin syringe

The tuberculin syringe holds up to 1 mL and is typically used for intradermal (ID) injections. It can also be used to give small doses, which may be required in pediatric and intensive care units.

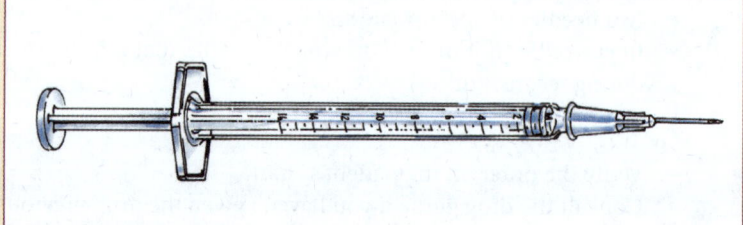

Unit-dose syringe

The unit-dose syringe is prefilled with a measured drug dose in a ready-to-dispense plastic cartridge. Some unit-dose syringes will require the addition of a needle.

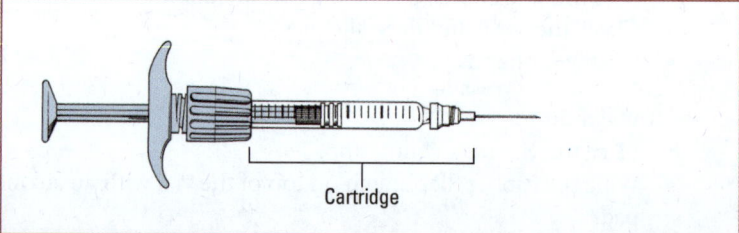

Cartridge

Selecting syringes and needles *(continued)*

Needles

Needle choice will depend on whether an ID, subcutaneous (sub-Q), or intramuscular (IM) injection is being given. Needles come in various lengths, diameters (or gauges), and bevel designs.

Intradermal needle

For an ID injection, select a needle 3/8 to 5/8 inch long and 25G in diameter, with a short bevel.

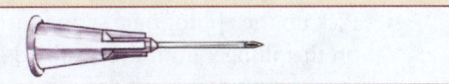

Subcutaneous needle

For a sub-Q injection, select a needle 5/8 to 7/8 inch long and 23G to 25G in diameter, with a medium bevel.

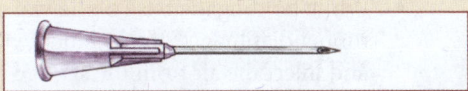

Intramuscular needle

For an IM injection, select a needle 1 to 3 inches long and 18G to 23G in diameter, with a medium bevel.

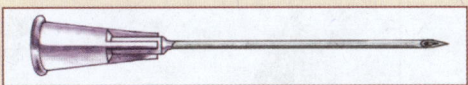

Shielded needle

To reduce the risk of needle-stick injury and the disease transmission that could result, a safety device built onto the syringe can be used to cover the needle when the injection is complete, thus eliminating the temptation to recap a used needle.

After the injection is complete, simply grasp the syringe flanges with one hand and push the shield forward with the other hand until it clicks, as shown below. The shield is now locked firmly in place over the needle. NOTE: There are several types of needle shields available. Ensure understanding of these safety devices before giving an injection.

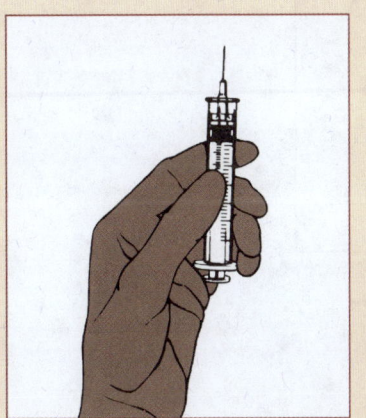
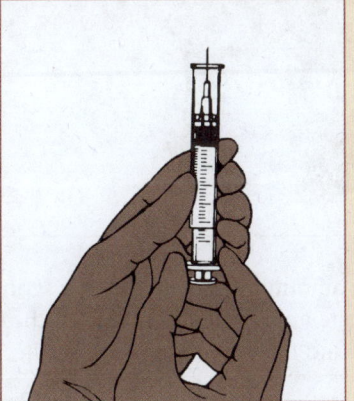
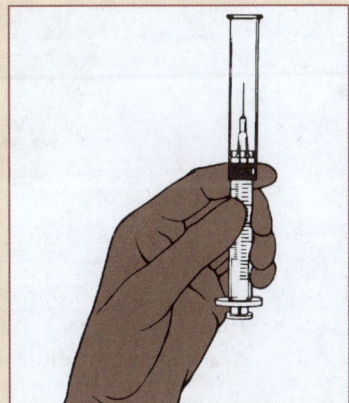

- Avoid rubbing the diaphragm vigorously because doing so can move bacteria from the nonsterile rim of the vial onto the diaphragm.
- Wipe the rubber diaphragm on the top of the diluent vial with a fresh alcohol pad.

Give it some space

- Pick up the appropriate syringe, uncap the needle, and pull back on the plunger until the air-filled space inside the syringe equals the amount of diluent desired.
- While holding the base of the vial to keep it steady, puncture the rubber diaphragm of the diluent vial with the needle, as shown, and inject the air from the syringe into the vial.

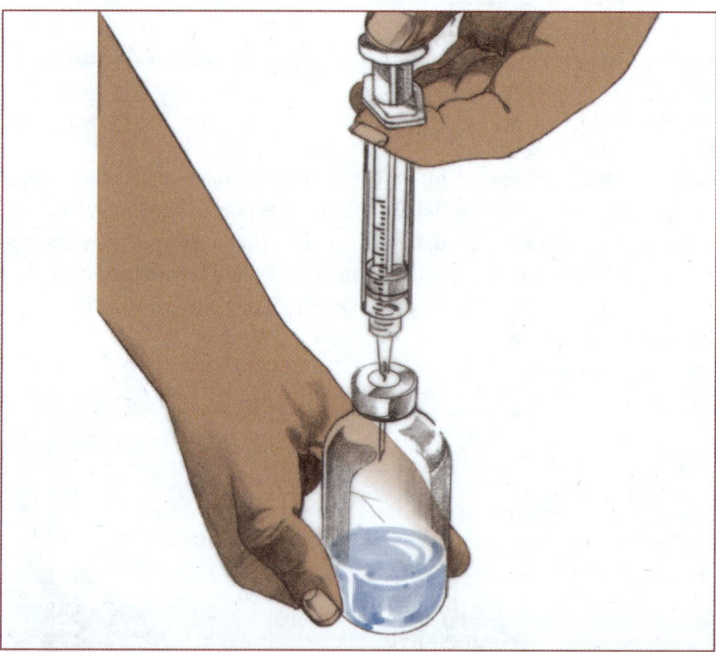

- Draw up the appropriate amount of diluent into the syringe.
- Turn to the drug vial. While holding the base to keep the vial steady, inject the diluent into it and withdraw the needle.

Gently roll

- Do not shake the vial; roll it in your hands to mix the drug and diluent thoroughly. Shaking the vial traps air in the drug.
- If the drug vial contains its own diluent compartment, remove the protective cap and depress the rubber plunger. This forces the lower stopper to fall to the bottom of the vial along with the diluent.

- If the drug must be drawn up through a filter needle, remove the original needle from the syringe, attach the filter needle, and then uncap it. If a filter needle is not necessary, simply leave the original needle on the syringe.

Pump up the volume

- Pull back on the plunger until the volume of air in the syringe equals the volume of drug to be given.
- Puncture the diaphragm of the drug vial and inject the air.
- Invert the vial, as shown below, and withdraw the amount of drug to be given.

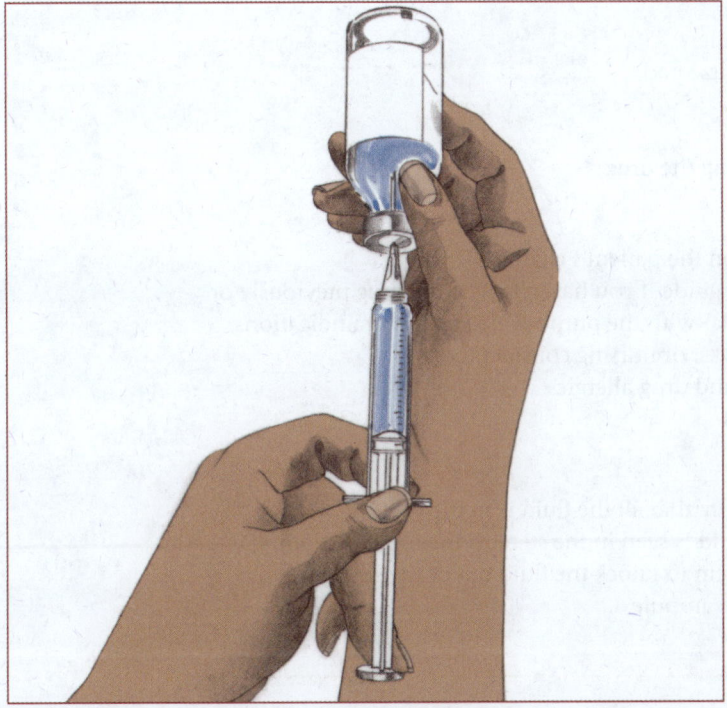

New needle needed

- Remove the needle from the syringe, and replace it with a new sterile needle. This is necessary because puncturing a rubber diaphragm can dull a needle and increase the pain of injection, and the drug stuck to the outside of the used needle could irritate the patient's tissues.
- Label the drug-filled syringe to finish preparing it for administration.

Practice pointers

- When inserting a needle through a rubber diaphragm, hold the needle bevel up and exert slight lateral pressure as the needle goes through the diaphragm. This technique helps to avoid cutting a piece of rubber out of the stopper and pushing it into the drug in the vial.

Withdrawing a drug from an ampule

Some drugs may be withdrawn from an ampule.

Supplies

- medication ampule
- dry 2 × 2-inch gauze pad
- syringe
- filter needle
- needle for injecting the drug

Getting ready

- Verify the order on the patient's chart.
- Consult the drug guide if you haven't given the drug previously or if you're unfamiliar with the purpose, dosage, contraindications, possible side effects, or nursing considerations.
- Check the MAR and drug allergies.
- Wash your hands.

How it's done

- Check to make sure that all the fluid is in the bottom of the ampule. If any fluid is seen in the stem or the top of the ampule, gently flick the stem to knock the fluid out of the stem and into the bottom of the ampule.

Bottom of the ampule

- When all the fluid is in the bottom of the ampule, wrap it in a dry 2 × 2-inch gauze pad so the pad covers the ampule's stem.
- Hold the body of the ampule with one hand and the top portion of the ampule between the thumb and the first two fingers of your other hand.
- Pointing the ampule away from you, snap off the top.
- With a filter needle on the syringe, aspirate the correct amount of drug from the open ampule. The filter needle strains out small pieces of glass that might have fallen into the drug (Taylor et al., 2023).

New needle needed (again)

- Replace the filter needle with a fresh needle appropriate for injecting the drug. Changing needles prevents excess drug on the outside of the filter needle from irritating the patient's tissues.
- Label the drug-filled syringe to finish preparing it for administration.

Practice pointers

- An opened ampule doesn't contain a vacuum, so air doesn't need to be injected as with a vial.

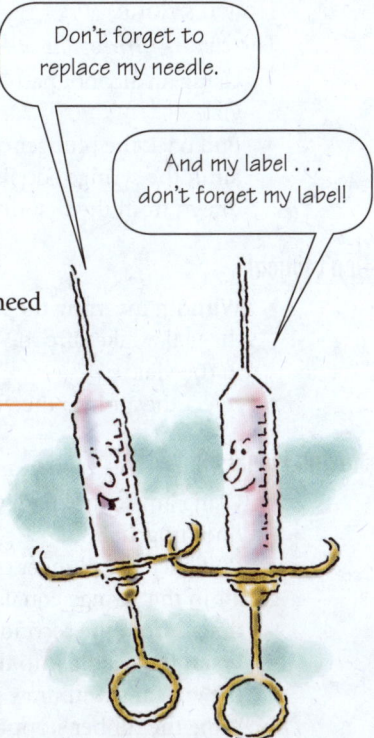

Don't forget to replace my needle.

And my label . . . don't forget my label!

Combining drugs in a syringe

Combining two drugs in one syringe or cartridge avoids the discomfort of two separate injections. Typically, drugs can be combined from:

- two multidose vials (as with regular and long-acting insulin, for example)
- one multidose vial and one ampule
- two ampules
- a multidose vial or an ampule into a partially filled cartridge injection system.

Bad combinations

Don't combine drugs in a syringe if the drugs are incompatible or if the combined doses exceed the amount of solution that can be absorbed from a single injection site.

Supplies

- drug vials or ampule
- alcohol pads
- syringe
- one or more needles of appropriate size

Getting ready

- Verify the order on the patient's chart.
- Consult the drug guide if you haven't given the drug previously or if you're unfamiliar with the purpose, dosage, contraindications, possible side effects, or nursing considerations.
- Check the MAR and drug allergies.
- Wash your hands.

How it's done

For two multidose vials

- Using an alcohol pad, wipe the rubber stopper on the first vial.
- Pull back the plunger of the syringe until the volume of air in the syringe equals the volume of drug to be withdrawn from the first drug vial.

Don't touch!

- Without inverting the first drug vial, insert the needle into the vial. Make sure the needle tip doesn't touch the liquid in the vial.
- Inject the air into the vial, and then withdraw the needle.

Moving to vial #2...

- Using an alcohol pad, wipe the rubber stopper on the second drug vial.
- Pull back the plunger of the syringe until the volume of air in the syringe equals the volume of drug to be withdrawn from the second vial.
- Insert the needle into the second vial, inject the air, invert the vial, and withdraw the correct amount of drug.
- Wipe the rubber stopper of the first vial again, insert the needle, invert the vial, and withdraw the correct amount of drug.

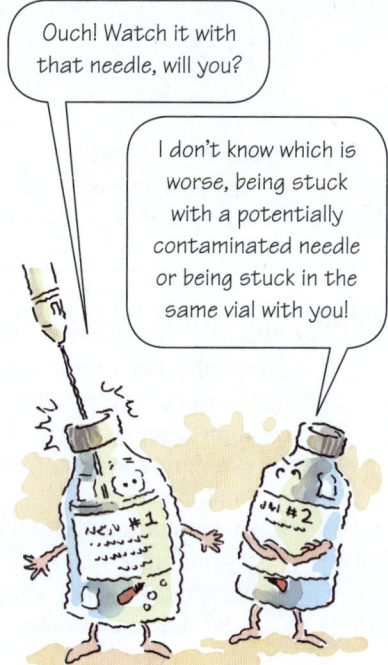

> Ouch! Watch it with that needle, will you?

> I don't know which is worse, being stuck with a potentially contaminated needle or being stuck in the same vial with you!

Change needles, if possible

- Ideally, to avoid contaminating the second drug drawn into the syringe, the needle should be changed on the syringe. In reality, this isn't always possible because many disposable syringes don't have removable needles.
- If possible, replace the needle with a fresh needle before drug administration.

For a multidose vial and ampule

- Wipe the vial's rubber stopper with an alcohol pad, inject an amount of air equal to the drug dose to be given, invert the vial, and withdraw the correct dose.
- Place the sterile cover back on the needle, and place the syringe on the counter.

Bottoming out

- Make sure all of the drug is in the bottom of the ampule, wrap the ampule with a dry 2 × 2-inch gauze pad, and snap the neck of the ampule away from your body.

- Replace the needle on the syringe with a filter needle, insert the needle into the ampule, and withdraw the correct drug dose into the syringe. Be careful not to touch the outside of the ampule with the needle.
- Change back to a regular needle to give the injection.

For two ampules

- Make sure all the fluid is in the bottom of the first ampule, wrap the ampule with a dry 2 × 2-inch gauze pad, and snap the neck of the ampule away from your body.
- Repeat this process for the second ampule.
- Use a filter needle to draw up the required amount of both drugs, one after the other.
- Change to a regular needle to give the injection.

For a cartridge injection system

- If the cartridge has a removable needle with a rubber stopper, gently remove the capped needle from the cartridge to expose the rubber stopper.
- Wipe the rubber stopper with an alcohol pad, and insert the needle of an empty syringe into the partly filled cartridge. Don't let the needle touch the drug inside the cartridge.

Equal volume

- Aspirate from the cartridge a volume of air equal to the volume of drug to be added to the cartridge, then withdraw the needle.
- Draw the correct amount of drug from a vial or an ampule into the syringe.

Rewipe

- Wipe the rubber stopper on the cartridge again, and insert the needle of the syringe into the cartridge.
- Inject the correct amount of compatible drug into the partly filled cartridge.
- Replace the needle on the cartridge using aseptic technique.

In addition...

- If the cartridge doesn't have a rubber stopper, a compatible drug can be added by holding the cartridge needle up, pulling back the plunger until it reaches a level equal to the combined drug volume, and then inserting the needle into an inverted, single-dose drug vial (after cleaning the diaphragm with an alcohol pad). Advance the needle until the tip is above the liquid in the vial. Inject into the vial an amount of air equal to the volume to be withdrawn from the vial, and then pull the needle into the liquid and withdraw the drug into the cartridge. Remove the needle from the vial, expel excess air, and replace the needle guard.

> Always make sure you know the correct amount of air to inject or solution to draw up before taking the plunge with that needle.

Irreconcilable differences

- After mixing drugs in a syringe or cartridge, check for signs of incompatibility, such as discoloration and precipitation.
- Label the drug-filled syringe to finish preparing it for administration.

Practice pointers

- Never combine drugs unless compatibility has been ensured.
- Although drug incompatibility usually causes a visible reaction (such as clouding, bubbling, or precipitation), it may not. Always check a reputable drug reference or ask a pharmacist if unsure about compatibility.

The clock may be ticking

- Some drugs should be given within 15 minutes after they're mixed; ask a pharmacist if unsure about timing.
- To reduce the risk of drug contamination, most facilities dispense parenteral drugs in single-dose vials. Insulin is the main exception. Check your facility's policy before mixing insulins.

Administering intradermal drugs

During intradermal (ID) drug administration, a small amount of liquid (usually 0.5 mL or less) is injected into the outer layers of a patient's skin. A substance administered in this way undergoes little systemic absorption.

Identifying ID

The ID route is used to deliver substances that test for allergies and tuberculosis (TB). It can also be employed to deliver a local anesthetic, such as lidocaine, before the patient undergoes a venipuncture procedure. Although the most common site for ID injection is the ventral forearm, other sites can be used. (See *Intradermal injection sites*.)

Giving an ID injection

ID injections may be used for the following purposes:
- TB testing
- allergy testing
- certain vaccines
- local anesthetics.

Intradermal injection sites

The most common ID injection site is the ventral forearm. Other sites (indicated by dotted areas in these illustrations) include the upper chest, upper arm, and shoulder blades. Skin in these areas is usually lightly pigmented, thinly keratinized, and relatively hairless, facilitating detection of adverse reactions.

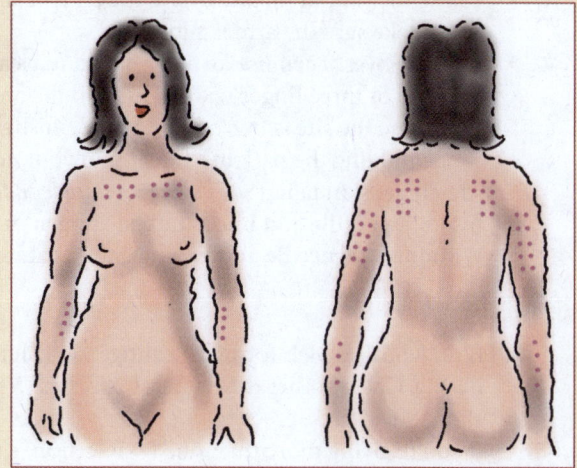

Supplies
- tuberculin syringe with a 26G or 27G needle
- ½- or ⅝-inch needle
- prescribed test antigen (or drug)
- gloves
- marking pen
- alcohol pads

Getting ready
- Verify the order on the patient's chart.
- Consult the drug guide if you haven't given the drug previously or if you're unfamiliar with the purpose, dosage, contraindications, possible side effects, or nursing considerations.
- Check the MAR and drug allergies.
- Check the drug's expiration date.
- Wash your hands.
- Confirm the patient's identity using at least two patient identifiers (not including the patient's room number).

Stand by, please
- Explain the procedure to the patient, and tell the patient to stay nearby for about 30 minutes after the time of injection in case the patient has a severe allergic reaction to it.

How it's done

- Select an injection site.
- To use the ventral forearm, have the patient sit up and extend one arm. Make sure the arm is supported.
- Put on gloves. Then use an alcohol pad to clean the ventral forearm two or three finger-widths distal to the antecubital space. Make sure the site is free of hair and blemishes. Let the skin air dry.
- While holding the patient's forearm in your nondominant hand, stretch the skin taut. (See *Giving an intradermal injection.*)
- Insert the needle and inject the test antigen or drug.
- Withdraw the needle at the same angle that it was inserted.

Missing wheals

- If no wheal or bleb forms, the antigen may have been injected too deeply. Give another dose at least 2 inches (5 cm) from the first site.
- If you're giving more than one ID injection, space them about 2 inches apart.

Keeping track

- Circle and label each test site with a pen so you can track the response to each substance given.
- Dispose of gloves, needles, and syringes according to standard precautions.

Practice pointers

- Be prepared to deal with a possible anaphylactic reaction. (See *Don't get caught off guard.*)

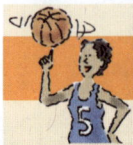

Stay on the ball

Giving an intradermal injection

To give an ID injection, first secure the forearm. Then insert the needle bevel up at a 10° to 15° angle so that it just punctures the skin's surface, as shown. The antigen should raise a small wheal or bleb as it is injected.

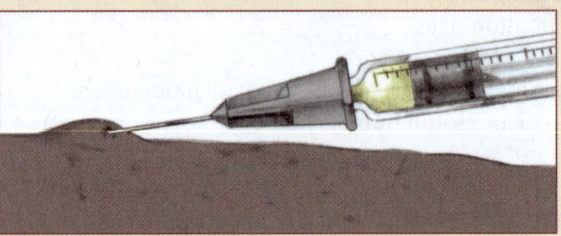

- Notify a health care provider immediately if an allergic reaction occurs.
- Don't rub the site after you give an ID injection. Doing so could irritate the underlying tissue and alter test results.
- Assess the patient's response to the skin testing in 24 to 48 hours.

Check the response

- When interpreting the patient's response, keep in mind that erythema without induration (a hard, raised area) isn't significant. If the test area is indurated, measure the diameter in millimeters (mm).
- Induration of more than 5 mm after a tuberculin test may indicate a positive test result. After allergy tests, induration and erythema of more than 3 mm may indicate a positive result. The larger the affected area, the stronger the allergic reaction.

> ### Don't get caught off guard
>
> A patient who's hypersensitive to the test antigen may have an anaphylactic reaction. Be prepared to inject epinephrine immediately and to perform emergency resuscitation procedures.

Administering subcutaneous drugs

During a subcutaneous (sub-Q) administration, a small amount of liquid drug (usually 0.5 to 2 mL) is injected into the subcutaneous tissue beneath the patient's skin. From there, the drug is absorbed slowly into nearby capillaries.

Steady and safe

Because of the slow absorption, a dose of concentrated drug delivered by sub-Q injection can have a longer duration of action than it would by other injection routes. Plus, sub-Q injection causes little tissue trauma and offers little risk of striking large blood vessels and nerves.

Subcutaneous contraindications

Typically, heparin and insulin are given by sub-Q injection. However, a sub-Q injection is contraindicated in areas that are inflamed, edematous, scarred, or covered by a mole, birthmark, or other lesion. It may also be contraindicated in patients with impaired coagulation.

Giving a subcutaneous injection

Sub-Q administration may be required for:
- heparin
- insulin
- ovulation-stimulating drugs (or fertility drugs).

Supplies

- prepared drug (with an appropriate syringe)
- needle of appropriate size (usually 25G to 27G and ⅝ or ½ inch long)
- gloves
- alcohol pad
- 2 × 2-inch gauze pad

For insulin administration

Insulin infusion pump or sub-Q injector is optional.
(See *Understanding insulin administration aids*.)

Understanding insulin administration aids

With recent advances in insulin administration, patients have insulin delivery options beyond standard sub-Q injections. These include insulin pens, injection ports, sub-Q infusion, or needle-free insulin delivery.

Insulin pen

An insulin pen is a small pen-like device containing a pre-filled insulin cartridge. The dose is given by dialing in the dose amount, attaching a disposable needle, and pressing a button, making this method easy and safe. Advanced technology has led to next-generation and now digitally connected pens. Next-generation pens launched the ability for pens to digitally store memory of previous doses. Connected pens advanced this technology to be shared via Bluetooth, with a smart device to store dosage information and guide future doses (Kesavadev et al., 2020).

Injection port

An injection port is a device that, once inserted and secured, allows insulin injections via syringe or insulin pen through the hub, eliminating needle sticks. The small needle used in the insertion device is removed after insertion, leaving a small, flexible cannula in the skin. The port can stay in place for up to 72 hours. The insertion site should be rotated every 2 to 3 days according to standard precautions. Teach the patient how to recognize and when to report possible problems with the device insertion site.

Subcutaneous infusion

In continuous sub-Q insulin infusion, the patient carries a portable infusion pump that holds insulin and is programmed to deliver precise insulin doses (both baseline and bolus) 24 hours a day. Some insulin pumps allow tracking of daily bolus doses, review of the last 12 alarms, and download of the device's long-term memory.

To deliver the infusion, the patient uses an infusion set, which usually includes an insertion device, a sub-Q needle, and a protective dressing. The patient inserts a 25G to 27G sub-Q needle into the abdomen, thigh, or arm according to the kit instructions. The insertion site should be rotated every 2 to 3 days according to standard precautions. Teach the patient how to recognize and when to report possible problems with the device insertion site.

A continuous insulin infusion pump can work in concert with a diabetes management program or phone application (app) and continuous glucose monitor. This combination is often referred to as an artificial pancreas because it mimics the function of a healthy pancreas (Kesavadev, et al., 2020).

Needle-free insulin delivery

There are two types of needle-free insulin delivery (Kesavadev et al., 2020):

- **A jet injection system** is a needle-free insulin delivery method using a device that looks something like a syringe without a needle. When the patient holds the device against the skin surface and discharges it, with the assistance of air pressure, a thin column of insulin penetrates the skin and disperses within the subcutaneous tissue.
- **An insulin inhaler** uses set-dose cartridges of powdered insulin. The patient selects the appropriate dose by choosing a cartridge or combination of cartridges. The cartridge is placed in the inhaler device, which creates access to the powder inside. The patient then inhales the powder, which is then absorbed in the lungs.

Getting ready

- Verify the order on the patient's chart.
- Consult the drug guide if you haven't given the drug previously or if you're unfamiliar with the purpose, dosage, contraindications, possible side effects, or nursing considerations.
- Check the MAR and drug allergies.
- Check the drug's color, clarity, and expiration date.
- Confirm the patient's identity using at least two patient identifiers (not including the patient's room number).
- Explain the procedure to the patient.
- Select an appropriate injection site. (See *Sub-Q injection sites.*)

Chill out

- Before giving the injection, you may apply a cold compress to the injection site to minimize pain.
- Wash your hands and put on gloves.

How it's done

- Position and drape the patient, if necessary.

Bubble trouble

- If giving insulin, gently invert and roll the vial to mix the drug. Don't shake the vial, because air bubbles could get into the syringe and reduce the dose given.

Sub-Q injection sites

Potential sub-Q injection sites (as indicated by the dotted areas in these illustrations) include the fat pads on the abdomen, upper hips, upper back, and lateral upper arms and thighs.

Preferred injection sites for insulin are the arms, abdomen, thighs, and buttocks. The preferred injection site for heparin is the lower abdominal fat pad, just below the umbilicus.

When repeated, rotate

For sub-Q injections administered repeatedly, such as insulin, rotate the injection sites. Choose one injection site in one area, move to a corresponding injection site in the next area, and so on. When returning to an area, choose a new site in that area.

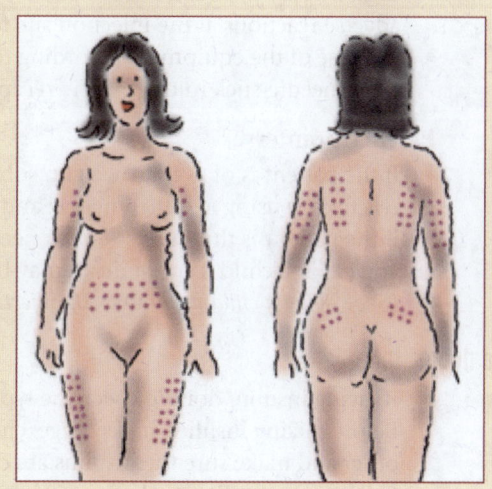

- Clean the injection site with an alcohol pad, starting at the center of the site and moving outward in a circular motion. Let the skin air dry to avoid stinging.
- Remove the protective needle sheath.

Hold the fat

- With your nondominant hand, grasp the skin around the injection site and firmly elevate the subcutaneous tissue to form a fat fold. If the patient is large, the skin may be spread taut rather than forming a fold. (See *Technique for sub-Q injections.*)
- Position the needle with the bevel up, and tell the patient they'll feel a prick.
- Insert the needle quickly at a 45° angle (90° angle for heparin).

Try not to be irritating

- Heparin should be given slowly over 30 seconds to reduce postinjection bruising (Medication administration: Subcutaneous injections, 2023).
- After injection, remove the needle gently but quickly at the same angle used for injection. However, when injecting heparin or insulin, leave the needle in place for 5 seconds and then withdraw it.
- Cover the injection site with a gauze pad, and DO NOT massage if administering heparin or insulin, because doing so may impact absorption or cause bruising.
- Document the medication given.

Just checking

- Check the injection site for bleeding or bruising. If bleeding continues, apply pressure. If a bruise develops, apply ice. Watch for adverse reactions at the injection site for 30 minutes.
- Dispose of the equipment according to standard precautions. To avoid needle-stick injuries, don't recap the needle.

Practice pointers

- If the patient is of average weight, subcutaneous tissue can be reached by using a ½-inch needle and inserting it at a 90° angle; if the patient is thin, use a ⅝-inch needle and insert it at a 45° angle. For a child, certain drugs may be given by the sub-Q route. (See *Giving a child a sub-Q or ID injection.*)

Do a double take

- If giving insulin, double-check the type, unit dose, and syringe. Before mixing insulins in a syringe, check the health care provider's order and make sure the insulins are compatible.
- Follow your facility's policy about which insulin to draw up first. Don't mix insulins of different purities or origins.

<aside>

Technique for sub-Q injections

Before giving a sub-Q injection, elevate the subcutaneous tissue at the site by grasping it firmly, as shown. The needle length and amount of subcutaneous tissue will determine the needle insertion angle (45° or 90° angle) to the skin surface. Some medications, such as heparin, should always be injected at a 90° angle.

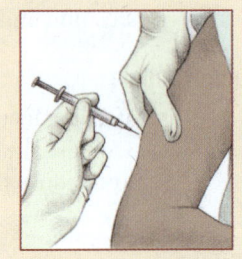

</aside>

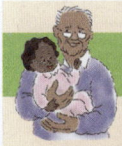

Ages and stages

Giving a child a sub-Q or ID injection

Certain drugs may be administered to children by the sub-Q or ID route. For example, insulin, hormone replacement, allergy desensitization, and some vaccines are given by sub-Q injection. Tuberculin testing, local anesthesia, and allergy testing are given by ID injection. The procedure for sub-Q or ID injection differs little from that used for an adult patient.

In a child, subcutaneous tissue can be reached by using a ⅝-inch needle and inserting it at a 45° angle.

Remember to rotate

- As with insulin, if giving repeated sub-Q injections, rotate the injection sites.
- Don't administer heparin injections within 2 inches (5 cm) of a scar, a bruise, the umbilicus or the belt line.
- Don't massage the site when giving insulin or heparin.
- Teach the patient the correct way to give a sub-Q injection if they need to self-administer insulin or other injections at home. (See *Teaching about sub-Q injections.*)
- Teach all patients, but especially older adults, how to use adherence aids. (See *Using adherence aids*, page 248.)

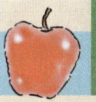

Education corner

Teaching about sub-Q injections

- If the patient will be giving their own sub-Q injections at home, teach them the correct way to perform the procedure. Send home written instructions to support teaching.
- Inform the patient that different brands of syringes have differing amounts of space between the bottom line and the needle. Suggest that the health care provider or pharmacist is notified if they change the brand of syringe used.

Administering intramuscular drugs

An intramuscular (IM) injection deposits a drug deep into muscle tissue that's richly supplied with blood. As a result, the injected drug moves rapidly into the systemic circulation. Other advantages include:

- bypassing damaging digestive enzymes
- relatively little pain (because muscle tissue contains few sensory nerves)
- delivery of a relatively large volume of the drug (the usual dose is 3 mL or less, but up to 5 mL may be given in a large muscle).

Be able to identify the candidate for IM

Children, older adults, or thin people may tolerate less than 2 mL. For some drugs, IM injections may be given using a Z-track technique or a needle-free injection system.

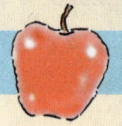

Using adherence aids

To help each patient safely comply with injectable drug therapy, a trained caregiver can premeasure doses for them using adherence aids, such as the ones shown here. Most pharmacies or community service agencies can supply similar aids.

Syringe-filling device

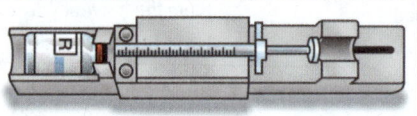

A syringe-filling device precisely measures insulin doses for a visually impaired person with diabetes. Designed for use with a disposable U-100 syringe and an insulin bottle, the device is set by the caregiver to accommodate the syringe's width. The patient then positions the plunger at the point determined by the dose and tightens the stop. When the device is set, they can draw up the precise dose ordered for each injection.

Drawbacks
The device has a few drawbacks:
• It can't be used if insulin must be mixed or if doses vary.

• The settings must be checked and adjusted whenever the syringe size or type is changed.
• The screws must be checked regularly because they loosen with repeated use.

Syringe scale magnifier

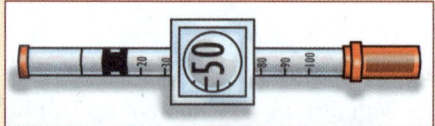

A syringe scale magnifier helps a visually impaired patient with diabetes read syringe markings, thereby enabling them to fill their own syringe. The plastic magnifier snaps onto the syringe barrel.

Drawbacks
This device may be impractical for a patient with arthritis who can't easily attach the magnifier to the syringe.

Giving an IM injection

Some drugs may be given intramuscularly, such as pain medications (opioids), antibiotics, vaccines, or hormones.

Reflection before injection

Some situations prevent IM administration of drugs. (See *Precautions for IM injections.*)

Supplies
• prescribed drug
• 1- to 5-mL syringe
• 18G to 25G needle (a lower gauge for a thicker drug) about 5/8 to 3 inches (2 to 7.5 cm) long, depending on the site used and the amount of fat present
• gloves

Precautions for IM injections

Before giving a patient an IM injection, remember these precautions:

• Don't give IM injections into inflamed, edematous, or irritated sites or sites with moles, birthmarks, scar tissue, or other lesions.

• IM injections may be contraindicated in patients who have impaired coagulation or conditions that hinder peripheral absorption, such as peripheral vascular disease, edema, and hypoperfusion, and during an acute myocardial infarction.

• Never give an IM injection into an immobile limb, because the drug will absorb poorly, and a sterile abscess could develop.

- alcohol pads or an alcohol pad and a 2 × 2-inch gauze pad
- a small bandage

Sold separately

The needle may be packaged separately, or it may come attached to the syringe. Choose a needle length that will deliver the medication deep into the muscle. This will vary based on the patient's size and amount of body fat. Usually, a 1½- to 2-inch needle will be used. All equipment must be sterile.

Getting ready

- Verify the order on the patient's chart.
- Consult the drug guide if you haven't given the drug previously or if you're unfamiliar with the purpose, dosage, contraindications, possible side effects, or nursing considerations.
- Check the MAR and drug allergies.
- Reconstitute the drug, if necessary; then, check the drug's color, clarity, and expiration date.
- Draw the correct amount into the syringe.
- Confirm the patient's identity using at least two patient identifiers (not including the patient's room number).
- Explain the procedure to the patient.
- Wash your hands.

Muscling up

- If the patient is an adult, consider using the ventrogluteal, vastus lateralis, or deltoid muscle. (It is recommended to not use other sites due to the risk of complications with nerves and blood vessels that could be present.) (See *Locating IM injection sites*, page 250.)
- If the patient is an infant or a child, consider using the vastus lateralis muscle. (See *IM injection sites in infants and children*, page 251.)
- If the patient is an older adult, additional points need to be considered. (See *IM injections in older adult patients*, page 252.)

Locating IM injection sites

The most common IM injection sites used in adults are discussed below.

Deltoid

Find the lower edge of the acromial process and the point on the lateral arm in line with the axilla. Insert the needle 1 to 2 inches (2.5 to 5 cm) below the acromial process, usually two or three finger widths, at a 90° angle or angled slightly toward the process.

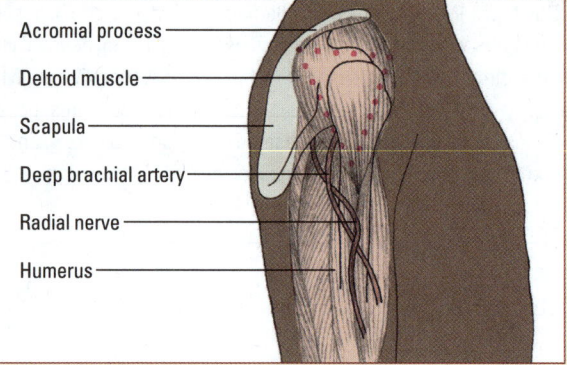

- Acromial process
- Deltoid muscle
- Scapula
- Deep brachial artery
- Radial nerve
- Humerus

Ventrogluteal

The greater trochanter of the femur should be located with the heel of the hand. Spread your index and middle fingers from the anterior superior iliac spine to as far along the iliac crest as you can reach. Insert the needle between the two fingers at a 90° angle to the muscle. (Remove your fingers before inserting the needle.)

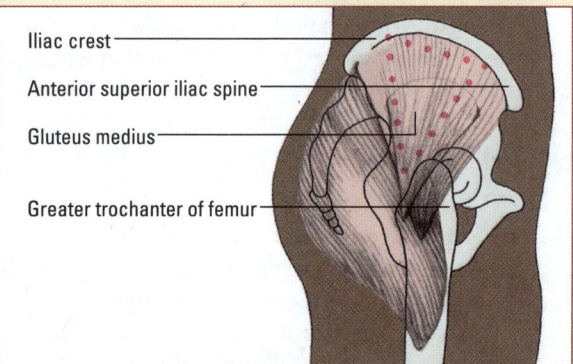

- Iliac crest
- Anterior superior iliac spine
- Gluteus medius
- Greater trochanter of femur

Vastus lateralis

Use the lateral muscle of the quadriceps group, from a handbreadth below the greater trochanter to a handbreadth above the knee. Insert the needle into the middle third of the muscle parallel to the surface on which the patient is lying. The muscle may need to be bunched before insertion.

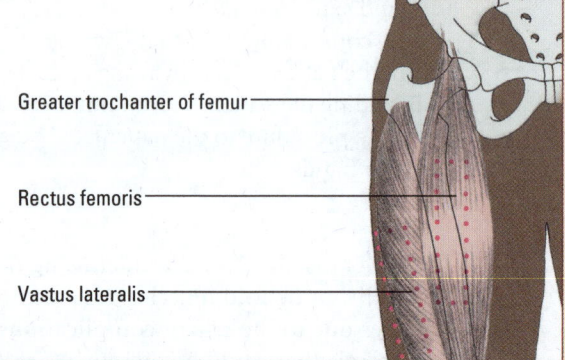

- Greater trochanter of femur
- Rectus femoris
- Vastus lateralis

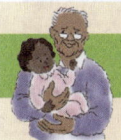

IM injection sites in infants and children

When selecting the best site for a child's IM injection, consider the child's age, weight, and muscular development; the amount of subcutaneous fat over the injection site; the type of drug being administered; and the drug's absorption rate.

Vastus lateralis injections

For a child younger than 3 years, the vastus lateralis muscle is typically used for an IM injection. Constituting the largest muscle mass in this age group, the vastus lateralis has few major blood vessels and nerves.

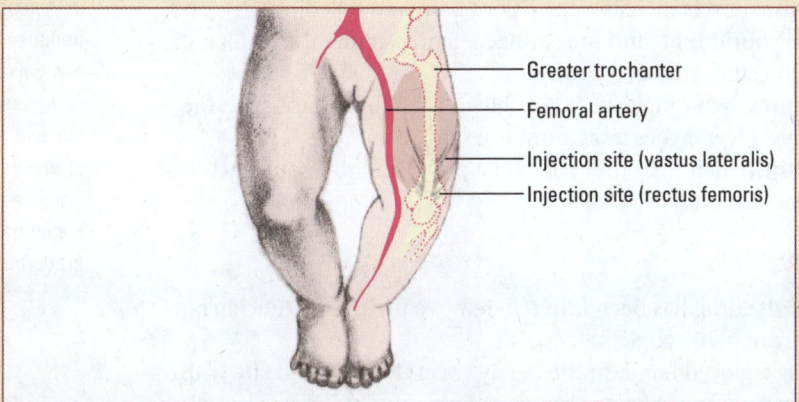

- Greater trochanter
- Femoral artery
- Injection site (vastus lateralis)
- Injection site (rectus femoris)

Ventrogluteal injections

For a child older than 3 years who has been walking for at least 1 year, the ventrogluteal muscle is typically used. This muscle is relatively free of major blood vessels and nerves.

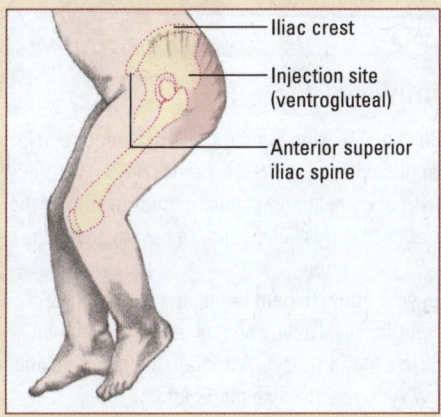

- Iliac crest
- Injection site (ventrogluteal)
- Anterior superior iliac spine

How it's done

- Position and drape the patient so you have easy access to the chosen site. Locate the specific insertion site, and choose the proper needle angle.
- Check the injection site to make sure it has no lumps, depressions, redness, warmth, or bruising.
- Put on gloves.
- Clean the site with an alcohol pad, starting at the center of the site and spiraling outward about 2 inches (5 cm). Let the skin air dry.
- Remove the needle cover, and expel all air bubbles from the syringe.
- Urge the patient to relax the muscle that will receive the injection. A tense muscle increases the risk of pain and bleeding.
- With your thumb and index finger, gently stretch the skin taut at the injection site.
- Position the syringe at a 90° angle to the skin surface, with the needle a few inches away from the skin.
- Tell the patient that they will feel a prick, and then quickly thrust the needle into the muscle.

Quickly yet gently

- After the drug has been injected, remove the needle quickly but gently, at a 90° angle.
- Using a gloved hand, immediately cover the injection site with a gauze pad. Applying pressure is not recommended due to leakage and damage to the tissue.

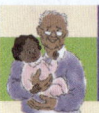

Ages and stages

IM injections in older adults

For older adults, who have less muscle mass, consider using a shorter needle for IM injections in the deltoid. Also, because this population typically has less subcutaneous tissue and more fat around the hips, abdomen, and thighs, consider using the vastus lateralis or ventrolateral area.

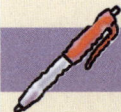

Take note!

Aspiration? It's complicated.

• Aspirating for blood before giving an injection is no longer standard practice unless the injection is to be given in the dorsogluteal site (Kim & De Jesus, 2022). This site is not recommended because of the risk of complications due to the proximity of the gluteal artery, but if no other appropriate site is possible, aspirate before giving the injection at this site. Here is how:

— While supporting the syringe with your nondominant hand, use your dominant hand to aspirate for blood. (Check your facility's policy on this protocol.) If blood appears in the syringe, the needle is in a blood vessel. Withdraw it, discard it, and prepare another injection with a new syringe and fresh medication.

— If no blood is aspirated, then inject the drug slowly and steadily into the muscle, allowing the muscle to distend and accept the drug gradually. Little or no resistance should be felt.

Inspection of injection

- Remove the gauze pad, and inspect the site for bleeding or bruising. If bleeding continues, apply pressure. If a bruise develops, apply ice. Watch for adverse reactions at the site for 30 minutes after the time of injection.
- Discard all equipment according to standard precautions.
- Document the medication.

Practice pointers

- If the patient complains of pain and anxiety from repeated IM injections, numb the site with ice or other cooling techniques for several seconds before giving the injection. Note that ice is not shown to be effective at reducing pain at injection sites for children (Hall et al., 2020).
- If more than 5 mL of drug needs to be injected, split it between two different sites.

A pinch of gentleness

- If the patient is extremely thin, pinch the muscle gently to elevate it, so the needle isn't pushed completely through the muscle.
- For an infant or toddler, use a 22G to 25G, ½- to 1-inch needle. Also, don't exceed recommended volumes when giving the injection. (See *Adapting injections for children.*)
- Older adult patients have a higher risk of hematoma and may need direct pressure over the puncture site for a longer time than usual.

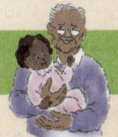

Ages and stages

Adapting injections for children

When giving an IM injection to a child, you'll need to adapt your approach to accommodate the child's age. This table serves as a guide for the appropriate site and needle size selection.

Age Group	Site and Needle Options
Newborns (0–28 days)	Vastus lateralis: 5/8-inch, 22–25 gauge
Infants (1–12 months) and toddlers (1–2 years)	Vastus lateralis: 1 inch, 22–25 gauge
Children (3–10 years)	Deltoid: 5/8 to 1 inch, 22–25 gauge Vastus lateralis: 1 inch, 22–25 gauge
Preteens and teens (11–18 years)	Deltoid: 5/8 to 1 inch, 22–25 gauge Vastus lateralis: 1 to 1 ½ inch, 22–25 gauge

Source: Wexler, D. (2020). Choosing proper needle length for vaccination of children and adults: what should you consider? Technically Speaking. https://www.immunize.org/technically-speaking/20200721.asp

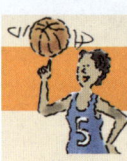

IM injection complications

Accidentally injecting concentrated or irritating medications into subcutaneous tissue or other areas where they can't be fully absorbed can cause sterile abscesses to develop.

In addition, failing to rotate sites in patients who require repeated injections can lead to deposits of unabsorbed medications. Such deposits can reduce the desired pharmacologic effect and may lead to abscess formation or tissue fibrosis.

Remember to rotate

- Rotate sites if the patient needs repeated injections.
- Prevent complications associated with IM injections. (See *IM injection complications.*)

Giving a Z-track injection

Z-track injection is a method of displacing the tissues before inserting the needle for an IM injection. Afterward, restoring the tissues to their normal positions traps the drug inside the muscle. The purpose of this technique is to reduce the risk of leakage or irritation to the subcutaneous tissue.

Supplies

- prescribed drug
- syringe of appropriate size
- two needles (one of which should be an appropriate length to administer the medication deep into the patient's muscle)
- alcohol pads
- 2 × 2-inch gauze pad
- gloves

Getting ready

- Verify the order on the patient's chart.
- Consult the drug guide if you haven't given the drug previously or if you're unfamiliar with the purpose, dosage, contraindications, possible side effects, or nursing considerations.
- Check the MAR and drug allergies.
- Reconstitute the drug as needed. Check the drug's color, clarity, and expiration date.
- Draw the correct amount into the syringe.

- After drawing up the ordered dose, replace the original needle with a sterile one that's an appropriate length for the patient.
- Confirm the patient's identity using at least two patient identifiers (not including the patient's room number).
- Explain the procedure to the patient.
- Wash your hands and put on gloves.

How it's done

- Select an injection site.
- Use an alcohol pad to clean the site, starting at the center and spiraling outward about 2 inches (5 cm). Let the skin air dry.

The straight skinny

- Place the index finger of one hand on the injection site, and drag the skin about 1 inch (2.5 cm) to one side.
- Insert the needle at a 90° angle into the site where the finger was originally placed.
- Inject the drug, and withdraw the needle.
- Then release the skin, allowing the displaced layers to return to their original positions. (See *Displacing the skin for Z-track injection.*)

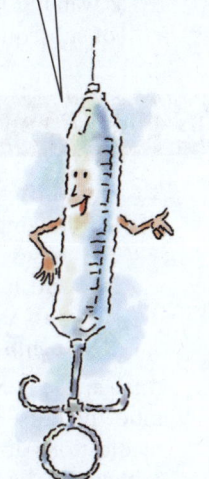

Administering using a Z-track helps the drugs to stay put!

Displacing the skin for Z-track injection

Discomfort and tissue irritation may result from drug leakage into subcutaneous tissue. Displacing the skin helps prevent these problems. By blocking the needle pathway after injection, the Z-track technique allows IM injection while minimizing the risk of subcutaneous irritation, staining, or leaking.

How to do it

To begin, place a finger on the skin surface, and pull the skin and subcutaneous layers out of alignment with the underlying muscle, as shown below. The skin should be moved about 1 inch (2.5 cm).

Insert the needle at a 90° angle at the site where the finger was initially placed, as shown below. Inject the drug and withdraw the needle.

Lastly, remove the finger from the skin surface, allowing the layers to return to their normal positions. The needle track (shown by the dotted line below) is now broken at the junction of each tissue layer, trapping the drug in the muscle.

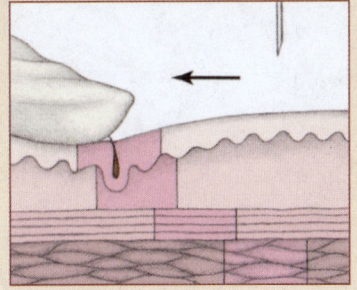
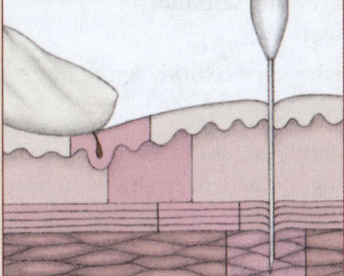
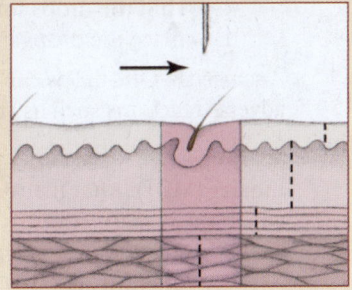

Practice pointers

- Never massage a Z-track injection site because this could cause irritation or force the drug into subcutaneous tissue.
- To increase the rate of absorption, encourage such physical activity as walking.
- For subsequent injections, alternate sites.

Quick quiz

1. Administering oral tablets through a gastric tube requires which of the following additional steps? (**Select all that apply.**)
   A. assess for gastric placement of the tube
   B. crush the tablets using an appropriate crushing device
   C. mix the crushed medications with normal saline
   D. confirm that the medications can be crushed

Answer: A, B, and D. Before giving an oral tablet through a gastric tube, the nurse must confirm that the tablets can be crushed; some medications do not have the intended effect if they are crushed. Tablets may be crushed using an appropriate crushing device and mixed with water for administration. Additionally, before giving any medications through a gastric tube, the placement of the tube must be verified, because it may have migrated.

2. The nurse is preparing to give a patient a dose of transdermal nitroglycerin. Which step should **NOT** be completed?
   A. Apply the prescribed amount of ointment to the measuring paper
   B. Wash the site with soap and warm water
   C. Remove any previously applied dose of the same drug
   D. Shave the site to remove excess hair

Answer: D. To remove excess hair, be sure to clip, not shave. Shaving can cause irritation, which could be exacerbated by the medication.

3. Before instilling otic medication drops, the nurse should:
   A. add dye to the drops to detect leakage
   B. warm the drops to body temperature
   C. chill the drops for a cooling sensation
   D. place the drops in a syringe

Answer: B. Otic drops can be warmed to body temperature to avoid adverse reactions such as vertigo or pain.

4. The nurse is teaching an adult patient to use a metered-dose inhaler (MDI). After instructing the patient to shake the canister well, which set of instructions is correct?
   A. Place your lips around the opening of the MDI. Compress the canister once to release the dose. Take three quick breaths.

B. Place your lips around the opening of the MDI. Compress the canister twice to release the dose, and breathe as deeply as possible.

C. Place your lips around the opening of the MDI. Compress the canister once to release the dose. Inhale slowly, then hold your breath for 10 seconds. Exhale slowly with pursed lips.

D. Place your lips around the opening of the MDI. Compress the canister twice to release the dose. Hold your breath for 5 seconds and exhale quickly and forcefully.

Answer: C. The patient should seal their lips around the mouthpiece of the MDI as they compress the canister only once. The patient should then inhale slowly, hold their breath for 10 seconds, and exhale slowly through pursed lips. This method provides an accurate dose as well as optimal drug absorption.

5. A drug is being administered to an adult patient from an ampule for intramuscular injection. What equipment will be needed?

A. Medication ampule, gauze pad, 3-mL syringe, filter needle, 1-inch needle for injecting the drug, alcohol pad, a small bandage

B. Medication ampule, gauze pad, 1-mL syringe, filter needle, 1-inch needle for injecting the drug, alcohol pad, a small bandage

C. Medication ampule, gauze pad, 5-mL syringe, 2-inch needle for injecting the drug, alcohol pad, a small bandage

D. Medication ampule, gauze pad, 1-mL syringe, 5/8-inch needle for injecting the drug, alcohol pad, a small bandage

Answer: A. The drug will be drawn up from an ampule, which means the ampule as well as a gauze pad, will be needed for protection. A filter needle will be needed to strain out glass particles when drawing up the drug. For administration, an alcohol pad will be required to clean the site. An intramuscular injection can be given in a 3- to 5-mL syringe with a 1- to 3-inch needle.

6. A nurse is administering 16 units of regular insulin to a patient with diabetes. Which means of administration are acceptable? (**Select all that apply**.)

A. Draw up 16 units of regular insulin in a 1-mL syringe. Inject the insulin intradermally.

B. Dial up 16 units on the patient's regular insulin pen. Attach the needle, and inject the insulin subcutaneously.

C. Draw up 16 units of regular insulin in an insulin syringe. Inject the insulin subcutaneously.

D. Draw up 16 units of regular insulin in a 1-mL syringe. Attach a 1-inch needle, and inject the insulin intramuscularly.

Answer: B and C. Insulin may be injected via an insulin pen or an insulin syringe. Insulin may also be administered in the following ways: infusion pump, injection port, and needle-free delivery.

Scoring

 If you answered all six questions correctly, sensational! Needle-less to say, you're in the top of your class!

 If you answered four to five questions correctly, great! You absorbed the material well.

 If you answered fewer than three questions correctly, it looks like you might need a shot in the arm. Review the chapter, and you'll soon feel sharp!

References

American Academy of Pediatrics (AAP). (2022). *How to give ear drops to a child.* https://www.healthychildren.org/English/safety-prevention/at-home/medication-safety/Pages/How-to-Give-Ear-Drops.aspx

American Lung Association (ALA). (2022). *How to use a metered-dose inhaler without a valved holding chamber or spacer.* https://www.lung.org/lung-health-diseases/lung-disease-lookup/asthma/treatment/devices/metered-dose-inhaler-chamber-spacer-mask

American Society of Ophthalmic Registered Nurses (ASORN). (2022). *ASORN recommended practice: Use of multi-dose medications.* https://asorn.org/assets/Use-of-Multi-dose-Medications.pdf

Gudgel D. T. (2021). *How to put in eye drops.* American Academy of Ophthalmology. https://www.aao.org/eye-health/treatments/how-to-put-in-eye-drops

Hall L. M., Ediriweera Y., Banks J., Nambiar A., & Heal C. (2020). Cooling to reduce the pain associated with vaccination: A systematic review. *Vaccine*, 38(51), 8082–8089. https://doi.org/10.1016/j.vaccine.2020.11.005

Jeong W. Y., Kwon M., Choi H. E., & Kim K. S. (2021). Recent advances in transdermal drug delivery systems: A review. *Biomaterials Research*, 25(1), 1–15. https://doi.org/10.1186/s40824-021-00226-6

Kc B., Khan G. M., & Shrestha N. (2020). Nasal spray use technique among patients attending the outpatient department of a tertiary care hospital, Gandaki Province, Nepal. *Integrated Pharmacy Research and Practice*, 9, 155–160. https://doi.org/10.2147/IPRP.S266191

Kesavadev J., Saboo B., Krishna M. B., & Krishnan G. (2020). Evolution of insulin delivery devices: From syringes, pens, and pumps to DIY artificial pancreas. *Diabetes Therapy*, 11(6), 1251–1269. https://doi.org/10.1007/s13300-020-00831-z

Kim J., & De Jesus O. (2022). *Medication routes of administration.* StatPearls. StatPearls Publishing. https://www.ncbi.nlm.nih.gov/books/NBK568677/

Medication administration: Subcutaneous injections. (2023). Elsevier - Clinical Skills. https://elsevier.health/en-US/preview/medication-administration-subcutaneous-injection-hhc

Pereira R. A., de Souza F. B., Rigobello M. C. G., Pereira J. R., da Costa L. R. M., & Gimenes F. R. E. (2020). Quality improvement programme reduces errors in oral medication preparation and administration through feeding tubes. *BMJ Open Quality*, 9(1), e000882. https://doi.org/10.1136/bmjoq-2019-000882

Smith L., Leggett C., & Borg C. (2022). Administration of medicines to children: A practical guide. *Australian Prescriber*, 45(6), 188–192. https://doi.org/10.18773/austprescr.2022.067

Taylor C., Lynn P., & Bartlett J. L. (2023). *Fundamentals of nursing* (10th ed.). Wolters Kluwer.

Usgaonkar U., Zambaulicar V., & Shetty A. (2021). Subjective and objective assessment of the eye drop instillation technique: A hospital-based cross-sectional study. *Indian Journal of Ophthalmology*, 69(10), 2638–2642. https://doi.org/10.4103/ijo.IJO_3333_20

Vallerand A. H., & Sanoski C. A. (2021). *Davis's drug guide for nurses* (17th ed.). F.A. Davis.

Wexler D. (2020). *Choosing proper needle length for vaccination of children and adults: What should you consider?* Technically Speaking. https://www.immunize.org/technically-speaking/20200721.asp

Chapter 11

Intravenous therapy

Just the facts

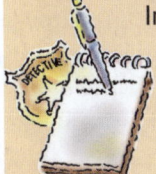

In this chapter, you'll learn:

♦ uses of IV therapy

♦ IV delivery methods

♦ IV infusion rates

♦ legal and professional standards governing the use of IV therapy

♦ patient teaching regarding IV therapy

♦ proper procedures for documenting IV therapy.

A look at IV therapy

Administration of fluids, medications, and blood products to patients is an essential nursing function. During intravenous (IV) therapy, liquid solutions are introduced directly into the patient's bloodstream.

IV therapy is used to:

* restore and maintain fluid and electrolyte balance
* provide medications and chemotherapeutic agents
* transfuse blood and blood products
* deliver parenteral nutrition and nutritional supplements.

Benefits of IV therapy

IV therapy has numerous benefits. For example, it can be used to administer fluids, drugs, nutrients, and other solutions when a patient can't take oral substances.

Accurate and fast

IV drug delivery also allows more accurate dosing. When a drug is administered via the IV route, it reaches the bloodstream immediately and begins to act almost instantaneously.

Disadvantages of IV therapy

Like other invasive procedures, IV therapy has its downside. Risks include:

- bleeding
- blood vessel damage
- infiltration (infusion of the IV solution into surrounding tissue rather than the blood vessel)
- infection
- overdose (because the response to IV drugs is more rapid)
- incompatibility when drugs and IV solutions are mixed
- adverse or allergic responses to infused substances.

Patient activity can also be problematic. Simple tasks, such as transferring to a chair, ambulating, and washing oneself, can become complicated when the patient must cope with IV poles, IV lines, and dressings. Finally, IV therapy is more costly than oral, subcutaneous, or intramuscular (IM) methods of delivering medications.

Fluids, electrolytes, and IV therapy

One of the primary objectives of IV therapy is to restore and maintain fluid and electrolyte balance. A quick review of some fluid and electrolyte basics will help set the stage for understanding how IV therapy works.

Water, water everywhere...

The human body is composed largely of liquid. These fluids account for about 60% of total body weight in an adult and about 80% of total body weight in an infant.

Solvents and solutes

Body fluids are composed of water (a solvent) and dissolved substances (solutes). The solutes in body fluids include electrolytes (such as sodium) and nonelectrolytes (such as proteins).

Fluid functions

Body fluids provide the following functions:

- regulation of body temperature
- transportation of nutrients throughout the body
- movement of cellular waste products to excretion sites.

Aim for the optimum

When fluid levels are optimal, the body performs swimmingly; however, when fluid levels deviate from an acceptable range, organs and systems can quickly become swamped or parched.

Inside and outside

Body fluids exist in two major compartments: inside the cells and outside the cells. Normally, the distribution of fluids between the two compartments is constant. Fluid is classified by whether it's inside or outside:

- intracellular fluid (ICF)—the fluid inside the cells, which is about 55% of the total body fluid
- extracellular fluid (ECF)—accounts for the rest of the body fluid.

The ABCs of ECF

ECF occurs in two forms: interstitial fluid (ISF) and intravascular fluid. ISF surrounds each cell of the body; even bone cells are bathed in it. Intravascular fluid is blood plasma, the liquid component of blood. It surrounds red blood cells and accounts for most of the blood volume.

In an adult, about 5% of body fluid is intravascular ECF; about 15% is interstitial ECF. Part of that interstitial ECF is transcellular fluid, which includes cerebrospinal fluid and lymph. Transcellular fluid contains secretions from the salivary glands, pancreas, liver, and sweat glands.

A balancing act

Maintaining fluid balance in the body involves the kidneys, heart, liver, adrenal and pituitary glands, and nervous system. This balancing act is affected by:

- fluid volume
- distribution of fluids in the body
- concentration of solutes in the fluid.

Gains = Losses

Every day, the body gains and loses fluid. To maintain fluid balance, the gains must equal the losses. (See *Daily fluid gains and losses*.)

Hormones at work

Fluid volume and concentration are regulated by the interaction of two hormones: antidiuretic hormone (ADH) and aldosterone. ADH, sometimes referred to as the *water-conserving hormone*, affects fluid volume and concentration by regulating water retention. It's secreted when plasma osmolarity increases or circulating blood volume decreases, and blood pressure drops. Aldosterone acts to

Daily fluid gains and losses

The body gains and loses fluid through several different processes. This illustration shows the main sites involved. The amounts shown apply to adults; infants exchange a greater amount of fluid than adults.

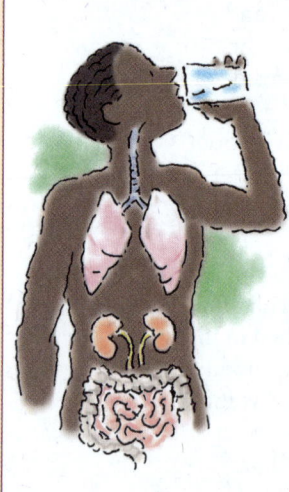

**Daily total intake —
2,400 to 3,200 mL**
- Liquids — 1,400 to 1,800 mL
- Water in foods (solid) — 700 to 1,000 mL
- Water of oxidation (combined water and oxygen in the respiratory system) —300 to 400 mL

**Daily total output —
2,400 to 3,200 mL**
- Lungs (respiration) — 600 to 800 mL
- Skin (perspiration) — 300 to 500 mL
- Kidneys (urine) — 1,400 to 1,800 mL
- Intestines (feces) — 100 mL

retain sodium and water. It's secreted when the serum sodium level is low, the potassium level is high, or the circulating volume of fluid decreases.

Thirsty?

The thirst mechanism (awareness of the desire to drink) also regulates water volume and participates with hormones in maintaining fluid balance. Thirst is experienced when water loss equals 2% of body weight or when osmolarity (solute concentration) increases by 2% to 3% (Lukitsch, 2023). Drinking water restores plasma volume and dilutes ECF osmolarity.

Picking out the baseline

It's important to establish the patient's baseline fluid status before starting fluid replacement therapy. During IV therapy, changes in fluid status alert the nurse to impending fluid imbalances. (See *Identifying fluid imbalances*, page 265.)

Identifying fluid imbalances

By carefully assessing a patient before and during IV therapy, fluid imbalances can be identified before serious complications develop. The following assessment findings and test results indicate fluid deficit or excess.

Fluid deficit
- Weight loss
- Increased, thready pulse rate
- Diminished blood pressure, commonly with orthostatic hypotension
- Decreased central venous pressure
- Sunken eyes, dry conjunctivae, decreased tearing
- Poor skin turgor (not a reliable sign in older adult patients)
- Pale, cool skin
- Poor capillary refill (more than 2 to 3 seconds)
- Lack of moisture in groin and axillae
- Thirst
- Decreased salivation
- Dry mouth
- Dry, cracked lips
- Furrows in the tongue
- Difficulty forming words (patient needs to moisten mouth first)
- Mental status changes
- Weakness
- Diminished urine output
- Increased hematocrit
- Increased serum electrolyte levels
- Increased blood urea nitrogen (BUN) levels
- Increased serum osmolarity

Fluid excess
- Weight gain
- Elevated blood pressure
- Bounding pulse that isn't easily obliterated
- Jugular vein distention
- Increased respiratory rate
- Dyspnea
- Moist crackles or rhonchi on auscultation
- Edema of dependent body parts; sacral edema in patients who are on bed rest; edema of feet and ankles in patients who are ambulatory
- Generalized edema
- Puffy eyelids
- Periorbital edema
- Slow emptying of hand veins when the arm is raised
- Decreased hematocrit
- Decreased serum electrolyte levels
- Decreased BUN levels
- Reduced serum osmolarity

Electrolytes

Electrolytes are a major component of body fluid. There are six major electrolytes:
- sodium
- potassium
- calcium
- chloride
- phosphorus
- magnesium.

All charged up

As the name implies, electrolytes are associated with electricity. These vital substances are chemical compounds that dissociate in solution into electrically charged particles called *ions*. Like wiring for the body, the electrical charges of ions conduct current that's necessary for normal cell function. (See *Understanding electrolytes*.)

Fluid and electrolyte balance

Fluids and electrolytes are usually discussed together, especially where IV therapy is concerned, because fluid balance and electrolyte balance are interdependent. Any change in one alters the other, and any solution given via IV can affect a patient's fluid and electrolyte balance.

Understanding electrolytes

Six major electrolytes play important roles in maintaining chemical balance: sodium, potassium, calcium, chloride, phosphorus, and magnesium. Electrolyte concentrations are expressed in milliequivalents per liter (mEq/L) and milligrams per deciliter (mg/dL).

Electrolyte	Principal functions	Signs and symptoms of imbalance
Calcium (Ca^{++})		
Major cation found in ECF of teeth and bones **Reference range:** 8.6 to 10.4 mg/dL	• Enhances bone strength and durability (along with P) • Helps maintain cell membrane structure, function, and permeability • Affects activation, excitation, and contraction of cardiac and skeletal muscles • Participates in neurotransmitter release at synapses • Helps activate specific steps in blood coagulation • Activates serum complement in immune system function	*Hypocalcemia:* muscle tremor; muscle cramps; tetany; tonic–clonic seizures; paresthesia; bleeding; arrhythmias; hypotension; numbness or tingling in fingers, toes, and area surrounding the mouth *Hypercalcemia:* lethargy, headache, muscle flaccidity, nausea, vomiting, anorexia, constipation, hypertension, polyuria
Chloride (Cl$^-$)		
Major anion found in ECF **Reference range:** 96 to 104 mEq/L	• Maintains serum osmolarity (along with Na$^-$) • Combines with major cations to create important compounds, such as sodium chloride (NaCl), hydrogen chloride (HCl), potassium chloride (KCl), and calcium chloride (CaCl$_2$)	*Hypochloremia:* increased muscle excitability, tetany, decreased respirations *Hyperchloremia:* stupor; rapid, deep breathing; muscle weakness

(Continued)

Understanding electrolytes *(continued)*

Electrolyte	Principal functions	Signs and symptoms of imbalance
Magnesium (Mg^{++})		
Major cation found in ICF (closely related to Ca^{++} and P) **Reference range**: 1.8 to 2.6 mg/dL with 33% bound protein and remainder as free cations	• Activates intracellular enzymes; active in carbohydrate and protein metabolism • Acts on myoneural vasodilation • Facilitates Na$^-$ and K$^+$ movement across all membranes • Influences Ca^{++} levels	***Hypomagnesemia:*** dizziness, confusion, seizures, tremor, leg and foot cramps, hyperirritability, arrhythmias, vasomotor changes, anorexia, nausea ***Hypermagnesemia:*** drowsiness; lethargy; coma; arrhythmias; hypotension; vague neuromuscular changes (such as tremor); vague GI symptoms (such as nausea); peripheral vasodilation; facial flushing; sense of warmth; slow, weak pulse
Phosphorus (P)		
Major anion found in ICF **Reference range**: 2.7 to 4.5 mg/dL	• Helps maintain bones and teeth • Helps maintain cell integrity • Plays a major role in acid–base balance (as a urinary buffer) • Promotes energy transfer to cells • Plays an essential role in muscle, red blood cell, and neurologic function	***Hypophosphatemia:*** paresthesia (circumoral and peripheral), lethargy, speech defects (such as stuttering or stammering), muscle pain and tenderness ***Hyperphosphatemia:*** renal failure, vague neuroexcitability to tetany and seizures, arrhythmias and muscle twitching with sudden rise in phosphate level
Potassium (K$^+$)		
Major cation in ICF **Reference range**: 3.5 to 5.0 mEq/L	• Maintains cell electroneutrality • Maintains cell osmolarity • Assists in conduction of nerve impulses • Directly affects cardiac muscle contraction • Plays a major role in acid–base balance	***Hypokalemia:*** decreased GI, skeletal muscle, and cardiac muscle function; decreased reflexes; rapid, weak, irregular pulse; muscle weakness or irritability; fatigue; decreased blood pressure; decreased bowel motility; paralytic ileus ***Hyperkalemia:*** cardiac irregularities, muscle weakness; nausea; diarrhea; oliguria; paresthesia (altered sensation) of the face, tongue, hands, and feet
Sodium (Na$^+$)		
Major cation in ECF **Reference range**: 136 to 145 mEq/L	• Maintains appropriate ECF osmolarity • Influences water distribution (with Cl$^-$) • Impacts concentration, excretion, and absorption of potassium and chloride • Helps regulate acid–base balance • Assists nerve- and muscle-fiber impulse transmission	***Hyponatremia:*** muscle weakness, muscle twitching, decreased skin turgor, headache, tremor, seizures, coma ***Hypernatremia:*** thirst; fever; flushed skin; oliguria; disorientation; dry, sticky membranes

Note: Reference ranges are from Fischbach et al. (2022).

Electrolyte balance

Not all electrolytes are distributed evenly. The major intracellular electrolytes are:

- potassium
- phosphorus.

The major extracellular electrolytes are:

- sodium
- chloride.

ICF and ECF contain different electrolytes because the cell membranes separating the two compartments have selective permeability, meaning only certain ions can cross those membranes. Although ICF and ECF contain different solutes, the concentration levels of the two fluids are about equal when balance is maintained.

Extra (cellular) credit

The two ECF components, ISF and intravascular fluid (plasma), have identical electrolyte compositions. Pores in the capillary walls allow electrolytes to move freely between the ISF and plasma, allowing for equal distribution of electrolytes in both substances.

The protein content of ISF and plasma differs, however. ISF doesn't contain proteins because protein molecules are too large to pass through capillary walls. Plasma has a high concentration of proteins.

Fluid movement

Fluid movement is another mechanism that regulates fluid and electrolyte balance.

Ebb and flow

Body fluids are in constant motion. Although separated by membranes, they continually move between the major fluid compartments. In addition to regulating fluid and electrolyte balance, this movement is how nutrients, waste products, and other substances get into and out of cells, organs, and systems.

Fluid movement is influenced by membrane permeability and colloid osmotic and hydrostatic pressures. Balance is maintained when solute and fluid molecules are distributed evenly on each side of the membrane. When this scale is tipped, these molecules are able to restore balance by crossing membranes as needed.

Solute and fluid molecules have several modes for moving through membranes. Solutes move between compartments mainly by:

- diffusion (passive transport)
- active transport.

Fluids (such as water) move between compartments by:

- osmosis
- capillary filtration and reabsorption.

Passive is popular

Most solutes move by diffusion. This means solute molecules move from areas of higher concentration to areas of lower concentration. This change is referred to as "moving down the concentration gradient." The result is an equal distribution of solute molecules. Because diffusion doesn't require energy, it's considered a form of passive transport.

Moving against the gradient

In contrast, during active transport, molecules move from areas of lower concentration to areas of higher concentration. This change, referred to as "moving against the concentration gradient," requires energy in the form of adenosine triphosphate.

In active transport, molecules are moved by physiologic pumps. The most well-known active transport pump is the sodium–potassium pump. It moves sodium ions out of cells to the ECF and potassium ions into cells from the ECF. This pump balances sodium and potassium concentrations.

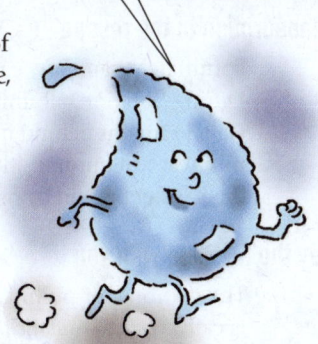

Water moves by osmosis—flowing passively across a membrane from an area of higher concentration to one of lower concentration.

Osmosis

Fluids (particularly water) move by osmosis. The movement of water is caused by the existence of a concentration gradient. Water flows passively across the membrane from an area of higher water concentration to an area of lower water concentration. This dilution process stops when the solute concentrations on both sides of the membrane are equal.

Osmosis between the ECF and ICF depends on the osmolarity (concentration) of the compartments. Normally, the osmotic (pulling) pressures of ECF and ICF are equal.

Equal, yet imbalanced

Osmosis can create a fluid imbalance between the ECF and ICF compartments, despite equal concentrations of solute, if the concentrations aren't optimal. This imbalance can cause complications such as tissue edema.

Up against the capillary wall

Of all the vessels in the vascular system, only capillaries have walls thin enough to let solutes pass. Water and solutes move across capillary walls through two opposing processes:
1. capillary filtration
2. capillary reabsorption.

From high to low

Filtration is the movement of substances from an area of high hydrostatic pressure to an area of lower hydrostatic pressure. (Hydrostatic pressure is the pressure at any level on water at rest due to the weight of water above it.) Capillary filtration forces fluid and solutes through capillary wall pores and into the ISF. Left unchecked, capillary filtration would cause plasma to move in only one direction: out of the capillaries. This movement would cause severe hypovolemia and shock.

Reabsorption to the rescue

Fortunately, capillary reabsorption keeps capillary filtration in check. During filtration, albumin (a protein that can't pass through capillary walls) remains behind in the diminishing volume of water. As the albumin concentration inside the capillaries increases, the albumin begins to draw water back in by osmosis. Water is thus reabsorbed by capillaries.

May the force be with you

The osmotic, or pulling, force of albumin in capillary reabsorption is called *colloid osmotic pressure* or *oncotic pressure*. As long as capillary blood pressure exceeds colloid osmotic pressure, water and diffusible solutes can leave the capillaries and circulate into the ISF. When capillary blood pressure falls below colloid osmotic pressure, water and diffusible solutes return to the capillaries.

Pressure points

In any capillary, blood pressure normally exceeds colloid osmotic pressure up to the vessel's midpoint and then falls below colloid osmotic pressure along the rest of the vessel. That's why capillary filtration takes place along the first half of a capillary and reabsorption occurs along the second half. As long as capillary blood pressure and plasma albumin levels remain normal, no net movement of water occurs. Water is equally lost and gained in this process.

Correcting imbalances

The impact an IV solution has on fluid compartments depends on the solution's osmolarity compared with serum osmolarity.

Osmolarity at parity?

Osmolarity is the concentration of a solution. It's expressed in milliosmoles of solute per liter of solution (mOsm/L). Normally, the serum has the same osmolarity as other body fluids, about 300 mOsm/L. A lower serum osmolarity suggests fluid overload; a higher serum osmolarity suggests hemoconcentration and dehydration.

Bring back the balance

The health care provider may order IV solutions to maintain or restore fluid balance. (See *Understanding IV solutions.*) There are three basic types of IV solutions:

- isotonic
- hypotonic
- hypertonic.

(See *Quick guide to IV solutions.*)

Isotonic solutions

An isotonic solution has the same osmolarity (or tonicity) as serum and other body fluids. Because the solution doesn't alter serum osmolarity, it stays where it's infused, inside the blood vessel (the intravascular compartment). The solution expands this compartment without pulling fluid from other compartments. One indication for an isotonic solution is hypotension due to hypovolemia. Common isotonic solutions include lactated Ringer and normal saline.

Understanding IV solutions

Solutions used for IV therapy may be isotonic, hypotonic, or hypertonic. The selection of the type of fluid given depends on the patient's needs and fluid status.

Isotonic solution	Hypotonic solution	Hypertonic solution

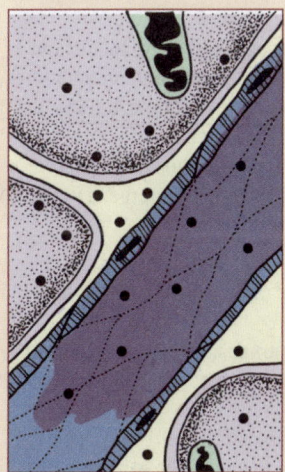 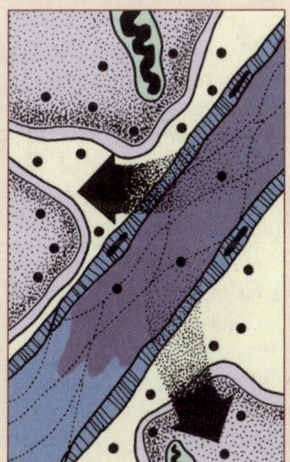 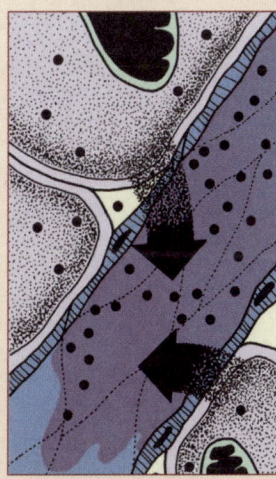

An isotonic solution has an osmolarity about equal to that of serum. Because it stays in the intravascular space, it expands the intravascular compartment.

A hypotonic solution has an osmolarity lower than that of serum. It shifts fluid out of the intravascular compartment, hydrating the cells and the interstitial compartments.

A hypertonic solution has an osmolarity higher than that of serum. It draws fluid into the intravascular compartment from the cells and the interstitial compartments.

Quick guide to IV solutions

A few common solutions can be used to illustrate the role of IV therapy in restoring and maintaining fluid and electrolyte balance. A solution is isotonic if its osmolarity falls within (or near) the normal range for serum (240 to 340 mOsm/L). A hypotonic solution has a lower osmolarity; a hypertonic solution, a higher osmolarity. This chart lists common examples of the three types of IV solutions and provides key considerations for administering them.

Solution	Examples	Nursing considerations
Isotonic	• Lactated Ringer (275 mOsm/L) • Ringer (275 mOsm/L) • Normal saline (308 mOsm/L) • Dextrose 5% in water (D_5W) (260 mOsm/L) • 5% albumin (308 mOsm/L) • Hetastarch (310 mOsm/L) • Normosol (295 mOsm/L)	• Closely monitor the patient for signs of fluid overload because isotonic solutions expand the intravascular compartment. This close monitoring is especially essential if the patient has hypertension or heart failure • Because the liver converts lactate to bicarbonate, don't give lactated Ringer solution if the patient's blood pH exceeds 7.5 • Avoid giving D_5W to a patient at risk for increased intracranial pressure (ICP) because it acts like a hypotonic solution. (Although usually considered isotonic, D_5W is actually isotonic only in the container. After administration, dextrose is quickly metabolized, leaving only water—a hypotonic fluid.) This phenomenon is particularly dangerous in premenopausal people assigned female at birth. Excessive infusion of D_5W in this population can lead to hyponatremia-associated encephalopathy
Hypotonic	• Half-normal saline (154 mOsm/L) • 0.33% sodium chloride (103 mOsm/L) • Dextrose 2.5% in water (126 mOsm/L)	• Administer cautiously. Hypotonic solutions cause a fluid shift from blood vessels into cells. This shift could cause cardiovascular collapse from intravascular fluid depletion and increased ICP from fluid shift into brain cells • Don't give hypotonic solutions to patients at risk for increased ICP from stroke, head trauma, or neurosurgery • Don't give hypotonic solutions to patients at risk for third-space fluid shifts, in which abnormal fluid shifts into the interstitial compartment or a body cavity (for example, patients suffering from burns, trauma, or low serum protein levels from malnutrition or liver disease) • Don't give hypotonic solutions to premenopausal people assigned female at birth, who are at risk of fluid shifts that could increase intracranial pressure
Hypertonic	• Dextrose 5% in half-normal saline (406 mOsm/L) • Dextrose 5% in quarter-normal saline (370 mOsm/L) • Dextrose 5% in normal saline (560 mOsm/L) • Dextrose 5% in lactated Ringer (575 mOsm/L) • 3% sodium chloride (1,025 mOsm/L) • 25% albumin (1,500 mOsm/L) • 7.5% sodium chloride (2,400 mOsm/L)	• Because hypertonic solutions greatly expand the intravascular compartment, administer them by IV pump and closely monitor the patient for circulatory overload • Hypertonic solutions pull fluid from the intracellular compartment, so don't give them to a patient with diabetic ketoacidosis (a condition that causes cellular dehydration) • Don't give hypertonic solutions to a patient with impaired heart or kidney function, due to a diminished ability to handle the extra fluid • Treat albumin as a blood product; therefore, it requires consent to infuse • Although usually considered hypertonic, D_5 1/2 NS and D_5 ¼ NS are hypertonic only for a short time. Soon after initiation of the infusion, the dextrose begins to be metabolized, leaving a solution with an osmolarity of an isotonic solution

Hypertonic solutions

A hypertonic solution has an osmolarity higher than serum osmolarity. When a patient receives a hypertonic IV solution, serum osmolarity initially increases, causing fluid to be pulled from the interstitial and intracellular compartments into the blood vessels.

When, why, and how to get hyper

Hypertonic solutions may be ordered for patients postoperatively because the shift of fluid into the blood vessels caused by a hypertonic solution has several beneficial effects for these patients. For example, it:

- reduces the risk of edema
- stabilizes blood pressure
- regulates urine output.

> A hypertonic solution can be beneficial postoperatively because it helps reduce edema, stabilize blood pressure, and regulate urine output.

Hypotonic solutions

A hypotonic solution has an osmolarity lower than serum osmolarity. When a patient receives a hypotonic solution, fluid shifts out of the blood vessels and into the cells and interstitial spaces, where osmolarity is higher. A hypotonic solution hydrates cells while reducing fluid in the circulatory system.

Hypotonic solutions may be ordered when diuretic therapy dehydrates cells or following the administration of some renal-damaging dyes used for radiological imaging. Other indications include hyperglycemic conditions, such as diabetic ketoacidosis and hyperosmolar hyperglycemic nonketotic syndrome. In these conditions, high serum glucose levels draw fluid out of cells.

Flood warning

Because hypotonic solutions flood cells, certain patients shouldn't receive them. Such patients include those with cerebral edema or increased intracranial pressure (or at risk for increased intracranial pressure). Premenopausal people assigned female at birth shouldn't receive hypotonic solutions because the increased ECF can cause further edema and tissue damage.

Additional uses of IV therapy

In addition to restoring and maintaining fluid and electrolyte balance, IV therapy is used to administer drugs, transfuse blood and blood products, and deliver parenteral nutrition. Because medications delivered via IV enter the bloodstream directly, it's essential that all steps of IV therapy be handled using strict aseptic technique.

Drug administration

The IV route provides a rapid, effective way of administering medications. Commonly infused drugs include antibiotics; thrombolytics; histamine-receptor antagonists; and antineoplastic, cardiovascular, and anticonvulsant drugs.

Drugs may be delivered long term by continuous infusion, over a short period, or directly as a single dose.

Three more rights

IV medications have three additional rights to consider before administration, as follows:

1. The nurse must check the rate of administration.
2. The nurse must check the compatibility of the medication with the fluid that it is being diluted with or infused into.
3. The nurse must check that the medication has been diluted to the recommended concentration.

Please pardon the interruption

If the patient is receiving a noncompatible solution that can be interrupted while the medication is being infused, the nurse can stop the primary solution, flush the IV with normal saline, administer the medication, flush the IV with normal saline, and then restart the primary infusion. This is called the SSASS technique for stop, saline, agent, saline, and start.

Blood administration

A nurse's responsibilities may include giving blood and blood components and monitoring patients receiving transfusion therapy. Blood products can be given through a peripheral or central IV line. Various blood products are given to:

- restore and maintain adequate circulatory volume
- prevent cardiogenic shock
- increase the blood's oxygen-carrying capacity
- maintain hemostasis.

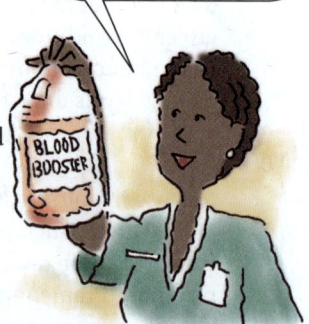

Nursing responsibilities include administration of blood and blood components and monitoring transfusion therapy.

Parts of the whole

Whole blood is composed of cellular elements and plasma. Cellular elements include:

- erythrocytes (red blood cells)
- leukocytes (white blood cells)
- thrombocytes (platelets).

Each of these elements is packaged separately for transfusion. Plasma may be delivered intact or separated into several components that may be given to correct various deficiencies. Whole blood transfusions are unnecessary unless the patient has lost massive quantities of blood (25% to 30%) in a short period.

Parenteral nutrition

When the patient cannot consume or tolerate nutrients in the stomach or intestines, parenteral nutrition provides essential nutrients to the blood, organs, and cells via the IV route. It isn't the same as a seven-course meal in a fine restaurant, but parenteral nutrition can contain the essence of a balanced diet.

Custom menu

Total parenteral nutrition (TPN) is customized for each patient. The ingredients in solutions developed for TPN are designed to meet a patient's energy and nutrient requirements, including:

- proteins
- carbohydrates
- fats
- electrolytes
- vitamins
- trace elements
- water.

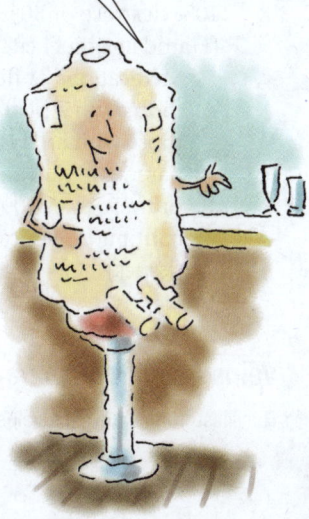

It may not be a gourmet meal, but TPN is packed with all the essential nutrients your patient needs.

Time for TPN?

TPN should be used only when the gastrointestinal (GI) tract is unable to absorb nutrients. A patient can receive TPN indefinitely; however, long-term TPN can cause liver damage.

PPN: A limited menu

Peripheral parenteral nutrition (PPN) is delivered by peripheral veins. PPN is used in limited nutritional therapy. The solution contains fewer nonprotein calories and lower amino acid concentrations than TPN solutions. The concentration of dextrose can be no higher than 10%. Solutions higher than 10% dextrose must be administered via a central line. PPN may also include lipid emulsions. A patient can receive PPN for approximately 3 weeks. It can be used to support the nutritional status of a patient who doesn't require total nutritional support. Complications associated with PPN include the risks of vein damage and infiltration (Berlana, 2022).

Tracking changes

When a patient is receiving parenteral nutrition, keep close track of changes in their fluid and electrolyte status and glucose levels. Assessment of the patient's response to the nutrient solution is also necessary to detect early signs of complications. These may include alterations in the pancreatic enzymes (lipase, amylase trypsin, and chymotrypsin), triglycerides, or albumin.

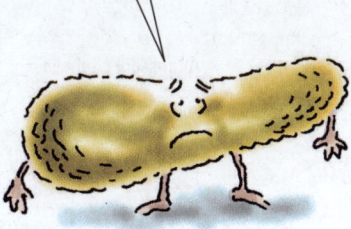

If your patient is receiving parenteral nutrition, please keep a close eye on my enzymes.

IV access and delivery

Depending in part on how concentrated an IV solution is, it may be delivered through a peripheral vein or a central vein. Usually, a low-concentration solution is infused through a peripheral vein in the arm or hand; a more concentrated solution (containing greater than 10% dextrose or 50% protein) must be given through a central vein (Hamdan & Puckett, 2023) (See *Veins used in IV therapy*.)

Medications or fluids that may be administered centrally include:

- those with a pH less than 5 or greater than 9
- those with an osmolarity greater than 500 mOsm/L
- parenteral nutrition formulas containing more than 10% dextrose or more than 50% protein
- continuous vesicant chemotherapy (chemotherapy that's toxic to tissues).

Veins used in IV therapy

This illustration shows the veins commonly used for peripheral and central venous therapy.

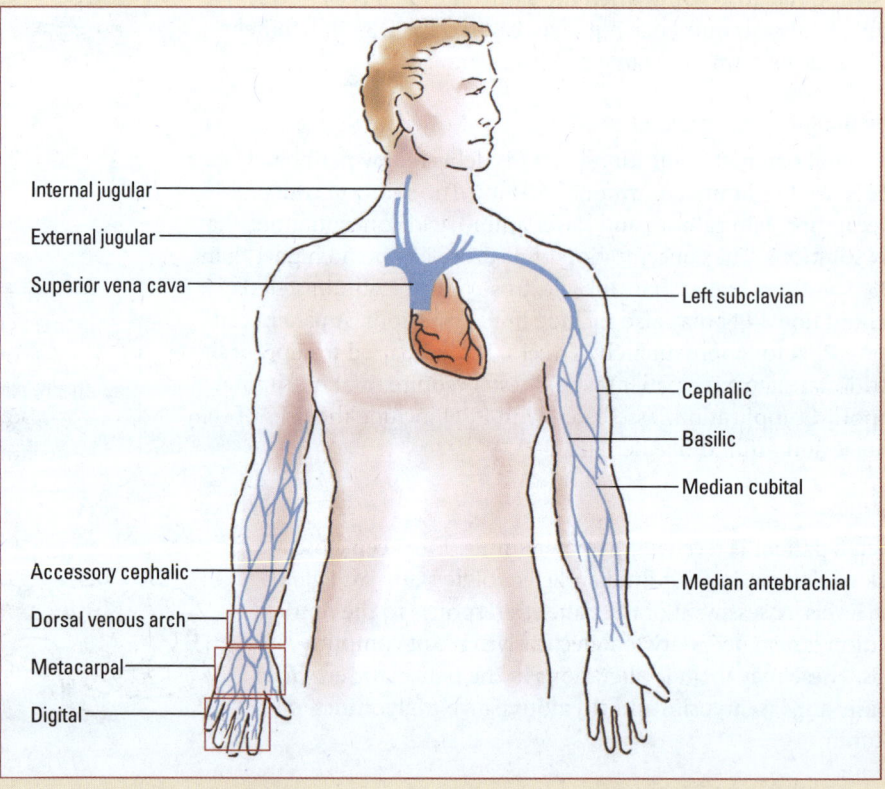

Venous access devices

IV therapy can be delivered via peripheral and central access devices. Peripheral access devices include:
- peripherally inserted angiocath
- peripherally inserted mid-line.
  Central access devices include:
- peripherally inserted central catheter (see illustration below)
- single- or multiple-lumen intrajugular and subclavian devices
- single- or multiple-lumen tunneled and implanted devices.

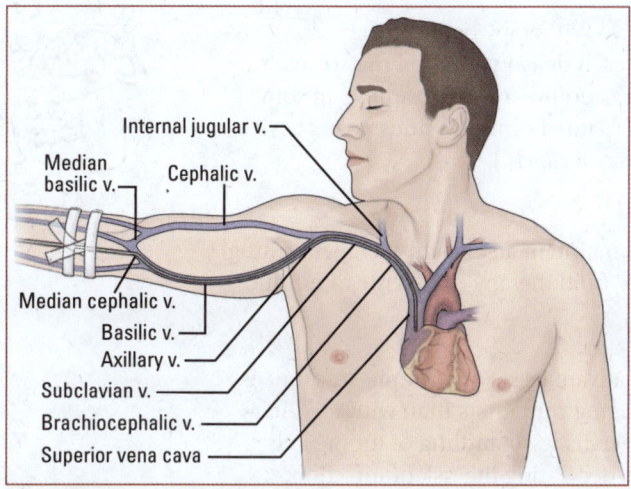

A peripherally inserted central catheter. (Reprinted with permission from Hinkle J. L., Cheever K. H., & Overbaugh K. (2022). *Brunner & Suddarth's Medical-Surgical Nursing* (15th ed., Fig. 12-6). Wolters Kluwer.)

To promote safety, needleless access ports are provided as saline locks and Y-ports on IV tubing. Needleless access reduces contaminated needle sticks (Gorski et al., 2021). Many facilities have a policy mandating that all needleless sites be covered with a chlorohexidine-impregnated cap when not in use to reduce the introduction of pathogens into the venous system.

Delivery methods

There are three basic methods for delivering IV therapy:
- continuous infusion (primary or drip)
- intermittent infusion (secondary or bolus)
- direct injection (IV push).

Setting the terms

Continuous IV therapy allows you to give a carefully regulated amount of fluid over a prolonged period. During intermittent IV therapy, a solution (commonly a medication) is given for shorter periods at set intervals. Direct injection (sometimes called *IV push*) is used to deliver a single dose (bolus) of a drug.

Making the right choice

The choice of IV delivery method depends not only on the purpose and duration of therapy but also on the patient's condition, age, and health history.

At times, a patient may receive IV therapy by more than one delivery method. Also, variations of each delivery method may be used, and some therapies require extra equipment. For example, in some long-term chemotherapy, an implanted central venous access device is needed. (See *Comparing IV delivery methods*.)

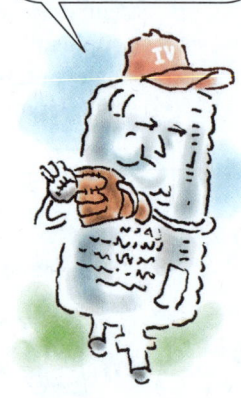

I always thought my delivery depended on my windup, pitch, and follow-through . . . gee, was I off base!

Continuous infusion

A continuous IV infusion helps maintain a constant therapeutic drug level. It's also used to provide IV fluid therapy or parenteral nutrition.

Upside...

Continuous IV infusion has its advantages. For example, less time is spent mixing solutions and hanging containers than with the intermittent method. In addition, there is less handling of tubing and access to the patient's IV device, decreasing the risk of infection.

...and downside

Continuous administration has some disadvantages, too. For example, the patient may become distressed if the equipment hinders mobility and interferes with other activities of daily living. Also, the drip rate must be carefully monitored to ensure that the IV fluid and medication don't infuse too rapidly or too slowly.

Intermittent infusion

The most common and flexible method of administering IV medications is by intermittent infusion.

On again, off again

In intermittent infusion, drugs are administered over a specified period at varying intervals, thereby maintaining therapeutic blood levels. A small volume (1 to 250 mL) may be delivered over several minutes or a few hours, depending on the infusion prescription. An intermittent infusion can be given through a primary line (the most common method) or a secondary line. The secondary line is usually connected or piggybacked into the primary line by way of a Y-site (a Y-shaped section of tubing with a self-sealing access port).

Comparing IV delivery methods

This chart lists the indications, advantages, and disadvantages of methods commonly used to administer IV medications.

Method and indications	Advantages	Disadvantages
Direct injection into a vein		
• Generally doesn't involve an administration set and is commonly referred to as *IV push* • When a nonirritating drug with a low risk of immediate adverse reactions is required for a patient with no other IV needs (e.g., single injection of furosemide, a diuretic)	• Eliminates the risk of complications from an implanted (indwelling) venous access device • Eliminates the inconvenience of an indwelling venous access device	• Requires venipuncture, which can cause patient anxiety • Requires two syringes—one to administer the medication and one to flush the vein after administration • Risks infiltration (puncture of the vein, allowing the solution to enter the surrounding tissue) from the steel needle • Risks phlebitis (inflammation within the vein) because many medications are irritants • Makes it impossible to dilute the drug or interrupt delivery when irritation occurs • In some states (depending on the state practice guidelines), can be given only by a specially certified nurse
Through an existing infusion line		
• When the patient requires immediate high blood levels of a medication (e.g., regular insulin, dextrose 50%, atropine, or antihistamines) • During emergencies, when the drug must be given quickly for immediate effect	• Doesn't require time or authorization to perform venipuncture because the vein is already accessed • Doesn't require an additional needle puncture, which can cause patient anxiety • Allows the use of an IV solution to test the patency of the venous access device before drug administration • Allows continued venous access in case of adverse reactions	• Carries the same inconveniences and complication risks as an indwelling venous access device
Intermittent infusion piggyback method		
• Requires connecting a second administration set to a primary line • Commonly used with drugs given over short periods at varying intervals (e.g., antibiotics and gastric secretion inhibitors)	• Avoids multiple intramuscular injections • Permits repeated administration of drugs through a single IV line • Provides high drug blood levels for short periods	• May cause periods when the drug level becomes too low to be clinically effective (e.g., when peak and trough times aren't considered in the medication order)

(Continued)

Comparing IV delivery methods (continued)

Method and indications	Advantages	Disadvantages
Saline lock		
• Allows for maintenance of venous access • When the patient requires constant venous access but not continuous infusion	• Provides venous access for patients with fluid restrictions • Allows better patient mobility between doses • Preserves veins by reducing frequent venipuncture • Lowers cost	• Requires close monitoring during administration so the device can be flushed on completion • Most commonly used in adults with peripheral IV access devices
Volume-control set		
• Has a medication chamber that allows it to deliver small doses over an extended period • When the patient requires a low volume of fluid	• Requires only one large-volume container and prevents fluid overload from runaway infusion	• May have high equipment costs • Carries a high contamination risk • Requires that the flow clamp be closed when the set empties (if set doesn't contain a membrane that blocks the air passage when it's empty)
Continuous infusion		
Through a primary line		
• When continuous serum levels are needed • When consistent fluid levels are needed	• Maintains steady serum levels • Lowers the risk of rapid shock and vein irritation from a large volume of fluid diluting the drug	• Increases the risk of incompatibility with drugs administered by piggyback infusion • Restricts patient mobility when the patient is connected to an IV system • Increases the risk of undetected infiltration because slow infusion makes it difficult to see swelling in the area of infiltration
Through a secondary line		
• A secondary infusion set is connected to a primary line • When the patient requires continuous infusion of two or more compatible admixtures administered at different rates • When there is a moderate to high chance of abruptly stopping one admixture without infusing the drug remaining in the IV tubing	• Permits the primary infusion and each secondary infusion to be given at different rates • Permits the primary line to be shut off and kept standing by to maintain venous access in case a secondary line must be abruptly stopped	• Eliminates the use of drugs with immediate incompatibility • Increases the risk of phlebitis or vein irritation from an increased number of drugs • Uses multiple IV systems (e.g., primary lines with secondary lines attached), which can create physical barriers to patient care and limit patient mobility, especially for those with electronic pumps or controllers

Direct injection

It could be said that IV therapy by direct injection gets right to the point. A vein can be accessed directly for a single dose of a prescribed drug or solution. The needle is then removed when the bolus is completed. A bolus injection may also be administered through an intermittent infusion device that's already in place.

Administration sets

It is important to select the correct administration set for a patient's infusion. The choice depends on the type of infusion to be provided, the infusion container, and whether a volume-control device is employed.

Vented and unvented

IV administration sets come in two forms: vented and unvented. The vented set is for containers that have no venting system (hard plastic containers or glass bottles). Flexible fluid containers don't require vented tubing.

Other features and options

IV administration sets come with various other features as well, including ports for infusing secondary medications and filters for blocking microbes, irritants, or large particles. The tubing also varies. Some types are designed to enhance the proper functioning of devices that help regulate the infusion rate. Other types of tubing are used specifically for continuous or intermittent infusion or for infusing parenteral nutrition and blood.

Infusion rates

A key aspect of administering IV therapy is maintaining accurate infusion rates for the solutions. If an infusion runs too fast or too slow, the patient may suffer complications, such as phlebitis, infiltration, circulatory overload (possibly leading to heart failure and pulmonary edema), and adverse drug reactions.

Volume-control devices and the correct administration set help prevent such complications. Use nonelectronic flow devices only for low-risk infusions where some variation in rate would not be dangerous. Nonelectronic flow devices include gravity infusion sets, manual flow regulators, and mechanical pumps. Infusions with higher risks should be infused using an electronic infusion pump (Gorski et al., 2021). The nurse can help reduce risks by being familiar with all of

Reading an IV order

Orders for IV therapy may be standardized for different illnesses and therapies or individualized for a particular patient. Some facility policies dictate an automatic stop order for IV fluids (for example, a stop order could specify that IV orders are good for 24 hours from the time they're written, unless otherwise specified).

It's complete

A complete order for IV therapy should specify:
- type and amount of solution
- additives and their concentrations (such as 10 mEq potassium chloride in 500 mL dextrose 5% in water)
- rate and volume of infusion
- duration of infusion.

When it isn't complete

If an order isn't complete or if the IV order is inappropriate because of the patient's condition, consult the health care provider.

the information in provider's orders and being able to recognize incomplete or incorrectly written orders for IV therapy. Lastly, it is essential for the nurse to be sure the fluids are infused at the recommended rate of administration for the medication (Gorski et al., 2021). (See *Reading an IV order*, page 282.)

Calculating gravity infusion rates

There are two basic types of infusion rates available with IV administration sets, and each set delivers a specific number of drops per milliliter (gtt/mL). Regardless of the type of set used, the formula for calculating infusion rates is the same. (See *Calculating gravity infusion rates*.)

Regulating infusion rates

When a patient's condition requires you to maintain precise IV infusion rates, use an infusion control device, such as:
- clamps
- volumetric pumps.

Are you using mL/h or gtt/minute??

When you regulate the IV infusion rate with a clamp, the rate is usually measured in drops per minute (gtt/minute). If using a pump, the infusion rate is measured in milliliters per hour (mL/h).

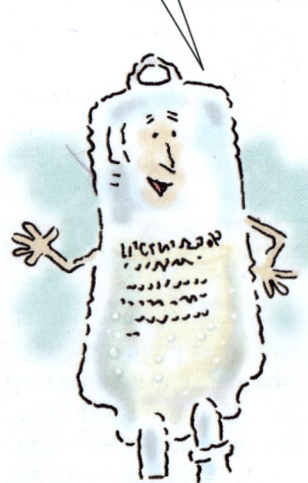

An infusion control device is an excellent way to regulate a patient's infusion rate, but close monitoring is still necessary.

Calculating gravity infusion rates

When calculating the infusion rate (drops per minute) of IV solutions infusing by gravity, remember that the number of drops required to deliver 1 mL varies with the type of administration set used and its manufacturer:

- Administration sets are of two types (see illustrations):
  - Macrodrip (the standard type) delivers 10, 15, or 20 gtt/mL
  - Microdrip usually delivers 60 gtt/mL.

- Manufacturers calibrate their devices differently, so be sure to look for the "drop factor"—expressed in drops per milliliter (or gtt/mL)—in the packaging that accompanies the set being used. (This packaging also has crucial information about such things as special infusions and blood transfusions.) When the device's drop factor is known, use the following formula to calculate specific infusion rates:

$$\frac{\text{volume of infusion (in milliliters)}}{\text{time of infusion (in minutes)}} \times \text{drop factor (in drops per milliliter)} = \text{infusion rate (in drops per minute)}$$

After you calculate the infusion rate for the set you're using, remove your watch and position it so you can see the watch and drip chamber side by side. Next, adjust the clamp to achieve the ordered infusion rate and count the drops for 1 full minute. Readjust the clamp as necessary and count the drops for another minute. Keep adjusting the clamp and counting the drops until the rate is correct.

Macrodrip

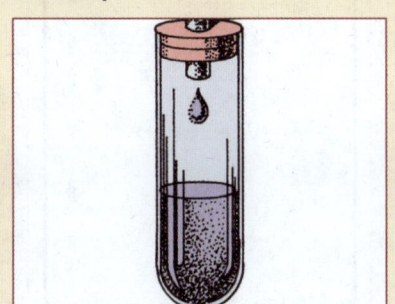

Microdrip

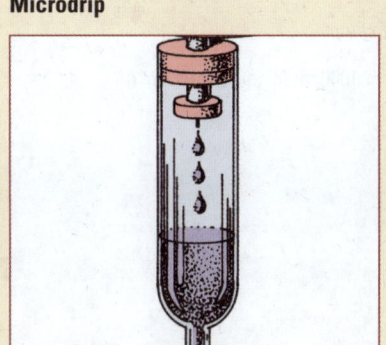

IV clamps

The infusion rate can be regulated with two types of clamps: screw and roller. The screw clamp offers greater accuracy, but the roller clamp, used for standard fluid therapy, is faster and easier to manipulate. A third type, the slide clamp, can stop or start the infusion but can't regulate the rate.

Pumps

New pumps are regularly developed; be sure to attend educational sessions to learn how to use them. Each facility should keep a file or database of instruction manuals (provided by the manufacturers) for each piece of equipment in use.

Calculating IV pump infusion rates

When using an infusion pump, most fluids are infused by milliliters per hour (mL/h). Below is an example of how to calculate fluid volume to be infused on a pump.

Health care provider's order: 1000 mL of 5% dextrose and 0.9% sodium chloride to infuse over 8 hours.

Step 1: Note the fluid available has the exact prescribed additives and strengths:

5% dextrose and 0.9% sodium chloride

Step 2: Infusion rate calculation for an infusion pump (mL/h):

Total volume/hours of infusion

Example:

1000 mL/8 hours = 125 mL/h

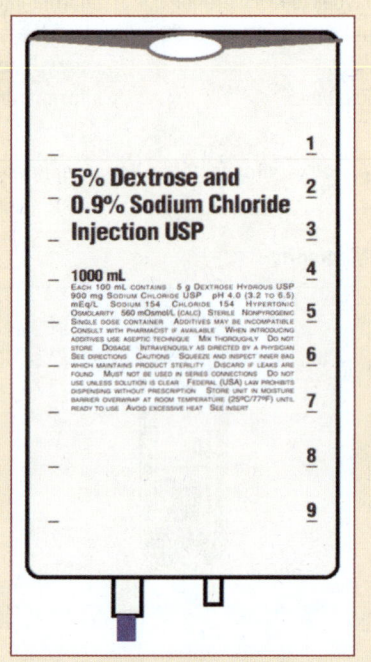

Factor these in

When using a clamp for infusion regulation, you must monitor the infusion rate closely and adjust as needed. Factors such as vein spasm, vein pressure changes, patient movement, manipulations of the clamp, and bent or kinked tubing can cause the rate to vary markedly. For easy monitoring, use a time tape, which marks the prescribed solution level at hourly intervals. (See *Using a time tape,* page 285.)

Other factors that affect infusion rate include the type of IV fluid and its viscosity, the height of the infusion container, the type of administration set, and the size and position of the venous access device.

Using a time tape

Here's a simple way to monitor IV infusion rate: Attach a piece of tape or a preprinted strip to the IV container; then, write hourly times on the tape or strip beginning with the time the solution was hung.

By comparing the actual time with the label time, you can quickly see if the rate needs to be adjusted. Remember that you should never increase IV infusion rates by more than 30% unless ordered by the health care provider.

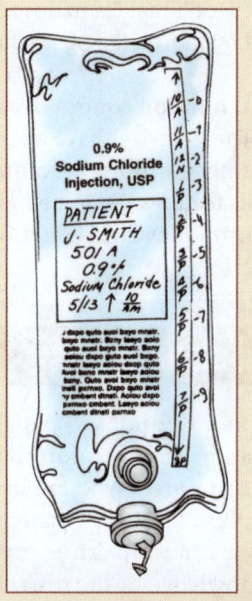

Checking infusion rates

Infusion rates can be fickle; they must be checked and adjusted regularly. The frequency with which infusion rates should be checked depends on the patient's condition and age and the solution or medication being administered.

Check and check again

A best practice is to check the IV infusion rate every time you're in a patient's room and after each position change, at a minimum. Assess the infusion rate more frequently for some patients, such as:

- critically ill patients
- patients with conditions that might be exacerbated by fluid overload
- pediatric patients
- older adult patients
- patients receiving a drug that can cause tissue damage if infiltration occurs.

When checking the infusion rate, inspect and palpate the IV insertion site and ask the patient how it feels.

Minor (not major) adjustments

If the infusion rate slows significantly, to get it back on schedule, adjust the rate slightly. Don't make a major adjustment, though. If the rate must be increased by more than 30%, check with the health care provider.

You should time an infusion control device or rate minder for 1 to 2 hours per shift. (These devices have an error rate ranging from 2% to 10%.) Before using any infusion control device, become thoroughly familiar with its features. Attend educational sessions and perform return demonstrations until you fully understand the new system.

Professional and legal standards

Administering drugs and solutions to patients is one of the most significant tasks nurses perform. Unfortunately, the number of lawsuits directed against nurses who are involved in IV therapy is increasing. For example, a 2021 systematic review reported that the leading causes of medication errors involving IV therapy were due to insufficient knowledge of the drug, failure to double-check high-alert medications, and calculation errors (Kuitunen et al., 2021).

Many lawsuits center on errors in infusion pump use. A 2021 study found that the use of smart infusion devices could have prevented between 8% and 13% of the errors (Jani et al., 2021). However, the use of these devices does not guarantee an error will not be made; the same study found that the use of the devices contributed to 9 of 66 errors (Jani et al., 2021). Strategies to reduce infusion errors include training on infusion therapy, including safe rates of administration, compatibility of medications, pump operation, monitoring practices, and high-alert medication recognition practices (Institute for Safe Medication Practices [ISMP], 2020).

IV therapy errors are some of the most common errors made by nurses. When such errors do occur, due to the rapid effect of IV therapy the adverse effects are frequently devastating. Lawsuits often result from the administration of the wrong medication dosage, inappropriate placement of an IV line, failure to monitor for adverse reactions, infiltration, dislodgment of IV equipment, unclear or missing documentation, and delays in notifying providers.

It's sobering to learn that a high percentage of lawsuits brought against nurses involve errors with IV administration.

Court cases involving IV therapy

Here are examples of lawsuits involving the more common causes of IV therapy errors.

Tales of a two-letter search

In Tennessee, a nurse was convicted of gross neglect of an impaired adult and negligent homicide when she accidentally administered vecuronium instead of Versed, the brand name for midazolam. This nurse's 75-year-old patient died when she received the powerful paralytic instead of the midazolam prescribed to relieve anxiety. The medication dispensing device the nurse used to access the drug was programmed with generic names only. The nurse searched for "VE" and selected the drug vecuronium that the search provided. When presented with a warning, the nurse completed a manual override to give the medication. Once the incorrect drug was given, the patient's respiratory system was paralyzed by the drug, leading to her death (Lusk et al., 2022). The nurse lost her license to practice and was given a 3-year probated sentence.

Be on high alert

In California, a nurse gave a 3,000 to 8,000 times higher dose of norepinephrine than prescribed (Rahhal, 2019), which resulted in the patient's death. The error was attributed to insufficient safeguards for high-alert medications, failure to double-check the dose with another nurse, and nursing inexperience. The patient's family received a nondisclosed amount in the settlement. The facility also was fined the maximum allowable amount of $75,000 by the California Department of Health.

IV line confusion

In Indiana, an internationally recognized medical researcher died when a nurse accidentally started the wrong IV infusion, infusing fentanyl instead of the patient's ordered hydration solution (Guglielmo, 2020). The hospital settled the case for a nondisclosed amount with the patient's family.

Striking a nerve

Several recent lawsuits have involved allegations that a nurse struck a patient's radial nerve during the insertion of an IV line. In California, a 29-year-old patient complained of burning pain when an IV was inserted before surgery. She asked that the IV be removed, but it was left in. The IV was removed during surgery, but the pain continued. She was later diagnosed with reflect sympathetic dystrophy as a result of the radial nerve being hit during the IV insertion. The patient sued, and the hospital argued that hitting a nerve was a reasonable risk of IV insertion; however, through arbitration, they agreed to pay a $155,000 settlement (Delegal & Gorrie, 2001).

Infiltration injury

IV infiltration occurs when the IV fluid leaks in the tissues around the IV site. Such injuries can cause compartment syndrome and may require emergency fasciotomy, skin grafts, and other surgery. Uncorrected compartment syndrome can progress to gangrene and may require significant surgical intervention. A patient in Georgia received $1.5 million after losing their thumb to this type of injury (Arenschield, 2019).

Wrong route

In Tennessee, a patient's family filed suit against a nurse who crushed the patient's oral medications and administered them intravenously instead of through the patient's gastrointestinal tube. The patient died within minutes of the mistake. The medical examiner listed the cause of death as "acute embolization of foreign material (crushed medications)." This suit remains in litigation (Satterfield, 2022).

Delays in monitoring, reporting, and documenting

Delays in recognizing the infiltration, stopping the infusion, and notifying the health care provider have also been cited in recent lawsuits, emphasizing the need for frequent assessment of IV sites and infusions.

Nursing responsibilities

Each nurse has a legal and ethical responsibility to their patients. The good news is that, if you honor these duties and the appropriate standards of care are met, these will serve as a strong foundation if a legal issue arises.

By becoming aware of professional standards and laws related to administering IV therapy, you can provide the best care for your patients and protect yourself legally. Professional and legal standards are defined by state nurse practice acts, federal regulations, and facility policies.

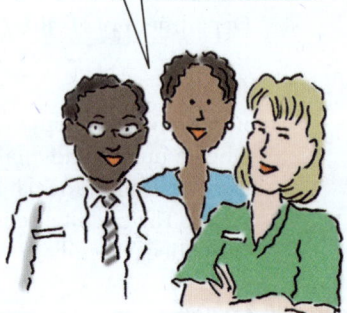

The bottom line is nurses should live up to professional standards and know legal and ethical responsibilities to better serve and protect patients.

State nurse practice acts

Each state has a nurse practice act that broadly defines the legal scope of nursing practice. Your state's nurse practice act is the most important law affecting your nursing practice.

Know your limits

Every nurse is expected to care for patients within defined limits. If a nurse gives care beyond those limits, the nurse becomes vulnerable to charges of violating the state nurse practice act. Copies of each state's nurse practice act can be found on each state nurses association's website or on the state board of nursing website.

Many states' nurse practice acts don't specifically address scope of practice regarding IV therapy by registered nurses (RNs). However, many nurse practice acts do address whether licensed practical nurses (LPNs) or licensed vocational nurses (LVNs) can administer IV therapy. It's important for LPNs and LVNs, as well as for the RNs who are supervising or training them, to be familiar with this information.

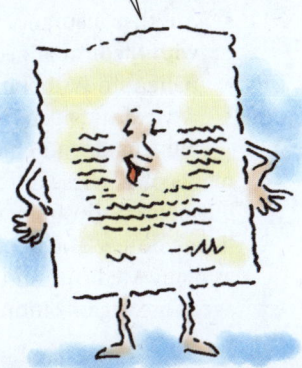

It's essential for you to become familiar with the legal scope and limitations regarding IV therapy in your state.

Federal regulations

The federal government issues regulations and establishes policies related to IV therapy administration. For example, it mandates adherence to standards of IV therapy practice for health care facilities so that they can be eligible to receive reimbursement under Medicare, Medicaid, and other programs.

Millions served

Medicare and Medicaid, the two major federal health care programs, serve about 150 million Americans (Centers for Medicare and Medicaid Services, 2023). They are run by the Health Care Financing Administration (HCFA), which is part of the US Department of Health and Human Services. HCFA formulates national Medicare policy, including policies related to IV therapy, but contracts with private insurance companies to oversee claims and make payment for services and supplies provided under Medicare. These agencies, in turn, enforce HCFA policy by accepting or denying claims for reimbursement. When reviewing claims, agencies may evaluate practices and quality of care, an important factor underlying the emphasis on proper documentation in health care.

Medicaid, which serves certain low-income people, is a state–federal partnership administered by a state agency. There are broad federal requirements for Medicaid, but states have a wide degree of flexibility to design their own programs.

One patient, many regulators

To be eligible for reimbursement, health care agencies must comply with the standards of a complex network of regulators. Consider, for example, a patient receiving IV medications at home with a reusable pump. This patient is primarily covered by Medicare with secondary Medicaid coverage. A variety of carriers, fiscal intermediaries, and agencies share responsibility for reimbursement and regulatory oversight of the patient's care:

- An insurance carrier contracts with Medicare to cover services such as refilling the pump.
- A separate insurance carrier (a durable medical equipment carrier designated by HCFA) covers administered drugs, the pump, and pump supplies.
- Another insurance carrier (called a *fiscal intermediary*) contracts with Medicare to cover preliminary in-hospital training of the patient in IV therapy techniques.
- A Medicaid agency also covers a portion of the patient's care. Nursing documentation must be complete to meet the requirements of all these different agencies. The underlying (although unstated) philosophy of these agencies is that "if it isn't documented, it isn't done." The regulatory network is becoming more complicated as many Medicare and Medicaid patients are being covered by managed care organizations that have their own rules and procedures.

Facility policy

Every health care facility has IV therapy policies for nurses. Such policies are required to obtain accreditation from The Joint Commission and other accrediting bodies. These policies can't go beyond what a state's nurse practice act permits, but they more specifically define the nurse's duties and responsibilities.

Awareness of facility policy is particularly important in rapidly developing areas of practice, such as home care, where the intensity of service and patient needs is increasing dramatically. For example, home health nurses must be acutely aware of patient and family education policies because infusion systems are being used in the home 24 hours per day without the presence of full-time nursing staff.

IV therapy standards of practice

The Infusion Nurses Society (INS) (2021) has developed a set of standards, the *Infusion Nursing Standards of Practice*, that are commonly used by committees developing facility policy. According to the INS, the goals of these standards are to promote safe IV therapy and protect patient rights (INS, 2021). These standards address all aspects of IV nursing. More information can be found at http://www.ins1.org.

Additionally, the Institute for Safe Medication Practices (ISMP) developed two sets of guidelines: the *Safe Practice Guidelines for Adult IV Push Medications* and the *Guidelines for Optimizing Safe*

Implementation and Use of the Smart Infusion Pumps (ISMP, 2015; 2020). The ISMP is a nonprofit organization dedicated to preventing medication errors. More information can be found at https://www.ismp.org/.

Documentation

IV therapy must be documented for several reasons. Proper documentation provides:

- an accurate description of care that can serve as legal protection (e.g., as evidence that a prescribed treatment was administered)
- a mechanism for recording and retrieving information
- a record for health care insurers of equipment and supplies used.

Documenting initiation of IV therapy

When you initiate IV therapy, it's important to include specific information about where the IV was started, what kind of equipment was used, and what solution was infused. After the IV therapy has been completed, you need to document the patient's response to the procedure and the therapy. (See *Documenting IV therapy*, page 292.)

Label that dressing...

In addition to documenting in the patient's EHR, label the dressing on the catheter insertion site. Whenever you change the dressing, label the new one. (See *How to label a dressing*.)

...and the container

The fluid container and tubing should also be labeled. For children, the volume-control set will also need to be labeled. In labeling the container and the set, follow your facility's policy and procedures. (See *How to label an IV bag*.)

Documenting IV maintenance

It's equally important to document how the IV site is maintained, including the conditions of the site; care that was provided; dressing, solution, tubing, or equipment changes made; and teaching provided. (See *Teaching about IV therapy*, page 293.)

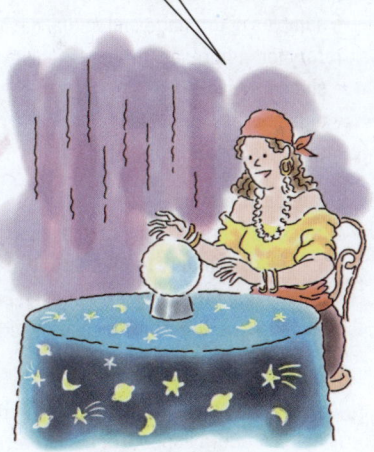

Be crystal clear when documenting how the IV site is maintained. If done correctly, I predict better nursing care!

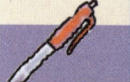

Take note!

Documenting IV therapy

Follow these tips to document IV site care, catheter removal, IV infusion, and other related care.

IV site care

When IV site care is completed, document the following:

- date and time of the dressing change
- condition of the insertion site, noting signs of
  - infection (redness and pain)
  - infiltration (coolness, blanching, or edema)
  - thrombophlebitis (redness, firmness, pain, or edema)
- care given and the type of dressing applied
- patient education provided.

If complications are present, document:

- name of the health care provider notified
- time of the notification
- specific orders given
- interventions
- the patient's response.

IV catheter removal

When an IV catheter is removed, document the following:

- date and time of removal
- condition of the catheter tip
- condition of the site
- drainage at the puncture site
- samples of drainage and actual device tip sent to laboratory for culture, according to facility policy
- site care given
- type of dressing applied
- patient education provided.

Barcode scanners

Barcode scanners (also referred to as barcode readers) are used to compare the IV therapy to the patient's identification and prescribed treatments. Errors are greatly reduced when these systems are used (INS, 2021).

Electronic health records

Within the electronic health record (EHR), the nurse is able to record aspects of the IV therapy to demonstrate effective monitoring and intervention. Nurses are expected to monitor IV infusions at least every 4 hours and more often if the infusion is high risk or the patient's condition is unstable (INS, 2021). To best employ EHR systems, you should record:

- infusion rate
- use of an electronic flow device or flow controller
- type of solution
- date and time of dressing and tubing changes.
- site condition
- patient response
- patient education
- any adverse effects you observe (if applicable)
- any adverse effects the patient reports (if applicable)

Intake and output sheets

When documenting intake and output of the IV therapy, follow these guidelines:

- If the patient is a child, note fluid levels on the IV containers hourly. If the patient is an adult, note these levels at least twice per shift.
- With children and critical care patients, record intake of all IV infusions, including fluids, medications, flush solutions, blood and blood products, and other infusions, every 1 to 2 hours.
- Document the total amount of each infusion and totals of all infusions at least every shift, so fluid balance can be monitored.
- Note output hourly or less often (but at least once each shift), depending on the patient's condition. Output includes urine, stool, vomitus, and gastric drainage. For an acutely ill or unstable patient, urine output may need to be assessed every 15 minutes.
- Read fluid levels from the infusion containers or electronic volume-control device to estimate the amounts infused and the amounts remaining to be infused.

Source: Infusion Nurses Society (INS). (2021). *Infusion therapy standards of practice* (8th ed.). https://www.ins1.org/publications/infusion-therapy-standards-of-practice/

How to label an IV bag

When an IV bag is labeled, be sure not to cover the name of the IV solution. To properly label an IV solution container, include (in addition to the time tape):
- patient's name, identification number, and room number
- date and time the container was hung
- any additives and their amounts
- rate at which the solution is to run
- date tubing should be changed
- expiration date and time of infusion
- nurse's name.

How to label a dressing

To label a new dressing over an IV site, include:
- date of insertion
- gauge and length of venipuncture device
- date and time of the dressing change
- nurse's initials.

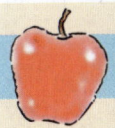

Education corner

Teaching about IV therapy

Although nurses are familiar with IV therapy, patients aren't. They may be apprehensive about the procedure and concerned that their condition requires increased intervention.

Teaching the patient and, when appropriate, family members will help them to relax and take the unknowns out of IV therapy.

Based on past experience

Begin by determining the patient's previous infusion experience, expectations, and knowledge of venipuncture and IV therapy. Then base the teaching content on these findings.

Patient education should include these steps:
- Describe the procedure. Tell the patient that IV means "inside the vein" and that a plastic catheter or needle will be placed in their vein.
- Explain that fluids containing certain nutrients or medications will flow from a bag or bottle through a length of tubing and then through the catheter or needle into the vein.
- Tell the patient how long the catheter or needle may stay in place, and explain that the health care provider will decide how much and what type of fluid and medication is needed.

The whole story

Give the patient as much information as possible. Consider providing pamphlets, sample catheters and IV equipment, slides, videos, and other appropriate information. Make sure to provide the whole story, including the following:
- Tell the patient they may feel transient pain as the needle goes in, the discomfort will stop when the catheter or needle is in place.
- Explain why IV therapy is needed and how the patient can help by holding still and not withdrawing if they feel pain when the needle is inserted.
- Explain that the IV fluids may feel cold at first, but the sensation should last only a few minutes.
- Instruct the patient to report any discomfort they feel after therapy begins.
- Explain activity restrictions such as those regarding bathing and ambulating.

Teaching about IV therapy *(continued)*

Easing anxiety

Give the patient time to express concerns and fears, and take the time to provide reassurance. Also, encourage the patient to use stress-reduction techniques such as deep, slow breathing. Allow the patient and their family to participate in the patient's care as much as possible.

But did they get it?

Make sure to evaluate how well the patient and family members understand the instruction and education.

Evaluate their understanding during teaching and when it's complete. Asking frequent questions and having the patient explain or demonstrate what has been taught helps to gauge understanding.

Don't forget to document

Document all teaching in the patient's records. Note what was taught and how well the patient understood it.

Quick quiz

1.   The nurse is caring for a patient with fluids running into a peripheral IV. On assessment, the IV insertion site is swollen, tender, and cool. The nurse recognizes that this patient's infusion has:
    A.   caused inflammation to the vein.
    B.   infiltrated into the surrounding tissues.
    C.   perforated the vein, causing a hematoma.
    D.   shifted from the cells to the interstitial area.

Answer: B. The angiocath is no longer in the vein; therefore, the fluid is infusing into the subcutaneous tissues.

2.   The nurse is caring for a patient experiencing low serum potassium (hypokalemia). The nurse knows which changes in the patient's condition can occur with hypokalemia?
    A.   Cardiac muscle excitability
    B.   Diarrhea and hyperactive bowel sounds
    C.   Leg cramping and muscle weakness
    D.   Poor skin turgor

Answer: C. The earliest and most frequent signs of hypokalemia are leg cramps, muscle weakness, and fatigue.

3.   A patient is receiving 5% dextrose and 0.9% sodium chloride IV for several hours. The nurse realizes this fluid will have which effect?
    A.   Decrease the patient's serum glucose level by diluting the glucose with sodium chloride.
    B.   Increase the patient's risk of experiencing hypernatremia, causing the patient to experience dehydration.
    C.   Move water from the circulatory system into the cells to replace the fluid loss in the cells.
    D.   Primarily replace intervascular volume but can pull water from the cells into the circulatory system.

Answer: D. The 5% dextrose and 0.9% sodium chloride is a hypertonic solution. Hypertonic solutions primarily replace intervascular volume but have some ability to pull water from the cells if the osmolality of the cells is lower than that of the solution.

4.   The nurse is preparing to administer cefazolin IV to a patient receiving lactated Ringer solution continuously. The nurse notes that cefazolin is not compatible with lactated Ringer solution. Which action should the nurse implement?

     A.   Ask the pharmacist to change the route to IM or PO instead of IV

     B.   Call the health care provider and have them change the antibiotic to one that is compatible.

     C.   Stop the primary solution temporarily, and flush with saline before and after the cefazolin is infused.

     D.   Wait until the primary solution is completely infused, then give the cefazolin before hanging another bag of the solution.

Answer: C. The nurse may stop the primary solution, flush with saline, give the agent, flush with saline again, and restart the lactated Ringer solution.

Scoring

☆☆☆   If you answered all four questions correctly, super! Your knowledge of IV therapy is diffuse.

  ☆☆   If you answered three questions correctly, bravo! You're no drip when it comes to IV therapy.

    ☆   If you answered fewer than three questions correctly, don't despair! Review the chapter for an infusion of IV know-how and try again.

References

Arenschield L. (2019). *'Be Nice' and document to prevent malpractice suits.* Medscape. https://www.medscape.com/viewarticle/913166

Berlana D. (2022). Parenteral nutrition overview. *Nutrients, 14*(21), 4480. https://doi.org/10.3390/nu14214480

Centers for Medicare and Medicaid Services (CMS). (2023). *CMS fast facts.* https://data.cms.gov/fact-sheet/cms-fast-facts

Delegal M. K. & Gorrie J. (2001). *Legal review and commentary: IV inserted to nerve results in radial nerve injury—$155,000 arbitration award.* https://www.reliasmedia.com/articles/62364-legal-review-amp-commentary-iv-inserted-to-nerve-results-in-radial-nerve-injury-155-000-arbitration-award

Fischbach T. F., Fischbach M. A., & Stout K. (2022). *Fischbach's: A manual of laboratory and diagnostic tests* (11th ed.). Wolters Kluwer.

Gorski L. A., Hadaway L., Hagle M. E., Broadhurst D., Clare S., Kleidon T., Meyer B. M., Nickel B., Rowley S., Sharpe E., & Alexander M. (2021). Infusion therapy standards of practice (8th ed.). *Journal of Infusion Therapy, 44*(1), S1. https://www.ins1.org

Guglielmo W. (2020). *Famous medical researcher dies after receiving wrong drug.* Medscape Nurses. https://www.medscape.com/viewarticle/943041

Hamdan M., & Puckett Y. (2023). *Total parenteral nutrition. StatPearls.* StatPearls Publishing. https://www.ncbi.nlm.nih.gov/books/NBK559036/

Infusion Nurses Society (INS). (2021). *Infusion therapy standards of practice* (8th ed.). https://www.ins1.org/publications/infusion-therapy-standards-of-practice/

Institute for Safe Medication Practices (ISMP). (2015). *Safe practice guidelines for adult IV push medications.* https://www.ismp.org/guidelines/iv-push

Institute for Safe Medication Practices (ISMP). (2020). *Guidelines for optimizing safe implementation and use of smart infusion pumps.* https://www.ismp.org/guidelines/safe-implementation-and-use-smart-pumps

Jani Y. H., Chumbley G. M., Furniss D., Blandford A., & Franklin B. (2021). The potential role of smart infusion devices in preventing or contributing to medication administration errors: A descriptive study of 2 data sets. *Journal of Patient Safety, 17*(8), e1894–e1900. https://doi.org/10.1097/PTS.0000000000000751

Kuitunen S., Niittynen I., Airaksinen M., & Holmström A. R. (2021). Systemic causes of in-hospital intravenous medication errors: A systematic review. *Journal of Patient Safety, 17*(8), e1660–e1668. https://doi.org/10.1097/PTS.000000000000000632

Lukitsch I. (2023). *Hypernatremia. Medscape.* https://emedicine.medscape.com/article/241094-overview

Lusk C., DeForest E., Segarra G., Neyens D. M., Abernathy J. H., & Catchpole K. (2022). Reconsidering the application of systems thinking in healthcare: The RaDonda Vaught case. *British Journal of Anaesthesia, 129*(3), e61–e62. https://doi.org/10.1016/j.bja.2022.05.023

Rahhal N. (2019). *Patient dies after nurse administered 8,000 times the prescribed dose of blood pressure medication. Daily Mail.* https://www.dailymail.co.uk/health/article-6573409/Patient-dies-nurse-administered-8-000-times-prescribed-dose-blood-pressure-medication.html

Satterfield J. (2022). *Knoxville hospital uses COVID-19 as liability shield for suit over fatal medical mistake. Tennessee Lookout.* https://tennesseelookout.com/2022/03/31/knoxville-hospital-uses-covid-as-liability-shield-for-suit-over-fatal-medical-mistake/

Part III

Physiologic needs

Chapter 12

Oxygenation

Just the facts

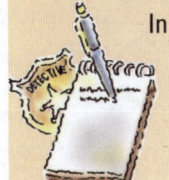

In this chapter, you'll learn:

◆ components that make up the respiratory system

◆ processes involved in respiration

◆ principles of acid–base balance

◆ treatments for respiratory disorders.

A look at the respiratory system

The respiratory system includes the airways, lungs, bony thorax, respiratory muscles, and central nervous system. They work together to deliver oxygen to the bloodstream and remove excess carbon dioxide from the body. Knowing the basic structures and functions of the respiratory system will help you perform a comprehensive respiratory assessment and recognize any abnormalities. (See *A close look at the respiratory system*, page 300.)

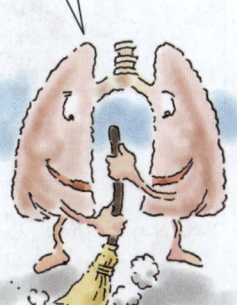

One of my main jobs is to get rid of excess carbon dioxide. Out you go, CO_2!!

Airways and lungs

The airways are divided into the upper and lower airways. The upper airways include the nasopharynx (nose), oropharynx (mouth), laryngopharynx, and larynx. Their purpose is to warm, filter, and humidify inhaled air. They also help make sound and send air to the lower airways.

Flap protection

The epiglottis is a flap of tissue that closes over the top of the larynx when the patient swallows. The epiglottis protects the patient from aspirating food or fluid into the lower airways.

Vocal point

The larynx is located at the top of the trachea and houses the vocal cords. It's the transition point between the upper and lower airways.

A close look at the respiratory system

The major structures of the upper and lower airways are illustrated below. The second illustration shows bronchioles and the alveolus, also called the *acinus*.

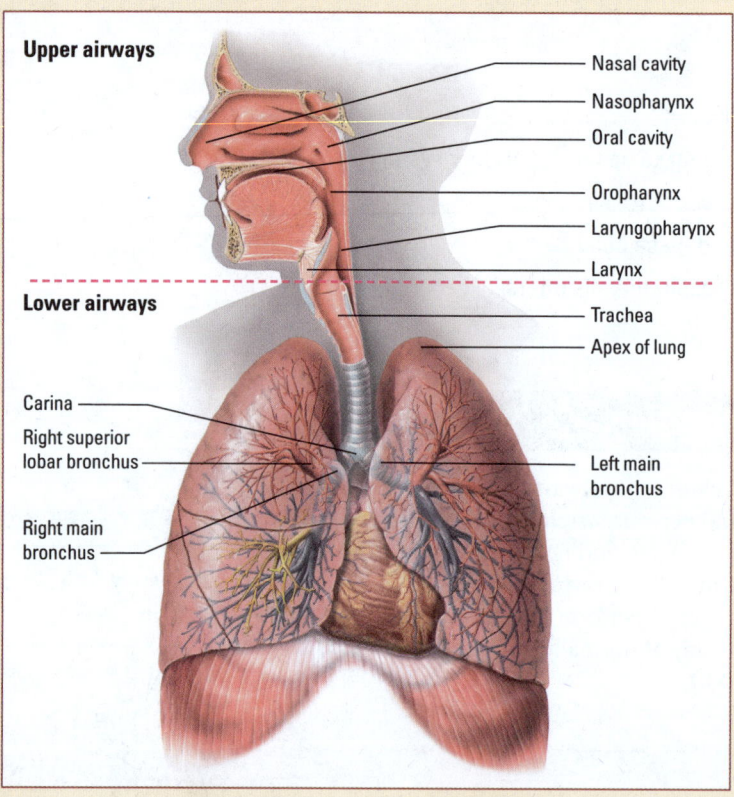

Upper airways
- Nasal cavity
- Nasopharynx
- Oral cavity
- Oropharynx
- Laryngopharynx
- Larynx

Lower airways
- Trachea
- Apex of lung
- Carina
- Right superior lobar bronchus
- Left main bronchus
- Right main bronchus

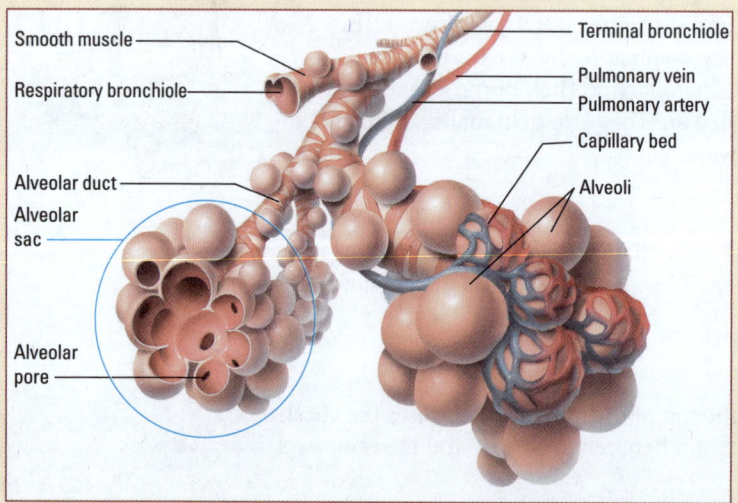

- Smooth muscle
- Respiratory bronchiole
- Terminal bronchiole
- Pulmonary vein
- Pulmonary artery
- Capillary bed
- Alveolar duct
- Alveoli
- Alveolar sac
- Alveolar pore

The lowdown on the lower airways

The lower airways begin with the trachea, which then divides into the right and left mainstem bronchi. The mainstem bronchi divide into the lobar bronchi, which are lined with mucus-producing ciliated epithelium, one of the lungs' major defense systems.

The lobar bronchi then divide into secondary bronchi, tertiary bronchi, terminal bronchioles, respiratory bronchioles, alveolar ducts, and finally, alveoli, the gas-exchange units of the lungs. An adult's lungs typically contain about 300 million alveoli (Khan & Lynch, 2023).

Lungs and lobes

Each lung is wrapped in a lining called the *visceral pleura*. The right lung is larger and has three lobes: upper, middle, and lower. The left lung is smaller and has only an upper and a lower lobe.

Smooth moves

The lungs share space in the thoracic cavity with the heart and great vessels, the trachea, the esophagus, and the bronchi. All areas of the thoracic cavity that come in contact with the lungs are lined with parietal pleura.

A small amount of fluid fills the area between the two layers of the pleura. This pleural fluid allows the layers to slide smoothly over each other as the chest expands and contracts. The parietal pleura also contain nerve endings that transmit pain signals when inflammation occurs.

Thorax

The bony thorax includes the clavicles, sternum, scapula, 12 sets of ribs, and 12 thoracic vertebrae.

Rack of ribs

Ribs consist of bone and cartilage and allow the chest to expand and contract during each breath. All ribs attach to the thoracic vertebrae. The first seven ribs also attach directly to the sternum. The 8th, 9th, and 10th ribs attach to the cartilage of the preceding rib. The 11th and 12th ribs are called *floating ribs* because they don't attach to anything in the anterior thorax.

Respiratory muscles

The diaphragm and the external intercostal muscles are the primary muscles used in breathing. They contract when the patient inhales and relax when the patient exhales.

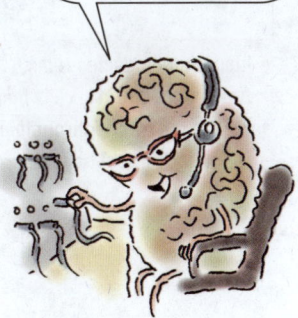

Yes, sir, it's the respiratory muscle again. It's asking whether you can slow the breathing rate just a tad . . . something about too much carbon dioxide in the CSF. Shall I put them through?

Message in a nerve

The respiratory center in the medulla initiates each breath by sending messages to the primary respiratory muscles over the phrenic nerve. Impulses from the phrenic nerve adjust the rate and depth of breathing, depending on the carbon dioxide and pH levels in the cerebrospinal fluid (CSF). (See *A close look at the mechanics of breathing*.)

Accessory to breathing

Other muscles, called *accessory muscles*, assist in breathing. Accessory inspiratory muscles include the trapezius, the sternocleidomastoid, and the scalene, which combine to elevate the scapula, clavicle, sternum, and upper ribs. That elevation expands the front-to-back diameter of the chest when use of the diaphragm and intercostal muscles isn't effective.

Expiration occurs when the diaphragm and external intercostal muscles relax. If the patient has an airway obstruction, they may also use the abdominal muscles and internal intercostal muscles to exhale.

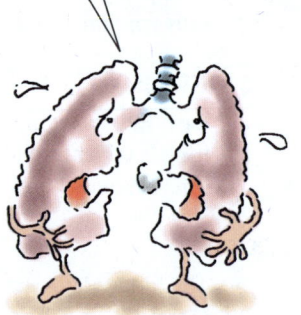

Where are the accessory muscles when you need them?!

A close look at the mechanics of breathing

These illustrations show how mechanical forces, such as the movement of the diaphragm and intercostal muscles, produce a breath. A plus sign (+) indicates positive pressure, and a minus sign (−) indicates negative pressure.

At rest

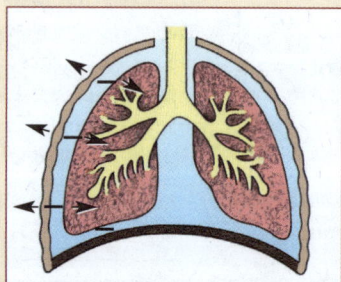

- Inspiratory muscles relax.
- Atmospheric pressure is maintained in the tracheobronchial tree.
- No air movement occurs.

Inhalation

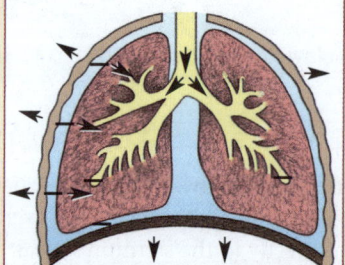

- Inspiratory muscles contract.
- The diaphragm descends and flattens.
- Negative alveolar pressure is maintained.
- Air moves into the lungs.

Exhalation

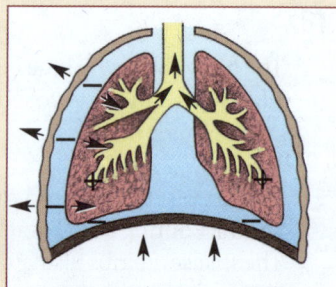

- Inspiratory muscles relax, causing lungs to recoil to their resting size and position.
- The diaphragm ascends, returning to its resting position.
- Positive alveolar pressure is maintained.
- Air moves out of the lungs.

Functions of the respiratory system

The functions of the respiratory system are respiration and ventilation to help maintain acid–base balance.

Respiration

Effective respiration requires gas exchange in the tissues (internal respiration) and in the lungs (external respiration). This exchange is vital to maintain adequate oxygenation and acid–base balance. Internal respiration occurs only through diffusion. External respiration occurs through three processes:

- Ventilation (gas distribution into and out of the pulmonary airways)
- Pulmonary perfusion (blood flow from the right side of the heart, through the pulmonary circulation, and into the left side of the heart)
- Diffusion (gas movement from an area of greater to lesser concentration through a semipermeable membrane)

Ventilation

Adequate ventilation depends on the nervous, musculoskeletal, and pulmonary systems for the requisite lung pressure changes. Any dysfunction in these systems increases the work of breathing, diminishing its effectiveness.

Nervous system influence

Although ventilation is largely involuntary, individuals can control its rate and depth. Involuntary breathing results from neurogenic stimulation of the respiratory center in the medulla and the pons of the brain stem. The medulla controls the rate and depth of respiration; the pons moderates the rhythm of the switch from inspiration to expiration. Specialized neurovascular tissue alters these phases of the breathing process automatically and instantaneously.

A special response

When carbon dioxide in the blood diffuses into the CSF, specialized tissue in the respiratory center of the brain stem responds. At the same time, peripheral chemoreceptors in the aortic arch and the bifurcation of the carotid arteries respond to reduced oxygen levels in the blood. When the carbon dioxide level rises or the oxygen level falls noticeably, the respiratory center of the medulla initiates respiration.

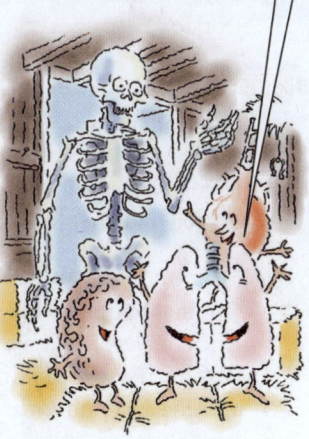

I bet with a little elbow grease and a couple more windows, we could turn this into the coolest respiration clubhouse!

Musculoskeletal influence

The adult thorax is a flexible structure. Its shape can be altered by contracting the chest muscles. The medulla controls ventilation primarily by stimulating contraction of the diaphragm and the external intercostal, the major muscles of breathing.

The diaphragm descends to expand the length of the chest cavity, whereas the external intercostal contracts to expand the anteroposterior and lateral chest diameter. These actions produce changes in intrapulmonary pressure that cause inspiration.

Pulmonary influence

During inspiration, air flows through the right and left mainstem bronchi. The airflow continues into the increasingly smaller bronchi, then into bronchioles, alveolar ducts, alveolar sacs, and finally reaches the alveolar membrane. Many factors can alter airflow distribution, including airflow pattern, volume, and location of the functional reserve capacity (air retained in the alveoli that prevents their collapse during respiration), the amount of intrapulmonary resistance, and the presence of lung disease.

The path of least resistance

If disrupted, airflow distribution will follow the path of least resistance. For example, an intrapulmonary obstruction or forced inspiration will cause an uneven distribution of air.

Active, then passive

Normal breathing requires active inspiration and passive expiration. Forced breathing, as in cases of emphysema, demands active inspiration and expiration. It activates accessory muscles of respiration, which require additional oxygen to work, resulting in less efficient ventilation with an increased workload.

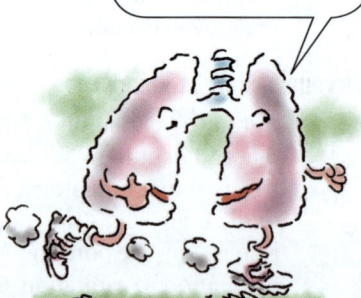

Just keep going. I'm sure we'll see the path of least resistance soon.

Noncompliance, resistance, fatigue—oh, my!

Other alterations in airflow, such as changes in compliance (dispensability of the lungs and thorax) and resistance (interference with airflow in the tracheobronchial tree), can also increase oxygen and energy demands and lead to respiratory muscle fatigue.

Pulmonary perfusion

Optimal pulmonary perfusion aids external respiration and promotes efficient alveolar gas exchange. However, factors that reduce blood flow, such as a cardiac output that's less than average (5 L/minute) and elevated pulmonary and systemic vascular resistance, can interfere with gas transport to the alveoli. Also, abnormal or insufficient hemo-globin (Hgb) picks up less oxygen than is needed for efficient gas exchange.

No uniformity

Gravity can affect oxygen and carbon dioxide transport by influencing pulmonary circulation. Gravity pulls more unoxygenated blood to the lower and middle lung lobes relative to the upper lobes, where most of the tidal volume also flows.

As a result, neither ventilation nor perfusion is uniform through-out the lung. Areas of the lung where perfusion and ventilation are similar have good ventilation–perfusion matching. In such areas, gas exchange is most efficient. Areas of the lung that demonstrate ventila-tion–perfusion inequality result in less efficient gas exchange.

Diffusion

In diffusion, molecules of oxygen and carbon dioxide move between the alveoli and the capillaries. Partial pressure (the pressure exerted by one gas in a mixture of gases) dictates the direction of movement, which is always from an area of greater concentration to one of lesser concentration.

Move it!

During diffusion, oxygen moves across the alveolar and capillary membranes, then dissolves in the plasma and passes through the red blood cell (RBC) membrane. Carbon dioxide moves in the opposite direction. (See *Exchanging gases*, page 306.)

Spaces in between

Successful diffusion requires an intact alveolocapillary membrane. The alveolar epithelium and the capillary endothelium are composed of a single layer of cells. Between these layers are minute interstitial spaces filled with elastin and collagen.

From the RBCs to the alveoli

Normally, oxygen and carbon dioxide move easily through all of these layers. Oxygen moves from the alveoli into the bloodstream, where it's taken up by Hgb in the RBCs. From there, it displaces carbon dioxide (the by-product of metabo-lism), which diffuses from the RBCs into the blood, and then it moves to the alveoli. Most transported oxygen binds with Hgb to form oxy-hemoglobin, while a small portion dissolves in the plasma (measur-able as the partial pressure of oxygen in arterial blood).

> *Where do you think you're going? Diffuse yourself in the opposite direction, buddy!*

Exchanging gases

Gas exchange occurs very rapidly in the millions of tiny, thin-membraned alveoli within the respiratory units. Inside these air sacs, oxygen from inhaled air diffuses into the blood while carbon dioxide diffuses from the blood into the air and is exhaled. Blood then circulates throughout the body, delivering oxygen and picking up carbon dioxide. Lastly, the blood returns to the lungs to be oxygenated again.

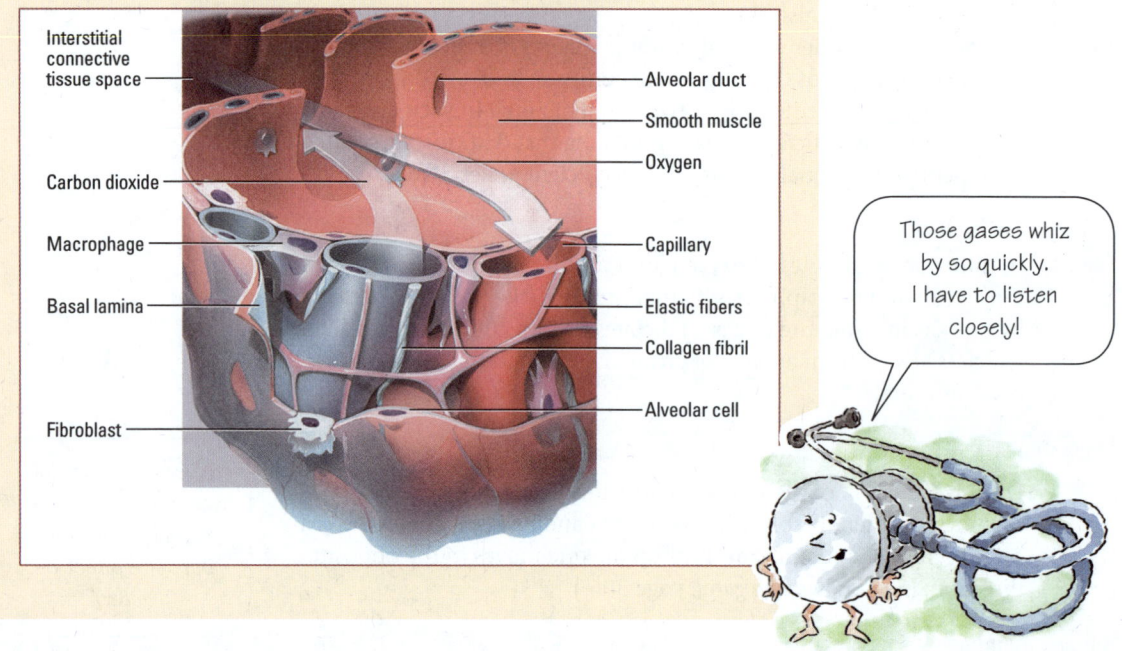

Interstitial connective tissue space

Carbon dioxide

Macrophage

Basal lamina

Fibroblast

Alveolar duct

Smooth muscle

Oxygen

Capillary

Elastic fibers

Collagen fibril

Alveolar cell

Those gases whiz by so quickly. I have to listen closely!

Up and down

After oxygen binds to Hgb, the RBCs travel to the tissues. At this point, the blood cells contain more oxygen, and the tissue cells contain more carbon dioxide. Internal respiration occurs during cellular diffusion, as RBCs release oxygen and absorb carbon dioxide. The RBCs then transport carbon dioxide back to the lungs for removal during expiration.

Acid–base balance

The lungs help maintain acid–base balance in the body by maintaining external and internal respiration. Oxygen collected in the lungs is transported to the tissues by the circulatory system, which exchanges it for the carbon dioxide produced by cellular metabolism. Because carbon dioxide is 20 times more soluble than oxygen, it dissolves in the blood, where most of it forms bicarbonate (base), and smaller amounts form carbonic acid (acid).

And back again

The lungs control bicarbonate levels by converting bicarbonate to carbon dioxide and water for excretion. In response to signals from the medulla, the lungs can change the rate and depth of ventilation.

Maintaining the balance

These changes maintain acid–base balance by adjusting the amount of carbon dioxide that's lost. For example, in metabolic alkalosis, which results from excess bicarbonate retention, the rate and depth of ventilation decrease so that carbon dioxide is retained. This increases carbonic acid levels. In metabolic acidosis (a condition resulting from excess acid retention or excess bicarbonate loss), the lungs increase the rate and depth of ventilation to exhale excess carbon dioxide, thereby reducing carbonic acid levels.

Broken balance beam

A patient with inadequately functioning lungs can experience acid–base imbalances. For example, hypoventilation (reduced rate and depth of ventilation) of the lungs, which results in carbon dioxide retention, causes respiratory acidosis. Conversely, hyperventilation (increased rate and depth of ventilation) of the lungs leads to increased exhalation of carbon dioxide and will result in respiratory alkalosis.

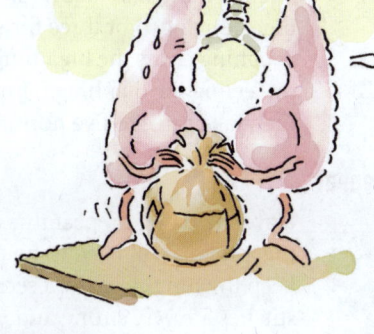

We're hyperventilating . . . if we just keep breathing slowly into the paper bag, we'll be OK.

Therapy for altered function

When altered respiratory function occurs, interventions such as coughing and deep breathing exercises, incentive spirometry, chest physiotherapy, and oxygen administration can enhance the patient's respiratory effort and improve oxygen status. Pulse oximetry allows monitoring of the patient's oxygen saturation. Surgical interventions, such as tracheostomy and chest tube insertion, can also improve oxygenation. Proper care of the patient during and after these procedures is vital.

Coughing exercises

Patients who are at risk for developing excess secretions should practice coughing exercises. However, some patients should not perform these exercises, such as those who have recently had ear or eye surgery or repair of a hiatal or large abdominal hernia. Also, patients who have undergone neurosurgery shouldn't practice coughing exercises postoperatively because doing so will cause intracranial pressure to rise.

If the patient's condition permits, instruct them to sit on the edge of the bed. Provide a small stool if their feet don't touch the floor. Instruct them to bend their legs and lean slightly forward.

Slow and deep

If the patient is scheduled for chest or abdominal surgery or has recently had such surgery, teach them how to splint the incision with a pillow before they cough. Instruct the patient to take a slow, deep breath; they should breathe in through the nose and concentrate on fully expanding the chest. Next, they should breathe out through the mouth and concentrate on feeling the chest sink downward and inward. Then they should take a second breath using the same method.

Once isn't enough

Then, tell them to take a third deep breath and hold it. They should then cough two or three times in a row (once is not enough). Repeated coughing clears the breathing passages. Encourage them to concentrate on feeling the diaphragm force out all the air in the chest. They should then take three to five normal breaths, exhale slowly, and relax.

Repeat

Have the patient repeat this entire exercise at least once. After surgery, this process will need to be performed at least every 2 hours to help keep the lungs free from secretions. Reassure the patient that the stitches are very strong and won't split during coughing.

Deep breathing exercises

Advise the patient that performing deep breathing exercises several times per hour helps keep the lungs fully expanded. To deep breathe correctly, the diaphragm and abdominal muscles must be used, not just the chest muscles. Tell the patient to practice the following exercise two or three times per day beginning a few days before surgery:

- Have the patient lie on their back in a comfortable position with one hand on the chest and the other over the upper abdomen. Teach them to relax and bend their knees slightly.
- Instruct the patient to exhale normally. The patient should then close their mouth and inhale deeply through the nose, concentrating on feeling the abdomen rise. They should hold their breath and count to five.
- Have the patient purse their lips as though about to whistle and then exhale completely through the mouth, without letting the checks puff out. The ribs should sink downward and inward.

After resting for several seconds, the patient should repeat this exercise 5 to 10 times. The patient can also change positions for every breath to help with lung expansion.

Incentive spirometry

Incentive spirometry involves using a breathing device to help the patient achieve maximal ventilation. The device measures the patient's inspiratory effort (flow rate) in cubic centimeters per second (mL/second). The device encourages the patient to take a deep breath and hold it for several seconds. This deep breath:

- increases lung volume
- boosts alveolar inflation
- promotes venous return
- loosens respiratory secretions

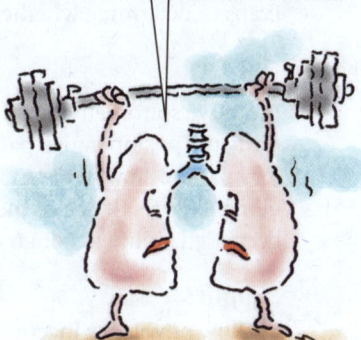

Any exercise that promises to get me back in shape is incentive enough for me.

Longer inflation, less collapse

This exercise establishes alveolar hyperinflation for a longer time than is possible with a normal deep breath, thus preventing and reversing the alveolar collapse that causes atelectasis and pneumonitis (Franklin & Anjum, 2023).

Visual feedback

Devices used for incentive spirometry provide a visual incentive to breathe deeply and encourage slow, sustained maximal inspiration. They can be divided into two types:

- **Flow incentive spirometer:** Used for patients at low risk for developing atelectasis
- **Volume incentive spirometer:** Used for patients at high risk for developing atelectasis (See *Types of spirometers.*)

Types of spirometers

Spirometers can be volume incentive or flow incentive.

Flow incentive spirometer

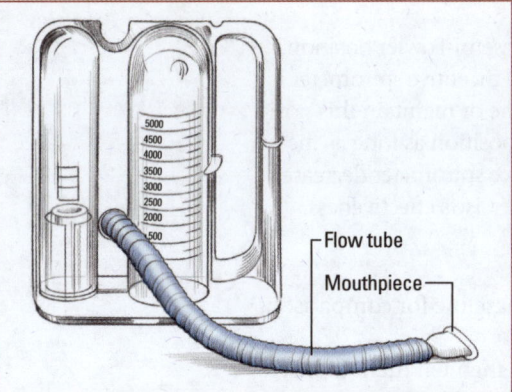

5000
4500
4000
3500
3000
2500
2000
1500

Flow tube

Mouthpiece

Volume incentive spirometer

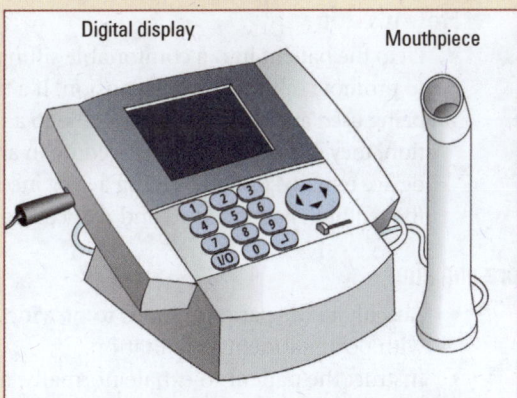

Digital display

Mouthpiece

Flow vs. Volume

Flow incentive spirometers contain plastic floats, which rise according to the amount of air the patient pulls through the device on inhalation. Volume incentive spirometers are activated when the patient inhales a certain volume of air. The device then estimates the amount of air inhaled. This device measures lung inflation more precisely and helps to determine whether the patient is inhaling adequately.

Benefits

Incentive spirometry benefits the patient on prolonged bed rest, especially the postoperative patient who may regain their normal respiratory pattern slowly due to factors like abdominal or thoracic surgery, being 65 years of age or older, inactivity, obesity, smoking, and decreased ability to cough effectively and expel lung secretions.

Supplies
- flow or volume incentive spirometer, as indicated, with sterile disposable tube and mouthpiece (The tube and mouthpiece are sterile on first use and clean on subsequent uses.)
- stethoscope
- watch

Getting ready
- Assemble the ordered equipment at the patient's bedside.
- Remove the sterile flow tube and mouthpiece from the package, and attach them to the device.
- Set the flow rate or volume goal as determined by the health care provider or respiratory therapist and based on the patient's preoperative performance.
- Explain the procedure to the patient, making sure they understand the importance of performing incentive spirometry regularly to maintain alveolar inflation.

How it's done
- Help the patient into a comfortable sitting or semi-Fowler position to promote optimal lung expansion. If a flow incentive spirometer is being used and the patient is unable to assume or maintain this position, they can perform the procedure in any position as long as the device remains upright. Tilting a flow incentive spirometer decreases the required patient effort and reduces the exercise's effectiveness.

Before and after
- Auscultate the patient's lungs to provide a baseline for comparison with posttreatment auscultation.
- Instruct the patient to exhale normally, and then tell them to insert the mouthpiece and close the lips tightly around it because a weak seal may alter flow or volume readings.

Sustained but maximal

- Tell the patient to inhale as slowly and as deeply as possible. If they have difficulty with this step, tell them to suck as they would through a straw but more slowly. Ask the patient to retain the entire volume of air they inhaled for 3 seconds or, if a device with a light indicator is being used, until the light turns off. This deep breath creates sustained transpulmonary pressure near the end of inspiration and is sometimes called *sustained maximal inspiration.*
- Tell the patient to remove the mouthpiece and exhale normally. Allow them to relax and take several normal breaths before attempting another breath with the spirometer. Repeat this sequence 5 to 10 times during every waking hour. Note tidal volumes.
- Patients who are postsurgical, especially with thoracic and abdominal surgeries, may need help with splinting wound areas with a pillow to help with pain control during incentive spirometry use.

Practice pointers

- Evaluate the patient's ability to cough effectively and encourage coughing after each effort, because deep lung inflation may loosen secretions and facilitate their removal. Observe any expectorated secretions.
- Auscultate the patient's lungs, and compare findings with the first auscultation.

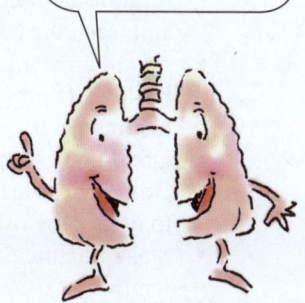

Remember to encourage the patient to cough. This helps loosen secretions.

Chest physiotherapy

Chest physiotherapy is usually performed with other treatments, such as suctioning, incentive spirometry, and administration of such medications as small-volume nebulizer aerosol treatments and expectorants.

Especially important for the patient who is confined to bed, chest physiotherapy improves secretion clearance and ventilation and helps prevent or treat atelectasis and pneumonia, which can hinder recovery. Chest physiotherapy procedures include:

- **percussion:** involves cupping the hands and fingers together and clapping them alternately (first one hand, then the other hand) over the patient's lung fields to loosen secretions (also achieved with the gentler technique of vibration)
- **vibration:** can be used with percussion or as an alternative to it in a patient who is frail, in pain, or recovering from thoracic surgery or trauma
- **postural drainage:** uses gravity to promote drainage of secretions from the lungs and bronchi into the trachea
- **deep breathing exercises:** help loosen secretions and promote more effective coughing
- **coughing:** helps clear secretions in the lungs, bronchi, and trachea and prevents aspiration

Supplies

- stethoscope
- pillows
- adjustable hospital bed
- emesis basin
- facial tissues
- suction equipment as needed
- equipment for oral care
- towel
- trash bag
- optional: sterile specimen container, supplemental oxygen

Getting ready

- Administer pain medication before the treatment (as ordered), and teach the patient to splint their incision.
- Auscultate the lungs to determine baseline status, and check the health care provider's order to determine which lung areas require treatment.
- Obtain pillows and a tilt board, if necessary.
- Don't schedule therapy immediately after a meal; wait 2 to 3 hours to reduce the risk of nausea and vomiting.
- Make sure the patient is adequately hydrated to facilitate removal of secretions.
- If ordered, administer bronchodilator and mist therapies before the treatment.
- Provide tissues, an emesis basin, and a cup for sputum.
- Set up suction equipment if the patient doesn't have an adequate cough to clear secretions.
- If they need oxygen therapy or are borderline hypoxemic without it, provide adequate flow rates of oxygen during therapy.

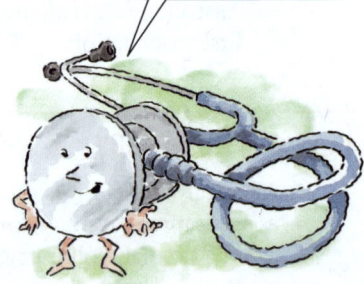

It's important for the patient to be well hydrated before beginning chest physiotherapy to facilitate the removal of secretions.

How it's done

- Position the patient as ordered. (The health care provider usually determines a position sequence after auscultation and chest x-ray review.) Be sure to position the patient so drainage is always oriented toward larger, more central airways.
- If the patient has a localized condition, such as pneumonia in a specific lobe, expect to start with that area first to avoid infecting uninvolved areas. If the patient has a diffuse disorder, such as bronchiectasis, expect to start with the lower lobes and work toward the upper ones. (See *Positioning the patient for postural drainage.*)

Positioning the patient for postural drainage

Postural drainage is most commonly required for the lower lobes of the lung. These illustrations show various postural drainage positions and the lung areas affected by each position.

Lower lobes: Posterior basal segments

Elevate the foot of the bed 30°. Have the patient lie prone with their head lowered. Position pillows under the chest and abdomen. Percuss the lower ribs on both sides of the spine.

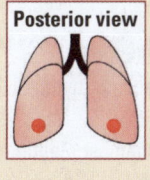

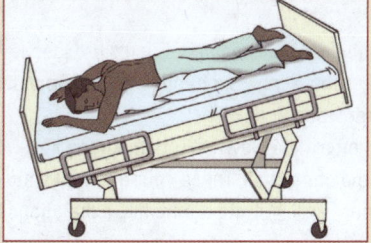

Lower lobes: Lateral basal segments

Elevate the foot of the bed 30°. Instruct the patient to lie on their abdomen with the head lowered and the upper leg flexed over a pillow for support. Then have them rotate a quarter turn upward. Percuss the lower ribs on the uppermost portion of the lateral chest wall.

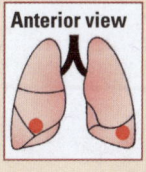

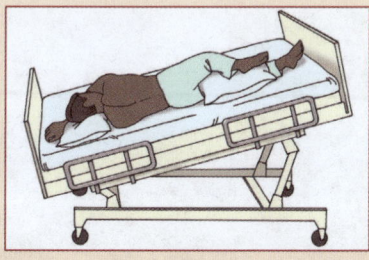

Lower lobes: Anterior basal segments

Elevate the foot of the bed 30°. Instruct the patient to lie on their side with their head lowered. Then place pillows as shown. Percuss with a slightly cupped hand over the lower ribs just beneath the axilla. If an acutely ill patient has trouble breathing in this position, adjust the bed to an angle they can tolerate before beginning percussion.

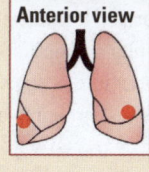

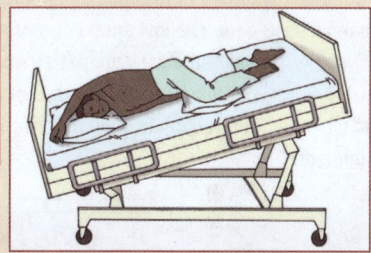

Lower lobes: Superior segments

With the bed flat, have the patient lie on their abdomen. Place two pillows under their hips. Percuss on both sides of the spine at the lower tip of the scapulae.

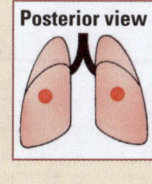

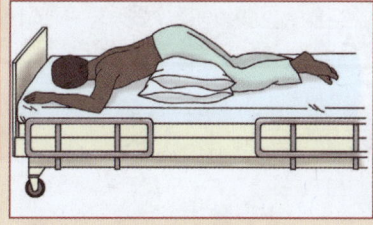

The percussion section

- Place your cupped hands against the patient's chest wall and rapidly flex and extend your wrists, generating a rhythmic, popping sound. (A hollow sound helps verify the correct performance of the technique.) (See *Performing percussion and vibration.*)
- Percuss each segment for a minimum of 3 minutes. The vibrations generated pass through the chest wall and help loosen secretions from the airways.

- Perform percussion throughout inspiration and expiration, and encourage the patient to take slow, deep breaths.
- Don't percuss over the spine, sternum, liver, kidneys, or (if the patient is a person assigned female at birth) the patient's breasts because this may cause trauma, especially in older adult patients.
- Percussion is painless when done properly, and the impact is diminished by a cushion of air formed in the cupped palm. This technique requires practice.

Performing percussion and vibration

To perform percussion, hold your hands in a cupped shape, with fingers flexed and thumbs pressed tightly against your index fingers. Percuss each segment for 1 to 2 minutes by alternating your hands against the patient in a rhythmic manner. Listen for a hollow sound on percussion to verify correct technique.

To perform vibration, ask the patient to inhale deeply and then exhale slowly through pursed lips. During exhalation, firmly press your fingers and the palms of your hands against the chest wall. Tense your arm and shoulder muscles in an isometric contraction to send fine vibrations through the chest wall. Vibrate during five exhalations over each chest segment.

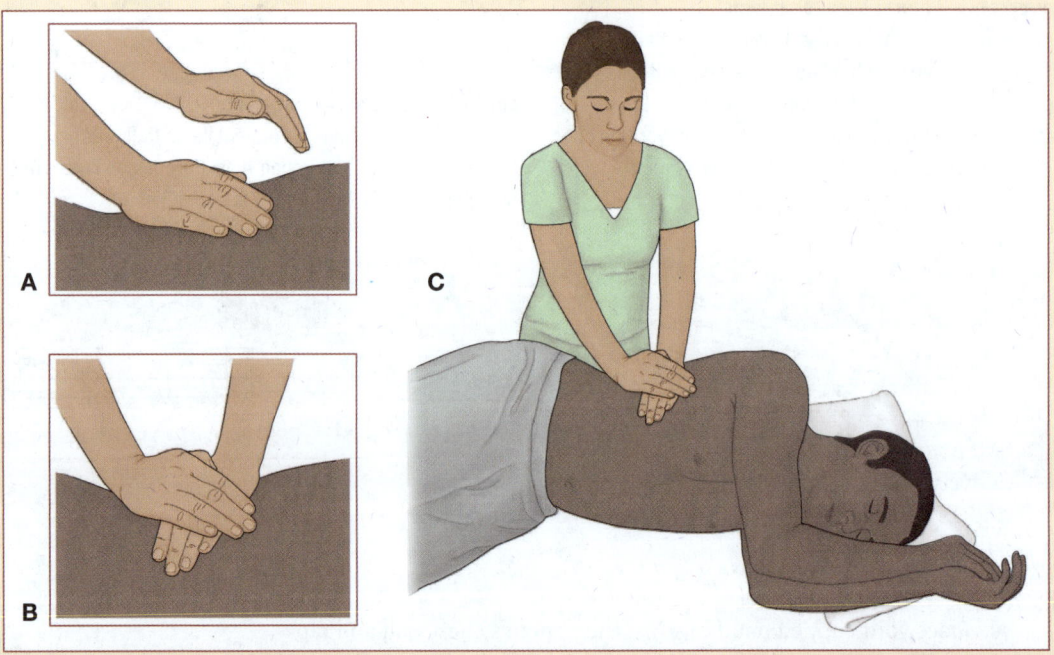

Percussion and vibration. A, Proper hand position for percussion. B, Proper hand position for vibration. C, Proper technique for vibration. The wrists and elbows remain stiff; the vibrating motion is produced by the shoulder muscles. (Adapted with permission from Hinkle, J. L., Cheever, K. H., & Overbaugh, K. (2022). *Brunner & Suddarth's Textbook of Medical-Surgical Nursing* (15th ed., Figure 20-7). Wolters Kluwer.)

Vibration

- Ask the patient to inhale deeply and then exhale slowly through pursed lips.
- During exhalation, firmly press your fingers and the palms of your hands against the chest wall. Tense the muscles of your arms and shoulders in an isometric contraction to send fine vibrations through the chest wall.
- Repeat vibration for five exhalations over each chest segment.
- If the technique is being performed correctly, a tremble should be heard in the patient's voice when they say "ah" on exhalation.

Practice pointers

- Evaluate the patient's tolerance for therapy, and make adjustments as needed. Watch for fatigue, and remember that the patient's ability to cough and breathe deeply diminishes as they tire.
- Assess for difficulty expectorating secretions. Use suction if the patient has an ineffective cough or a diminished gag reflex.
- Provide oral hygiene after therapy; secretions may taste foul or have an unpleasant odor.
- Be aware that postural drainage positions can cause nausea, dizziness, dyspnea, and hypoxemia.
- Patients with chronic bronchitis, bronchiectasis, or cystic fibrosis may need chest physiotherapy at home.

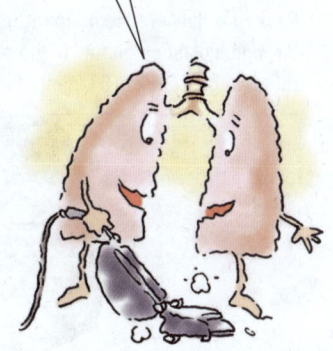

Percussion and vibration help to clean me up and make me feel brand new!

Oxygen therapy

In oxygen therapy, oxygen is delivered by mask, nasal prongs, nasal catheter, or transtracheal catheter to prevent or reverse hypoxemia and reduce the work of breathing. Possible causes of hypoxemia include chronic obstructive pulmonary disease, pneumonia, heart failure, and myocardial infarction. (See *Oxygen delivery systems.*) Oxygen delivery differs significantly among flow-adjustable mask devices. An understanding of the oxygen delivery capabilities of each mask type will help with the selection of the best mask to meet patients' oxygen requirements.

Fully equipped

The equipment depends on the patient's age and condition as well as the required fraction of inspired oxygen (FiO_2). High-flow systems, such as a Venturi mask and ventilators, deliver a precisely controlled air–oxygen mixture. Low-flow systems, such as nasal prongs, a nasal catheter, a simple mask, a partial rebreather mask, and a

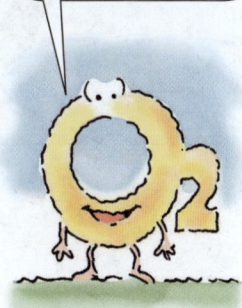

I get excited when I think about all the ways I can be delivered to a patient!

Oxygen delivery systems

Patients may receive oxygen through one of several administration systems, including a nasal cannula, a simple mask, a partial rebreather mask, a nonrebreather mask, a Venturi mask, a continuous positive airway pressure (CPAP) mask, aerosols, and transtracheal oxygen.

Nasal cannula

Oxygen is delivered in concentrations of less than 40% through a plastic cannula in the patient's nostrils. Flow rates range from 2 to 6 L/minute.

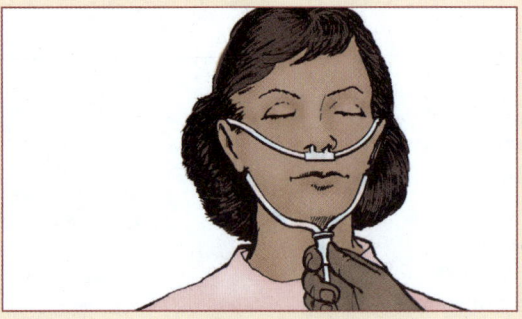

Simple mask

Oxygen flows through an entry port at the bottom of the mask and exits through large holes on the sides of the mask. It delivers oxygen in concentrations of around 40% and should be used with a flow rate of 5 to 8 L/minute.

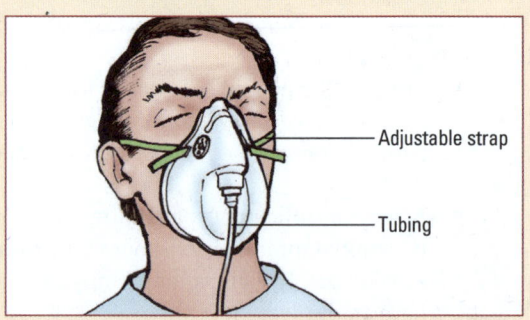

Adjustable strap

Tubing

High-flow nasal cannula

Similar to the nasal cannula, oxygen is delivered through a specially designed plastic cannula placed in the patient's nostrils. Oxygen is delivered at flow rates (~30 L/minute) that exceed the inspiratory pressure of the patient. This process allows the delivery of increased levels of fraction of inspired oxygen (FiO_2) while allowing the patient to eat and talk.

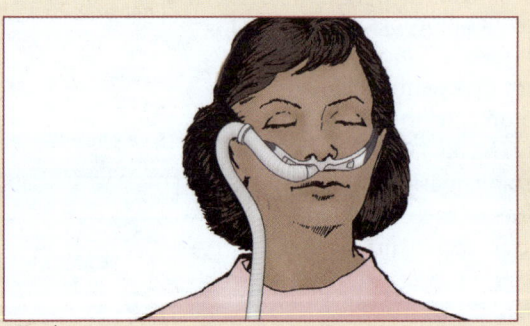

Partial rebreather mask

The patient inspires oxygen from a reservoir bag along with atmospheric air and oxygen from the mask. The first third of exhaled tidal volume enters the bag; the rest exits the mask. Because air entering the reservoir bag comes from the trachea and bronchi, where no gas exchange occurs, the patient rebreathes the oxygenated air they just exhaled. With this partial rebreather mask, oxygen can be administered in concentrations of 40% to 60%.

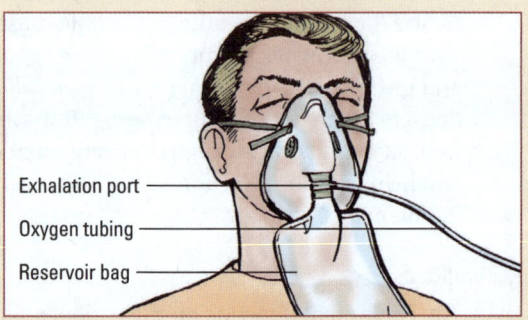

Exhalation port

Oxygen tubing

Reservoir bag

Oxygen delivery systems *(continued)*

Nonrebreather mask

On inhalation, the one-way inspiratory valve opens, directing oxygen from a reservoir bag into the mask. On exhalation, gas exits the mask through the one-way expiratory valves and enters the atmosphere. The patient breathes air only from the bag. This type of mask delivers the highest possible oxygen concentration (60% to 90%) short of intubation and mechanical ventilation.

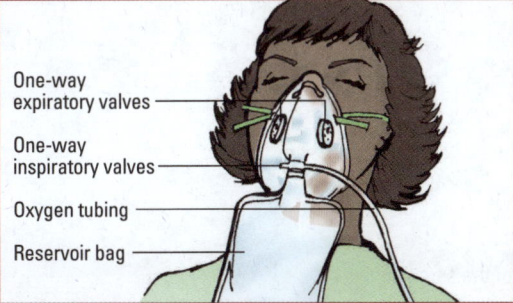

One-way expiratory valves

One-way inspiratory valves

Oxygen tubing

Reservoir bag

Venturi mask

The mask is connected to a Venturi device, which mixes a specific volume of air and oxygen. It delivers highly accurate oxygen concentration despite the patient's respiratory pattern.

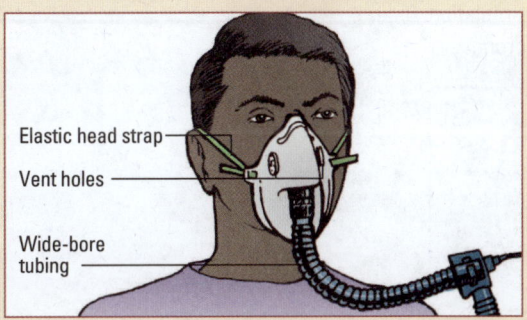

Elastic head strap

Vent holes

Wide-bore tubing

Aerosols

A face mask, hood, tent, or tracheostomy tube or collar is connected to wide-bore tubing that receives aerosolized oxygen from a jet nebulizer. An aerosol delivers high-humidity oxygen.

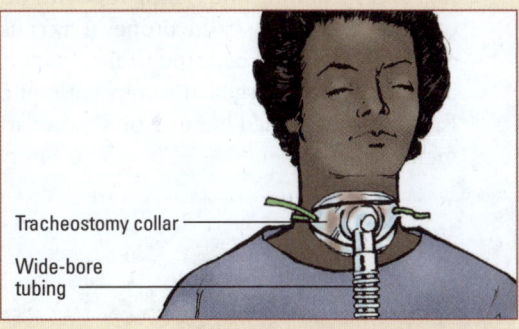

Tracheostomy collar

Wide-bore tubing

CPAP mask

This system allows the spontaneously breathing patient to receive CPAP with or without an artificial airway.

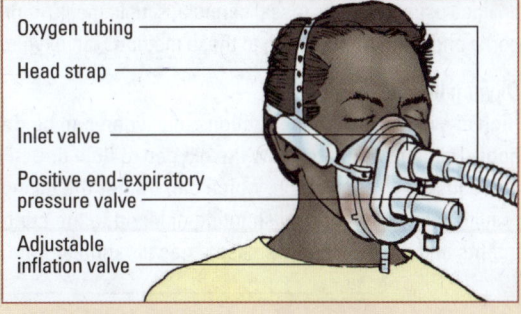

Oxygen tubing

Head strap

Inlet valve

Positive end-expiratory pressure valve

Adjustable inflation valve

Transtracheal oxygen

The patient receives oxygen through a catheter inserted into the base of their neck in a simple outpatient procedure.

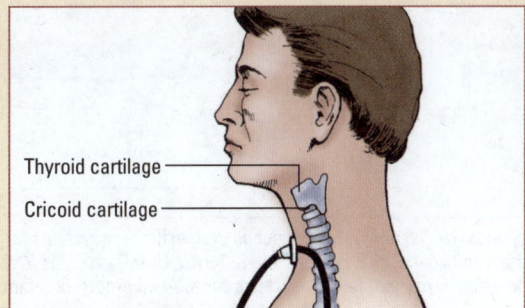

Thyroid cartilage

Cricoid cartilage

Source: Weekley, M. S. & Bland, L. E. (2022). *Oxygen administration*. StatPearls. https://www.ncbi.nlm.nih.gov/books/NBK551617/

nonrebreather mask, allow variation in the oxygen percentage delivered based on the patient's respiratory pattern. Children and infants don't tolerate masks. (See *Oxygen delivery in children.*)

Compare and contrast

Nasal prongs deliver oxygen at flow rates ranging from 0.5 to 6 L/minute. Inexpensive and easy to use, the prongs permit talking, eating, and suctioning, interfering less with the patient's activities than other devices. Even so, the prongs may cause nasal drying and can't deliver high oxygen concentrations. In contrast, a nasal catheter can deliver low-flow oxygen at somewhat higher concentrations, but it isn't commonly used because of discomfort and drying of the mucous membranes.

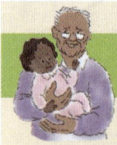

Ages and stages

Oxygen delivery in children

Oxygen delivery to children can be accomplished using many of the same delivery devices used for adults (nasal cannula, simple mask, nonrebreathers, etc.). For newborns and infants, in addition to these methods, an oxygen hood can be used.

Oxygen hood

High as well as low concentrations of oxygen can be delivered by an oxygen hood. Remember not to allow the oxygen to flow directly on the infant's face. This can cause cold stimulation, which can trigger the diving reflex. The diving reflex results in bradycardia and shunting of blood to the central circulation. Older infants and children can also use a nasal cannula or nasal prongs.

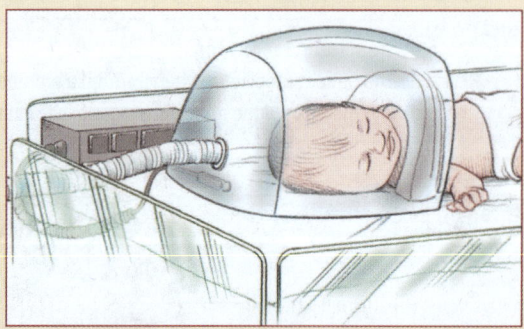

Source: Nagler, J. (2021). Continuous oxygen delivery systems for the acute care of infants, children, and adults. In: P. Parsons and S. Torrey, UpToDate. https://www.uptodate.com/contents/continuous-oxygen-delivery-systems-for-the-acute-care-of-infants-children-and-adults#H11

New flow

Over the past 2 decades, a less invasive option for high-flow oxygen has emerged. Originally used to treat apnea in premature infants, a high-flow nasal cannula (HFNC) was developed to deliver a high flow of oxygen (~30 L/minute) with proper heat and humidification to patients. HFNC uses a specially designed nasal cannula to deliver oxygen while allowing the patient to talk and eat. This delivery method has become increasingly popular for respiratory failure and was used often during the COVID-19 pandemic to support patients (Spicuzza & Schisano, 2020).

Chronic oxygen therapy

Masks deliver up to 100% oxygen concentrations but can't be used to deliver controlled oxygen concentrations. In addition, they may fit poorly, causing discomfort, and must be removed to eat. Transtracheal oxygen catheters, used for patients requiring chronic oxygen therapy, permit highly efficient oxygen delivery and increased mobility with portable oxygen systems while avoiding the adverse effects of nasal delivery systems. Even so, they may become a source of infection and require close monitoring and follow-up after insertion as well as daily maintenance care.

Supplies

The equipment depends on the type of delivery system ordered by the health care provider. Equipment includes selections from the following list:

- oxygen source (wall unit, cylinder, liquid tank, or concentrator)
- flow meter
- adapter (if using a wall unit) or pressure reduction gauge (if using a cylinder)
- sterile humidity bottle and adapters
- sterile distilled water
- OXYGEN PRECAUTIONS sign
- appropriate oxygen delivery system (for low flow and variable oxygen concentrations, a nasal cannula, HFNC, a simple mask, a partial rebreather mask, or a nonrebreather mask; or a Venturi mask, an aerosol mask, a T tube, or a tracheostomy collar)
- small diameter and large diameter connection tubing
- water-soluble lubricant
- gauze pads and tape (for oxygen masks)
- jet adapter for Venturi mask (if adding humidity)
- optional: oxygen analyzer

Getting ready

- To help prevent fire, instruct the patient, their roommates, and any visitors not to use heating pads, curling irons, electric razors, hair dryers, or other equipment near the oxygen source. Place an OXYGEN PRECAUTIONS sign on the outside of the patient's door. (See *Oxygen precautions.*)

- Perform a cardiopulmonary assessment, and check that a baseline arterial blood gas (ABG) or oximetry value has been obtained.

How it's done

- Check the patency of the patient's nostrils. (A mask may be necessary if the nostrils are blocked.) Consult the health care provider if a change in administration route is necessary.
- Assemble the equipment, check the connections, and turn on the oxygen source. Make sure the humidifier bubbles and oxygen flows through the prongs, catheter, or mask.
- Set the flow rate as ordered. If necessary, have the respiratory care practitioner check the flow meter for accuracy.

Practice pointers

- Periodically perform a cardiopulmonary assessment for the patient receiving any form of oxygen therapy.
- Perform a skin assessment to assure the patient is not experiencing any skin breakdown from contact with the oxygen therapy device.
- If the patient is on bed rest, change their position frequently to ensure adequate ventilation and circulation.
- Provide good skin care to prevent irritation and breakdown caused by the tubing, prongs, or mask.

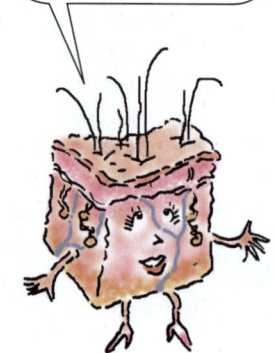

Don't forget basic position changes for patients on bed rest. Practice good skin care to prevent irritation and breakdown caused by oxygen devices.

Oxygen precautions

When a patient is prescribed oxygen therapy, it is important that they understand there are precautions due to its ability to support combustion. Here are the guidelines that should be followed in the hospital and at home:

1. Do not smoke, and do not allow others to smoke around you.
2. Heat and flame sources should be kept at least five feet away from oxygen equipment.
3. Hair dryers, curling irons, heating pads, and electric razors should not be used during oxygen therapy.
4. Do not use aerosol sprays, oil-based creams, or alcohol-based products near oxygen concentrators.
5. Have a fire extinguisher nearby to extinguish a fire quickly if it occurs.

Source: American Lung Association. (2024). Oxygen therapy: Using oxygen safely. https://www. lung.org/lung-health-diseases/lung-procedures-and-tests/oxygen-therapy/using-oxygen-safely

To humidify or not to humidify…

- Be sure to humidify oxygen flow exceeding 3 L/minute to help prevent drying of mucous membranes. However, don't add humidity when using a Venturi mask because water can block the Venturi jets.
- Assess for signs of hypoxia, including decreased level of consciousness (LOC), tachycardia, arrhythmias, diaphoresis, restlessness, altered blood pressure or respiratory rate, clammy skin, and cyanosis. If these occur, notify the health care provider, obtain a pulse oximetry reading, and check the oxygen delivery equipment to see whether it's malfunctioning. Be especially alert for changes in respiratory status when oxygen therapy is changed or discontinued.

Check those valves

- If the patient is using a nonrebreather mask, periodically check the valves to see that the mask is functioning properly. If the valves stick closed, it will cause the patient to inhale carbon dioxide and not receive adequate oxygen. If the mask is not functioning correctly, replace the mask.
- If the patient receives high oxygen concentrations (exceeding 50%) for more than 24 hours, ask the patient if they are experiencing burning, substernal chest pain, dyspnea, and dry cough, which are symptoms of oxygen toxicity. Atelectasis and pulmonary edema may also occur.

Take a deep breath and cough

- Encourage coughing and deep breathing to help prevent atelectasis. Frequently monitor ABG levels, pulse oximetry values, or both, and reduce oxygen concentrations as soon as ABG results or pulse oximetry values indicate it's feasible.
- Use a low flow rate if the patient has chronic pulmonary disease. However, don't use a simple face mask because low flow rates won't flush carbon dioxide from the mask, and the patient will rebreathe carbon dioxide. Watch for alterations in LOC, heart rate, and respiratory rate.

Go home with the flow

- If the patient needs oxygen at home, the health care provider will order the flow rate, the number of hours per day to be used, and the conditions of use.
- Several types of delivery systems are available, including a tank, concentrator, and liquid oxygen system. The system chosen depends on the patient's needs and the availability and cost of each system. Make sure the patient can use the prescribed system safely and effectively. The patient will need regular follow-up care to evaluate their response to therapy.

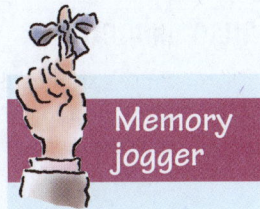

Memory jogger

If hypoxia is suspected, check for **high, low, clammy, and blue**:

↑ heart rate, respiratory rate, and restlessness

↓ level of consciousness

Clammy, diaphoretic skin

Blue coloring of skin, specifically around the lips or in nail beds (cyanosis)

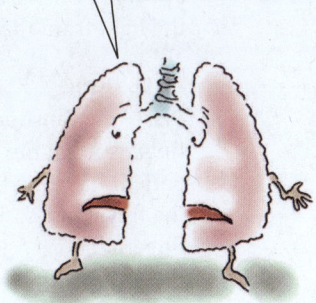

Be aware that too much oxygen can cause oxygen toxicity, with such symptoms as burning, substernal chest pain, and dyspnea.

Pulse oximetry

Pulse oximetry is a noninvasive way to monitor a patient's oxygen saturation to determine how well the patient's lungs are delivering oxygen to their blood. It can be performed continuously or intermittently.

Light reading

In pulse oximetry, two diodes send red and infrared light through a pulsating arterial vascular bed such as the one in the fingertip. A photodetector slipped over the finger measures the transmitted light as it passes through the vascular bed, detects the relative amount of color absorbed by arterial blood, and calculates the exact mix of venous oxygen saturation without interference from surrounding venous blood, skin, connective tissue, or bone (Torp et al., 2022). (See *How oximetry works.*)

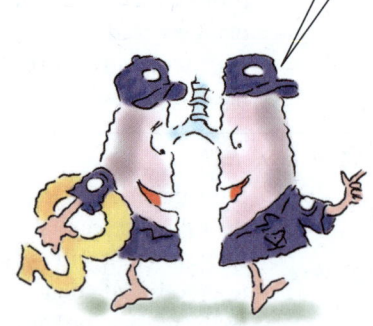

Pulse oximetry measures how well I deliver oxygen to the blood. I try to be right on time every time with my deliveries!

Symbolically speaking

Pulse oximetry usually denotes arterial saturation values with the symbol SpO_2. Invasively measured arterial oxygen saturation values, such as from ABG analysis, are denoted by the symbol SaO_2.

Supplies
- pulse oximetry
- alcohol pads
- nail polish remover, if necessary

Getting ready
- Review the manufacturer's directions for assembling the oximeter.
- Select a finger for the test. Although the index finger is commonly used, a smaller finger may be selected if the patient's fingers are too large for the equipment.
- Make sure the patient isn't wearing false fingernails, and remove any nail polish from the test finger, because it may alter or absorb the light from the pulse oximeter.

How it's done
- Place the transducer (photodetector) probe over the patient's finger so that the light beam sensors oppose each other. If the patient has long fingernails, position the probe perpendicular to the finger, if possible, or (with the patient's permission) clip the fingernails.

How oximetry works

Pulse oximetry allows noninvasive monitoring of a patient's arterial oxygen saturation (SaO_2) levels by measuring the absorption (amplitude) of light waves as they pass through areas of the body that are highly perfused by arterial blood. Oximetry also monitors pulse rate and amplitude.

Light-emitting diodes in a transducer (photodetector) attached to the patient's body (shown below on the index finger) send red and infrared light beams through tissue. The photodetector records the relative amount of each color absorbed by arterial blood and transmits the data to a monitor, which displays the information with each heartbeat. If the SaO_2 level or pulse rate varies from preset limits, the monitor triggers visual and audible alarms.

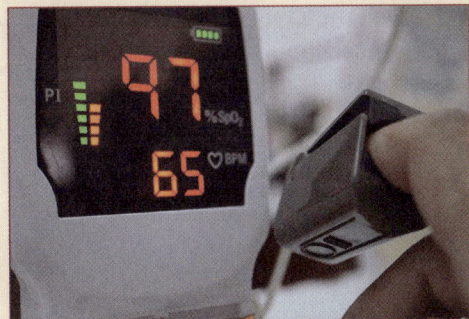

(Shutterstock/toysf400)

Source: Torp, K. D., Modi, P., & Simon, L. V. (2022). *Pulse oximetry*. StatPearls. https://www.ncbi.nlm.nih.gov/books/NBK470348/

Be level with the heart

- Always position the patient's hand at heart level to eliminate venous pulsations and to promote accurate readings. (See *Pediatric pulse oximetry.*)
- Turn on the power switch. If the device isn't working properly, a beep will sound, a display will light momentarily, the pulse searchlight will flash. If the device is working properly, the SpO_2 and pulse rate displays will show stationary zeroes. After four to six heartbeats, the SpO_2 and the pulse rate displays will supply information with each heartbeat, and the pulse amplitude indicator will begin tracking the pulse.

Practice pointers

If oximetry has been performed properly, readings are typically accurate. However, factors such as low body temperature and low blood pressure may interfere with accuracy (Torp et al., 2022). It is especially

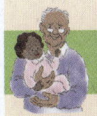

Ages and stages

Pediatric pulse oximetry

If arterial oxygen saturation is being measured in a neonate or a small infant, wrap the oximeter's probe around the infant's foot so that light beams and detectors oppose each other. For a large infant, use a probe that fits on the great toe, and secure it to the foot.

important to acknowledge that pulse oximetry may overestimate the SpO_2, of a patient with darker skin, because this may impact care (Cabanas et al., 2022).

Detour over the bridge

- If the patient has compromised circulation in their extremities, a photodetector can be placed across the bridge of the nose.
- If an automatic blood pressure cuff is used on the same extremity that's used for measuring SpO_2, the cuff will interfere with SpO_2 readings during inflation.

Problem solving

- Normal SpO_2 levels for pulse oximetry are 95% to 100% for adults and 93.8% to 100% by 1 hour after birth for healthy, full-term neonates. Oxygen saturation of less than 90% indicates hypoxemia, which warrants intervention (Torp et al., 2022) and notification of the health care provider. (See *Documenting pulse oximetry*.)

Take note!

Documenting pulse oximetry

Document the procedure, including the date, time, procedure type, oximetric measurement, and actions taken. Record the readings on appropriate flowcharts, if indicated.

Tracheostomy care

A tracheotomy may be performed in an emergency situation or after careful preparation. It may be a permanent measure or a temporary therapy. No matter the circumstances, tracheostomy care always has the following goals:

- to ensure airway patency by keeping the tube free from mucus buildup
- to maintain mucous membrane and skin integrity
- to prevent infection
- to provide psychological support

Simple, medium, and complex

The patient may have one of the following types of tracheostomy tube:

- **Uncuffed tube:** This type of tube may be plastic, polyvinyl chloride, or metal. It comes in various sizes, lengths, and styles depending on the patient's needs. It allows air to flow freely around the tracheostomy tube and through the larynx, reducing the risk of tracheal damage.
- **Fenestrated tube:** This type of tube allows speech to be possible through the upper airway when the external opening is capped and the cuff is deflated. Mechanical ventilation is possible with the inner cannula in place and the cuff inflated.
- **Cuffed tube:** This type of tube is made of plastic or polyvinyl chloride and is disposable. The cuff and the tube won't separate

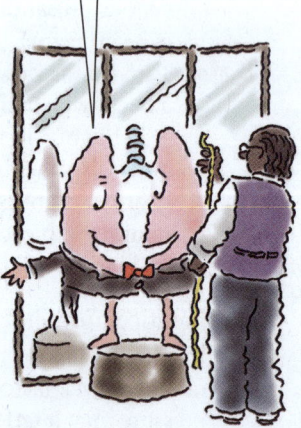

I think I like a little more cuff showing.

accidentally inside the trachea because the cuff is bonded to the tube. Also, it doesn't require periodic deflating to lower pressure because cuff pressure is low and evenly distributed against the tracheal wall. Although cuffed tubes may cost more than other tubes, they reduce the risk of tracheal damage. (See *Comparing tracheostomy tubes*.)

Comparing tracheostomy tubes

Tracheostomy tubes are made of plastic or metal and come in uncuffed, cuffed, or fenestrated varieties. Tube selection depends on the patient's condition and the health care provider's preference. It is important to be familiar with the advantages and disadvantages of these commonly used tracheostomy tubes.

Uncuffed
(plastic or metal)

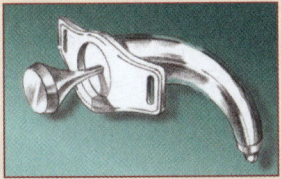

Advantages
• Free flow of air around tube and through larynx
• Reduced risk of tracheal damage
• Mechanical ventilation possible in patient with neuromuscular disease

Disadvantages
• Increased risk of aspiration in adults due to lack of cuff
• Adapter possibly needed for ventilation

Plastic cuffed
(low pressure and high volume)

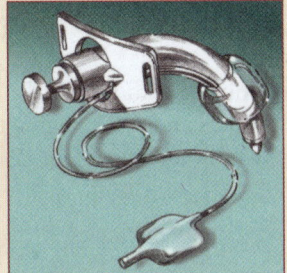

Advantages
• Disposable
• Cuff bonded to tube (won't detach accidentally inside trachea)
• Low cuff pressure that's evenly distributed against tracheal wall (no need to deflate periodically to lower pressure)
• Reduced risk of tracheal damage

Disadvantages
• Possibly more expensive than other tubes

Fenestrated

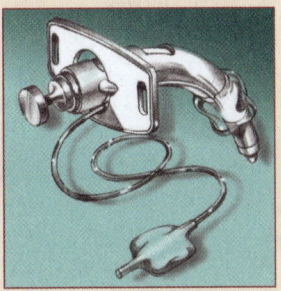

Advantages
• Speech possible through upper airway when external opening is capped and cuff is deflated
• Breathing by mechanical ventilation possible with inner cannula in place and cuff inflated
• Easy removal of inner cannula for cleaning

Disadvantages
• Possible occlusion of fenestration
• Possible dislodgment of inner cannula
• Cap removal necessary before inflating cuff

Source: Pruitt, B. (2022). *Tracheostomy care and the respiratory therapist.* RT Magazine. https://rtmagazine.com/department-management/clinical/tracheostomy-care-and-the-respiratory-therapist/

Keeping it clean

To prevent infection, tracheostomy care should be performed using an aseptic technique until the stoma has healed. For recently performed tracheotomies, use sterile gloves for all manipulations at the tracheostomy site. When the stoma has healed, clean gloves may be substituted for sterile ones.

Supplies

For aseptic stoma and outer cannula care

- waterproof trash bag
- two sterile solution containers
- normal saline solution
- hydrogen peroxide
- sterile cotton-tipped applicators
- sterile 4 × 4-in gauze pads
- sterile gloves
- prepackaged sterile tracheostomy dressing (or 4 × 4-in gauze pad)
- equipment and supplies for suctioning and mouth care
- materials as needed for cuff procedures and for changing tracheostomy ties (see the below sections on these topics)

For aseptic inner cannula care

All of the preceding equipment plus:

- prepackaged commercial tracheostomy care set or sterile forceps
- sterile nylon brush
- sterile, 6-in (15.2-cm) pipe cleaners
- clean gloves
- a third sterile solution container
- a disposable temporary inner cannula (for a patient on a ventilator)

For changing tracheostomy ties

- a 30-in (76.2-cm) length of tracheostomy twill tape or prepackaged disposable trach ties
- bandage scissors
- sterile gloves
- hemostat

For emergency tracheostomy tube replacement

- sterile tracheal dilator or sterile hemostat
- sterile obturator that fits the tracheostomy tube in use
- extra sterile tracheostomy tube and obturator in an appropriate size
- suction equipment and supplies

In plain sight

Keep these supplies in the patient's room at all times for easy access in case of an emergency. Consider taping an emergency sterile tracheostomy tube in a sterile wrapper to the head of the bed for easy access.

For cuff procedures
- 5- or 10-mL syringe
- padded hemostat
- stethoscope

Getting ready
- Wash your hands, and assemble all equipment and supplies in the patient's room. Open the waterproof trash bag, and place it next to the workspace to avoid reaching across the sterile field or the patient's stoma when discarding soiled items.

Set the table

- Establish a sterile field near the patient's bed (usually on the over-bed table), and place equipment and supplies on it. Pour normal saline solution, hydrogen peroxide, or a mixture of equal parts of both solutions into one of the sterile solution containers; then, pour normal saline solution into the second sterile container for rinsing.

For the inner

- For inner cannula care, a third sterile solution container may be used to hold the gauze pads and cotton-tipped applicators saturated with cleaning solution. If the disposable inner cannula is being replaced, open the package containing the new inner cannula while maintaining sterile technique. Obtain or prepare new tracheostomy ties, if indicated.

How it's done
- Assess the patient's condition to determine their need for care.
- Explain the procedure to the patient, even if they are unresponsive. Provide privacy.
- Place the patient in semi-Fowler position (unless it's contraindicated) to decrease abdominal pressure on the diaphragm and to promote lung expansion.
- Remove humidification or ventilation devices.
- Using sterile technique, suction the entire length of the tracheostomy tube to clear the airway of any secretions that may hinder oxygenation. (See the "Tracheal suction" section, which begins on page 334.)
- Reconnect the patient to the humidifier or ventilator, if necessary.

Cleaning a stoma and outer cannula

- Wash hands.
- Put on sterile gloves if not already in place.
- Saturate a cotton-tipped applicator or sterile gauze pad with the cleaning solution. Squeeze out the excess liquid to prevent accidental aspiration. Then, wipe the patient's neck under the tracheostomy tube flanges and twill tapes.
- Use more pads or cotton-tipped applicators to clean the stoma site and the tube's flanges. Wipe only once with each pad or applicator, and then discard it to prevent contamination of a clean area with a soiled pad.
- Rinse debris and peroxide (if used) with one or more sterile 4 × 4-in gauze pads dampened in normal saline solution. Dry the area thoroughly with additional sterile gauze pads, then apply a new sterile tracheostomy dressing.
- Remove and discard gloves.
- Wash hands.

Cleaning a nondisposable inner cannula

- Wash hands.
- Put on sterile gloves.

Remove and discard

- Remove and discard the patient's tracheostomy dressing, and disconnect the ventilator or humidification device. Unlock the tracheostomy tube's inner cannula by rotating it counterclockwise. Place the inner cannula in the container of hydrogen peroxide.

Scrub-a-dub-dub

- Working quickly with a sterile hand scrub the cannula with the sterile nylon brush. If the brush doesn't slide easily into the cannula, use a sterile pipe cleaner.
- Immerse the cannula in the container of normal saline solution, and agitate it for about 10 seconds to rinse it thoroughly.
- Inspect the cannula for cleanliness. Repeat the cleaning process, if necessary. Once it's clean, tap it gently against the inside edge of the sterile container to remove excess liquid and prevent aspiration. Don't dry the outer surface, because a thin film of moisture acts as a lubricant during insertion.
- Reinsert the inner cannula into the patient's tracheostomy tube. Lock it in place, and then gently pull on it to make sure it's positioned securely. Reconnect the mechanical ventilator. Apply a new sterile tracheostomy dressing.

- If the patient can't tolerate being disconnected from the ventilator for the time it takes to clean the inner cannula, replace the existing inner cannula with a clean one and reattach the mechanical ventilator. Then clean the cannula just removed from the patient, and store it in a sterile container for the next time.

Caring for a disposable inner cannula

- Wash hands and put on clean gloves.
- Remove the patient's inner cannula. After evaluating the secretions in the cannula, discard the cannula.
- Pick up the new inner cannula, touching only the outer locking portion. Insert the cannula into the tracheostomy and, following the manufacturer's instructions, lock it securely.

Changing tracheostomy ties

- Obtain assistance from another nurse or a respiratory therapist because of the risk of accidental tube expulsion during this procedure. Patient movement or coughing can dislodge the tube.
- Wash your hands thoroughly, and put on sterile gloves if you aren't already wearing them.
- If commercially packaged tracheostomy ties aren't being used, prepare new ties from a 30 in (76.2 cm) length of twill tape by folding one end back 1 in (2.5 cm) on itself. Then, with the bandage scissors, cut a ½ in (1.3 cm) slit down the center of the tape from the folded edge.
- Prepare the other end of the tape the same way.

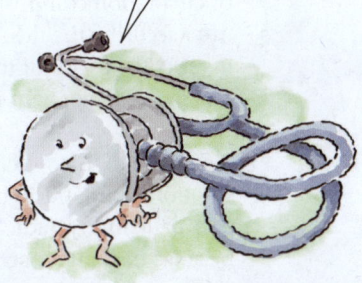

Always enlist the help of another nurse or a respiratory therapist before changing tracheostomy ties.

Cut to order

- Hold both ends together and, using scissors, cut the resulting circle of tape so that one piece is approximately 10 in (25 cm) long and the other is about 20 in (51 cm) long.
- Help the patient into a semi-Fowler position, if possible.
- After the assistant puts on gloves, instruct them to hold the tracheostomy tube in place to prevent its expulsion during replacement of the ties. If the procedure is performed without assistance, to prevent tube expulsion, fasten the clean ties in place before removing the old ties.
- With the assistant's gloved fingers holding the tracheostomy tube in place, cut the soiled tracheostomy ties with the bandage scissors, or untie them and discard the ties. Be careful not to cut the tube of the pilot balloon.

Thread and tie

- Thread the slit end of one new tie a short distance through the eye of one tracheostomy tube flange from the underside; use the hemostat, if needed, to pull the tie through. Then, thread the other end of the tie completely through the slit end, and pull it taut so it loops firmly through the flange. This avoids knots that can cause throat discomfort, tissue irritation, pressure, and necrosis on the patient's neck.
- Fasten the second tie to the opposite flange in the same manner.

Know the knots

- Instruct the patient to flex their neck while the ties are brought around to the side, and tie them together with a square knot. Flexion produces the same neck circumference as coughing and helps prevent an overly tight tie. Instruct the assistant to place one finger under the tapes as they are tied to ensure that they're tight enough to avoid slippage but loose enough to prevent choking or jugular vein constriction. Tight ties can also cause skin breakdown or circulation compromise.
- After securing the ties, cut off the excess tape with the scissors and instruct the assistant to release the tracheostomy tube.
- Make sure the patient is comfortable and can reach the call button easily.
- Because neck diameter can increase from swelling and cause constriction, check tracheostomy tie tension often on patients with traumatic injury, radical neck dissection, or cardiac failure.
- Because ties can loosen and cause tube dislodgment, frequently check patients who are restless or neonatal patients (who have delicate equipment, arms and fingers that they cannot control, and smaller airways).

Concluding tracheostomy care

- Replace the humidification device.
- Provide oral care as needed to prevent the oral cavity from becoming dry and malodorous or from developing sores from encrusted secretions.

Look closely

- Observe soiled dressings and suctioned secretions for amount, color, consistency, and odor.
- Properly clean or dispose of all equipment, supplies, solutions, and trash according to facility policy.
- Take off and discard gloves. Wash hands.

- Make sure the patient is comfortable.
- Make sure all necessary supplies are readily available at the bedside.
- Repeat the procedure as needed and ordered. Change the dressing as often as necessary regardless of whether the entire cleaning procedure is performed, because a wet dressing with exudate or secretions predisposes the patient to skin excoriation, breakdown, and infection.

Deflating and inflating a tracheostomy cuff

- Read the cuff manufacturer's instructions; cuff types and procedures vary widely.
- Assess the patient's condition, explain the procedure to them, and be reassuring. Wash your hands thoroughly.

Sit up…

- Help the patient into semi-Fowler position, if possible, or place them in a supine position *so* secretions above the cuff site will be pushed up into their mouth if they are receiving positive-pressure ventilation.

…and suction

- Suction the oropharyngeal cavity to prevent pooled secretions from descending into the trachea after cuff deflation.
- If a hemostat is present, release the padded hemostat clamping the cuff inflation tubing.

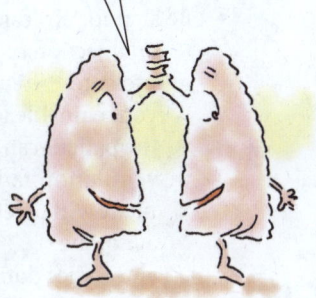

Don't forget to suction the oropharyngeal cavity to prevent secretions from descending after cuff deflation.

Slowly deflate…

- Insert a 5- or 10-mL syringe into the cuff pilot balloon, and very slowly withdraw all air from the cuff. Leave the syringe attached to the tubing for later reinflation of the cuff. Slow deflation allows positive lung pressure to push secretions upward from the bronchi. Cuff deflation may also stimulate the patient's cough reflex, producing additional secretions.
- Remove any ventilation device. Suction the lower airways through any existing tube to remove all secretions. Then reconnect the patient to the ventilation device.
- Maintain cuff deflation for the prescribed time. Observe the patient for adequate ventilation, and suction as necessary. If the patient has difficulty breathing, reinflate the cuff immediately by depressing the syringe plunger very slowly. Inject the least amount of air necessary to achieve an adequate tracheal seal.

...then pump back up

- If the cuff is being inflated using cuff pressure measurement, be careful not to exceed 25 mm Hg. Note the exact amount of air needed to inflate the cuff. If the pressure exceeds 25 mm Hg, notify the health care provider because you may need to change to a larger size tube, use higher inflation pressures, or permit a larger air leak. The recommended cuff pressure is between 20 and 30 mm Hg (Pruitt, 2022).
- After you've inflated the cuff, if the tubing doesn't have a one-way valve at the end, clamp the inflation line with a padded hemostat (to protect the tubing) and remove the syringe.

No sounds allowed

- Check for a minimal-leak cuff seal. You shouldn't feel air coming from the patient's mouth, nose, or tracheostomy site, and a conscious patient shouldn't be able to speak.
- Be alert for air leaks from the cuff itself. Suspect a leak if:
  ○ an injection of air fails to inflate the cuff or increase cuff pressure
  ○ you're unable to inject the amount of air withdrawn
  ○ the patient can speak
  ○ ventilation fails to maintain adequate respiratory movement with pressures or volumes previously considered adequate
  ○ air escapes during the ventilator's inspiratory cycle.
- Make sure the patient is comfortable.
- Properly clean or dispose of all equipment, supplies, and trash according to facility policy.
- Replenish any used supplies, and make sure all necessary emergency supplies are at the bedside.

Practice pointers

- Make sure the patient can easily reach the call button and communication aids.
- Keep appropriate equipment at the patient's bedside for immediate use in an emergency.
- Follow facility policy regarding the procedure if a tracheostomy tube is expelled or if the outer cannula becomes blocked. Use extreme caution when attempting to reinsert an expelled tracheostomy tube because of the risk of tracheal trauma, perforation, compression, and asphyxiation.

What *not* to do

- Refrain from changing tracheostomy ties unnecessarily during the immediate postoperative period before the stoma track is well formed (usually 4 days) to avoid accidental dislodgment and expulsion of the tube. Unless secretions or drainage are a problem, ties can be changed once per day.

Class time

- If the patient is being discharged with a tracheostomy, start self-care teaching as soon as they are receptive. Teach the patient how to change and clean the tube.
- Assess for complications, which can occur within the first 48 hours after tracheostomy tube insertion. Complications can include:
  - hemorrhage at the operative site
  - bleeding or edema in tracheal tissue, causing airway obstruction
  - aspiration of secretions
  - introduction of air into the pleural cavity, causing pneumothorax
  - hypoxia or acidosis, triggering cardiac arrest
  - introduction of air into surrounding tissues, causing subcutaneous emphysema. (See *Documenting tracheostomy care.*)

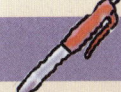

Take note!

Documenting tracheostomy care

When tracheostomy care is complete, be sure to document:
- date and time of the procedure
- type of procedure
- amount, consistency, color, and odor of secretions
- stoma and skin condition
- patient's respiratory status
- tracheostomy tube changes made by the health care provider
- duration of cuff deflation
- amount of cuff inflation
- cuff pressure readings, with patient's body position during reading
- complications and nursing actions taken
- patient's tolerance of the procedure
- patient or family teaching provided

Tracheal suction

Tracheal suction involves the removal of secretions from the trachea or bronchi by means of a catheter inserted through the mouth or nose, a tracheal stoma, a tracheostomy tube, or an endotracheal (ET) tube.

Say no to pneumonia

In addition to removing secretions, tracheal suctioning also stimulates the cough reflex. This procedure helps maintain a patent airway to promote optimal exchange of oxygen and carbon dioxide and to prevent pneumonia that results from pooling of secretions (Hanlon, 2019). Performed as frequently as the patient's condition warrants, tracheal suction calls for strict aseptic technique.

Supplies
- oxygen source (wall or portable unit, and handheld resuscitation bag with a mask, 15-mm adapter, or positive end-expiratory pressure [PEEP] valve, if indicated)
- wall or portable suction apparatus
- collection container
- connecting tube
- suction catheter kit or sterile suction catheter, one sterile glove, one clean glove, and a disposable sterile solution container
- gown
- mask
- goggles
- 1 L bottle of sterile water or normal saline solution
- sterile water-soluble lubricant (for nasal insertion)
- syringe for deflating the cuff of the ET or tracheostomy tube
- optional: sterile towel

Getting ready
- Choose the correct suction catheter. The diameter should be no larger than half the inside diameter of the tracheostomy or ET tube to minimize hypoxia during suctioning. Place the suction apparatus on the overbed table or bedside stand.
- Attach the collection container to the suction unit and the connecting tube to the collection container. Label and date the normal saline solution or sterile water. Put on gown, mask, and goggles.

How it's done
- Before suctioning, determine whether the facility requires a health care provider's order and obtain one, if necessary.
- Assess the patient's vital signs, breath sounds, and general appearance to establish a baseline for comparison after

suctioning. Review the patient's ABG values and oxygen saturation levels, if available. If nasotracheal suctioning is being performed, check the patient's history for a deviated septum, nasal polyps, nasal obstruction, nasal trauma, epistaxis, or mucosal swelling.
- Wash your hands. Explain the procedure to the patient even if they're unresponsive.

Positioned to cough

- Unless contraindicated, place the patient in semi-Fowler or high-Fowler position to promote lung expansion and productive coughing.
- Set the suction pressure according to facility policy. Typically, pressure may be set under 200 mm Hg for adult patients and under 120 mm Hg for pediatric patients (Blakeman et al., 2022); higher pressures may cause traumatic injury. Occlude the suction port to assess suction pressure.

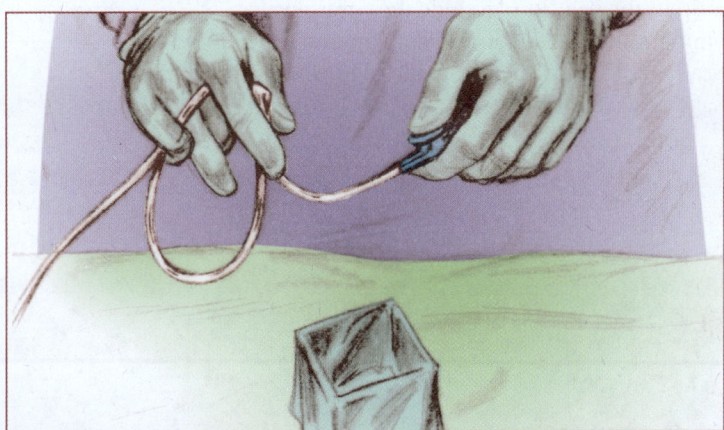

- Remove the top from the normal saline solution or water bottle.
- Open the package containing the sterile solution container.
- Using aseptic technique, open the kit and put on gloves; alternatively, open the suction catheter and gloves, place the nonsterile glove on your nondominant hand, and place the sterile glove on your dominant hand.
- Use your nondominant (nonsterile) hand to pour the normal saline solution or sterile water into the solution container.
- Place a small amount of lubricant on the sterile area to facilitate passage of the catheter during nasotracheal suctioning.
- Place a sterile towel over the patient's chest, if desired, to provide an additional sterile area.

One hand does this...

Using sterile technique, unwrap the catheter. Keep it coiled so it can't touch a nonsterile object. Use your nonsterile hand to attach the tubing to the catheter.

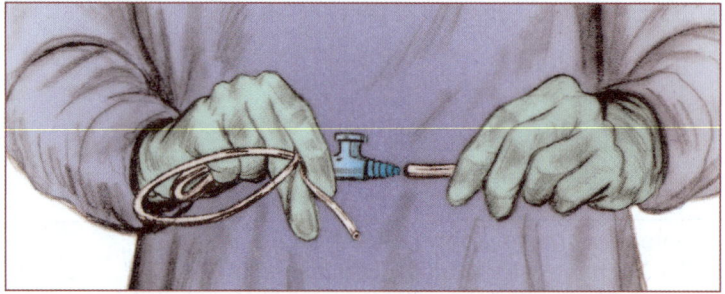

- Dip the catheter tip in the saline solution to lubricate the outside of the catheter and to reduce tissue trauma during insertion.
- With the catheter tip in the solution, occlude the control valve with your nondominant thumb. Suction a small amount of solution through the catheter to lubricate the inside of it, which will facilitate the passage of secretions.

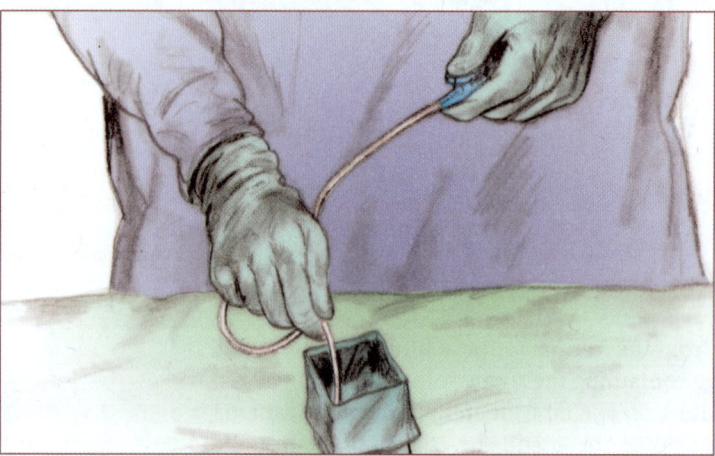

- For nasal insertion of the catheter, lubricate the tip of the catheter with the sterile, water-soluble lubricant to reduce tissue trauma during insertion.
- If the patient isn't intubated or is intubated but isn't receiving supplemental oxygen or aerosol, instruct them to take three to six deep breaths to help minimize or prevent hypoxia during suctioning.

Add oxygen?

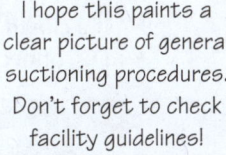

- If the patient isn't intubated but is receiving oxygen, evaluate their need for preoxygenation. If indicated, instruct them to take three to six deep breaths while using the supplemental oxygen. (If needed, the patient may continue to receive supplemental oxygen during suctioning by leaving the nasal cannula in one nostril or by keeping the oxygen mask over the mouth.)
- If the patient is being mechanically ventilated, preoxygenate them using a handheld resuscitation bag, by adjusting the sigh mode on the ventilator, or by adjusting the FiO_2 to 0.1. To use the resuscitation bag, set the oxygen flow meter at 15 L/minute, disconnect the patient from the ventilator, and deliver three to six breaths with the resuscitation bag (Blakeman et al., 2022).

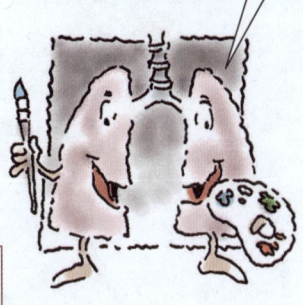

I hope this paints a clear picture of general suctioning procedures. Don't forget to check facility guidelines!

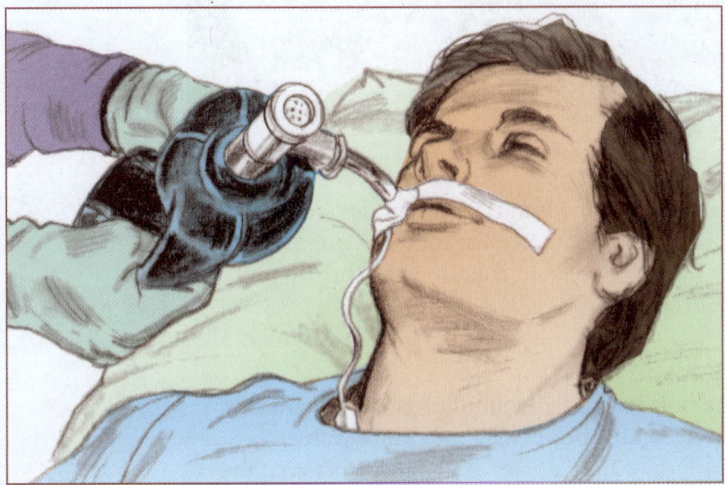

- If the patient is being maintained on PEEP, evaluate the need to use a resuscitation bag with a PEEP valve.

Nasotracheal insertion in a nonintubated patient

- Disconnect the oxygen from the patient, if applicable.
- Raise the tip of the patient's nose to straighten the passageway and to facilitate catheter insertion.
- Insert the catheter into the patient's nostril while gently rolling it to help it advance through the turbinate.
- Ask the patient to inhale. As the patient inhales, quickly advance the catheter as far as possible. To avoid oxygen loss and tissue trauma, don't apply suction during insertion.
- If the patient coughs as the catheter passes through the larynx, briefly hold the catheter still, and then resume advancement when the patient inhales.

Insertion in an intubated patient

- If a closed system is used, see *Closed tracheal suctioning*, page 339.
- Disconnect the patient from the ventilator.

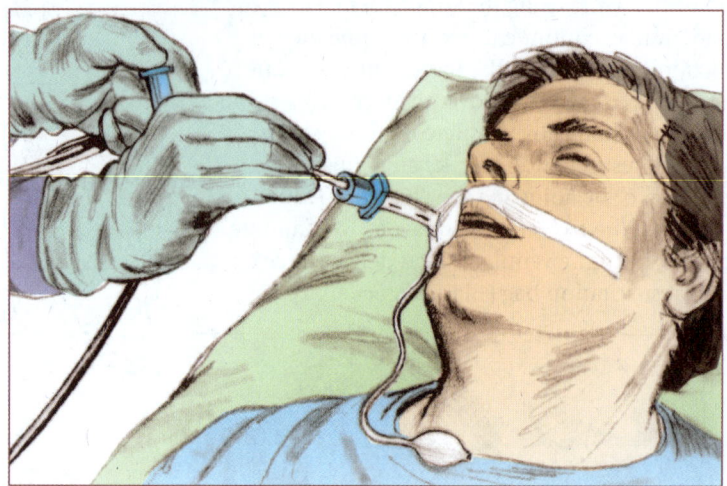

- Using sterile technique, gently insert the suction catheter into the artificial airway. Advance the catheter, without applying suction, until resistance is met. If the patient coughs, pause briefly, and then resume advancement.

Suctioning the patient

- After inserting the catheter, apply suction intermittently by removing and replacing the thumb over the control valve. Simultaneously withdraw the catheter as you roll it between the thumb and forefinger of the other hand. This rotating motion prevents the catheter from pulling tissue into the tube as it exits, preventing tissue trauma. To prevent hypoxia, never suction more than 10 seconds at a time.
- If the patient is intubated, stabilize the tip of the ET tube as the catheter is withdrawn to prevent mucous membrane irritation or accidental extubation.

May the source be with you

- If applicable, resume oxygen delivery by reconnecting the source of oxygen or ventilation and hyperoxygenating the patient's lungs before continuing to prevent or relieve hypoxia.
- Observe the patient, and allow them to rest for a few minutes before the next suctioning.

Closed tracheal suctioning

The closed tracheal suction system can ease removal of secretions and reduce patient complications. Consisting of a sterile suction catheter in a clear plastic sleeve, the system permits the patient to remain connected to the ventilator during suctioning. As a result, the patient can maintain the tidal volume, oxygen concentration, and PEEP delivered by the ventilator while being suctioned, which reduces the occurrence of suction-induced hypoxemia.

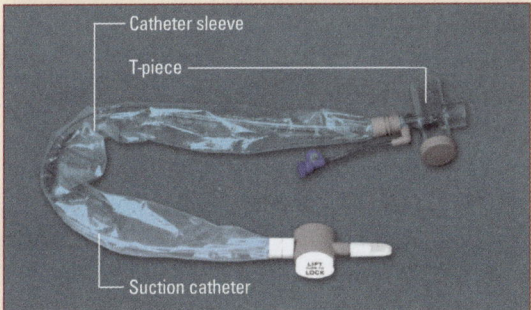

Catheter sleeve
T-piece
Suction catheter

Another advantage of this system is a reduced risk of infection, even when the same catheter is used many times. Because the catheter remains in a protective sleeve, gloves aren't required; however, they're still recommended. The caregiver doesn't need to touch the catheter, and the ventilator circuit remains closed.

Implementation

To perform the procedure, gather a closed suction control valve, a T-piece to connect the artificial airway to the ventilator breathing circuit, and a catheter sleeve that encloses the catheter and has connections at each end for the control valve and the T-piece. Put on personal protective equipment, if you haven't already done so. Then, follow these steps:

• Remove the closed suction system from its wrapping. Attach the control valve to the connecting tubing.

• Depress the thumb suction control valve, and keep it depressed while setting the suction pressure to the desired level.

• Connect the T-piece to the ventilator breathing circuit, making sure that the irrigation port is closed; then, connect the T-piece to the patient's endotracheal or tracheostomy tube (as shown below).

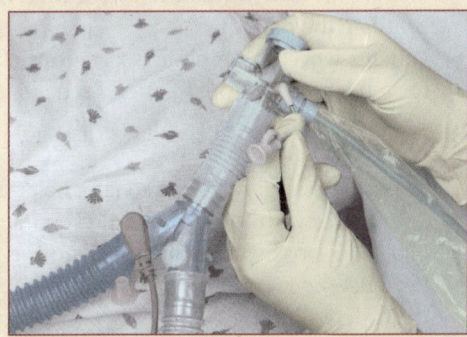

• With one hand keeping the T-piece parallel to the patient's chin, use the thumb and index finger of the other hand to advance the catheter through the tube and into the patient's tracheobronchial tree (as shown below). It may be necessary to retract the catheter sleeve as the catheter is gently advanced.

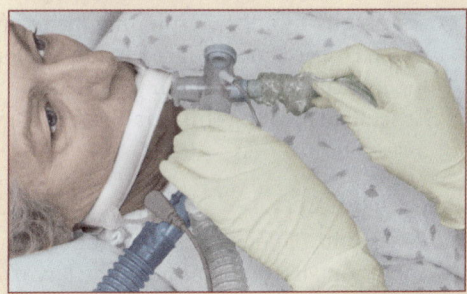

• While continuing to hold the T-piece and control valve, apply intermittent suction, and withdraw the catheter until it reaches its fully extended length in the sleeve. Repeat the procedure as necessary.

• After suctioning is complete, flush the catheter by maintaining suction while slowly introducing normal saline solution or sterile water into the irrigation port.

• Place the thumb control valve in the off position.

• Dispose of and replace the suction equipment and supplies according to facility policy.

• Change the closed suction system every 24 hours to minimize the risk of infection.

Source: Blakeman, T., Scott, J., Yoder, M., Capellari, E., & Strickland, S. (2022). American Association for Respiratory Care clinical guidelines: Artificial airway suctioning. *Respiratory Care*, 67(2), 258–271.

Taking the secret out of secretions

- Observe the secretions. If they're thick, clear the catheter periodically by dipping the tip in the saline solution and applying suction. If the patient's heart rate and rhythm are being monitored, observe for arrhythmias. If arrhythmias occur, stop suctioning and ventilate the patient.
- Patients who can't mobilize secretions effectively may need to perform tracheal suctioning after discharge.

After suctioning

- After suctioning, hyperoxygenate the patient being maintained on a ventilator with the handheld resuscitation bag by adjusting the FiO_2 to 0.1 or by using the ventilator's sigh mode.
- Readjust the FiO_2 and, for ventilated patients, the tidal volume to the ordered settings.
- After suctioning the lower airways, assess the patient's need for upper airway suctioning. If the cuff of the ET or tracheostomy tube is inflated, suction the upper airway before deflating the cuff with a syringe. Always change the catheter and sterile glove before resuctioning the lower airways to avoid introducing microorganisms into the lower airways (Pasrija & Hall, 2023).
- Discard the gloves, gown, mask, goggles, and catheter. Clear the connecting tubing by aspirating the remaining saline solution or water. Discard and replace suction equipment and supplies according to facility policy. Wash your hands.
- Auscultate the lungs bilaterally and take vital signs, if indicated, to assess effectiveness.

Practice pointers

- Raising the patient's nose into the sniffing position (if the patient's condition allows) helps align the larynx and pharynx and may facilitate passing the catheter during nasotracheal suctioning.
- To prevent damage to the suction machine, don't allow the collection container on the machine to become more than three-quarters full.
- Assess the patient for complications of tracheal suctioning. (See *Complications of tracheal suctioning*, page 341, for details.)
- Document the procedure according to facility policy. (See *Documenting tracheal suctioning*, page 341.)

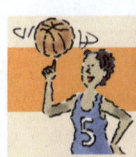

Complications of tracheal suctioning

Common complications of tracheal suctioning include:
- hypoxemia and dyspnea from removal of oxygen along with secretions
- altered respiratory patterns from anxiety
- cardiac arrhythmias from hypoxia and vagus nerve stimulation
- tracheal or bronchial trauma from traumatic or prolonged suctioning
- in patients with compromised cardiovascular or pulmonary status: hypoxemia, arrhythmias, hypertension, and hypotension
- in patients with a history of nasopharyngeal bleeding, those receiving anticoagulants, those who have undergone a recent tracheostomy, and those with blood dyscrasias: bleeding
- in patients with increased ICP: a further rise in intracranial pressure (ICP)

Rare complications
- Rare complications of suctioning include laryngospasm and bronchospasm. If either occurs, disconnect the suction catheter from the connecting tubing and let the catheter act as an airway. It is essential to plan ahead with the health care provider to reduce the risk of these complications.

Source: Pasrija, D., & Hall, C. A. (2023). *Airway suctioning*. StatPearls. https://www.ncbi.nlm.nih.gov/books/NBK557386/

Documenting tracheal suctioning

Be sure to document:
- date and time of the procedure
- suctioning technique used
- reason for suctioning
- amount, color, consistency, and odor of secretions
- complications and nursing actions taken
- patient's tolerance of the procedure

Thoracic drainage

Thoracic drainage, also known as a *chest tube thoracostomy*, uses gravity (and occasionally suction) to restore negative pressure, to remove material that collects in the pleural cavity, or to expand a partially or totally collapsed lung (Shlamovitz, 2020). An underwater seal in the drainage system allows air and fluid to escape from the pleural cavity but doesn't allow air to reenter. Insertion of a chest tube is always completed by a specially trained health care provider; however, nurses often monitor and care for these systems after placement.

Rare sighting

The drainage apparatus is a self-contained, disposable system that collects drainage, creates a water seal, and controls suction. (See *Closed chest drainage systems*, page 342.)

Supplies
- closed chest drainage system (which can function as a gravity drainage system or be connected to suction to enhance chest drainage)
- sterile distilled water (usually 1 L)
- adhesive tape

- sterile clear plastic tubing
- bottle or system rack
- two rubber-tipped Kelly clamps
- sterile 50-mL catheter-tip syringe
- suction source, if ordered
- pain medication, if ordered

Getting ready

Check the health care provider's order to determine the type of drainage system to be used and specific procedure details. If appropriate, request the drainage system and suction system from the central supply department. Collect the appropriate equipment, and take it to the patient's bedside.

How it's done

- Explain the procedure to the patient, and wash your hands.
- To avoid introducing pathogens into the pleural space, maintain sterile technique throughout the entire procedure and whenever changes in the system are made or any of the connections are altered.

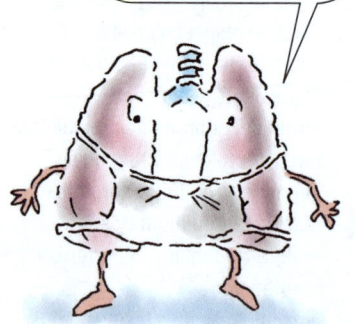

When performing thoracic drainage, maintain sterile technique to prevent pathogens from entering the pleural space.

Closed chest drainage systems

One-piece, disposable plastic drainage systems contain three chambers. The drainage chamber is on the right and has three calibrated columns that display the amount of drainage collected. When the first column fills, drainage carries over into the second column and, when that fills, into the third column. The water-seal chamber is located in the center. The suction-control chamber on the left is filled with water to achieve various suction levels. Rubber diaphragms are provided at the rear of the device to change the water level or to remove samples of drainage. A positive pressure relief valve at the top of the water-seal chamber vents excess pressure into the atmosphere, preventing pressure buildup.

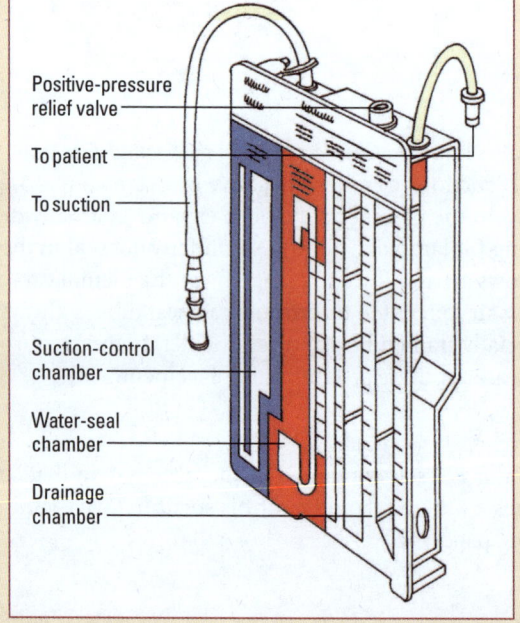

Positive-pressure relief valve

To patient

To suction

Suction-control chamber

Water-seal chamber

Drainage chamber

Setting up a commercially prepared disposable system

Open the packaged system, and place it on the floor in the rack supplied by the manufacturer to avoid accidentally knocking it over or dislodging the components. After the system is prepared, it may be hung from the side of the patient's bed.

Just add water

- Remove the plastic connector from the short tube attached to the water-seal chamber. Using a 50–mL catheter-tip syringe, instill sterile distilled water into the water-seal chamber until it reaches the 2-cm mark or the mark specified by the manufacturer.
- If suction is ordered, remove the cap (also called the *muffler* or the *atmosphere vent cover*) on the suction-control chamber to open the vent. Next, instill sterile distilled water until it reaches the 20-cm mark or the ordered level, and recap the suction-control chamber.
- Using the long tube, connect the patient's chest tube to the closed drainage collection chamber. Secure the connection with tape.
- Connect the short tube on the drainage system to the suction source, and turn on the suction. Gentle bubbling should begin in the suction chamber, indicating that the correct suction level has been reached.

Managing closed chest underwater-seal drainage

- Frequently note the character, consistency, and amount of drainage in the drainage collection chamber.
- Mark the drainage level in the drainage collection chamber by noting the time and date at the drainage level on the chamber every 8 hours (or more often if there's a large amount of drainage).

Look for the level

- Check the water level in the water-seal chamber every 8 hours. If necessary, carefully add sterile distilled water until the level reaches the 2-cm mark indicated on the water-seal chamber of the commercial system.
- Check for fluctuation in the water-seal chamber as the patient breathes. Normal fluctuations of 2 to 4 in (5 to 10 cm) reflect pressure changes in the pleural space during the respiration cycle. To check for fluctuation when a suction system is being used, momentarily disconnect the suction system so the air vent is opened, and observe for fluctuation.

Bubbles, bubbles everywhere

- Check for intermittent bubbling in the water-seal chamber. Bubbling occurs normally when the system is removing air from the pleural cavity. If bubbling isn't readily apparent during quiet breathing,

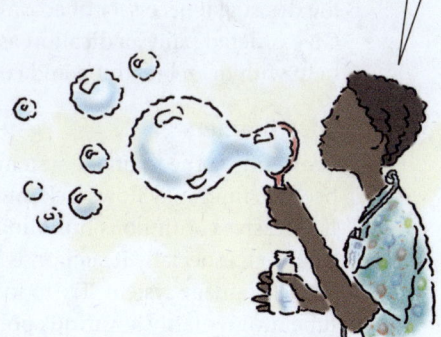

The amount of bubbling is a sign of how efficiently air is being removed from the pleural cavity.

have the patient take a deep breath or cough. The absence of bubbling indicates that the pleural space has been sealed.

- Check the water level in the suction-control chamber. Detach the chamber from the suction source; when bubbling ceases, observe the water level. If necessary, add sterile distilled water to bring the level to the 20-cm line or as ordered.
- Check for gentle bubbling in the suction-control chamber because it indicates that the proper suction level has been reached. Vigorous bubbling in this chamber increases the rate of water evaporation.
- Periodically check that the air vent in the system is working properly. Occlusion of the air vent results in a buildup of pressure in the system that could cause the patient to develop a tension pneumothorax.

Always ready to clamp down

- Be sure to keep two rubber-tipped clamps at the bedside to clamp the chest tube if the system cracks or to locate an air leak in the system. (See *Clamping alert.*)
- Encourage the patient to frequently cough and deep breathe to help drain the pleural space and to expand the lungs.
- Tell the patient to sit upright for optimal lung expansion and to splint the insertion site while coughing to minimize pain.
- Check the rate and quality of the patient's respirations and auscultate their lungs periodically to assess air exchange in the affected lung. Diminished or absent breath sounds may indicate that the lung hasn't expanded.

Cause for alarm

- Tell the patient to report breathing difficulty immediately. Notify the health care provider immediately if the patient develops cyanosis, rapid or shallow breathing, subcutaneous emphysema, chest pain, or excessive bleeding.
- Check the chest tube dressing as indicated by the provider and facility policy. Palpate the area surrounding the dressing for crepitus or subcutaneous emphysema, which indicates that air is leaking into the subcutaneous tissue surrounding the insertion site. Change the dressing if necessary or according to facility policy.
- Give ordered pain medication as needed for comfort and to help with deep breathing and coughing.

Practice pointers

- Avoid lifting the drainage system above the patient's chest, because fluid may flow back into the pleural space.
- If excessive continuous bubbling is present in the water-seal chamber, especially if suction is being used, rule out a leak in the drainage system. Try to locate the leak by clamping the tube momentarily at various points along its length. Begin clamping at the tube's proximal end, and work down toward

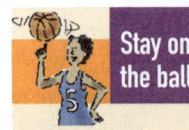

Stay on the ball

Clamping alert

Never leave a chest tube clamped for longer than 1 minute. Keeping it clamped too long may cause a tension pneumothorax from the pressure that builds up when air and fluid can't escape.

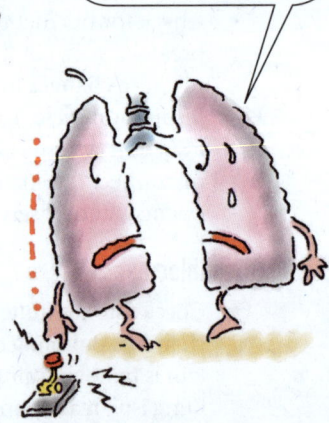

Alert the health care provider immediately if the patient develops breathing difficulty or signs of complications.

the drainage system, paying special attention to the seal around the connections. If a connection is loose, push it back together and tape it securely. The bubbling will stop when a clamp is placed between the air leak and the water seal. If the entire length of the tube is clamped and the bubbling doesn't stop, the drainage unit may be cracked and needs replacement (Roebker et al., 2023).

- If the drainage collection chamber fills, replace it. To do this, double-clamp the tube close to the insertion site (use two clamps facing in opposite directions), exchange the system, remove the clamps, and retape the bottle connection.

What if it cracks?

- If the commercially prepared system cracks, prepare a new unit to replace it. After doing so, clamp the chest tube momentarily with the two rubber-tipped clamps at the bedside (placed there at the time of tube insertion). Place the clamps close to each other near the insertion site; they should face in opposite directions *to provide a more complete seal.* Observe the patient for altered respirations while the tube is clamped. Then replace the damaged equipment.
- Tension pneumothorax is a medical emergency that may result from excessive accumulation of air, drainage, or both. A tension pneumothorax can exert pressure on the heart and aorta, causing a precipitous fall in cardiac output (Sahota & Sayad, 2024).

> Investigate any excessive bubbling or suspected cracks promptly to rule out problems that can lead to tension pneumothorax.

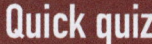

Quick quiz

1. When preparing to suction a patient, the nurse knows that all EXCEPT which of the following should be done?

  A. Apply suction intermittently as the catheter is removed.
  B. Suction the patient for no longer than 10 seconds at a time.
  C. Oxygenate the patient's lungs before and after suctioning.
  D. Apply suction continuously as the catheter is inserted.

Answer: D. Suctioning while inserting the catheter will be uncomfortable for the patient and may decrease oxygen levels.

2. A nurse is assisting a patient with breathing exercises and treatments. To help the patient with the achievement of maximal ventilation, what would be the best technique or treatment to teach the patient?

  A. Puffing breathing
  B. Box breathing
  C. Use of an incentive spirometer
  D. Use of a turbo inhaler

Answer: C. An incentive spirometer helps achieve maximal ventilation by inducing the patient to take a deep breath and hold it. Incentive spirometry is a lung expansion technique that uses sustained maximal inspiration. It can help to improve ventilation–perfusion mismatch, optimize oxygenation via splinting, and prevent the collapse of alveoli.

3. Which type of tracheostomy tube is associated with a lower risk of damage to the trachea?
   A. Uncuffed tube
   B. Cuffed tube
   C. Fenestrated tube
   D. Two-piece tube

Answer: B. Cuffed tubes do not require periodic deflating to lower pressure because cuff pressure is low and evenly distributed against the tracheal wall. Because of that even distribution of pressure, there is decreased risk of tracheal damage. In addition, the cuff and the tube will not separate accidentally inside the trachea because the cuff is bonded to the tube.

4. When performing chest physiotherapy, the nurse asks the patient to say "ah" and hears a tremble in their voice. Which technique is the nurse using to produce this effect?
   A. Percussion
   B. Postural drainage
   C. Vibration
   D. Deep breathing exercises

Answer: C. Vibration, which can be used with percussion or as an alternative to it in a patient who is frail, in pain, or recovering from thoracic surgery or trauma, produces a tremble in the patient's voice when they say "ah" on exhalation.

Scoring

 If you answered all four questions correctly, congrats! Your brain is saturated with knowledge of oxygenation.

If you answered three questions correctly, good job! Your knowledge of oxygenation is perfusing nicely.

If you answered fewer than three questions correctly, don't despair! Take a deep breath to reoxygenate those tissues, and try again.

References

American Lung Association. (2024). Oxygen therapy: Using oxygen safely. https://www.lung.org/lung-health-diseases/lung-procedures-and-tests/oxygen-therapy/using-oxygen-safely

Blakeman, T., Scott, J., Yoder, M., Capellari, E., & Strickland, S. (2022). AARC clinical practice guidelines: Artificial airway suctioning. *Respiratory Care, 67*(2), 258–271.

Cabanas, A. M., Fuentes-Guajardo, M., Latorre, K., León, D., & Martín-Escudero, P. (2022). Skin pigmentation influence on pulse oximetry accuracy: A systematic review and bibliometric analysis. *Sensors, 22*(9), 3402. https://doi.org/10.3390/s22093402

Franklin, E., & Anjum, F. (2023). *Incentive spirometer and inspiratory muscle training.* StatPearls. https://www.ncbi.nlm.nih.gov/books/NBK572114/

Hanlon, P. (2019). *Preventing lung infections via airway suction.* RT Magazine. https://rtmagazine.com/department-management/clinical/preventing-lung-infections-via-airway-suction/

Khan, Y., & Lynch, D. (2023). *Histology, lung.* StatPearls. https://www.ncbi.nlm.nih.gov/books/NBK534789/

Nagler, J. (2021). *Continuous oxygen delivery systems for the acute care of infants, children, and adults.* In Parsons, P. and Torrey, S., UpToDate. https://www.uptodate.com/contents/continuous-oxygen-delivery-systems-for-the-acute-care-of-infants-children-and-adults#H11

Pasrija, D., & Hall, C. A. (2023). *Airway suctioning.* StatPearls. https://www.ncbi.nlm.nih.gov/books/NBK557386/

Pruitt, B. (2022). *Tracheostomy care and the respiratory therapist.* RT Magazine. https://rtmagazine.com/department-management/clinical/tracheostomy-care-and-the-respiratory-therapist/

Roebker, J., Kord, A., Chan, K., Rao, R., & Ray, C. E.Jr., Ristagno, R (2023). Chest tube placement and management: A practical review. *Seminars in Interventional Radiology, 40*(2), 231–239. https://doi.org/10.1055/s-0043-1768680

Sahota, R., & Sayad, E. (2024). *Tension pneumothrorax.* StatPearls. https://www.ncbi.nlm.nih.gov/books/NBK559090/

Shlamovitz, G. Z. (2020). *Tube thoracostomy.* Medscape. https://emedicine.medscape.com/article/80678

Spicuzza, L., & Schisano, M. (2020). High-flow nasal cannula oxygen therapy as an emerging option for respiratory failure: the present and the future. *Therapeutic Advances in Chronic Disease, 11*, 2040622320920106. https://doi.org/10.1177/2040622320920106

Torp, K. D., Modi, P., & Simon, L. V. (2022). *Pulse oximetry.* StatPearls. https://www.ncbi.nlm.nih.gov/books/NBK470348/

Weekley, M. S., & Bland, L. E. (2022). *Oxygen administration.* StatPearls. https://www.ncbi.nlm.nih.gov/books/NBK551617/

Chapter 13

Self-care and hygiene[*]

Just the facts

In this chapter, you'll learn:

♦ various methods for determining a patient's ability to perform activities of daily living
♦ factors that affect self-care
♦ ways that hygiene affects health
♦ common hygiene practices.

Learning about self-care and hygiene

Hygiene means performing practices that promote health through personal cleanliness. Hygiene practices include bathing, cleaning and maintaining fingernails and toenails, shampooing and grooming hair, oral care, feeding, and toileting. Hygiene also refers to caring for assistive devices, including hearing aids, eyeglasses, contacts, and dental appliances such as dentures and removable dental bridges.

Hygiene practices and a person's ability to perform them are influenced by many factors. Age, gender, personal preferences, socioeconomic status, and religious or cultural practices commonly affect a person's approach to self-care. Personal care needs can also be affected by physical limitations, body image, or changes in health status. Although nurses need to be mindful of how these factors affect self-care, they should encourage patients to perform hygiene and self-care whenever possible.

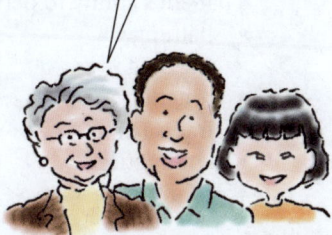

Hygiene practices can vary because of age, gender, religion, culture, physical limitations, and changes in health.

Promoting independence

The inability to perform self-care and attend to hygiene needs can be extremely embarrassing as well as frustrating, especially for adult

---

[*]Note: In this chapter, the term "male" refers to a person assigned male at birth, and the term "female" refers to a person assigned female at birth.

patients. A young child is accustomed to having an adult help with brushing teeth, combing hair, toileting, or bathing, but an adult may feel a loss of dignity and independence when needing assistance. Emotional well-being and health status can be enhanced with the ability to independently perform self-care and hygiene procedures. Promoting independence and helping patients to learn or relearn self-care activities is a primary goal of nursing.

Normal self-care patterns

Daily self-care and hygiene routines are largely based on personal and cultural preferences. Many patients are accustomed to a morning routine of rising from sleep, then brushing their teeth, bathing, and dressing. The morning routine may also include shaving or trimming facial hair, or application of makeup.

Establish a routine

When a patient experiences illness and hospitalization, daily practices and routines are often affected. The nurse can assess a patient's needs and abilities by establishing a routine similar to normal self-care practices. By observing the patient's abilities to perform routine self-care, the nurse can determine in which areas the patient may need assistance.

Assessing the ability to perform activities of daily living

The Katz index is a widely used tool for evaluating a patient's ability to perform daily personal care activities (McCabe, 2023). The tool ranks a patient's ability to perform six functions:
- bathing
- dressing
- toileting
- transfer
- continence
- feeding.

Factors affecting self-care

Many factors can affect a patient's ability to perform self-care and hygiene, including:
- vision impairment
- activity intolerance or weakness from a past medical condition or a current illness

- mental impairment or a psychiatric condition that alters cognitive ability
- pain or discomfort from surgery or disease
- neuromuscular impairment such as a stroke
- skeletal impairment, such as a fracture or joint replacement
- medically prescribed activity restriction, such as a pregnant patient on bedrest
- therapeutic procedure that restrains physical activity, such as a cast application or an intravenous infusion that restricts movement
- environmental barriers, such as financial restraints that may prevent the patient from affording shampoo, shaving supplies, or clean clothes, or the resources to wash them
- psychological barriers such as a reluctance to ask for help.

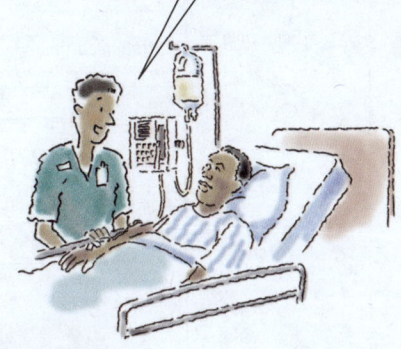

Many factors can impact a person's ability to perform self-care practices.

Hygiene and the body

Most hygiene practices help to maintain or restore healthy skin, mucous membranes, hair, and nails.

The integumentary system

The skin, also called the *integumentary system*, covers the internal structures of the body, protecting them from the external world. Intact, healthy skin is important for preventing infection. Regular bathing removes excess oil, perspiration, and bacteria from the skin surface.

Functions of skin

The skin is the body's largest organ and carries out several important functions, including:

- protecting the tissues from trauma and bacteria
- preventing the loss of water and electrolytes from the body
- sensing temperature, pain, touch, and pressure
- regulating body temperature through sweat production and evaporation
- synthesizing vitamin D
- promoting wound repair by allowing cell replacement of surface wounds.

What's in your skin

This cross-section of the skin illustrates major skin structures.

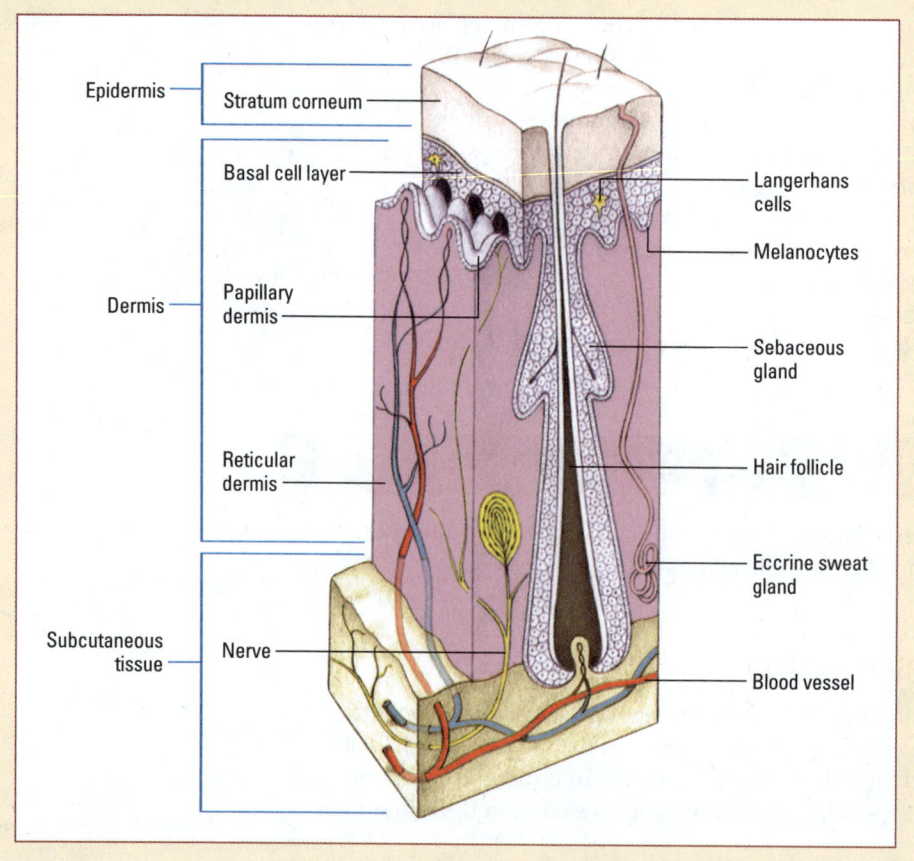

Epidermis — Stratum corneum

Basal cell layer

Langerhans cells

Melanocytes

Dermis

Papillary dermis

Sebaceous gland

Reticular dermis

Hair follicle

Eccrine sweat gland

Subcutaneous tissue

Nerve

Blood vessel

Layers of the skin

The skin consists of two distinct layers: the epidermis and the dermis. Subcutaneous tissue lies beneath these layers. The epidermis—the outer layer—is made of squamous epithelial tissue; it is thin and contains no blood vessels. The two major layers of the epidermis are the stratum corneum—the most superficial layer—and the deeper basal cell layer, or stratum germinativum. (See *What's in your skin.*)

Cell movement

The stratum corneum is made up of cells that form in the basal cell layer, then migrate to the skin's outer surface, and die as they reach the surface. However, because epidermal regeneration is continuous, new cells are constantly being produced.

The colors of skin

The basal cell layer contains melanocytes, which produce melanin and are responsible for skin color. Hormones, the environment, and heredity influence melanocyte production. Because melanocyte production is greater in some people than in others, skin color varies considerably.

Laying it on thick

The dermis—the thick, deeper layer of the skin—consists of connective tissue and an extracellular material called *matrix*, which contributes to the skin's strength and pliability. Blood vessels, lymphatic vessels, nerves, and hair follicles are located in the dermis, as are sweat and sebaceous glands. The dermis is well supplied with blood to deliver nutrition to the epidermis. In addition, wound healing and infection control take place in the dermis.

Give the glands a hand!

Sebaceous glands, found primarily in the skin of the scalp, face, upper body, and genital region, are part of the same structure that contains the hair follicles. Their main function is to produce sebum, which is secreted onto the skin or into the hair follicle to make the hair shiny and pliant.

There are two types of sweat glands:

- *Eccrine glands* are located over most of the body. In response to thermal stress, eccrine glands produce a watery fluid that helps regulate body temperature. Eccrine glands in the palms and soles secrete fluid in response to emotional stress.
- *Apocrine glands* secrete a milky substance and open into the hair follicle. They're located mainly in the axillae and the genital areas. Inadequate hygiene allows bacteria to break down the fluid, causing body odor.

Hair

Hair is formed from keratin and produced by matrix cells in the dermal layer. Each hair lies in a hair follicle and receives nourishment from a papilla, a loop of capillaries at the base of the follicle. At the lower end of the hair shaft is the hair bulb. The hair bulb contains melanocytes, which determine hair color.

Each hair is attached at the base to a smooth muscle called the *arrector pili*. This muscle contracts during emotional stress or exposure to cold and elevates the hair, causing goose bumps.

Hair today, gone tomorrow

As a person ages, melanocyte function declines, producing light or gray hair, and the hair follicle itself becomes drier as sebaceous gland function decreases. Hair growth declines, so the amount of body hair decreases. Balding, which is genetically determined in younger individuals, occurs in many people as a normal result of aging.

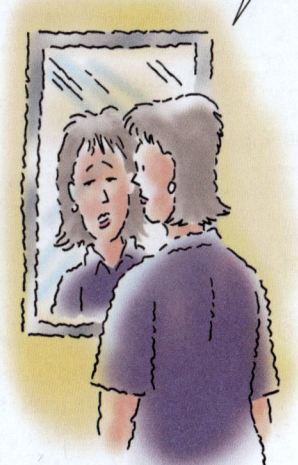

Changes in hair color and growth associated with aging can impact body image.

Nails

Nails are formed when epidermal cells are converted into hard plates of keratin. The nails are made up of the nail root (or nail matrix), nail plate, nail bed, lunula, nail folds, and cuticle.

What's on the plate?

The nail plate is the visible, hardened layer that covers the fingertip. The plate is clear, with fine longitudinal ridges. The pink color results from blood vessels underlying vascular epithelial cells.

What is the matrix?

The nail matrix is the site of nail growth and is protected by the cuticle. At the end of the matrix is the white, crescent-shaped area, the lunula, which extends beyond the cuticle.

Not hard as nails anymore

As adults age, nail growth slows, and the nails become brittle and thin. Longitudinal ridges in the nail plate become more pronounced, making the nails prone to splitting. Also, the nails lose their luster and become yellowed.

Oral cavity

The mouth (also called the *buccal cavity* or *oral cavity*) contains glands that secrete saliva to moisten food for mechanical breakdown. Proper hygiene practices in the care of mucous membranes and teeth contribute to optimal health.

Teeth

Teeth are considered accessory digestive organs. Upper teeth are anchored in the alveoli (sockets) of the left and right maxillae; lower teeth, in the alveoli of the mandible. Teeth consist of enamel, dentin, and pulp.

Those pearly whites

All exposed surfaces of the teeth are covered with enamel, the hardest tissue of the body. Enamel protects the underlying layers from food acids, heat, and cold. Enamel is shiny, hard, nonliving tissue that can't repair itself after being damaged.

Second hardest

The second hardest tissue in the body, dentin, is the yellow substance under tooth enamel. Dentin is composed of millions of tiny canals that contain nerve fibers and cells. It has a slight flexibility, which protects teeth from breaking during chewing.

Performing hygiene practices

Deep inside

Pulp is the innermost part of the tooth. It holds tiny nerves and blood vessels. The root canal is a conduit for nerve vessels between the tooth socket and the pulp area. A thin protective layer of cementum covers each tooth root. Cementum is similar to bone; it's alive and can repair itself.

Performing hygiene practices

Hygiene practices help maintain personal cleanliness and healthy integumentary structures. Most patients routinely perform bathing, shaving, brushing the teeth, shampooing, and caring for nails. Always ask the patient their personal hygiene practices before planning care.

Giving a bed bath

A bed bath is often provided to patients who are on bedrest or who are unable to get in the shower. A complete bed bath cleans the skin, stimulates circulation, provides mild exercise, and promotes comfort. Bathing also allows the nurse to assess the patient's skin condition, joint mobility, and muscle strength (Konya et al., 2021). Depending on their overall condition and duration of hospitalization, the patient may have a complete or partial bath daily. A partial bath—including hands, face, axillae, back, genitalia, and anal region—may be more appropriate than a complete bath for someone with dry, fragile skin or extreme weakness. It also can be given to supplement a complete bath when a patient has diaphoresis or incontinence.

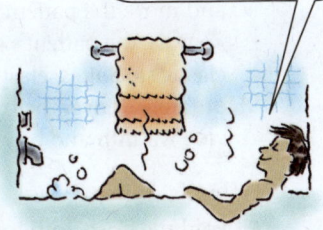

Most people routinely perform bathing and other hygiene practices. Another added benefit of a warm bath includes relaxation!

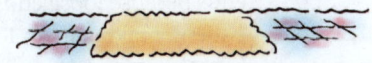

Supplies
- bath basin
- bath blanket
- soap
- towel and washcloth
- skin lotion
- gloves
- deodorant
- optional: bath oil, perineal pad, abdominal (ABD) pad, and linen-saver pad

Getting ready
- Adjust the temperature of the patient's room, and close any doors or windows to prevent drafts.

- Determine the patient's preference for soap or other hygiene aids, because some patients are allergic to soap or prefer bath oil or lotions. Assemble the equipment on an overbed table or bedside stand.

Communication points

- Tell the patient they'll be getting a bath, and provide privacy. If the patient's condition permits, encourage them to assist with bathing to provide exercise and to promote independence.
- Fill the bath basin two-thirds full of warm water (about 115 °F [46 °C]), and bring it to the patient's bedside. If a bath thermometer isn't available, test the water temperature carefully to avoid scalding or chilling the patient; the water should feel comfortably warm.
- If the bed will be changed after the bath, remove the top linen. If not, fanfold it to the foot of the bed.
- Raise the patient's bed to a comfortable working height to avoid back strain. Offer the bedpan or urinal prior to beginning.
- Put on gloves. Position the patient supine, if possible, and move the patient close to you.
- Remove the patient's gown and other articles, such as elastic stockings, elastic bandages, and restraints (as ordered). Cover the patient with a bath blanket to provide warmth and privacy.

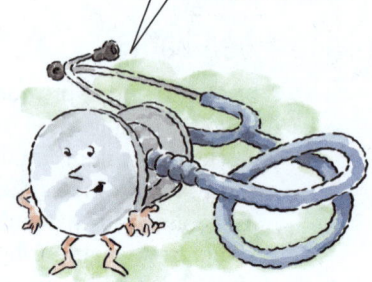

Try to get your patient to help with their bath. This is one way to provide exercise and promote independence.

How it's done

- Fold the washcloth into a mitt on your hand so there are no loose ends because loose ends can cool quickly and drag across the patient, making them feel cold and uncomfortable. (See *Making a washcloth mitt*, page 9.)

Chin up

- Place a towel under the patient's chin. To wash the face, begin with the eyes, working from the inner to the outer canthus without soap. Use a separate section of the washcloth for each eye to avoid spreading ocular infection.
- Apply soap to the cloth, and wash the rest of the face, ears, and neck, using firm, gentle strokes. Rinse thoroughly because residual soap can cause itching and dryness. Then dry the area thoroughly, taking special care in skin folds and creases. Observe the skin for irritation, scaling, or other abnormalities.

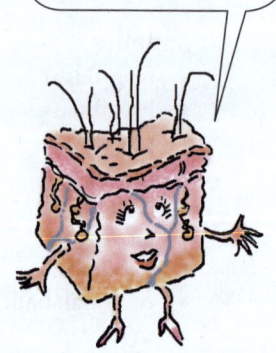

Observe the skin for irritation, scaling, or other abnormalities.

Making a washcloth mitt

Follow these steps to fold a washcloth into a mitt so that there are no loose ends to drag across the patient's skin. Loose ends cool quickly and can chill the patient.

Fold the washcloth in thirds over your hand, as shown below.

Straighten the folded washcloth, as shown.

Fold the ends over your hand, and tuck the loose ends of the washcloth over your palm.

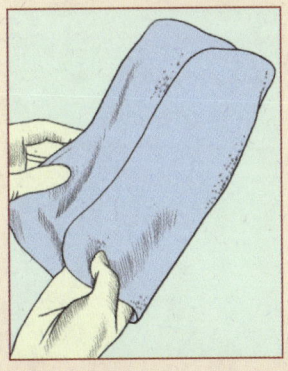 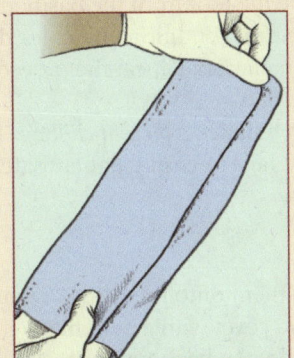 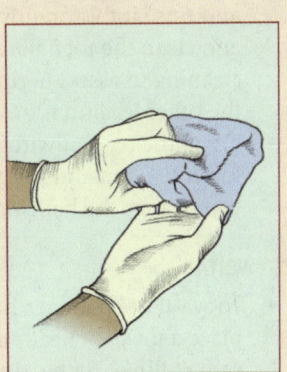

One side at a time

- Turn down the bath blanket, and drape the patient's chest with a bath towel (uncover one side of the chest at a time, beginning with the far side). While washing, rinsing, and drying the chest and axillae, observe the patient's respirations. Use firm strokes. Apply deodorant if tolerated by the patient.
- Place a bath towel beneath the patient's arm farthest from you. Then bathe the arm, using long, smooth strokes and moving from wrist to shoulder to stimulate venous circulation.

Manicure, anyone?

- If possible, soak the patient's hand in the basin to remove dirt and to soften nails. Clean the patient's fingernails, if necessary. Observe the color of the hand and nail beds to assess peripheral circulation. Follow the same procedure for the other arm and hand.
- Turn down the bath blanket to expose the patient's abdomen and groin, keeping a bath towel across the chest to prevent chills. Bathe, rinse, and dry the abdomen and groin while checking for abdominal distention or tenderness. Then turn back the bath blanket to cover the patient's chest and abdomen.

- Uncover the leg farthest from you, and place a bath towel under it. Use a bath sheet to cover the perineum. Flex this leg and bathe it, moving from ankle to hip to stimulate venous circulation. Rinse and dry the leg.

Ah, a foot soak!

- If possible, place a basin on the patient's bed, flex the leg at the knee, and place the foot in the basin. Soak the foot, and then wash and rinse it thoroughly. Remove the foot from the basin, dry it, and clean the toenails. Observe skin condition and color during cleaning to assess peripheral circulation. Repeat the procedure for the other leg and foot.
- Cover the patient with the bath blanket *to prevent chilling.* Then lower the bed and raise the side rails to ensure patient safety while you change the bath water.

Keep them warm!

- To wash the patient's back, roll them onto their side or stomach, place a towel beneath them, and cover with a bath blanket to prevent chilling. Bathe, rinse, and dry the back and buttocks.

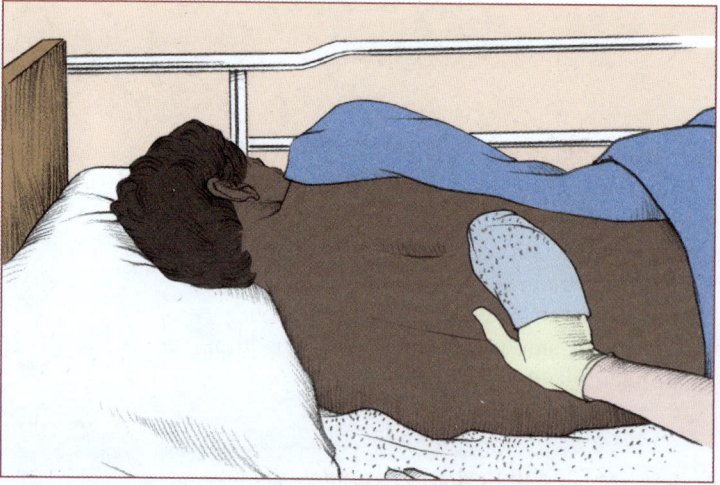

- Massage the patient's back with lotion, paying special attention to bony prominences. Check for redness, abrasions, and pressure injuries. Do not massage reddened, bony prominences, because this can lead to further tissue damage.
- Bathe the anal area from front to back to avoid contaminating the perineum. Rinse and dry the area well.

Remember, front to back

- After lowering the bed and raising the side rails to ensure the patient's safety, change the bath water again. Then, turn the patient on their back and bathe the genital area thoroughly but gently, using a different section of the washcloth for each downward stroke. Bathe from front to back, avoiding the anal area. Rinse thoroughly and pat dry.
- If applicable, perform indwelling urinary catheter care. Apply perineal pads or scrotal supports as needed.

Dressed to heal

- Dress the patient in a clean gown, and reapply elastic bandages, elastic stockings, or other items removed before the bath.
- Remake the bed or change the linens, and remove the bath blanket.
- Place a bath towel beneath the patient's head to catch loose hair, and then brush and comb their hair.
- Return the bed to its original position, and make the patient comfortable.
- Carry soiled linens to the hamper with outstretched arms. To avoid spreading microorganisms, don't let soiled linens touch personal clothing. Remove gloves.

Practice pointers

- Change the water as often as necessary to keep it warm and clean.
- Remove and dispose of gloves appropriately. Wash your hands.

Additional considerations

- Carefully dry creased skinfold areas—for example, under breasts; in the groin area; and between fingers, toes, and buttocks. If not contraindicated, consider a light dusting of these areas with talcum powder to reduce friction.
- Massage the patient's back while applying lotion. Warm the lotion before using it for back massage because cold lotion can startle the patient and induce muscle tension and vasoconstriction. (See the *Providing back care* section on page 362.)
- A bag bath involves the use of 8 to 10 premoistened, warmed, disposable cloths contained in a plastic bag or a prepackaged pouch. The cloths contain a no-rinse surfactant instead of soap. Prior to use, the cloths are warmed in a microwave or a special warming unit supplied by the manufacturer. A separate cloth is used to wash each part of the body. A bag bath saves time compared with the conventional bed bath because no rinsing is required (Goldenhart & Hassan, 2022).

- To improve circulation, maintain joint mobility, and preserve muscle tone, move the body joints through their full range of motion during the bath.
- If the patient is incontinent, loosely tuck an ABD pad between their buttocks and place a linen-saver pad under them to absorb fecal drainage. Together, these pads will help prevent skin irritation and reduce the number of linen changes.

Performing perineal care

Perineal care, which includes care of the external genitalia and the anal area, should be performed during the daily bath and, if necessary, at bedtime and after urination and bowel movements. The procedure promotes cleanliness and prevents infection. It also removes irritating and odorous secretions, such as smegma, a cheese-like substance that collects under the foreskin of the penis and on the inner surface of the labia. For the patient with perineal skin breakdown, frequent bathing followed by application of an ointment or cream aids healing (Cowdell et al., 2020).

Standard precautions must be followed when providing perineal care, with due consideration given to the patient's privacy.

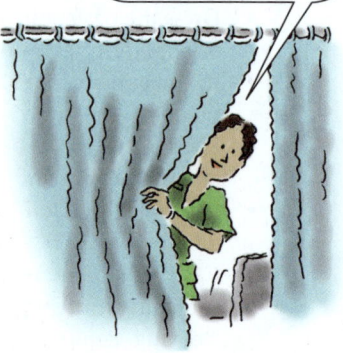

It's important to maintain the patient's privacy during bath time.

Supplies
- gloves
- washcloths
- clean basin
- mild soap
- bath towel
- bath blanket
- toilet tissue
- linen-saver pad
- optional: trash bag, bedpan, perineal bottle, antiseptic soap, petroleum jelly, zinc oxide cream, vitamin A and D ointment, and an ABD pad

Following genital or rectal surgery, sterile supplies (including sterile gloves, gauze, and cotton balls) may be needed.

Getting ready
- Obtain ointment or cream, as needed. Fill the basin two-thirds full with warm water. Also fill the perineal bottle with warm water, if needed.
- Assemble equipment at the patient's bedside, and provide privacy.
- Wash hands thoroughly, put on gloves, and explain to the patient what you're about to do.

How it's done

- Adjust the bed to a comfortable working height to prevent back strain, and lower the head of the bed, if the patient's condition allows. Lower the side rail closest to you.
- Provide privacy and help the patient to a supine position. Place a linen-saver pad under the patient's buttocks to protect the bed from stains and moisture.

Perineal care for the female patient

- To minimize the patient's exposure and embarrassment, place the bath blanket over them, with corners head to foot and side to side. Wrap each leg with a side corner, tucking it under the hip. Then fold back the corner between the legs to expose the perineum.
- Ask the patient to bend their knees slightly and to spread legs apart. Separate the labia with one hand and wash with the other, using gentle downward strokes from the front to the back of the perineum to prevent intestinal organisms from contaminating the urethra or vagina. Avoid the area around the anus, and use a clean section of washcloth for each stroke by folding each used section inward. This prevents the spread of contaminated secretions or discharge.

Rinse and pat dry

- Using a clean washcloth, rinse thoroughly from front to back, because soap residue can cause skin irritation. Pat the area dry with a bath towel, because moisture can also cause skin irritation and discomfort.
- Apply ordered ointments or creams.
- Turn the patient on their side to Sims position, if possible, to expose the anal area.
- Clean, rinse, and dry the anal area, starting at the posterior vaginal opening and wiping from front to back.
- Apply ordered ointments or creams.

Perineal care for the male patient

- Drape the patient's legs to minimize exposure and embarrassment, and expose the genital area.
- Hold the shaft of the penis with one hand and wash with the other, beginning at the tip and working in a circular motion from the center to the periphery to avoid introducing microorganisms into the urethra. Use a clean section of washcloth for each stroke to prevent the spread of contaminated secretions or discharge.
- Rinse thoroughly, using the same circular motion.

Retract and replace

- For the uncircumcised patient, gently retract the foreskin and clean beneath it. Rinse well, but don't dry, because moisture provides lubrication and prevents friction when replacing the foreskin. Replace the foreskin to avoid constriction of the penis, which causes edema and tissue damage.
- Wash the rest of the penis, using downward strokes toward the scrotum. Rinse well and pat dry with a bath towel.
- Clean the top and sides of the scrotum; then, rinse thoroughly and pat dry. Handle the scrotum gently to avoid causing discomfort.
- Turn the patient on their side. Clean the bottom of the scrotum and the anal area. Rinse well and pat dry.

After providing perineal care

- Reposition the patient and make them comfortable. Remove the bath blanket and linen-saver pad, and then replace the bed linens.
- Clean and return the basin, and dispose of soiled articles, including gloves. Wash hands.

Practice pointers

- Give perineal care in a matter-of-fact way to minimize embarrassment.
- If the patient is incontinent, first remove excess feces with toilet tissue. Then position them on a bedpan, and add a small amount of antiseptic soap to a perineal bottle to eliminate odor. Irrigate the perineal area to remove any remaining fecal matter.
- After cleaning the perineum, apply ointment or cream (petroleum jelly, zinc oxide cream, or vitamin A and D ointment) to prevent skin breakdown by providing a barrier between the skin and excretions.
- To reduce the number of linen changes, tuck an ABD pad between the patient's buttocks to absorb oozing feces.

Providing back care

Regular bathing and massage of the neck, back, buttocks, and upper arms promotes patient relaxation and allows assessment of skin condition. Particularly important for the patient who is bedridden, massage causes cutaneous vasodilation, helping to prevent pressure injuries caused by prolonged pressure on bony prominences or by perspiration. Although you can perform gentle back massage after a patient has a myocardial infarction, it may be contraindicated in those with rib fractures, surgical incisions, or other recent traumatic injury to the back.

Supplies

- basin
- soap
- bath blanket
- bath towel
- washcloth
- back lotion with lanolin base
- gloves, if the patient has open lesions or has been incontinent
- optional: talcum powder

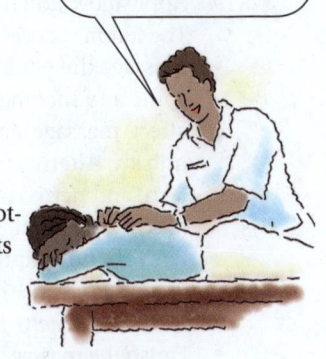

Application of warmed lotion prevents chilling or startling the patient.

Getting ready

- Fill the basin two-thirds full with warm water. Place the lotion bottle in the basin to warm it. Application of warmed lotion prevents chilling or startling the patient, thereby reducing muscle tension and vasoconstriction.

How it's done

- Assemble the equipment at the patient's bedside.
- Explain the procedure to the patient, and provide privacy. Ask them to tell you if you're applying too much or too little pressure.
- Adjust the bed to a comfortable working height, and lower the head of the bed, if the patient's condition allows. Wash hands and put on gloves, if applicable. Lower the side rail closest to you.

Position the patient

- Place the patient in the prone position, if possible, or on their side. Position them along the edge of the bed nearest you to prevent back strain.
- Untie the patient's gown, and expose the back, shoulders, and buttocks. Then drape the patient with a bath blanket to prevent chills and to minimize exposure. Place a bath towel next to or under their side to protect bed linens from moisture.

While bathing the patient, be sure to assess the skin and bony prominences.

Make a mitt

- Fold the washcloth around your hand to form a mitt. This prevents the loose ends of the cloth from dripping water onto the patient and keeps the cloth warm longer.
- Work up a lather with soap. Using long, firm strokes, bathe the patient's back, beginning at the neck and shoulders and moving downward to the buttocks.

Rinse and dry

- Rinse and dry well, because moisture trapped between the buttocks can cause chafing and predispose the patient to pressure injuries.
- While giving back care, closely examine the patient's skin, especially the bony prominences of the shoulders, the scapulae, and the coccyx, for redness or abrasions.

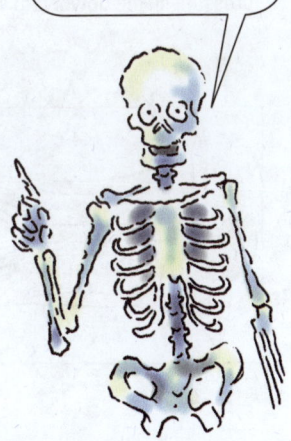

Moisturize first, then massage

- Remove the warmed lotion bottle from the basin, and pour a small amount of lotion into your palm. Rub your hands together to distribute the lotion.
- Apply the lotion to the patient's back, using long, firm strokes. The lotion reduces friction, making back massage easier.
- Massage the patient's back, beginning at the base of the spine and moving upward to the shoulders. For a relaxing effect, massage slowly; for a stimulating effect, massage quickly. Alternate the three basic strokes: effleurage, friction, and pétrissage. (See *How to give a back massage.*) Add lotion as needed, keeping one hand on the patient's back to avoid interrupting the massage.
- Compress, squeeze, and lift the trapezius muscle *to help relax the patient.*
- Finish the massage by using long, firm strokes, and blot any excess lotion from the patient's back with a towel. Then, retie the patient's gown and straighten or change the bed linens, as needed.

> When providing a back massage, always choose an appropriate lotion, and warm it in a basin of water first.

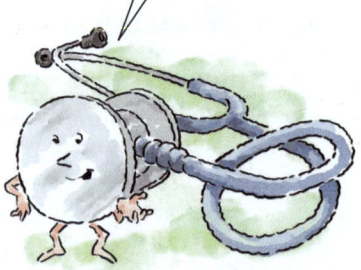

How to give a back massage

Three strokes commonly used during back massage are effleurage, friction, and pétrissage. Start with effleurage and then go on to friction and pétrissage. Perform each stroke at least six times before moving on to the next, and then repeat the whole series if desired.

When performing effleurage and friction, keep your hands parallel to the vertebrae to avoid tickling the patient. For all three strokes, maintain a regular rhythm and steady contact with the patient's back to help them relax.

Effleurage

Using your palm, stroke from the buttocks up to the shoulders, over the upper arms, and back to the buttocks (as shown below). Use slightly less pressure on the downward strokes.

Friction

Use circular thumb strokes to move from buttocks to shoulders; then, using a smooth stroke, return to the buttocks (as shown below).

Pétrissage

Using your thumb to oppose your fingers, knead and stroke half the back and upper arms, starting at the buttocks and moving toward the shoulder (as shown below). Then knead and stroke the other half of the back, rhythmically alternating your hands.

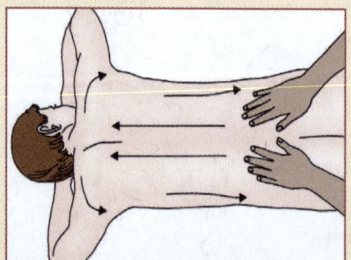
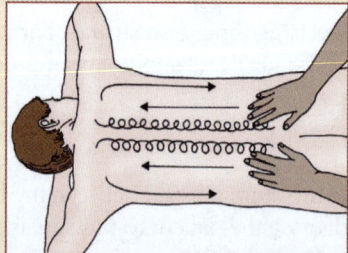
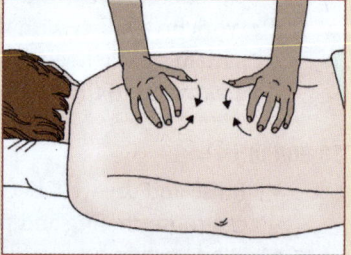

After care

- Return the bed to its original position, and make the patient comfortable. Empty and clean the basin.
- Dispose of gloves, if used, and return equipment to the appropriate storage area. Wash hands.

Practice pointers

- Before giving back care, assess the patient's body structure and skin condition, and tailor the duration and intensity of the massage accordingly.
- If the patient has oily skin, instead of using the usual lotion, substitute a talcum powder or lotion of the patient's choice. However, to avoid aspiration, don't use powder if the patient has an endotracheal or tracheal tube in place.
- Don't massage the patient's legs unless ordered, because massage can dislodge a blood clot, causing an embolus.
- Give special attention to bony prominences, because pressure injuries are common in these areas. Do not massage reddened, bony prominences.

Keep the powder and the lotion separate

- Avoid using powder and lotion together, because doing so may lead to skin maceration.
- Develop a turning schedule, and provide back care at each position change.

Performing hair care

Hair care includes combing, brushing, and shampooing. Combing and brushing stimulate scalp circulation, remove dead cells and debris, and distribute hair oils to produce a healthy sheen. Shampooing removes dirt and old oils and helps prevent skin irritation. Hair care also enhances self-esteem and body image. Ask the patient about their usual hair hygiene routine.

Frequency

Frequency of hair care depends on the length and texture of the patient's hair, the duration of hospitalization, and the patient's condition. Usually, hair should be combed and brushed daily and shampooed according to the patient's normal routine. Typically, no more than 1 week should elapse between washings. Shampooing is contraindicated in patients with recent craniotomy, depressed skull fracture, conditions necessitating intracranial pressure monitoring, or other cranial involvement.

Supplies

- comb and brush
- hand towel
- liquid shampoo (or mild soap)
- washcloth
- three bath towels
- two bath blankets
- plastic shampoo basin
- two large pitchers or other large containers
- linen-saver pads
- optional: gloves, hair conditioner or rinse, alcohol, oil, hair ties, footstool, drawsheet

The comb and brush should be clean. If necessary, wash them in hot, soapy water. The comb should have dull, even teeth to prevent scratching the scalp. The brush should have stiff bristles to enhance vigorous brushing and stimulation of circulation.

Getting ready

Combing and brushing

- Tell the patient they will have their hair brushed. If possible, encourage them to do it by themselves, assisting as needed.
- Adjust the bed to a comfortable working height to prevent back strain. If the patient's condition allows, help them to a sitting position by raising the head of the bed.
- Provide privacy, and drape a bath towel over the patient's pillow and shoulders to catch loose hair and dirt. Put on gloves.

Shampooing the hair of a patient who is bedridden

- Before shampooing the patient's hair, adjust room temperature and eliminate drafts to prevent chilling the patient. Next, obtain a shampoo tray or devise a trough, if necessary.
- Assemble the equipment on the patient's bedside stand.
- Cover the patient with a bath blanket. Then, fanfold the linens to the foot of the bed, or remove them if they're scheduled to be changed.
- Fill large pitchers or containers with comfortably warm water and place them on the overbed table.
- Lower the head of the bed until it's horizontal, and remove the patient's pillow, if the patient's condition allows. Lower the side rail closest to you.

A blanket buffer

- Fold the second bath blanket, and tuck it under the patient's shoulders to improve water drainage.
- Cover the bath blanket and the head of the bed with a linen-saver pad to protect them from moisture.

- Place a bath towel and linen-saver pad together, and position them around the patient's neck and over their shoulders to protect the patient from moisture and to pad their neck against the pressure of the shampoo tray.
- Place the shampoo tray under the patient's head, with their neck in the U-shaped opening. Arrange the bath blanket and towel so the patient is comfortable.

Watch the water!

- Adjust the shampoo tray to carry wastewater away from the patient's head. Tuck a folded towel or drawsheet under the opposite side of the shampoo tray to promote drainage, if necessary. Put on gloves.

How it's done
Combing and brushing

- For short hair, comb and brush one side at a time. For long or curly hair, turn the patient's head away from you, and then part the hair down the middle from front to back. If the hair is tangled, rub alcohol or oil on the hair strands to loosen them. Comb and vigorously brush the hair on the side facing you. Then turn the patient's head, and comb and brush the opposite side.

Easy does it

- Part hair into small sections for easier handling. Comb one section at a time, working from the ends toward the scalp to remove tangles. Anchor each section of hair above the area being combed to avoid hurting the patient. After combing, brush vigorously. Avoid shaking the patient's head when brushing.

Braids, bangs, or barrettes?

- Style the hair as the patient prefers. Braiding long or curly hair helps prevent snarling. To braid, part hair down the middle of the scalp and begin braiding near the face. To avoid patient discomfort, don't braid too tightly. Fasten the ends of the braids with hair ties. Pin the braids across the top of the patient's head or let them hang, as the patient desires, so the finished braids don't press against the patient's scalp.
- After styling the hair, carefully remove the towel by folding it inward to prevent loose hairs and debris from falling onto the pillow or into the patient's bed.

Shampooing the hair of a patient who is bedridden

- Before shampooing, place cotton in the patient's ears to prevent moisture from collecting in them.

Rinse well

- Fill the small pitcher or beaker by dipping it into the large pitcher. Carefully pour water over the patient's hair. To avoid spills, don't overfill the shampoo tray.

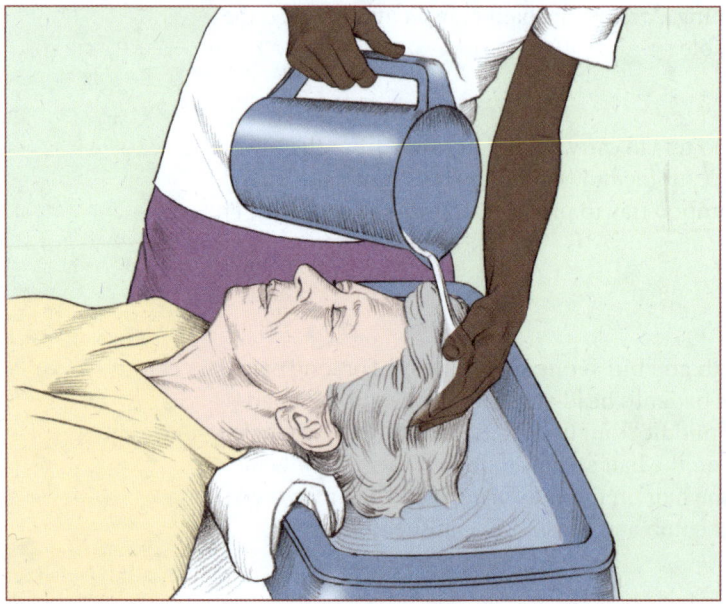

- Then, with your fingertips, rub shampoo into the patient's hair. Massage the scalp well to emulsify hair oils. Vigorous rubbing stimulates the scalp and also helps the patient relax. Don't hyperextend the neck or shake the head.
- Using the small pitcher or beaker, pour water over the patient's hair until it's free of shampoo. Then reapply shampoo and rinse again. Apply conditioner or a rinse, if desired.

That's a wrap!

- Remove the shampoo tray, and wrap the patient's hair in a towel. Remove the linen-saver pad from the bed, and return the bed to its original position.
- Dry the patient's hair by gently rubbing it with a towel. Then comb, brush, and style it.
- Remake the bed or change the linens, if needed, and remove the bath blanket.
- Reposition the patient comfortably.
- Remove and empty the pail. Clean the shampoo tray, and return it to storage. Remove pitchers from the bedside, and return the shampoo to the bedside stand.
- Remove gloves and wash hands.

Practice pointers

- When giving hair care, check the patient's scalp carefully for signs of scalp disorders, head lice, or skin breakdown, particularly if the patient is bedridden. Make sure each patient has their own comb and brush to avoid cross-contamination.
- If you don't have a shampoo tray and can't devise a trough, place pillows under the patient's shoulders to elevate their head, and use a basin. Because a standard basin doesn't have a drainage spout, empty it frequently to prevent overflow.

Shaving a patient

Performed with a straight, safety, or electric razor, shaving is part of the male patient's usual daily care. In addition to reducing bacterial growth on the face, shaving promotes patient comfort by removing whiskers that can itch and irritate the skin and produce an unkempt appearance. Shaving may also foster positive self-esteem.

Shaving can foster self-esteem, promote comfort, and reduce bacterial growth on the face.

When to use an electric razor

Because nicks and cuts are most common with use of a straight or safety razor, shaving with an electric razor is indicated for the patient with a clotting disorder or the patient undergoing anticoagulant therapy. Shaving may be contraindicated in the patient with a facial skin disorder or wound.

Supplies
For a straight or safety razor
- shaving kit containing a straight razor or a safety razor, and a soap container
- gloves
- soap or shaving cream
- towel and washcloth
- basin
- optional: aftershave lotion, talcum powder

For an electric razor
- bath towel
- optional: preshave lotions or creams, and aftershave lotions, mirror, and grounded three-pronged plug

Getting ready
- With a straight or a safety razor, make sure the blade is sharp, clean, even, and rust-free. If necessary, insert a new blade securely into the razor. A razor may be used more than once, but only by

the same patient. If the patient is bedridden, assemble the equipment on the bedside stand or overbed table; if the patient is ambulatory, assemble it at the sink. When the patient is ready to shave, fill the basin or sink with warm water.

Safety

- If using an electric razor, check the cord for fraying or other damage that could create an electrical hazard. If the razor isn't double insulated or battery operated, use a grounded three-pronged plug. Examine the razor head for sharp edges and dirt. Read the manufacturer's instructions, if available, and assemble the equipment at the bedside.

Privacy, please

- Tell the patient that you're going to shave them and provide privacy. To promote independence, ask them to assist as much as possible.
- Unless contraindicated, place the conscious patient in high-Fowler or semi-Fowler position. If the patient is unconscious, elevate their head to prevent soap and water from running behind it.
- Direct bright light onto the patient's face but not into their eyes.

How it's done
Using a straight or safety razor

- Drape a bath towel around the patient's shoulders, and tuck it under their chin to protect the bed from moisture and to catch falling whiskers.

Stay sharp

- Put on gloves, and fill the basin with warm water. Using the washcloth, wet the patient's facial hair with warm water. Let the warm cloth soak the areas with facial hair for at least 1 minute to soften whiskers.
- Apply shaving cream to the whiskers. Or, if using soap, rub to form a lather.
- Gently stretch the patient's skin taut with one hand and shave with the other, holding the razor firmly. Ask the patient to puff their cheeks or turn their head, as necessary, to shave hard-to-reach areas.
- To reduce skin irritation and help prevent nicks and cuts, begin at the sideburns and work toward the chin using short, firm, downward strokes in the direction of hair growth.

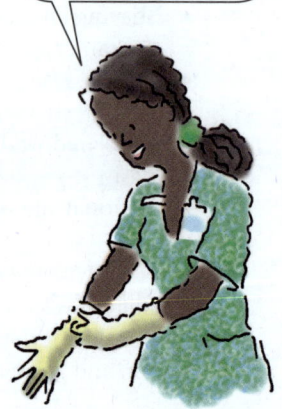

Shaving involves the use of sharp instruments and the potential for blood exposure . . . so don't forget the gloves!

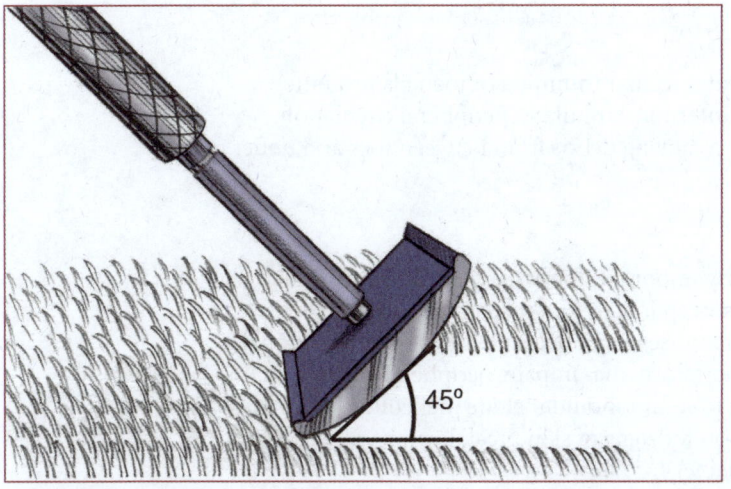

45°

- Rinse the razor often to remove whiskers. Apply more warm water or shaving cream to the face, as needed, to maintain adequate lather.

Smooth as a baby's bottom

- Shave across the chin and up the neck and throat. To avoid skin irritation, use short, gentle strokes for the neck and the area around the nose and mouth.
- Change the water, and rinse any remaining lather and whiskers from the patient's face. Then dry the face with a bath towel and, if the patient desires, apply aftershave lotion or talcum powder.
- Rinse the razor and basin, and then return the razor to its storage area.

Using an electric razor

- Plug in the razor and apply preshave lotion, if available, to remove skin oils. If the razor head is adjustable, select the appropriate setting.
- Using a circular motion and pressing the razor firmly against the skin, shave each area of the patient's face until smooth.
- If the patient desires, apply talcum powder or aftershave lotion.
- Clean the razor head, and return the razor to its storage area.

Practice pointers

- If the patient is conscious, find out their usual shaving routine. Although shaving in the direction of hair growth is most common, the patient may prefer the opposite direction.

No sharing of razors

- To prevent cross-contamination, don't interchange patients' shaving equipment.
- Shaving may be contraindicated if the patient is on anticoagulant therapy (e.g., after tissue plasminogen activator or heparin infusion). Check the facility's policy.

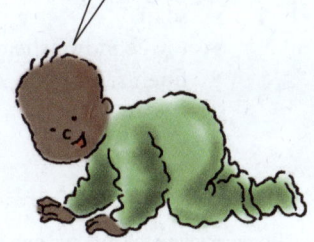

Done correctly, shaving should leave the patient's face smooth as a baby's bottom.

Performing foot care

Daily bathing of feet and regular trimming of toenails promotes cleanliness, prevents infection, stimulates peripheral circulation, and controls odor by removing debris from between toes and under toenails.

Foot care is important!

Foot care is particularly important for patients who are bedridden and those especially susceptible to foot infection, such as patients with peripheral vascular disease, diabetes mellitus, poor nutritional status, arthritis, or a condition that impairs peripheral circulation. In such patients, proper foot care should include meticulous cleanliness and regular observation for signs of skin breakdown. (See *Foot care for patients who have diabetes*.)

Supplies
- bath blanket
- large basin
- soap
- towel and washcloth
- linen-saver pad

Foot care for patients who have diabetes

Because diabetes mellitus can reduce blood supply to the feet, normally minor foot injuries can lead to dangerous infection. When caring for a patient who has diabetes, keep these foot care guidelines in mind:
- Exercising the feet daily can help improve circulation. While the patient is sitting on the edge of the bed, ask them to point toes upward, then downward, 10 times. Then have them make a circle with the toes of each foot 10 times.
- The shoes of a patient with diabetes must fit properly. Instruct the patient to break in new shoes gradually by initially wearing them for 30 minutes and then increasing wearing time by 30 minutes each day. Also tell them to check old shoes frequently for rough spots in the lining; if these develop. the shoes should be discarded.
- Tell the patient to wear clean socks daily and to avoid socks with holes; darned spots; or rough, irritating seams.
- Advise the patient to see a health care provider if they have corns or calluses.
- Tell the patient to wear warm socks or slippers and to use extra blankets to avoid cold feet. The patient should not use heating pads and hot water bottles, because these can cause burns.
- Teach the patient to regularly inspect the skin on the feet for cuts; cracks; blisters; and red, swollen areas. Even slight cuts on the feet should receive a health care provider's attention. As a first-aid measure, tell them to wash the cut thoroughly and to apply a mild antiseptic. Urge the patient to avoid harsh antiseptics, such as iodine, because they can damage tissue.
- Advise the patient to avoid tight-fitting garments or activities that can decrease circulation. They should especially avoid sitting with their knees crossed, picking at sores or rough spots on their feet, walking barefoot, or applying adhesive tape to the skin on their feet.

- pillow
- gloves, if the patient has open lesions
- optional: gauze pads and heel protectors, cotton balls, lotion, water-absorbent powder, and bath thermometer

Getting ready
- Fill the basin halfway with warm water. Test water temperature with a bath thermometer, because patients with diminished peripheral sensation could burn their feet in excessively hot water (over 105 °F [40.6 °C]) without feeling any warning pain. If a bath thermometer isn't available, test the water by inserting your elbow. The water temperature should feel comfortably warm.
- Assemble equipment at the patient's bedside. Wash hands, and put on gloves.

Foot care
- Tell the patient that you'll be washing their feet and providing foot care.
- Cover the patient with a bath blanket. Fanfold the top linen to the foot of the bed.
- Place a linen-saver pad and a towel under the patient's feet to keep the bottom linen dry. Then position the basin on the pad.

Pressure free
- Insert a pillow beneath the patient's knee to provide support, and cushion the rim of the basin with the edge of the towel *to prevent pressure.*

How it's done
- Immerse one foot in the basin, wash it with soap, and allow it to soak for about 10 minutes. Soaking softens the skin and toenails, loosens debris under toenails, and comforts and refreshes the patient.
- After soaking the foot, rinse it with a washcloth, remove it from the basin, and place it on the towel.

Soft–cloth touch
- To prevent skin breakdown, dry the foot thoroughly, especially between the toes. Blot gently to dry, because harsh rubbing may damage the skin.
- Empty the basin, refill it with warm water, and clean and soak the other foot.

Putting your best foot forward
- While the second foot is soaking, give the first one a pedicure. Using the cotton-tipped applicator, carefully clean the toenails.

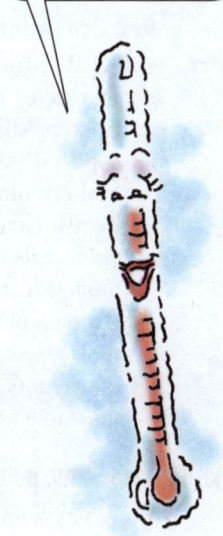

Remember that a patient with diminished peripheral sensation can burn their feet in hot water without feeling any warning pain. Always test bath water first.

- Consult a podiatrist if nails need trimming.
- Rinse the foot that has been soaking, and dry it thoroughly.

Final touches

- Apply lotion (Goldenhart & Hassan, 2022) to moisten dry skin, or lightly dust water-absorbent powder between the toes to absorb moisture.
- Remove and clean all equipment. Dispose of gloves and wash hands.

Practice pointers

- While providing foot care, observe the color, shape, and texture of the toenails. If there is redness, drying, cracking, blisters, discoloration, or other signs of traumatic injury, especially in patients with impaired peripheral circulation and/or diabetes, notify the health care provider. *Because such patients are vulnerable to infection and gangrene, they need prompt treatment.*
- If a patient's toenail grows inward at the corners, tuck a wisp of cotton under it to relieve pressure on the toe. Refer the patient with ingrown toenails to a podiatrist.

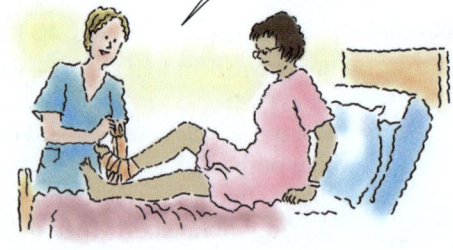

Redness, drying, cracking, blisters, discoloration, or any evidence of traumatic injury to the feet could be a sign of infection or gangrene and should be reported to a healthcare provider.

Tailoring care to the patient who is bedridden

- When giving the patient who is bedridden foot care, perform range-of-motion exercises unless contraindicated to stimulate circulation and prevent foot contractures and muscle atrophy. Tuck folded 2 × 2″ gauze pads between overlapping toes to protect the skin from the toenails. Apply heel protectors to prevent skin breakdown.

A clean mouth is a healthy mouth, and that means being able to enjoy eating all types of food.

Performing mouth care

Given in the morning, at bedtime, or after meals, mouth care entails brushing and flossing the teeth and inspecting the mouth. Mouth care removes soft plaque deposits and calculus from the teeth, cleans and massages the gums, reduces mouth odor, and helps prevent infection. A patient's comfort and self-esteem are increased by freshening their mouth. Appreciation of food is enhanced, thereby aiding appetite and nutrition.

A mouthful of attention

Although an ambulatory patient can usually perform mouth care alone, a patient who is bedridden may require partial or full assistance. A comatose patient requires use of

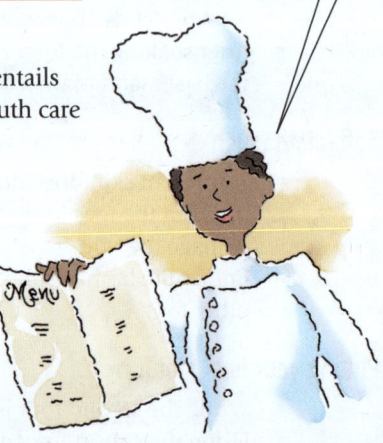

suction equipment to prevent aspiration during oral care. Frequency of oral care should be based on the patient's abilities, level of consciousness, and the facility's policy. Typically, a patient who is independent, or one who needs some assistance, should be encouraged to perform oral care twice a day (CDC, 2023).

Supplies
- towel or facial tissues
- emesis basin
- mouthwash
- toothbrush and toothpaste
- pitcher and glass
- dental floss
- optional: oral irrigating device, trash bag, small mirror, drinking straw

For a patient who is unconscious or debilitated
- Linen-saver pad
- hydrogen peroxide
- cotton-tipped mouth swab
- along with a cotton-tipped mouth swab a foam swab may also be used to cleanse
- oral suction equipment or gauze pads
- optional: mouth-care kit, tongue blade, 4 × 4″ gauze pads, and adhesive tape

Getting ready
- Fill a pitcher with water, and bring it and other equipment to the patient's bedside.
- If using oral suction equipment, connect the tubing to the suction bottle and suction catheter, insert the plug into an outlet, and check for correct operation.
- If necessary, devise a bite block to protect yourself from being bitten during the procedure: Wrap a gauze pad over the end of a tongue blade, fold the edge in, and secure it with adhesive tape.
- Wash hands thoroughly, put on gloves, explain the procedure to the patient, and provide privacy.

How it's done
- If the patient is bedridden but capable of self-care, encourage them to perform their own mouth care.
- If the patient's condition allows, place the patient in Fowler position. Place the overbed table in front of them, and arrange the equipment on it. Open the table and set up the built-in mirror, if available, or position a small mirror on the table.
- Drape a towel over the patient's chest to protect their gown. Ask them to floss teeth while looking into the mirror.

Inspecting the technique

- Observe the patient to make sure they are flossing correctly, and correct their technique if necessary.
- Instruct them to wrap the floss around the second or third finger of each hand. Starting with the back teeth and without injuring the gums, they should insert the floss as far as possible into the space between each pair of teeth. Then they should clean the surfaces of adjacent teeth by pulling the floss up and down against the side of each tooth. After the patient flosses a pair of teeth, remind them to use a clean 1″ (2.5 cm) section of floss for the next pair.

After the floss

- After the patient flosses, mix mouthwash and water in a glass (or a mixture of half peroxide and half water), place a straw in it, and position the emesis basin nearby.
- Instruct the patient to brush teeth and gums while looking in the mirror. Encourage rinsing frequently during brushing, and provide facial tissues to wipe the mouth.

Performing mouth care for the patient

- If the patient is comatose or conscious but incapable of self-care, perform mouth care for them. If they wear dentures, clean them thoroughly. (See *Dealing with dentures*, page 377.) Some patients may benefit from using an oral irrigating device.

Prepping the patient

- Raise the bed to a comfortable working height to prevent back strain. Then lower the head of the bed, and position the patient on their side, with the face extended over the edge of the pillow to facilitate drainage and prevent fluid aspiration.
- Arrange the equipment on the overbed table or bedside stand, including the oral suction equipment, if necessary. Turn on the machine. If a suction machine isn't available, wipe the inside of the patient's mouth frequently with a gauze pad.
- Place a linen-saver pad under the patient's chin and an emesis basin near their cheek to absorb or catch drainage.

Lubricate as needed

- Lubricate the patient's lips with petroleum jelly to prevent dryness and cracking. Reapply lubricant, as needed, during oral care.
- If necessary, insert the bite block to hold the patient's mouth open during oral care. *Caution: Never place your fingers in the patient's mouth unless a bite block is in place.*

Watch your patient closely to make sure they are flossing correctly, and correct their technique if necessary.

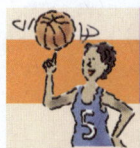

Dealing with dentures

Dentures require proper care to remove soft plaque deposits and calculus and to reduce mouth odor. Such care involves removing and rinsing dentures after meals, daily brushing and removal of tenacious deposits, and soaking in a commercial denture cleaner. Dentures must be removed from the comatose or presurgical patient to prevent possible airway obstruction.

Equipment and preparation
Start by assembling the following equipment at the patient's bedside:
- emesis basin
- labeled denture cup
- toothbrush or denture brush
- gloves
- toothpaste or commercial denture cleaner
- paper towel
- cotton-tipped mouth swab and/or a foam swab
- mouthwash
- gauze
- optional: adhesive denture liner

Removing dentures
- Wash hands and put on gloves.
- To remove a full upper denture, grasp the front and palatal surfaces of the denture with your thumb and forefinger. Position the index finger of your opposite hand over the upper border of the denture, and press to break the seal between denture and palate. Grasp the denture with gauze, because saliva can make it slippery.
- To remove a full lower denture, grasp the front and lingual surfaces of the denture with your thumb and index finger and gently lift up.
- To remove partial dentures, first ask the patient or caregiver how the prosthesis is retained and how to remove it. If the partial denture is held in place with clips or snaps, then exert equal pressure on the border of each side of the denture. Avoid lifting the clasps, which can easily bend or break.

Oral and denture care
- After removing dentures, place them in a properly labeled denture cup. Add warm water and a commercial denture cleaner to remove stains and hardened deposits. Follow package directions. Avoid soaking dentures in mouthwash containing alcohol, because it may damage a soft liner.
- Instruct the patient to rinse with mouthwash to remove food particles and to reduce mouth odor. Then stroke the palate, buccal surfaces, gums, and tongue with a soft toothbrush or cotton-tipped mouth swab to clean the mucosa and stimulate circulation. Check for irritated areas or sores, because they may indicate a poorly fitting denture.
- Carry the denture cup, emesis basin, toothbrush, and toothpaste to the sink. After lining the basin with a paper towel, fill it with water to cushion the dentures in case you drop them. Hold the dentures over the basin, wet them with warm water, and apply toothpaste to a denture brush or long-bristled toothbrush. Clean the dentures using only moderate pressure to prevent scratches and using warm water to prevent distortion.
- Clean the denture cup, and place the dentures in it. Rinse the brush, and clean and dry the emesis basin. Return all equipment to the patient's bedside stand.

Wearing dentures
- If the patient desires, apply adhesive liner to the dentures; this provides a strong seal that promotes patient comfort by improving the fit of the dentures. Moisten the dentures with water, if necessary, to reduce friction and ease insertion.
- Encourage the patient to wear dentures to facilitate eating and speaking and to prevent changes in the gum line that may affect denture fit.

Flossing and rinsing

- Using a dental floss holder, hold the floss against each tooth and direct it as close to the gum as possible without injuring the sensitive tissues around the tooth.
- After flossing the patient's teeth, mix mouthwash and water in a glass, and place the straw in it.

Brushing them clean

- Wet the toothbrush with water. If necessary, use hot water to soften the bristles. Apply toothpaste.
- Brush the patient's lower teeth from the gum line up; the upper teeth, from the gum line down.

Covering all the angles

- Place the brush at a 45° angle to the gum line, and press the bristles gently into the gingival sulcus. Using short, gentle strokes to prevent gum damage, brush the buccal surfaces (toward the cheek) and the lingual surfaces (toward the tongue) of the bottom teeth; use just the tip of the brush for the lingual surfaces of the front teeth. Using the same technique, brush the buccal and lingual surfaces of the top teeth. Brush the biting surfaces of the bottom and top teeth using a back-and-forth motion.
- Hold the emesis basin steady under the patient's cheek, and wipe the mouth and cheeks with facial tissues as needed.

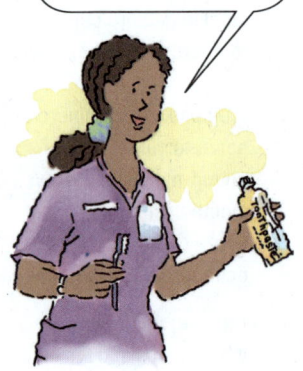

Follow the proper brushing technique, and use gentle strokes to prevent damaging tooth and gum surfaces.

Swabbing the deck clean

- After brushing the patient's teeth, dip a cotton-tipped mouth swab into the mouthwash solution (or a mixture of half peroxide and half water). Press the swab against the side of the glass to remove excess moisture. Gently stroke the gums, buccal surfaces, palate, and tongue to clean the mucosa and stimulate circulation.

After mouth care

- Assess the patient's mouth for cleanliness and tooth and tissue condition.
- Rinse the toothbrush, and clean the emesis basin and glass.
- Empty and clean the suction bottle, if used, and place a clean suction catheter on the tubing.
- Return reusable equipment to the appropriate storage location, and discard disposable equipment in the trash bag. Remove gloves and wash hands.

Practice pointers

- Use cotton-tipped mouth swabs and/or a foam swab to clean the teeth of a patient with sensitive gums. These swabs produce less friction than a toothbrush; however, they don't clean as well.
- If the patient is breathing through their mouth or receiving oxygen therapy, moisten the mouth and lips regularly with mineral oil or water.

Making an unoccupied bed

Daily changing and periodic straightening of bed linens promotes patient comfort and prevents skin breakdown. When preceded by hand washing, performed using clean technique, and followed by proper handling and disposal of soiled linens, this procedure helps control hospital-acquired (also referred to as nosocomial) infections.

Supplies

- two sheets (one fitted, if available)
- pillowcase
- bedspread
- optional: gloves, bath blanket, laundry bag, linen-saver pads, and drawsheet

Getting ready

- Obtain clean linen, which should be folded in half lengthwise and then folded again. The bottom sheet should be folded so that the rough side of the hem is face down when placed on the bed to help prevent skin irritation caused by the rough hem edge rubbing against the patient's heels. The top sheet should be folded similarly so that the smooth side of the hem is face up when folded over the spread, giving the bed a finished appearance and protecting the patient's skin.
- Wash your hands thoroughly, put on gloves, and bring clean linen to the patient's bedside. If the patient is present, tell them that you're going to change the bed. Help them to a chair, if necessary.
- Move any furniture away from the bed to provide ample working space.
- Lower the head of the bed to make the mattress level and to ensure tight-fitting, wrinkle-free linens. Then raise the bed to a comfortable working height to prevent back strain. Make sure the wheels of the bed are locked.

How it's done

- When stripping the bed, watch for any belongings that may have fallen among the linens.
- Remove the pillowcase and place it in the laundry bag or hook it over the back of a chair and use it as a laundry bag. Set the pillow aside.

- Lift the mattress edge slightly and work around the bed, untucking the linens. If planning to reuse the top linens, fold the top hem of the spread down to the bottom hem. Then pick up the hemmed corners, fold the spread into quarters, and hang it over the back of the chair. Otherwise, carefully remove and place the top linens in the laundry bag or pillowcase. To avoid spreading microorganisms, don't fan the linens, hold them against personal clothing, or place them on the floor.
- Remove the soiled bottom linens, and place them in the laundry bag.
- If the mattress has slid downward, push it to the head of the bed. *Adjusting it after bed making loosens the linens.*
- Place the bottom sheet with its center fold in the middle of the mattress. For a fitted sheet, secure the top and bottom corners over the mattress corners on the side of the bed nearest you. For a flat sheet, align the end of the sheet with the foot of the mattress, and miter the top corner to keep the sheet firmly tucked under the mattress.

Miter this

- To miter the corner, first tuck the top end of the sheet evenly under the mattress at the head of the bed. Then lift the side edge of the sheet about 12" (30 cm) from the mattress corner and hold it at a right angle to the mattress. Tuck in the bottom edge of the sheet hanging below the mattress. Lastly, drop the top edge and tuck it under the mattress, as shown below.

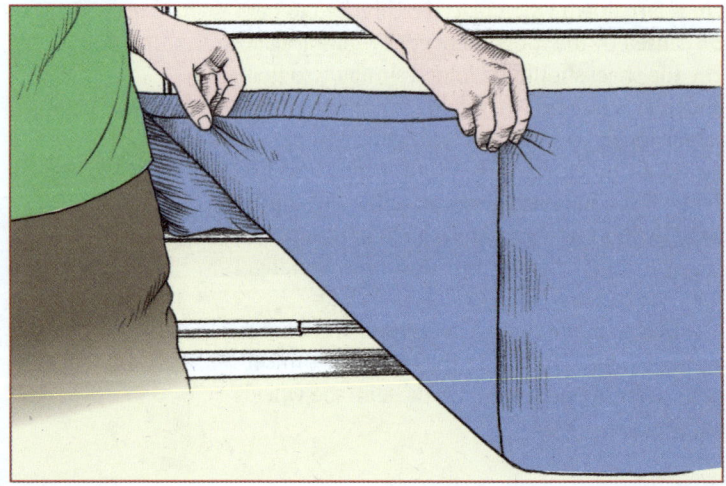

To "tuck" or "no-tuck"

- After tucking under one side of the bottom sheet, place the drawsheet (if needed) about 15 in (38 cm) from the top of the bed, with its center fold in the middle of the bed. Then tuck in the entire edge of the drawsheet on that side of the bed.
- Place the top sheet with its center fold in the middle of the bed and its wide hem even with the top of the bed. Position the rough side of the hem face up so that the smooth side shows after folding. Allow enough sheet at the top of the bed to form a cuff over the spread.
- Place the spread over the top sheet, with its center fold in the middle of the bed.

Heel and "toe"

- Make a 3-in (7.6 cm) toe pleat, or vertical tuck, in the top linens to allow room for the patient's feet and to prevent pressure that can cause discomfort, skin breakdown, and footdrop.
- Tuck the top sheet, and spread it under the foot of the mattress. Then miter the bottom corners.
- Move to the opposite side of the bed, and repeat the procedure.

Who "taut" you that?

- After fitting all corners of the bottom sheet or tucking them under the mattress, pull the sheet at an angle from the head toward the foot of the bed. *Pulling the sheet tightens the linens, making the bottom sheet taut and wrinkle-free, promoting patient comfort.*
- Fold the top sheet over the spread at the head of the bed to form a cuff and give the bed a finished appearance. When making an open bed, fanfold the top linens to the foot of the bed. If a linen-saver pad is needed, place it on top of the bottom sheets.

"Seams" like a good plan

- Slip the pillow into a clean case, tucking in the corners. Then place the pillow with its seam toward the top of the bed to prevent it from rubbing against the patient's neck, which would cause irritation, and its open edge facing away from the door to give the bed a finished appearance.
- Lower the bed, making sure the wheels remain locked to ensure the patient's safety.
- Assist the patient in returning to bed.

Getting carried away

- Return furniture to its proper place, and place the call button within the patient's easy reach. Carry away soiled linens in outstretched arms to avoid contaminating personal clothing.
- After disposing of the linens, remove gloves (if used) and wash hands thoroughly to prevent the spread of microorganisms.

Practice pointers

- Because a hospital mattress is usually covered with plastic to protect it and to facilitate cleaning between patients, a flat bottom sheet tends to loosen and become untucked. Use a fitted sheet, if available, to prevent this.
- If a fitted sheet isn't available, the top corners of a flat sheet may be tied together under the top of the mattress to prevent the sheet from becoming dislodged.
- A bath blanket placed on top of the mattress, under the bottom sheet, helps to absorb moisture and prevent dislodgment of the bottom sheet.

Making an occupied bed

For the patient who is bedridden, daily linen changes promote comfort and help prevent skin breakdown and hospital-acquired infection. Such changes necessitate the use of side rails to prevent the patient from rolling out of bed and, depending on the patient's condition, the use of a turning sheet to move them from side to side.

It takes two

Making an occupied bed may require more than one person. It also entails loosening the bottom sheet on one side and fanfolding it to the center of the mattress instead of loosening the bottom sheet on both sides and removing it, as in an unoccupied bed. Also, the foundation of the bed must be made before the top sheet is applied instead of both the foundation and top being made on one side before being completed on the other side.

Supplies

- two sheets (one fitted, if available)
- pillowcase
- one or two drawsheets
- bedspread
- one or two bath blankets
- optional: gloves, laundry bag, and linen-saver pad

Getting ready

- Obtain clean linen and make sure it's folded properly, as for an unoccupied bed.

Keep it clean

- Wash hands, put on gloves, and bring clean linen to the patient's room.
- Identify the patient and tell them you'll be changing the bed linens. Explain how they can help if they are able, adjusting the plan according to their abilities and needs. Provide privacy.
- Move any furniture away from the bed to ensure ample working space.

Raising the bar

- Raise the side rail on the far side of the bed to prevent falls. Adjust the bed to a comfortable working height to prevent back strain. Make sure the wheels are locked.
- If the patient's condition allows, lower the head of the bed to ensure tight-fitting, wrinkle-free linens.

How it's done

- When stripping the bed, watch for belongings among the linens.
- Cover the patient with a bath blanket to avoid exposure and provide warmth and privacy. Then fanfold the top sheet and spread from beneath the bath blanket, and bring them back over the blanket.
- Loosen the top linens at the foot of the bed, and remove them separately. If reusing the top linens, fold each piece and hang it over the back of the chair. Otherwise, place it in the laundry bag. To avoid dispersing microorganisms, don't fan the linens, hold them against your clothing, or place them on the floor.
- If the mattress slides down when the head of the bed is raised, pull it up again. *Adjusting the mattress after the bed is made loosens the linens.* If the patient is able, ask them to grasp the head of the bed and pull with you; otherwise, ask a coworker for help.

Side to side

- Roll the patient to the far side of the bed, and turn the pillow lengthwise under their head *to support the neck*. Ask the patient to help (if they can) by grasping the far side rail as they turn so that they are positioned at the far side of the bed.
- Loosen the soiled bottom linens on the side of the bed nearest you. Then roll the linens toward the patient's back in the middle of the bed, as shown on the next page.

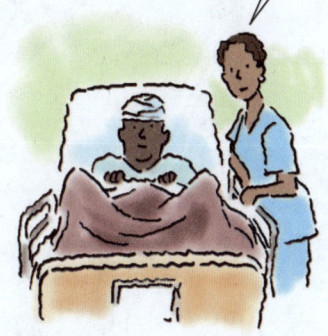

Tell the patient that you'll be changing the bed linens, and explain how they can help if they are able.

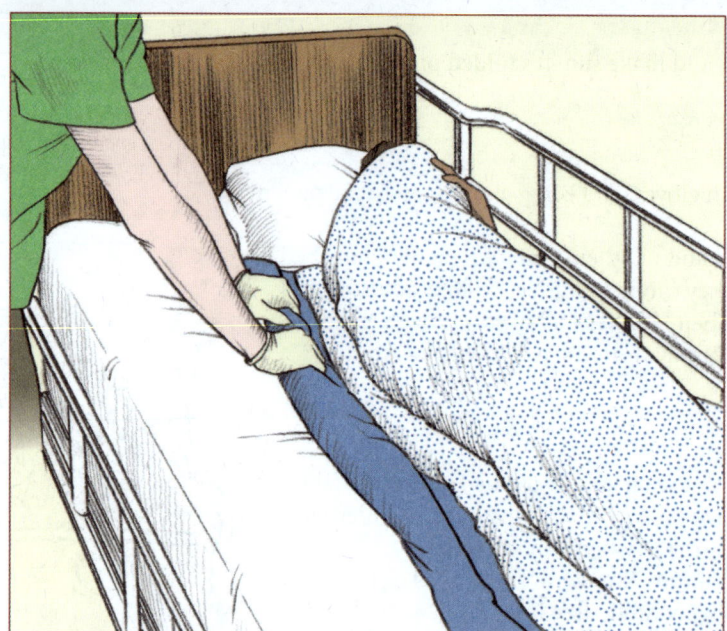

- Place a clean bottom sheet on the bed, with its center fold in the middle of the mattress. For a fitted sheet, secure the top and bottom corners over the side of the mattress nearest you. For a flat sheet, place its end even with the foot of the mattress. Miter the top corner as you would for an unoccupied bed to keep linens firmly tucked under the mattress, preventing wrinkling.

A center fold

- Fanfold the remaining clean bottom sheet toward the patient, and place the drawsheet, if needed, about 15 in (38 cm) from the top of the bed, with its center fold in the middle of the mattress. Tuck in the entire edge of the drawsheet on the side nearest you. Fanfold the remaining drawsheet toward the patient. Make sure the edge faces away from you.
- If necessary, position a linen-saver pad on the drawsheet to absorb excretions or surgical drainage, and fanfold it toward the patient.
- Raise the other side rail, and roll the patient to the clean side of the bed.

Loosen and remove

- Move to the unfinished side of the bed and lower the side rail nearest you. Then loosen and remove the soiled bottom linens separately and place them in the laundry bag.
- Pull the clean bottom sheet taut. Secure the fitted sheet, or place the end of a flat sheet even with the foot of the bed, and miter

the top corner. Pull the drawsheet taut and tuck it in. Unfold and smooth the linen-saver pad, if used.

- Assist the patient to the supine position, if their condition allows.
- Remove the soiled pillowcase, and place it in the laundry bag. Then slip the pillow into a clean pillowcase, tucking its corners well into the case to ensure a smooth fit. Place the pillow beneath the patient's head, with its seam toward the top of the bed to prevent it from rubbing against the patient's neck, which would cause irritation. Place the pillow's open edge away from the door to give the bed a finished appearance.

No "cuff" links

- Unfold the clean top sheet over the patient with the rough side of the hem facing away from the bed to avoid irritating the patient's skin. Make sure there is enough sheet available to form a cuff over the spread.
- Remove the bath blanket from beneath the sheet, and center the spread over the top sheet.

Be kind to your patient's feet

- Make a 3-in (7.6 cm) toe pleat, or vertical tuck, in the top linens to allow room for the patient's feet and to prevent pressure that can cause discomfort, skin breakdown, and footdrop.
- Tuck the top sheet and spread under the foot of the bed, and miter the bottom corners. Fold the top sheet over the spread to give the bed a finished appearance.

At the end

- Raise the head of the bed to a comfortable position, make sure both side rails are raised, and then lower the bed and lock its wheels to ensure the patient's safety. Assess the patient's body alignment and their mental and emotional status.
- Place the call button within the patient's easy reach. Remove the laundry bag from the room.
- Remove and discard gloves and wash hands to prevent the spread of hospital-acquired infections.

Practice pointers

- Use a fitted sheet, when available, because a flat sheet slips out from under the mattress easily, especially if the mattress is plastic coated.
- Prevent the patient from sliding down in bed by tucking a tightly rolled pillow under the top linens at the foot of the bed.
- For the patient who is bedridden or has diaphoresis, fold a bath blanket in half lengthwise and place it between the bottom sheet and the plastic mattress cover; the blanket acts as a cushion and

helps absorb moisture. To help prevent sheet burns on the heels and bony prominences, center a bath blanket or sheepskin over the bottom sheet, and tuck the blanket under the mattress.

Turning and positioning

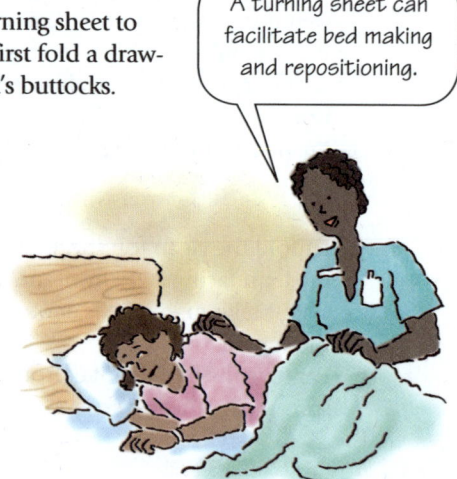

A turning sheet can facilitate bed making and repositioning.

- If the patient isn't able to move or turn, devise a turning sheet to facilitate bed making and repositioning. To do so, first fold a draw-sheet or bath blanket and place it under the patient's buttocks. Make sure the sheet extends from the shoulders to the knees so that it supports most of the patient's weight. Roll the sides of the sheet to form handles as close to the patient as possible.
- Next, ask a coworker to help you lift and move the patient. When lifting a patient, make sure both rolled handles are equidistant from the patient. Each nurse should take one of the handles, and both nurses should lift at the same time, taking care not to drag the patient because this can promote back injury for the nurses. With one person holding each side of the sheet, moving the patient without wrinkling the bottom linens is possible.

Turn the tables

- To turn the patient alone, stand at the side of the bed. Turn the patient toward the rail, and, if they are able, ask them to grasp the opposite rolled edge of the turning sheet. Pull the rolled edge carefully toward you and turn the patient.

Quick quiz

1. What layer of the skin determines skin coloration?
   A. The epidermis
   B. The dermis
   C. The subcutaneous tissue
   D. The basal cell layer

Answer: D. The basal cell layer contains melanocytes, which produce melanin. Melanin is responsible for skin color.

2. When performing denture care, which of the following can be done to provide patient comfort?
   A. Soak dentures in mouthwash after cleaning
   B. Warm dentures to room temperature
   C. Apply adhesive liner or gel to dentures before replacing them in patient's mouth
   D. Use an ADA-approved toothbrush while cleaning dentures

Answer: C. Applying an adhesive liner or gel product to the dentures provides a strong seal that promotes patient comfort by improving the fit of the dentures.

3. While performing foot care, you notice the patient's toenail growing inward at the corners. What intervention should you perform?
    A. Tuck a wisp of cotton under it to relieve pressure on the toe
    B. Let the nail grow without intervention
    C. Remove the ingrowing nail with nail clippers
    D. Apply antibiotic ointment to prevent infection

Answer: A. Tuck a wisp of cotton under the toenail. This prevents pressure on the toe and may prevent an acute ingrown toenail and risk of infection.

4. Your patient is at high risk for bleeding. While performing facial hygiene, what changes would need to be considered?
    A. Use a safety razor while shaving the patient
    B. Use an electric razor
    C. Use a straight razor
    D. Administer vitamin K before shaving to reduce bleeding risk

Answer: B. An electric razor is less likely to nick and cut the skin, making this a safer option for a patient using anticoagulants.

Scoring

 If you answered all four questions correctly, congratulations! You really cleaned up!

If you answered three questions correctly, great! You're fundamentally prepared to take care of yourself.

If you answered fewer than three questions correctly, don't despair! Just review the chapter, and you'll be a whiz at patient care in no time.

References

Centers for Disease Control and Prevention. (2023). Oral health in healthcare settings to prevent pneumonia toolkit. https://www.cdc.gov/hai/prevent/Oral-Health-Toolkit.html#:~:text=For%20most%20patients%2C%20oral%20care,%2C%20desensitizing%2C%20non%2Dfoaming

Cowdell, F., Jadotte, Y. T., Ersser, S. J., Danby, S., Lawton, S., Roberts, A., & Dyson, J. (2020). Hygiene and emollient interventions for maintaining skin integrity in older people in hospital and residential care settings. *Cochrane Database of Systematic Reviews*, 1(1), CD011377. https://doi.org/10.1002/14651858.CD011377.pub2

Goldenhart, A., & Hassan, N. (2022). *Assisting patients with personal hygiene*. [Updated 2022 Sep 26]. In *StatPearls* [Internet]. StatPearls Publishing. https://www.ncbi.nlm.nih.gov/books/NBK563155/

Konya, I., Nishiya, K., & Yano, R. (2021). Effectiveness of bed bath methods for skin integrity, skin cleanliness and comfort enhancement in adults: A systematic review. *Nursing Open, 8*(5), 2284–2300. https://doi.org/10.1002/nop2.836

McCabe, D. (2023). *Katz index of independence in activities of daily living (ADL)*. Hartford Institute of Geriatric Nursing. https://hign.org/consultgeri/try-this-series/katz-index-independence-activities-daily-living-adl

Chapter 14

Mobility, activity, and exercise

Just the facts

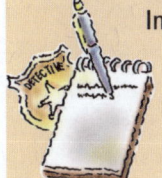

In this chapter, you'll learn:

◆ factors that affect musculoskeletal functioning

◆ proper patient positioning

◆ use of alignment and pressure-reducing devices

◆ methods of transferring a patient

◆ crutch walking and walker use

◆ range-of-motion exercises.

A look at mobility, activity, and exercise

Mobility is defined as an individual's ability to move freely and interact with the environment. A patient's mobility or ability to move and be active affects their physical and emotional well-being. Mobility is essential to function well and live independently. Many adults experience changes to mobility with age. However, younger patients can also be affected by immobility from prolonged bed rest due to the physical restraints secondary to fractures or traction, or from loss of strength due to illness.

Actively active

Activity keeps the mind and body active. Musculoskeletal inactivity or immobility adversely affects all body systems. Exercise—even passive range-of-motion (ROM) exercises—helps prevent muscle atrophy, prevent muscle contractures, and maintain circulation. Exercise increases muscle strength, tone, and mass. It also enhances the condition of other body systems.

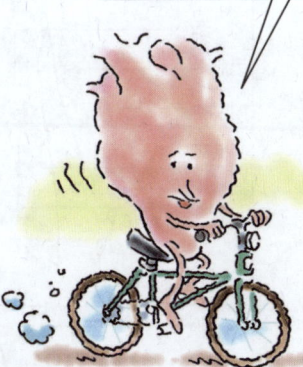

Exercise helps maintain circulation.

A look at the musculoskeletal system

Muscles, bones, joints, tendons, and ligaments give the human body its shape and ability to be mobile, perform such activities as those of daily living, and exercise. The three main components of the musculoskeletal system are:

- bones
- joints
- muscles

Bones

The 206 bones of the skeleton form the body's framework, supporting and protecting organs and tissues. The bones also serve as storage sites for minerals and contain bone marrow, the primary site for blood production. (See *A close look at the skeletal system*.)

A close look at the skeletal system

Of the 206 bones in the human skeletal system, 80 form the axial skeleton (skull, facial bones, vertebrae, ribs, sternum, and hyoid bone) and 126 form the appendicular skeleton (arms, legs, shoulders, and pelvis). Shown here are the body's major bones.

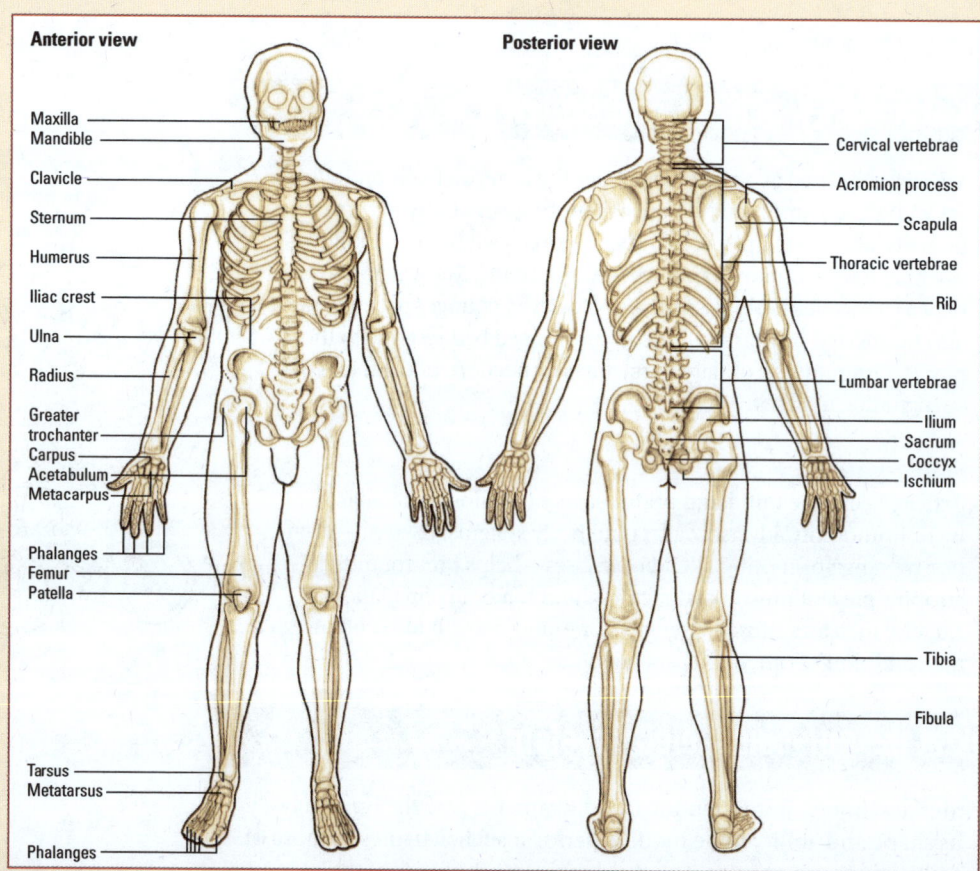

Anterior view

Maxilla
Mandible
Clavicle
Sternum
Humerus
Iliac crest
Ulna
Radius
Greater trochanter
Carpus
Acetabulum
Metacarpus
Phalanges
Femur
Patella
Tarsus
Metatarsus
Phalanges

Posterior view

Cervical vertebrae
Acromion process
Scapula
Thoracic vertebrae
Rib
Lumbar vertebrae
Ilium
Sacrum
Coccyx
Ischium
Tibia
Fibula

Joints

The junction of two or more bones is called a *joint*. Joints stabilize the bones and allow a specific type of movement. The two types of joints are:

- synovial
- nonsynovial

Synovial

Synovial joints move freely; the bones are separate from each other and meet in a cavity filled with synovial fluid, a lubricant. In synovial joints, a layer of resilient cartilage covers the surfaces of opposing bones. This cartilage cushions the bones and allows full joint movement by making the surfaces of the bones smooth. These joints are surrounded by a fibrous capsule that stabilizes the joint structures. The capsule also surrounds the joint's ligaments—the tough, fibrous bands that join one bone to another.

Synovial joints come in several types, including ball-and-socket joints and hinge joints. Ball-and-socket joints—the shoulders and hips being the only examples of this type—enable flexion, extension, adduction, and abduction. These joints also rotate in their sockets and are assessed by their degree of internal and external rotation. Hinge joints, such as the knee and elbow, typically move in flexion and extension only. (See *Synovial joint.*)

Nonsynovial

In nonsynovial joints, the bones are connected by fibrous tissue, also called *cartilage*. The bones may be immovable, such as the sutures in the skull, or slightly movable, such as the vertebrae of the spinal column.

Muscles

Muscles are groups of contractile cells or fibers that effect movement of an organ or a part of the body. Skeletal muscles, the focus of this chapter, contract and produce skeletal movement when they receive a stimulus from the central nervous system (CNS). The CNS is responsible for involuntary and voluntary muscle function. Tendons, the tough fibrous portions of muscle, attach the muscles to bone. Loss of muscle is common with aging and disuse. Osteoarthritis (OA) is the most common joint problem experienced as part of aging. The Centers for Disease Control and Prevention predicts that by the year 2040, 78 million adults over the age of 18 will have a diagnosis of OA (CDC, 2021; Joint Health, 2023).

Synovial joint

Normally, bones fit together. Cartilage—a smooth, fibrous tissue—cushions the end of each bone, and synovial fluid fills the joint space. This fluid lubricates the joint and eases movement, much as the brake fluid functions in a car.

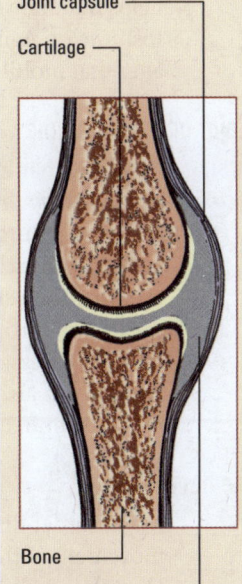

Joint capsule

Cartilage

Bone

Joint space filled with synovial fluid

Where would we be without bursae?

Bursae are sacs filled with friction-reducing synovial fluid; they're located in areas of high friction such as the knee. Bursae enable adjacent muscles or muscles and tendons to glide smoothly over each other during movement.

Factors affecting musculoskeletal function

When an individual has limited mobility and movement, their health can deteriorate, and multiple complications can occur. The signs and symptoms of inactivity, commonly described as *disuse syndrome*, can include decreased muscle strength and tone, lack of coordination, altered gait, falls, decreased joint flexibility, pain on movement, and decreased activity tolerance.

Lifestyle and habits can affect a person's mobility. Regular exercise helps maintain musculoskeletal functioning and mobility. (National Institute on Aging, 2020). Inactivity due to age, disease, or trauma can alter that mobility.

Major or minor trauma

Anything that interferes with bone resiliency and strength or muscle strength may impair the musculoskeletal system's capacity to assist mobility. Trauma can result in injury to tendons, ligaments, joints, bones, or muscles. This damage can be minor or major and can affect mobility for a short time or for a longer time if it involves a dislocated joint, broken bone, torn tendon, or joint replacement.

Such diseases as rheumatoid arthritis (RA), osteoporosis, gout, and OA can also limit mobility. Bone tumors can cause pain and may require amputation of the affected limbs.

The nerves have it

Any disorder that impairs the nervous system's ability to control movement of the muscles and coordination hinders mobility. Disorders such as muscular dystrophy, Parkinson disease, and multiple sclerosis slowly erode and destroy the patient's capacity for coordinated movement.

Two or four

Brain or spinal cord injuries can result in a severed or severely damaged spinal cord, causing paralysis below the injury site. Decreased motor and sensory function to the legs is referred to as *paraplegia,* and paralysis of the arms and the legs is called *quadriplegia.*

O₂ needed

Oxygen is needed for the muscles to function properly. Any disease that limits the oxygen supply affects muscle contraction and movement. Lung conditions reduce the amount of oxygen delivered to the cells, including skeletal muscles.

Ouch! That hurts!

Activity intolerance may be associated with pain or edema. Alternatively, the patient's activity may be severely restricted by such conditions as fractures requiring skeletal traction, RA, vertebral fractures, neurogenic arthropathy, Paget disease, muscular dystrophy, and other disorders.

Treating immobility

Impaired physical mobility is related to many musculoskeletal disorders that involve joint inflammation as well as fractures, bone disorders, and other disorders that cause decreased mobility.

Proper positioning

Proper positioning and alignment and pressure-reducing devices help maintain correct body positioning and prevent complications that can occur with prolonged bed rest. (See *Positioning patients*, page 394.) When a patient is weak, in pain, frail, paralyzed, immobilized, or unconscious, they can't readily position and reposition themselves. Thus, assistance to help or provide position changes may be needed. Assessing the skin and providing skin care before and after repositioning is also important.

Change is good

Frequent position changes help prevent muscle discomfort, damage to superficial nerves and blood vessels, prolonged pressure resulting in pressure injuries, and muscle contractures.

Using alignment and pressure-reducing devices

Alignment and pressure-reducing devices include protective boots to protect the heels and help prevent skin breakdown and footdrop; abduction pillows to help prevent internal hip rotation after femoral fracture, hip fracture, or surgery; trochanter rolls to help prevent external hip rotation; and hand rolls to help prevent hand contractures.

Positioning patients

Dorsal recumbent position

In the dorsal recumbent (or *supine*) position, the patient is placed on their back with the knees slightly flexed. Place a pillow beneath the head for comfort. This position immobilizes the spine. It's commonly used for a spinal cord injury, urinary catheter insertion, or a vaginal examination.

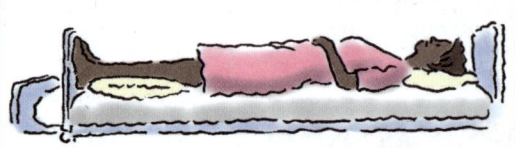

Semi-Fowler position

For semi-Fowler position, elevate the head of the bed to 30° and raise the bed section under the patient's knees, flexing the knees slightly. This position promotes drainage, cardiac output, and ventilation. It also prevents aspiration of food and secretions. Like Fowler position, it's commonly used for a patient who has a head injury, increased intracranial pressure, or dyspnea; has undergone abdominal surgery, cranial surgery, thyroidectomy, or eye surgery; or is vomiting.

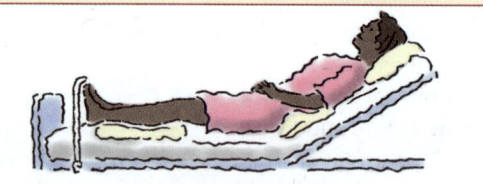

Prone position

The prone position is used to promote gas exchange and enable examination of the back. It's accomplished by placing the patient on their stomach with the head turned to one side and positioning the arms at the side or above the head. Make sure that the legs are extended. This position is commonly used for immobilization, acute respiratory distress syndrome, and after lumbar puncture or a myelogram.

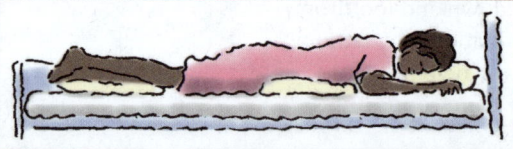

Lateral position

The lateral (or *side-lying*) position promotes safety and prevents atelectasis, pressure injuries, and aspiration of food and secretions. Place the patient on their side, with the weight supported mostly by the lateral aspect of the lower scapula and the lower ilium. Support this position by placing pillows as needed. This position is commonly used for administering an enema or a suppository and for a patient who has undergone abdominal surgery, is in a coma, or has pressure injuries.

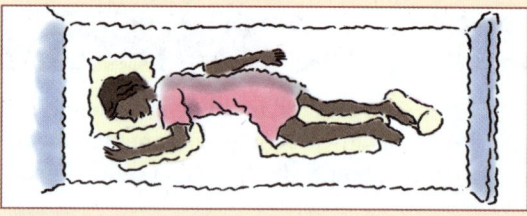

Sims position

Also called a *semi-prone position*, Sims position enables examination of the back and rectum and can help prevent atelectasis and pressure injuries. Position the patient on their side with a small pillow placed beneath the head. Flex one knee toward the abdomen, with the other knee only slightly flexed. Place one arm behind the body and the other in a comfortable position. Support the patient in this position with pillows as needed. Sims position is commonly used for a patient who has sustained rectal injuries or is in a coma.

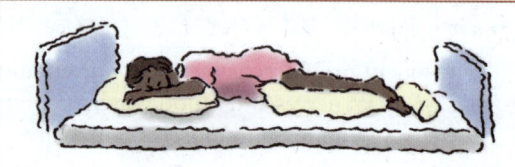

Several of these devices—protective boots, trochanter rolls, and hand rolls—are especially useful when caring for patients who have a loss of sensation, mobility, or consciousness or following a neuromuscular incident such as stroke.

Supplies

- protective boots
- abduction pillow
- trochanter rolls
- hand rolls (See *Common preventive devices*, page 396.)

Getting ready

If you're using a device that's available in different sizes, select the appropriate size for the patient.

How it's done

- Explain the purpose and steps of the procedure to the patient.

Applying a protective boot

- Open the slit on the superior surface of the boot. Then place the patient's foot in the boot and fasten the ankle and foot straps. If the patient is positioned laterally, you may apply the boot only to the bottom foot and support the flexed top foot with a pillow.
- If appropriate, insert the other foot in the second boot.
- Position the patient's legs in alignment to prevent strain on hip ligaments and pressure on bony prominences.

Applying an abduction pillow

- Place the patient in a supine position and put the pillow between their legs. Slide the pillow toward the groin so that it touches the legs all along their length.
- Place the upper part of both legs in the pillow's lateral indentations, and secure the straps to prevent the pillow from slipping.

Applying a trochanter roll

- Place one roll on the outside of the thigh from the iliac crest to midthigh. Then place another roll along the other thigh. Make sure neither roll extends as far as the knee to avoid peroneal nerve compression and palsy, which can lead to footdrop.
- If you've fashioned trochanter rolls from a towel or rolled sheet, leave several inches unrolled and tuck this part under the patient's thigh to hold the device in place and maintain the patient's position.

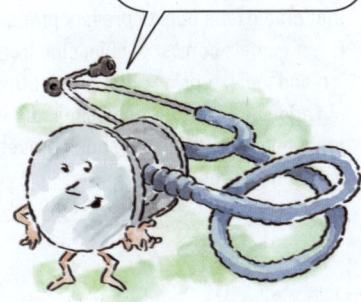

A disorder affecting the nervous system can impair a person's ability to coordinate movement.

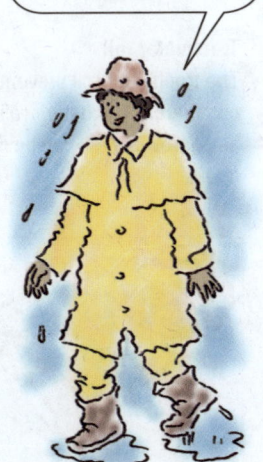

Protective boots protect the heels and prevent skin breakdown and footdrop.

Common preventive devices

These illustrations show different devices used to reduce pressure or help maintain positioning, depending on the patient's needs.

Protective boot

The protective boot prevents footdrop and skin breakdown. Some protective boots are made of soft material that cradles the heel to prevent pressure on the heel. Other models consist of aluminum frames with fleece lining and toe extensions that protect the toes and prevent hip adduction. High-topped sneakers may be used to help prevent footdrop, but they don't prevent external hip rotation or heel pressure.

Abduction pillow

The abduction pillow prevents internal hip rotation. It's a wedge-shaped piece of sponge rubber with lateral indentations for the patient's thighs. Its straps wrap around the thighs to maintain correct positioning. Although a properly shaped bed pillow may temporarily substitute for the commercial abduction pillow, it's difficult to apply and fails to maintain the correct lateral alignment.

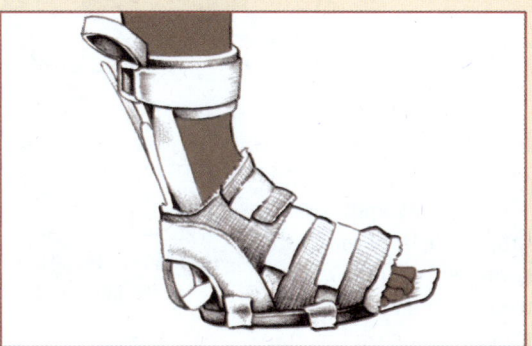

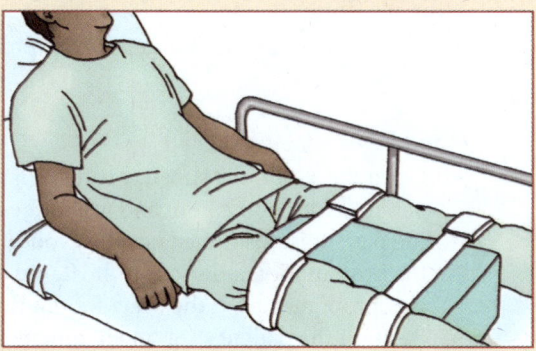

Trochanter roll

The trochanter roll prevents external hip rotation. The commercial trochanter roll is made of sponge rubber; an improvised roll can be made from a rolled blanket or towel.

Hand roll

The hand roll prevents hand contractures. It's available in hard and soft materials and is held in place by fixed or adjustable straps. A hand roll can be improvised from a rolled washcloth secured with roller gauze and adhesive tape.

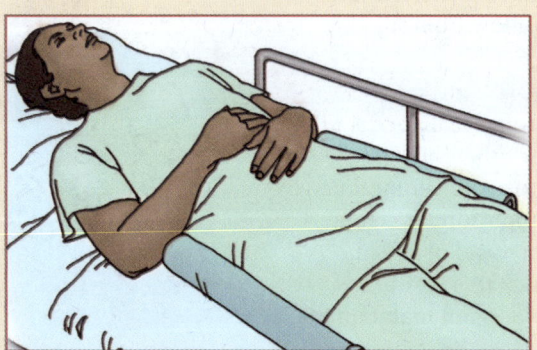

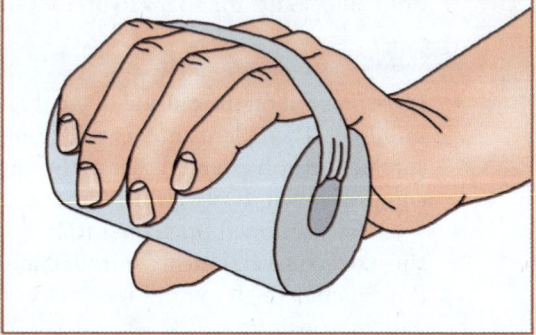

Applying a hand roll

- Place one roll in the patient's hand. This will help maintain the neutral position. Then secure the strap, if present, or apply roller gauze and secure with hypoallergenic or adhesive tape.
- Place another roll in the other hand.
- Remember that the use of assistive devices doesn't preclude regularly scheduled patient positioning, ROM exercises, and skin care.
- Contractures and pressure injuries may occur with the use of a hand roll and, possibly, with other assistive devices. To avoid these problems, remove a soft hand roll every 4 hours (every 2 hours if the patient has hand spasticity); remove a hard hand roll every 2 hours.

Ambulating patients

Many patient care activities require the nurse to push, pull, lift, and carry. By using proper body mechanics, the nurse can avoid musculoskeletal injury and fatigue and reduce the risk of injuring patients.

Using proper body mechanics

Correct body mechanics can be summed up in three principles:
- Keep a low center of gravity by flexing the hips and knees instead of bending at the waist to distribute weight evenly between the upper and lower body and maintain balance.
- Create a wide base of support by spreading your feet apart to provide lateral stability and lower your body's center of gravity.
- Maintain proper body alignment and keep your body's center of gravity directly over the base of support by moving your feet rather than twisting and bending at the waist.

Do it right

In addition to the three basic principles, follow the directions below to push, pull, stoop, lift, and carry correctly.

Pushing and pulling correctly
- Stand close to the object, and place one foot slightly ahead of the other, as in a walking position. Tighten your leg muscles and set your pelvis by simultaneously contracting your abdominal and gluteal muscles.
- To push, place your hands on the object and flex your elbows. Lean into the object by shifting weight from your back leg to your front leg, and apply smooth, continuous pressure.

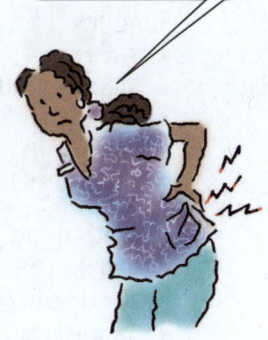

Spare your back. Know the proper way to lift, push, pull, and carry!

- To pull, grasp the object and flex your elbows. Lean away from the object by shifting weight from your front leg to your back leg. Pull smoothly, avoiding sudden, jerky movements.
- After you've started to move the object, keep it in motion; stopping and starting uses more energy.

Stooping correctly

- Stand with your feet 10" to 12" (25 to 30 cm) apart and one foot slightly ahead of the other to widen the base of support.
- Lower yourself by flexing your knees and place more weight on the front foot than on the back foot. Keep your upper body straight by not bending at the waist.
- To stand up again, straighten your knees and keep your back straight.

Lifting and carrying correctly

- Assume the stooping position directly in front of the object to minimize back flexion and avoid spinal rotation when lifting.
- Grasp the object, and tighten your abdominal muscles.
- Stand up by straightening your knees, using your leg and hip muscles. Always keep your back straight to maintain a fixed center of gravity.
- Carry the object close to your body at waist height—near the body's center of gravity—to avoid straining your back muscles. (See *Transfer tips.*)

Transfer from bed to stretcher

Transfer from bed to stretcher, one of the most common transfers, can require the help of one or more coworkers, depending on the patient's size and condition and the primary nurse's physical ability. Techniques for achieving this transfer include the straight lift, carry lift, lift sheet, and sliding board.

Supplies

- stretcher
- sliding board or lift sheet, if necessary

Getting ready

Adjust the bed to the same height as the stretcher.

How it's done

- Tell the patient that you're going to move them from the bed to the stretcher, and place them in the supine position.
- Instruct team members to remove watches and rings. This will prevent scratching the patient during transfer.

Transfer tips

When transferring a patient or performing other care activities, remember these tips:
- Wear shoes with low heels, flexible nonslip soles, and closed backs to promote correct body alignment, facilitate proper body mechanics, and prevent accidents.
- When possible, pull rather than push an object, because elbow flexors are stronger than extensors.
- When doing heavy lifting or moving, remember to use assistive or mechanical devices, if available, or obtain assistance from coworkers; know your limitations and use sound judgment.

Four-person straight lift

- Place the stretcher parallel to the bed, and lock the wheels of both to ensure patient safety.

Get into position

- Stand at the center of the stretcher, and have another team member stand at the patient's head. The two other team members should stand next to the bed on the other side—one at the center and the other at the patient's feet.
- Slide your arms, palms up, under the patient while the other team members do the same. In this position, you and the team member directly opposite to you support the patient's buttocks and hips; the team member at the head of the bed supports the patient's head and shoulders; and the one at the foot supports the patient's legs and feet.

One, two, three

- On a count of three, you and your team members lift the patient several inches, move them onto the stretcher, and slide your arms out from under them. Keep movements smooth to minimize patient discomfort and avoid muscle strain by team members.
- Position the patient comfortably on the stretcher, apply safety straps, and raise and secure the side rails.

Four-person carry lift

- Place the stretcher perpendicular to the bed, with the head of the stretcher at the foot of the bed. Lock the bed and the stretcher wheels to ensure patient safety.
- Raise the bed to a comfortable working height.

Top to bottom, tallest to shortest

- Line up all four team members on the same side of the bed as the stretcher. Place the tallest member at the patient's head and the shortest at their feet. The member at the patient's head is the team leader and gives the lift signals.
- The team leader will tell the team members to flex their knees and slide their hands, palms up, under the patient until they rest securely on their upper arms.
- Make sure the patient is adequately supported at the head and shoulders, buttocks and hips, and legs and feet.

Reduce the strain

- On a count of three, the team members straighten their knees and roll the patient onto their side, against the team members' chests.

This reduces strain on the team members and allows them to hold the patient for several minutes, if necessary.

- Together, the team members step back, with the member supporting the feet moving the farthest.

On the count of three

- The team members move forward to the stretcher's edge and, on a count of three, lower the patient onto the stretcher by bending at the knees and sliding their arms out from under the patient.
- Position the patient comfortably on the stretcher, apply safety straps, and raise and secure the side rails.

Four-person lift sheet transfer

- Position the bed, stretcher, and team members for the straight lift.

Make it close to the patient

- Instruct the team to hold the edges of the sheet under the patient, grasping them close to the patient to obtain a firm grip, provide stability, and spare the patient feelings of instability.

One smooth, continuous motion

- On a count of three, the team members lift or slide the patient onto the stretcher in one smooth, continuous motion to avoid muscle strain and minimize patient discomfort.
- Position the patient comfortably on the stretcher, apply safety straps, and raise and secure the side rails.

Sliding board transfer

- Place the stretcher parallel to the bed, and lock the wheels of both to ensure patient safety.
- Stand next to the bed, and instruct a coworker to stand next to the stretcher.
- Reach over the patient and pull the far side of the bed sheet toward you to turn the patient slightly on their side.

Bridging the gap

- Instruct your coworker to place the sliding board beneath the patient, making sure the board bridges the gap between the stretcher and the bed.
- Ease the patient onto the sliding board, and release the sheet.

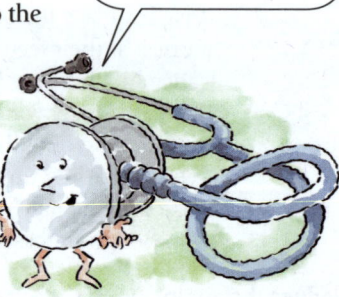

Make sure you apply safety straps and secure the side rails after any patient transfer.

Making the transfer

- Instruct your coworker to grasp the near side of the sheet at the patient's hips and shoulders and to pull them onto the stretcher in a smooth, continuous motion. Then have the coworker reach over the patient, grasp the far side of the sheet, and logroll the patient toward them.

Getting the patient settled

- Remove the sliding board as your coworker returns the patient to the supine position.
- Position the patient comfortably on the stretcher, apply safety straps, and raise and secure the side rails.

Special circumstances

If the patient is obese

- When transferring from the bed to the stretcher, lift and move the patient with obesity, in increments, to the edge of the bed. After resting for a few seconds, lift them onto the stretcher.
- Depending on the patient's size and condition, lift sheet transfer can require two or more people.
- If available, consider using a mechanical lift to transfer the patient. (See *Using a mechanical lift,* page 402.)

If the patient can bear weight

- Two or three coworkers can perform a transfer if the patient can bear weight on their arms or legs. One can support the buttocks and guide the patient, another can stabilize the stretcher by leaning over it and guiding the patient into position, and a third can transfer any attached equipment. If a team member isn't available to guide equipment, move IV lines and other tubing first to make sure they're out of the way and not in danger of pulling loose, or disconnect the tubes if possible.

If the patient is light

- Three coworkers can perform the carry lift if the patient is light, but no matter how many team members are present, one must stabilize the patient's head if they aren't able to support it themselves, have cervical instability or injury, or have undergone surgery.
- Document the time and type of transfer in your notes. Complete other required forms as necessary.

Using a mechanical lift

Training and practice are necessary before using a mechanical lift. Know the type of lift and how to operate the equipment before using. Prepare the equipment before use to ensure the battery is charged and the equipment is operable. Assess the patient's physical capabilities and mental status, and review their medical condition to ensure the correct lift and sling is selected so as not to make the patient's condition worse.

Assess the patient's size and weight to ensure the correct sling is selected. Position the center of the sling under the patient's spine. After placing the patient in the supine position in the center of the sling, position the hydraulic lift above them (as shown below). Then attach the chains to the hooks on the sling.

Turn the lift handle clockwise to raise the patient to the sitting position. If they are positioned properly, continue to raise them until they are suspended just above the bed.

After positioning the patient above the wheelchair, turn the lift handle counterclockwise to lower them onto the seat. When the chains become slack, stop turning and unhook the sling from the lift.

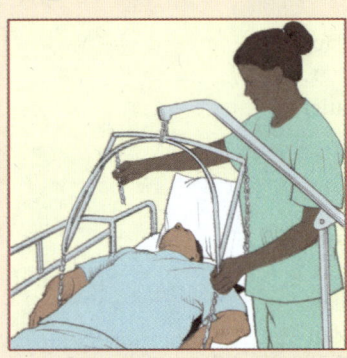 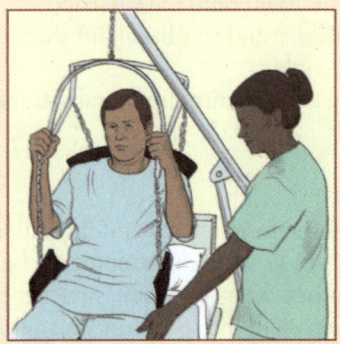 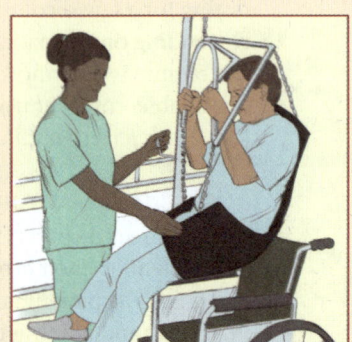

Transfer from bed to wheelchair

For a patient with diminished or absent lower body sensation or one-sided weakness, immobility, or injury, transfer from bed to wheelchair may require partial support to full assistance—initially by at least two people. After transfer, proper positioning helps prevent excessive pressure on bony prominences, which predisposes the patient to skin breakdown.

Supplies

- wheelchair with locks (or sturdy chair)
- pajama bottoms (or robe)
- shoes or slippers with nonslip soles
- optional: transfer board if appropriate

Getting ready

- Explain the procedure to the patient and demonstrate the patient's role. (See *Teaching the patient to use a transfer board.*)
- Place the wheelchair parallel to the bed, facing the foot of the bed, and lock its wheels. Make sure the bed wheels are also locked. Raise the footrests to avoid them interfering with the transfer.

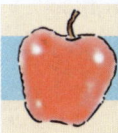

Education corner

Teaching the patient to use a transfer board

For the patient who isn't able to stand, a transfer board allows safe transfer from bed to wheelchair. To help the patient perform this transfer, take these steps:

- Explain the procedure to the patient, and then demonstrate it. They may eventually become proficient enough to transfer with or without supervision.
- Help the patient put on pajama bottoms or a robe and shoes or slippers.
- Angle the wheelchair slightly facing the foot of the bed. Lock the wheels, and remove the armrest closest to the patient. Make sure the bed is flat, and adjust its height so that it's level with the wheelchair seat.
- Assist the patient to a sitting position on the edge of the bed, with feet resting on the floor. Make sure the front edge of the wheelchair seat is aligned with the back of the patient's knees (as shown below left). Depending on the patient, they may find it easier to transfer to an even surface or to a slightly lower surface.
- Ask the patient to lean away from the wheelchair while you slide one end of the transfer board under them.

- Then place the other end of the transfer board on the wheelchair seat, and help the patient return to the upright position.
- Stand in front of the patient to prevent them from sliding forward. Tell them to push down with both arms, lifting the buttocks up and onto the transfer board. Have them repeat this maneuver, edging along the board, until seated in the wheelchair. If they aren't able to use their arms to help with the transfer, stand in front of the patient, put your arms around them, and—if they can—have the patient put their arms around you. Gradually slide them across the board until safely in the chair (as shown below right).
- Then remove the transfer board, replace the wheelchair armrest, and reposition the patient in the chair.

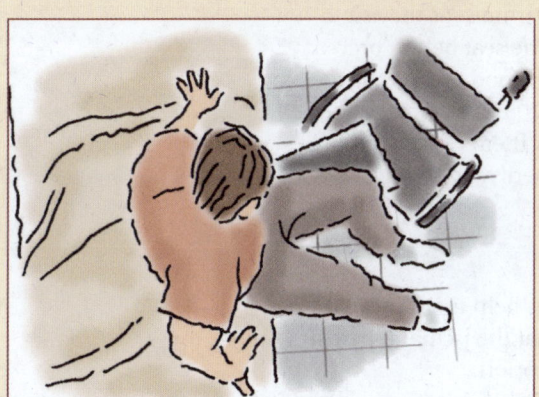

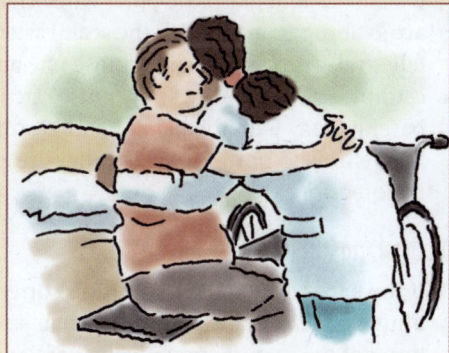

Check the vitals

- Check the patient's pulse rate and blood pressure when they are in a supine position to obtain a baseline. Assist the patient with putting on pajama bottoms and slippers or shoes with nonslip soles to prevent falls.

How it's done

- Raise the head of the bed, and allow the patient to rest briefly to adjust to posture changes. Then bring them to the dangling position. Recheck their pulse rate and blood pressure if you suspect cardiovascular instability, and don't proceed until the patient is stabilized to prevent falls.

Out of the bed...

- Tell the patient to move toward the edge of the bed and, if possible, to place feet flat on the floor. Stand in front of the patient, blocking the toes with your feet and their knees with yours to prevent the knees from buckling.
- Flex your knees slightly, place your arms around the patient's waist, and tell them to place their hands on the edge of the bed. Avoid bending at your waist to prevent back strain.
- Ask the patient to push off the bed and to support as much of their own weight as possible. At the same time, straighten your knees and hips, raising the patient as you straighten your body.
- Supporting the patient as needed, pivot toward the wheelchair, keeping your knees next to theirs. Tell them to grasp the farthest armrest of the wheelchair with their closest hand.

...and into the chair

- Help the patient lower themselves into the wheelchair by flexing your hips and knees but not your back. Instruct the patient to reach back and grasp the other wheelchair armrest as they sit to avoid abrupt contact with the seat. Fasten the seat belt to prevent falls and, if necessary, check pulse rate and blood pressure to assess cardiovascular stability. If the pulse rate is 20 beats or more above baseline, stay with the patient and monitor them closely until the rate returns to normal because they are experiencing orthostatic hypotension.

Position, position, position

- If the patient isn't able to position correctly, help them move their buttocks against the back of the chair so that the ischial tuberosities, not the sacrum, provide the base of support.
- Place the patient's feet flat on the footrests, pointed straight ahead.
- Position the knees and hips with the correct amount of flexion and in appropriate alignment.

- If appropriate, use elevating leg rests to flex the patient's hips at more than 90°; this position relieves pressure on the popliteal space and places more weight on the ischial tuberosities.
- Position the patient's arms on the wheelchair's armrests with shoulders abducted, elbows slightly flexed, forearms pronated, and wrists and hands in the neutral position.
- If necessary, support or elevate their hands and forearms with a pillow.
- If the patient starts to fall during transfer, ease them to the closest surface. *Never stretch to finish the transfer. Doing so can cause loss of balance, falls, muscle strain, and other injuries to you and the patient.*

Compensating for weakness

- If the patient has one-sided weakness, follow the preceding steps, but place the wheelchair on their unaffected side. Instruct them to pivot and bear as much weight as possible on the unaffected side. Support the affected side because the patient will tend to lean to this side. If the patient is hemiplegic, use pillows to support the affected side to prevent slumping in the wheelchair.

Crutch walking

Crutches remove weight from one or both legs, enabling the patient to support themselves with their hands and arms. Typically prescribed for a patient with lower extremity injury or weakness, crutches require balance, stamina, and upper body strength for successful use. Crutch selection and walking gait depend on the patient's condition. A patient who isn't able to use crutches may be able to use a walker.

Supplies
- crutches with axillary pads, handgrips, and rubber suction tips
- optional: walking belt

Getting ready
- Choose the appropriate crutches, and then adjust their height with the patient standing or, if necessary, recumbent. (See *Selecting and fitting a crutch,* page 406.)
- Consult with the patient's healthcare provider and physical therapist to coordinate rehabilitation orders and teaching.

How it's done
- Describe the gait that should be used with crutches and explain the reason for this gait type. Then demonstrate the gait as necessary. Have the patient give a return demonstration.

Selecting and fitting a crutch

When fitting a patient for a crutch, selecting the right type of crutch is the first step. Three types of crutches are commonly used:

• Standard aluminum or wooden crutches are used by the patient with a sprain, strain, or cast. They require stamina, balance, and upper body strength.

• Aluminum forearm crutches are used by the paraplegic or other patient using the swing-through gait. They have a collar that fits around the forearm and a horizontal handgrip that provides support.

• Platform crutches are used by the arthritic patient who has an upper extremity deficit that prevents weight bearing through the wrist. They provide padded surfaces for the upper extremities.

The right fit

If the patient is using a standard aluminum or wooden crutch, it must fit properly. To fit the crutch to the patient, position the crutch so that it extends from a point 4″ to 6″ (10 to 15 cm) to the side of, and 4″ to 6″ in front of, the patient's feet to 1½″ to 2″ (4 to 5 cm) below the axillae (about the width of two fingers). Then adjust the handgrips so that the patient's elbows are flexed at a 15° angle when they are standing with the crutches in the resting position.

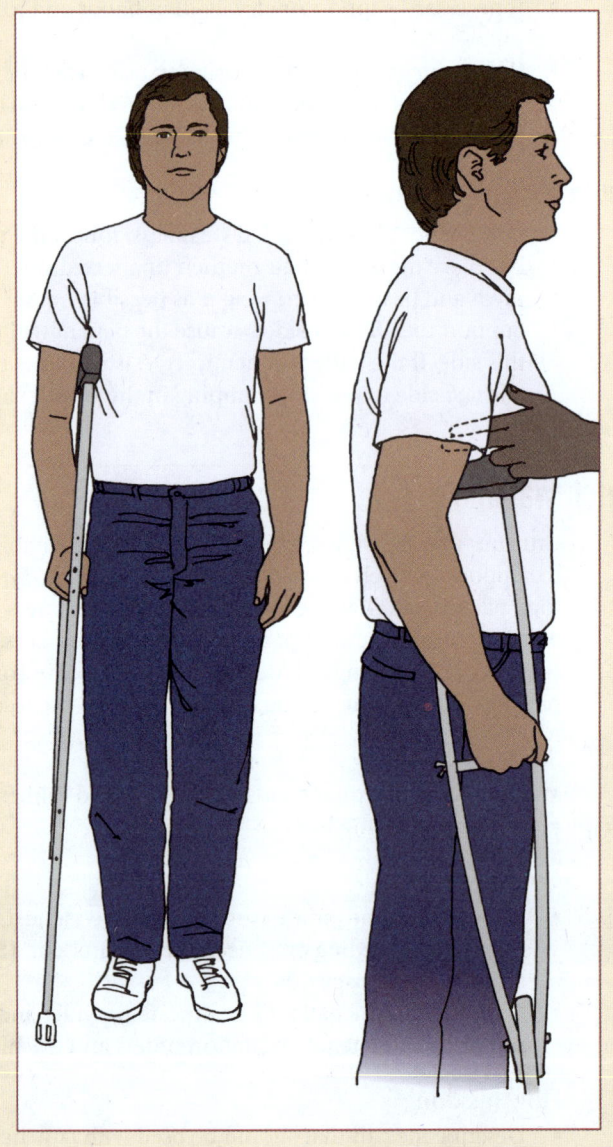

- Place a walking belt around the patient's waist, if necessary, to help prevent falls. Tell the patient to position the crutches and shift their weight from side to side. Then place them in front of a full-length mirror to facilitate learning and coordination.

Four point
- Teach the four-point gait to the patient who can bear weight on both legs. Although this is the safest gait because three points are always in contact with the floor, it requires greater coordination than others because of the constant weight shifting. Use this sequence: right crutch, left foot, left crutch, right foot. Suggest counting to help develop rhythm, and make sure each short step is of equal length. If the patient gains proficiency at this gait, teach them the faster two-point gait.

Three point
- Teach the three-point gait to the patient who can bear only partial or no weight on one leg. Instruct them to advance both crutches 6″ to 8″ (15 to 20 cm) along with the involved leg. Then tell them to bring the uninvolved leg forward and to bear the bulk of the weight on the crutches but some of it on the involved leg, if possible. Stress the importance of taking steps of equal length and duration with no pauses.
- Teach the swing-to or swing-through gaits—the fastest gaits—to the patient with complete paralysis of the hips and legs. Instruct them to advance both crutches simultaneously and to swing the legs parallel to (swing-to) or beyond (swing-through) the crutches.
- To teach the patient who uses crutches to get up from a chair, tell them to hold both crutches in one hand, with the tips resting firmly on the floor. Then instruct them to push up from the chair with the free hand, supporting themselves with the crutches.
- To sit down, the patient reverses the process: Instruct them to support themselves with the crutches in one hand and lower themselves with the other.
- To teach the patient to ascend stairs using the three-point gait, tell them to lead with the uninvolved leg and follow with both the crutches and the involved leg. To descend stairs, they should lead with the crutches and the involved leg and follow with the uninvolved leg.

Two point
- Teach the two-point gait to the patient with weak legs but good coordination and arm strength. This is the most natural crutch-walking gait because it mimics walking, with alternating swings of the arms and legs. Instruct the patient to advance the right crutch and left foot simultaneously, followed by the left crutch and right foot.

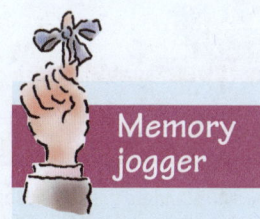

Memory jogger

To help your patient using the three-point gait to climb stairs, teach them to remember "**The good goes up; the bad goes down.**" Going up, they should lead with the uninvolved leg, and going down, they should lead with the involved leg and the crutches.

Arms and shoulders

- Encourage arm- and shoulder-strengthening exercises to prepare the patient for crutch walking. If possible, consult physical therapy to teach the patient two techniques—one fast and one slow—and teach the patient to alternate between them to prevent excessive muscle fatigue and to enable an easier transition to walking.

Using a walker

A walker consists of a metal frame with handgrips and four legs that buttresses the patient on three sides; one side remains open. Because this device provides greater stability and security than other ambulatory aids, it's recommended for the patient who may not be able to use crutches or a cane due to insufficient strength and balance or those who have weakness and require frequent periods of rest (Sehgal et al., 2021).

Attachments for standard walkers and modified walkers help meet special needs. For example, a walker may have a platform added to support an injured arm.

Supplies

- walker
- platform or wheel attachments, as necessary (See *Types of walkers.*)

Types of walkers

Various types of walkers are available.

Standard walker

The standard walker is used by the patient with unilateral or bilateral weakness or an inability to bear weight on one leg. It requires arm strength and balance.

Platform attachments

Platform attachments may be added to a standard walker for the patient with arthritic arms or a casted arm who isn't able to bear weight directly on the hand, wrist, or forearm.

Got wheels

With the approval of the healthcare provider, wheels may be placed on the front legs of the standard walker to allow the patient with very weak legs or who is poorly coordinated to roll the device forward instead of lifting it. The rolling walker has four wheels and may also have a seat. However, wheels aren't commonly applied because they pose a safety hazard.

Getting ready

- Obtain the appropriate walker with the advice of a physical therapist, and adjust it to the patient's height: The patient's elbows should be flexed at a 15° angle when standing comfortably within the walker with their hands on the grips.
- To adjust the walker, turn it upside down, and change the leg length by pushing in the button on each shaft and releasing it when the leg is in the correct position.
- Make sure the walker is level before the patient attempts to use it.

How it's done

- Help the patient stand within the walker, and instruct them to hold the handgrips firmly and equally. Stand behind the patient, closer to the involved leg.
- If the patient has one-sided leg weakness, tell them to advance the walker 6″ to 8″ (15 to 20 cm), step forward with the involved leg, and follow with the uninvolved leg, supporting themselves on their arms. Encourage them to take equal strides. If they have equal strength in both legs, instruct them to advance the walker 6″ to 8″ and step forward with either leg. If they aren't able to use one leg, tell them to advance the walker 6″ to 8″ and swing onto it, supporting their weight on their arms.

Four-point gait

- If the patient is using a wheeled walker, reinforce the physical therapist's instructions.
- Teach the patient how to sit down and get up from a chair safely. (See *Teaching safe use of a walker*, page 410.)
- If the patient starts to fall, support their hips and shoulders to help them maintain an upright position, if possible. If unsuccessful, ease them slowly to the closest surface—bed, floor, or chair.

Helping patients exercise

Exercise maintains or increases muscle strength and endurance and helps maintain cardiopulmonary function. Because an immobilized patient may not be able to perform exercises by themselves, learning how to assist a patient in exercise is an essential part of proper care and health promotion.

Passive then active

Passive ROM exercises help prevent deterioration of the muscles and tissues of a patient who isn't able to independently perform exercise. If the patient later gains strength and no longer needs passive exercise, they can perform isometric or active ROM exercises.

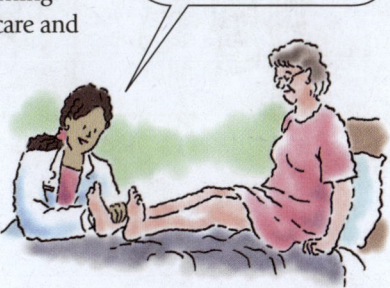

> Passive ROM exercises help prevent deterioration of muscles and tissues. Later, the patient may be able to perform isometric or active ROM exercises.

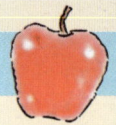

Teaching safe use of a walker

To teach a patient how to sit down and get up safely using a walker, follow the steps outlined here.

Sitting down

• Tell the patient to stand with the back of the stronger leg against the front of the chair, the weaker leg slightly off the floor, and the walker directly in front.

• Tell them to grasp the armrests on the chair one arm at a time while supporting most of the weight on the stronger leg. (In the illustrations below, the patient has left leg weakness.)

• Tell the patient to lower themselves into the chair and slide backward. After they're seated, they should place the walker beside the chair.

Getting up

• After bringing the walker to the front of the chair, tell the patient to slide forward in the chair. Placing the back of their stronger leg against the seat, they should then advance the weaker leg.

• Next, with both hands on the armrests, the patient can push themselves to a standing position. Supporting themselves with the stronger leg and the opposite hand, the patient should grasp the walker's handgrip with the free hand.

• Then the patient should grasp the free handgrip with the other hand.

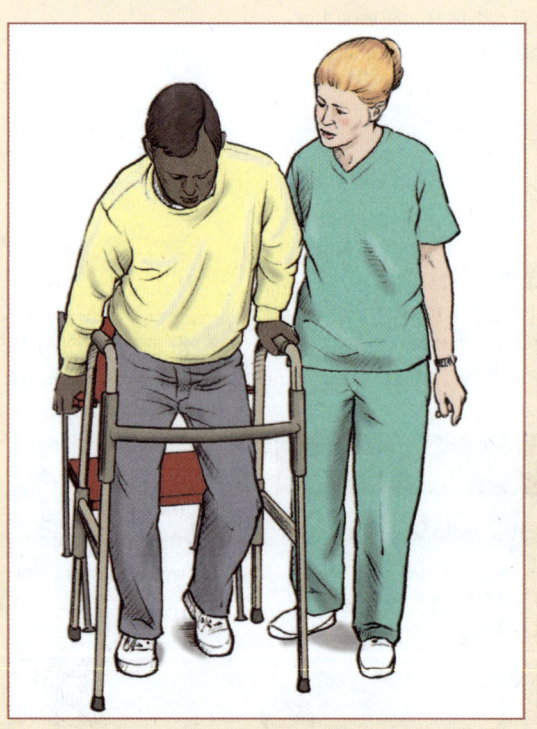

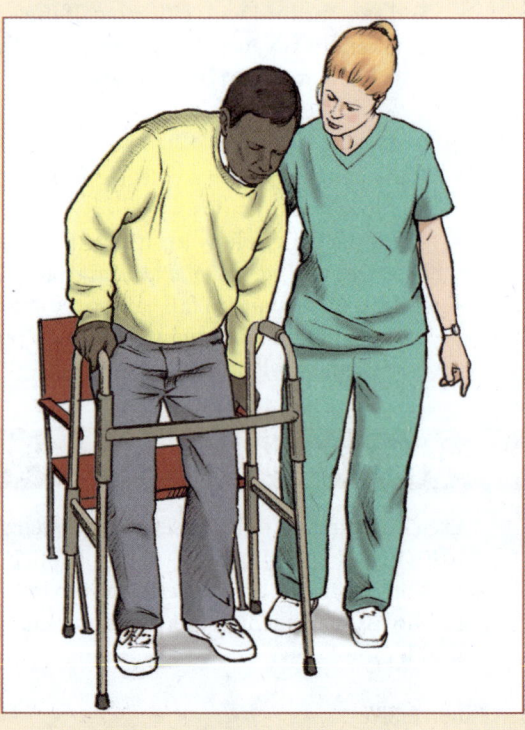

Passive ROM exercises

Passive ROM exercises improve or maintain joint mobility and help prevent contractures. Performed by a nurse, a physical therapist, or a caregiver of the patient's choosing, these exercises are indicated for the patient with temporary or permanent loss of mobility, sensation, or consciousness. Passive ROM exercises require recognition of the patient's limits of motion and support of all joints during movement.

Just say no

Passive ROM exercises are contraindicated in patients with septic joints, acute thrombophlebitis, severe arthritic joint inflammation, or recent trauma with possible hidden fractures or internal injuries.

Equal opportunity exercises

The exercises discussed here don't have to be performed in the order given or all at once. The exercises can be scheduled over the course of a day, whenever the patient is in the most convenient position. Remember to perform all exercises slowly, gently, and to the end of the normal ROM or to the point of pain, but no further. (See *Types of joint motion*, page 412.)

Getting ready

- Determine the joints that need ROM exercises, and consult the healthcare provider or physical therapist about limitations or precautions for specific exercises.
- Before beginning, raise the bed to a comfortable working height.

How it's done

Use the following steps to perform ROM on the patient's neck, shoulder, elbow, forearm, wrist, fingers and thumb, hip and knee, ankle, and toes.

Exercising the neck

- Support the patient's head with your hands and extend the neck, flex the chin to the chest, and tilt the head laterally toward each shoulder.
- Rotate the head from right to left.

Exercising the shoulder

- Support the patient's arm in an extended, neutral position; then extend the forearm and flex it back. Abduct the arm outward from the side of the body, and adduct it back to the side.
- Rotate the patient's shoulder so that the arm crosses midline, and bend the elbow so that the hand touches the opposite shoulder and then the mattress of the bed for complete internal rotation.
- Return the shoulder to a neutral position and, with the elbow bent, push the arm backward so that the back of the hand touches the mattress for complete external rotation.

Types of joint motion

These illustrations show various areas of the body and what types of movements their joints allow.

Circumduction

Moving in a circular manner

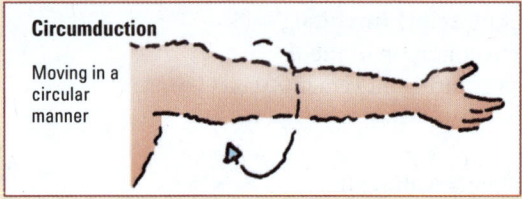

Flexion
Bending, decreasing the joint angle

Extension
Straightening, increasing the joint angle

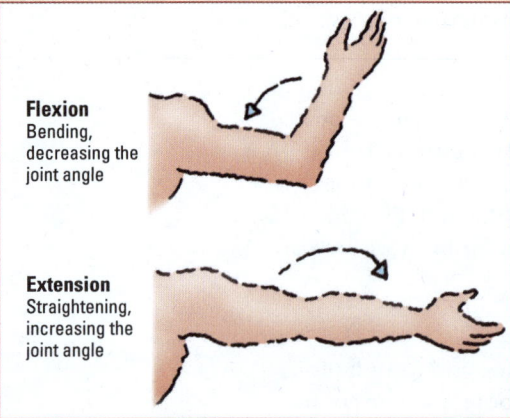

Abduction
Moving away from midline

Adduction
Moving toward midline

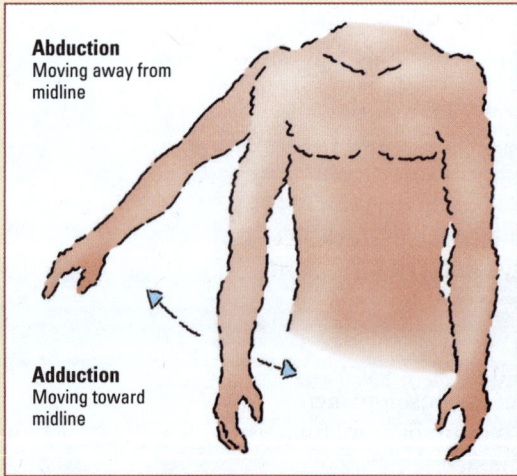

Retraction and protraction
Moving backward and forward

Pronation
Turning downward

Supination
Turning upward

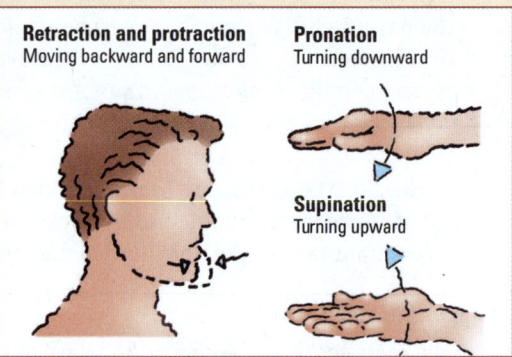

Internal rotation
Turning toward midline

External rotation
Turning away from midline

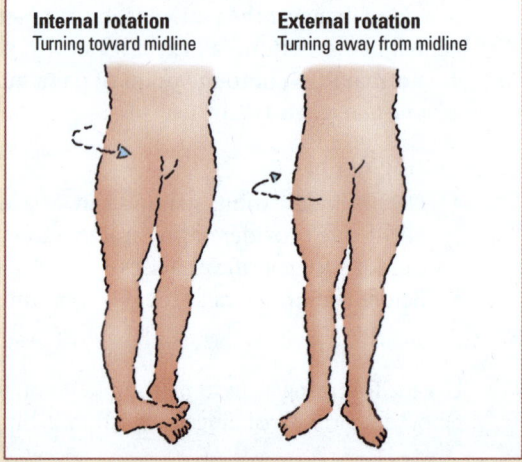

Eversion
Turning outward

Inversion
Turning inward

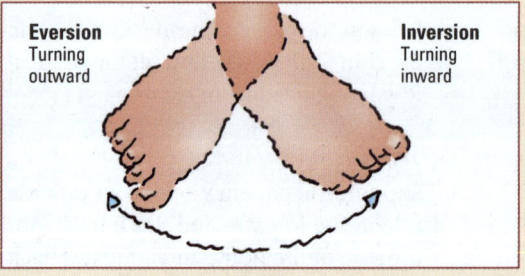

Exercising the elbow

- Place the patient's arm at the side with palm facing up.
- Flex and extend the arm at the elbow.

Exercising the forearm

- Stabilize the patient's elbow, and then twist the hand to bring the palm up (supination).
- Twist it back again to bring the palm down (pronation).

Exercising the wrist

- Stabilize the patient's forearm, and flex and extend the wrist. Then rock the hand sideways for lateral flexion, and rotate the hand in a circular motion.

Exercising the fingers and thumb

- Extend the patient's fingers, and then flex the hand into a fist; repeat extension and flexion of each joint of each finger and thumb separately.
- Spread two adjoining fingers apart (abduction), and then bring them together (adduction).
- Oppose each fingertip to the thumb, and rotate the thumb and each finger in a circle.

Exercising the hip and knee

- Extend the patient's leg, and then bend the hip and knee toward the chest, allowing full joint flexion.
- Next, move the straight leg sideways, out and away from the other leg (abduction), and then back, over, and across it (adduction).
- Rotate the straight leg internally toward the midline, then externally away from the midline.

Exercising the ankle

- Bend the patient's foot so that the toes push upward (dorsiflexion), and then bend the foot so that the toes push downward (plantar flexion).
- Rotate the ankle in a circular motion.
- Invert the ankle so that the sole of the foot faces the midline, and then evert the ankle so that the sole faces away from the midline.

Exercising the toes

- Flex the patient's toes toward the sole, and then extend them back toward the top of the foot.
- Spread two adjoining toes apart (abduction), and bring them together (adduction).

Time is of the essence

- Joints begin to stiffen within 24 hours of disuse; therefore, passive ROM exercises should be started as soon as possible, and performed at least once per shift, particularly while bathing or turning the patient. Use proper body mechanics, and repeat each exercise at least three times.

Get the family involved

- If the patient requires long-term rehabilitation after discharge, consult a physical therapist, and teach a family member or caregiver to perform passive ROM exercises. (See *Documenting passive ROM exercises.*)

Isometric and active ROM exercises

Patients on prolonged bed rest or with limited activity without profound weakness can also be taught to perform ROM exercises on their own (called *active ROM*) or they may benefit from isometric exercises. (See *Learning about isometric exercises*, page 415.)

Take note!

Documenting passive ROM exercises

To document passive ROM exercises, include in the notes:
- which joints were exercised
- patient's tolerance of the exercises
- edema or pressure areas
- pain from the exercises
- ROM limitation

Learning about isometric exercises

A patient can strengthen and increase muscle tone by contracting muscles against resistance (from other muscles or from a stationary object, such as a bed or wall) without joint movement. These exercises require only a comfortable position—standing, sitting, or lying down—and proper body alignment. For each exercise, instruct the patient to hold each contraction for 2 to 5 seconds and to repeat it three to four times daily.

Neck rotators

The patient places the heel of the hand above one ear. Then they push the head toward the hand as forcefully as possible, without moving the head, neck, or arm. The patient repeats the exercise on the other side.

Neck flexors

The patient places both palms on the forehead. Without moving the neck, they push the head forward while resisting with the palms.

Neck extensors

The patient clasps the fingers behind the head, and then pushes the head against the clasped hands without moving the neck.

Shoulder elevators

Holding the right arm straight down at the side, the patient grasps the right wrist with the left hand. They then try to shrug the right shoulder but prevent it from moving by holding the arm in place. Repeat this exercise, alternating arms.

Shoulder, chest, and scapular musculature

The patient places the right fist in the left palm and raises both arms to shoulder height. They push the fist into the palm as forcefully as possible without moving either arm. Then, with the arms in the same position, they clasp the fingers and try to pull the hands apart. Repeat the pattern, beginning with the left fist in the right palm.

Elbow flexors and extensors

With the right elbow bent 90° and the right palm facing upward, the patient places the left fist against the right palm. Then they try to bend the right elbow further while resisting with the left fist. Repeat the pattern, bending the left elbow.

Abdomen

The patient assumes a sitting position and bends slightly forward, with the hands in front of the middle of the thighs. Then they try to bend forward further, resisting by pressing the palms against the thighs.

Alternatively, in the supine position, clasp the hands behind the head. Then raise the shoulders about 1″ (2.5 cm), holding this position for a few seconds.

Back extensors

In a sitting position, the patient bends forward and places the hands under the buttocks. They try to stand up, resisting with both hands.

Hip abductors

While standing, the patient squeezes the inner thighs together as tightly as possible. Placing a pillow between the knees supplies resistance and increases the effectiveness of this exercise.

Hip extensors

The patient squeezes the buttocks together as tightly as possible.

Knee extensors

The patient straightens the knee fully, then vigorously tightens the muscle above the knee so that it moves the kneecap upward. Repeat this exercise, alternating legs.

Ankle flexors and extensors

The patient pulls the toes upward, holding briefly, then pushes them down as far as possible, again holding briefly.

Quick quiz

1. Ball-and-socket joint examples include:
   A. neck and vertebrae.
   B. knees and elbows.
   C. shoulders and hips.
   D. wrists and thumbs.

Answer: C. The shoulders and hips are examples of ball-and-socket joints.

2. A patient isn't able to move their right arm away from the midline. This is documented as impaired:
   A. supination.
   B. abduction.
   C. adduction.
   D. rotation.

Answer: B. Abduction is the ability to move a limb away from the midline.

3. Which patient position is best for eating a meal in bed?
   A. Fowler
   B. Lateral
   C. Prone
   D. Supine

Answer: A. In Fowler position, the head of the bed is elevated to 45°, and the bed section under the patient's knees is also raised to flex the knees slightly. This would be ideal for allowing the patient to eat without risk of aspiration.

4. Which assistive device should a patient with weak gait and poor upper body strength use?
   A. Cane
   B. Walker
   C. Wheelchair
   D. Crutches

Answer: B. A walker is the safest option for a person with weak gait and poor upper body strength.

Scoring

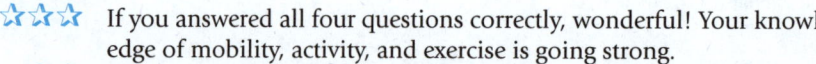

⭐⭐⭐ If you answered all four questions correctly, wonderful! Your knowledge of mobility, activity, and exercise is going strong.

⭐⭐ If you answered three questions correctly, great! Your brain exercises are really paying off.

⭐ If you answered fewer than three questions correctly, don't fret! Do some extra ROM (reading on mobility) and try again!

References

Centers for Disease Control. (2021, October 12). Arthritis. Retrieved from https://www.cdc.gov/arthritis/data_statistics/arthritis-related-stats.htm

Joint health guide: Improve mobility and ease inflammation. (2023). Retrieved from https://1md.org/article/joint-health-101-1md

National Institute on Aging. (2020). *Maintaining mobility and preventing disability are key to living independently as we age.* https://www.nia.nih.gov/news/maintaining-mobility-and-preventing-disability-are-key-living-independently-we-age

Sehgal, M., Jacobs, J., & Biggs, W. (2021). Mobility assistive device use in older adults. *American Family Physician, 103*(12), 737–744.

Chapter 15

Skin integrity and wound healing

Just the facts

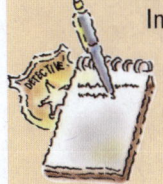

In this chapter, you'll learn:

◆ layers and functions of the skin

◆ types of wounds

◆ phases of wound healing

◆ ways to classify wounds according to age, depth, and color

◆ basic wound care assessment and treatment

◆ pressure injury prevention, care, and treatment.

A look at the skin

The skin, or *integumentary system*, is the largest organ in the body. It accounts for about 6 to 8 lb (2.5 to 3.5 kg) of a person's body weight and has a surface area of more than 20 ft². The thickest skin is located on the hands and the soles of the feet; the thinnest skin, around the eyes and over the tympanic membranes in the ear (McNichol et al., 2022).

Skin basics

Skin is made up of distinct layers that function as a single unit. The outermost layer, which is actually a layer of dead cells, is completely replaced every 4 to 6 weeks by cells that migrate to the surface from the layers beneath. The living cells in the skin receive oxygen and nutrients through an extensive network of small blood vessels. In fact, every square inch of skin contains more than 158 blood vessels!

Up close and personal

Skin protects the body by acting as a barrier between internal structures and the external world. Skin also stands between each of us and the social world around us, so it's no wonder that the condition and characteristics of a person's skin impact self-image. When a person has healthy skin, unblemished skin with good tone (firmness) and color, they feel better about themselves. Skin also reflects the body's general physical health and can be physical manifestation of internal pathologies. For example, the skin may look bluish if blood oxygen levels are low, liver disease can turn the skin yellow, and the skin can appear flushed or red if a person has a fever (Norris, 2025).

Surgery, accidents, or sun

Any damage to the skin is considered a wound. Wounds can result from planned events, such as surgery, or unplanned events, including accidents such as a fall from a bike; they can also be caused by exposure to the environment (the ultraviolet [UV] rays in sunlight can cause skin damage), and even by prolonged pressure to the skin surface (McNichol et al., 2022).

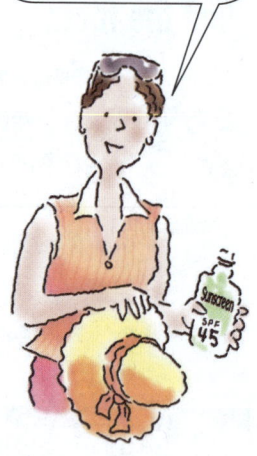

Bad burns from UV rays are wounds, too. Make sure you wear sunscreen and protect your skin!

Layers of the skin

Skin has two main layers: the *epidermis* and the *dermis*, which function as one interrelated unit. A layer of subcutaneous fatty connective tissue, sometimes called the *hypodermis*, lies beneath these layers. The following structural networks, which are stabilized by hair and sweat gland ducts, exist within the epidermis and dermis:

- collagen fibers
- elastic fibers
- small blood vessels
- nerve fibrils
- lymphatics

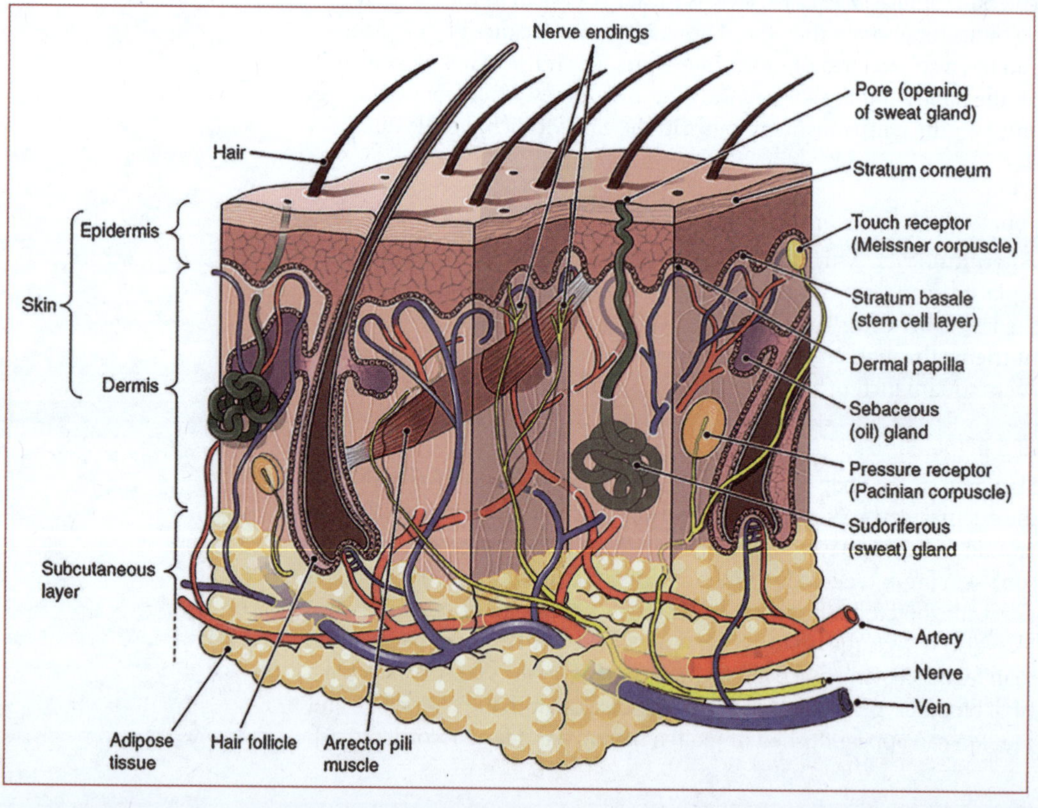

Nerve endings

Hair

Epidermis

Skin

Dermis

Subcutaneous layer

Adipose tissue   Hair follicle   Arrector pili muscle

Pore (opening of sweat gland)

Stratum corneum

Touch receptor (Meissner corpuscle)

Stratum basale (stem cell layer)

Dermal papilla

Sebaceous (oil) gland

Pressure receptor (Pacinian corpuscle)

Sudoriferous (sweat) gland

Artery

Nerve

Vein

Epidermis

The epidermis is the outermost of the skin's two main layers. It varies in thickness from about 0.1 mm thick on the eyelids to as much as 1 mm thick on the palms and soles. The epidermis is slightly acidic, with an average pH of 5.5. This is a really important point, because the skin's acidity is protective and, when altered, may lead to skin breakdown. Covering the epidermis is the keratinized epithelium, a layer of cells that migrate up from the underlying dermis and die upon reaching the surface. These cells are continuously generated and replaced. The keratinized epithelium is supported by the dermis and underlying connective tissue (McNichol et al., 2022).

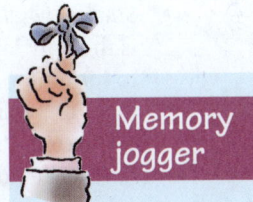

Memory jogger

Remember the order of the skin's layers by thinking of the prefix **epi-**, which means "upon." Therefore, the **epi**dermis is upon, or on top of, the dermis.

In living color

The epidermis also contains melanocytes (cells that produce the brown pigment melanin), which give skin and hair their colors. The more melanin produced by melanocytes, the darker the skin. Skin color varies from one person to the next, but it can also vary from one area of skin on the body to another. The hypothalamus regulates melanin production by secreting melanocyte-stimulating hormone.

Layer upon layer

The epidermis is divided into five distinct layers. Each layer's name reflects its structure or its function. Here's a look at them from the outside in:

- *Stratum corneum* (horny layer) is the superficial layer of dead skin cells, the skin layer that's in contact with the environment. It has an acid mantle that helps protect the body from some fungi and bacteria. Cells in this layer are shed daily and replaced with cells from the layer beneath it, the stratum lucidum. In such diseases as eczema and psoriasis, the stratum corneum may become abnormally thick and irritate skin structures and peripheral nerves (Yousef et al., 2023).
- *Stratum lucidum* (clear layer) is a single layer of cells that forms a transitional boundary between the stratum corneum above and stratum granulosum below. This layer is most evident in areas where skin is thickest, as on the soles of the feet. It appears to be absent in areas where skin is especially thin, as on the eyelids. Although cells in this layer lack active nuclei, this is an area of intense enzyme activity that prepares cells for the stratum corneum.
- *Stratum granulosum* (granular layer) is three to five cells thick and is characterized by flat cells with active nuclei. Experts believe this layer aids keratin formation and acts as a glue, keeping the cells stuck together (Yousef et al., 2023).
- *Stratum spinosum* is the area in which cells begin to flatten as they migrate toward the skin surface.

- *Stratum basale* or *stratum germinativum* is only one cell thick and is the only layer of the epidermis in which cells undergo mitosis to form new cells. The stratum basale forms the dermoepidermal junction, which is the area where the epidermis and dermis are connected. Protrusions of this layer (called *rete pegs* or *epidermal ridges*) extend down into the dermis, where they're surrounded by vascularized dermal papillae. This unique structure supports the epidermis and facilitates the exchange of fluids and cells between the skin layers.

Dermis

The dermis is a thick, deep layer of skin composed of collagen, elastin fibers, and an extracellular matrix; all these components contribute to the skin's strength and pliability. Collagen fibers give skin its strength, and elastin fibers provide elasticity. The meshing of collagen and elastin determines the skin's physical characteristics. (See *Structural supports: Collagen and elastin*.)

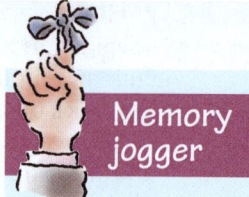

Memory jogger

To remember the order of the five layers of the epidermis, think, "**C**ontiguous **L**ayers **G**enerate **S**kin **B**arriers." The first letter of each of these words will remind you that the epidermis consists of the strata:

Corneum

Lucidum

Granulosum

Spinosum

Basale

Structural supports: Collagen and elastin

Normally, skin returns to its original position after it's pulled on due to the actions of the connective tissues collagen and elastin, two key components of the skin. Collagen and elastin work together to support the dermis and give skin its physical characteristics.

Collagen

Collagen fibers form tightly woven networks in the papillary layer of the dermis. These fibers are relatively inextensible and nonelastic and, therefore, give the dermis high tensile strength. In addition, collagen constitutes approximately 70% of the skin's dry weight and is the skin's principal structural body protein.

Elastin

Elastin is made up of wavy fibers that intertwine with collagen in horizontal arrangements at the lower dermis and vertical arrangements at the epidermal margin. Elastin makes skin pliable and is the structural protein that enables extensibility in the dermis.

Seeing the effects of age

As a person ages, collagen and elastin fibers break down, causing the fine lines and wrinkles that are associated with aging to develop. Extensive exposure to sunlight accelerates this breakdown process. Deep wrinkles are caused by changes in facial muscles. Over time, laughing, crying, smiling, and frowning cause facial muscles to thicken and eventually cause wrinkles in the overlying skin.

Source: Yousef, H., Ajhajj, M., & Sharma, S. (2023). *Anatomy, skin (integument), epidermis.* StatPearls. https://www.ncbi.nlm.nih.gov/books/NBK470464/.

In addition, the dermis contains:

- blood vessels and lymphatic vessels, which transport oxygen and nutrients to cells and remove waste products
- nerve fibers and hair follicles, which contribute to skin sensation, temperature regulation, and excretion and absorption through the skin
- fibroblast cells, which are important in the production of collagen and elastin (McNichol et al., 2022; Norris, 2025).

Laying it on thick

The dermis is composed of two layers of connective tissue:

- *Papillary dermis*, the outermost layer, is composed of collagen and reticular fibers, which are important in healing wounds. Capillaries in the papillary dermis carry the nourishment needed for metabolic activity.
- *Reticular dermis,* the innermost layer, is formed by thick networks of collagen bundles that anchor it to the subcutaneous tissue and underlying support structures, such as fasciae, muscle, and bone.

Sebaceous and sweat glands

Although sebaceous glands and sweat glands appear to originate in the dermis, they're actually appendages of the epidermis that extend downward into the dermis.

Give the glands a hand!

Sebaceous glands, found primarily in the skin of the scalp, face, upper body, and genital region, are part of the same structure that contains hair follicles. These saclike glands produce sebum, a fatty substance that lubricates and softens the skin.

Sweat glands are tightly coiled tubular glands; the average person has roughly 2.6 million of them. They're present throughout the body in varying amounts. The palms and soles have many, but the external ear, lip margins, nail beds, and glans penis have none. The secreting portion of the sweat gland originates in the dermis and the outlet is on the surface of the skin. The sympathetic nervous system regulates the production of sweat, which, in turn, helps control body temperature (Yousef et al., 2023).

There are two types of sweat glands:

- *Eccrine* glands are active at birth and are found throughout the body. They're most dense on the palms, the soles of the feet, and the forehead. These glands connect to the skin's surface through pores and produce sweat that lacks proteins and fatty acids. Eccrine glands are smaller than apocrine glands.
- *Apocrine* glands begin to function at puberty. (See *Oh no, BO!*) These glands open into hair follicles; therefore, most are found in areas where hair typically grows, such as the scalp, the groin,

Oh no, BO!

The sweat produced by apocrine glands contains the same water, sodium, and chloride found in the sweat produced by eccrine glands. However, it also contains proteins and fatty acids. The unpleasant body odor (BO) associated with sweat comes from the interaction of bacteria with these proteins and fatty acids.

and the axillary region. The coiled secreting portion of the gland lies deep in the dermis (deeper than eccrine glands), and a duct connects it to the upper portion of the hair follicle. The sweat produced by apocrine glands contains water, sodium, chloride, proteins, and fatty acids. It's thicker than the sweat produced by eccrine glands and has a milky white or yellowish tinge. (See *Oh no, BO!*)

Subcutaneous tissue

The subcutaneous tissue, or *hypodermis*, is a subdermal (below the skin) layer of loose connective tissue that contains major blood vessels, lymph vessels, and nerves. Subcutaneous tissue:

- has a high proportion of fat cells and contains fewer small blood vessels than the dermis
- varies in thickness depending on body type and location
- constitutes about 15% to 20% of a man's weight and approximately 20% to 25% of a woman's weight
- insulates the body
- absorbs shocks to the skeletal system
- helps skin move easily over underlying structures

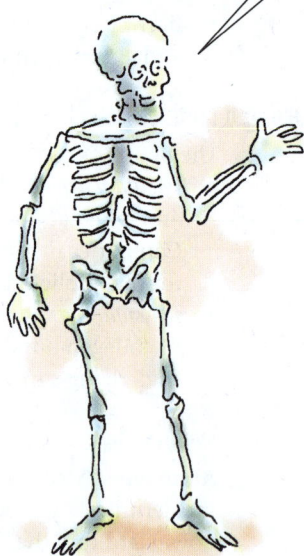

It's a little chilly without any subcutaneous tissue!

Blood supply

The skin receives its blood supply through vessels that originate in the underlying muscle tissue. Here, arteries branch into smaller vessels, which then branch into the network of capillaries that permeate the dermis and subcutaneous tissue. Body temperature is regulated by the increase and decrease of blood supply to the skin; this mechanism is extremely effective (Yousef et al., 2023).

The thin and thinner of it

Within the vascular system, only capillaries have walls thin enough (typically only a single layer of endothelial cells) to let solutes pass through. These thin walls allow nutrients and oxygen to pass from the bloodstream into the interstitial space around skin cells. At the same time, waste products pass into the capillaries and are carried away.

Lymphatic system

The skin's lymphatic system helps remove waste products from the dermis.

Go with the flow

Lymphatic vessels, or *lymphatics* for short, are similar to capillaries in that they're thin-walled, permeable vessels. However, lymphatics aren't part of the blood circulatory system. Instead, the lymphatics belong to a separate system that removes proteins, large waste products, and excess fluids from the interstitial spaces in skin and transports them to the venous circulation. The lymphatics merge into two main trunks, the thoracic duct and the right lymphatic duct, which empty into the junction of the subclavian and internal jugular veins.

Functions of the skin

The skin performs or participates in a host of vital functions, including:

- protection
- sensory perception
- thermoregulation
- excretion
- metabolism
- absorption
- social communication

Damage to the skin impairs its ability to carry out these important functions.

Protection

The skin acts as a physical barrier to microorganisms and foreign matter, protecting the body against infection. It also protects underlying tissue and structures from mechanical injury. Consider the feet for a moment. As a person walks or runs, the soles of the feet withstand a tremendous amount of force, yet the underlying tissue and bone structures remain unharmed.

The skin also helps maintain a stable environment inside the body by preventing the loss of water, electrolytes, proteins, and other substances. Any damage (any wound) jeopardizes this protection. However, when damaged, skin goes into repair mode to restore protection by stepping up the normal process of cell replacement.

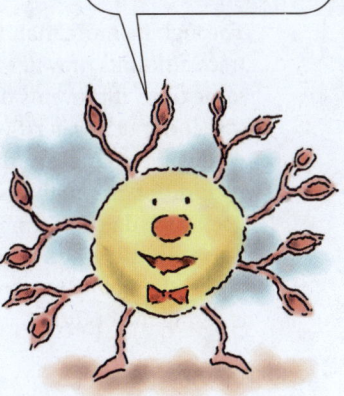

My sensory nerve fibers make you aware of pain, pressure, heat, and cold.

Sensory perception

Nerve endings in the skin allow a person literally to touch the world around them. Sensory nerve fibers originate in the nerve roots along the spine and supply specific areas of the skin known as *dermatomes*. Dermatomes are used to document sensory function. This same network helps a person avoid injury by making them aware of pain, pressure, heat, and cold (Norris, 2025).

Just sensational

Sensory nerves exist throughout the skin; however, some areas are more sensitive than others—for example, the fingertips are more sensitive than the back. Sensation allows us to identify potential dangers and avoid injury. Any loss or reduction of sensation, local or general, increases the chance of injury.

Thermoregulation

Thermoregulation, or control of body temperature, involves the concerted effort of nerves, blood vessels, and eccrine glands in the dermis.

Warming up

When skin is exposed to cold or internal body temperature falls, blood vessels constrict, reducing blood flow and thereby conserving body heat.

Cooling down

Similarly, if skin becomes too hot or internal body temperature rises, small arteries within the skin dilate, increasing the blood flow, and sweat production increases to promote cooling.

Excretion

Unlikely as it may seem, the skin is an excretory organ. Excretion through the skin plays an important role in thermoregulation, electrolyte balance, and hydration. In addition, sebum excretion helps maintain the skin's integrity and suppleness.

Water works

Through its more than two million pores, skin efficiently transmits trace amounts of water and body wastes to the environment. At the same time, it prevents dehydration by ensuring that the body doesn't lose too much water. Sweat carries water and salt to the skin surface, where it evaporates, aiding thermoregulation and electrolyte balance. In addition, a small amount of water evaporates directly from the skin itself each day. A normal adult loses about 500 mL of water a day this way. Although the skin is busy regulating fluids that are leaving the body, it's equally busy preventing unwanted or dangerous fluids from entering the body.

Metabolism

Skin also helps maintain the mineralization of bones and teeth. A photochemical reaction in the skin produces vitamin D, which is crucial to the metabolism of calcium and phosphate. These minerals, in turn, play a central role in the health of bones and teeth.

Let the sunshine in

When skin is exposed to sunlight—the UV spectrum in sunlight, to be specific—vitamin D is synthesized in a photochemical reaction. Keep in mind, however, that although sunlight can be beneficial, overexposure to UV light causes skin damage that reduces its ability to function properly and can lead to some forms of cancer.

Absorption

Some drugs and toxic substances (e.g., pesticides) can be absorbed directly through the skin and into the bloodstream. This process has been used to treat certain disorders via skin patch drug delivery systems. Although one of the best-known examples of this method is the patch used in some nicotine withdrawal programs, this technology is also used to administer forms of hormone therapy, nitroglycerin, steroids, and pain medications.

Social communication

A commonly overlooked but important function of the skin is its role in self-esteem development and social communication. Every time a person looks in the mirror, they decide whether they like what they see. Although bone structure, body type, teeth, and hair all have an impact, the condition and characteristics of skin can have a significant impact on a person's self-esteem. Skin also conveys information to the people around us. Embarrassment can result in blushing, and a stressful situation can lead to increased sweat production.

Virtually every face-to-face interpersonal exchange includes nonverbal language, including facial expression and body posture. Skin characteristics, which are visible at all times, and level of self-esteem have an impact on how a person communicates verbally and nonverbally and how a listener receives the person communicating.

A look at wound healing

Any break in the skin is considered a wound. Wounds can result from a planned event, such as surgery, or from an unexpected event, such as an accident, trauma, or exposure to pressure, heat, sun, or chemicals. Tissue damage in wounds varies widely, from a superficial break in the epithelium to deep trauma that involves the muscle and bone.

A wound is described as "dirty" if it may contain bacteria or debris. Trauma typically produces dirty wounds. A wound is described as "clean" if it is free of bacteria or debris. An example of a "clean" wound is a wound produced by surgery. The rate of recovery is influenced by the extent and type of damage incurred as well as other intrinsic factors, such as patient circulation, nutrition, hydration, and the presence of a chronic illness. However, regardless of the cause of a wound, the healing process is similar.

Types of wound healing

Wounds are classified by the way the wound closes. A wound can close by primary intention, secondary intention, or tertiary intention.

Primary intention

Primary healing involves reepithelialization, in which the skin's outer layer grows closed. Cells grow in from the margins of the wound and out from epithelial cells lining the hair follicles and sweat glands.

Just a scratch

Wounds that heal through primary intention are, most commonly, wounds that involve only the epidermis and don't involve the loss of tissue—for example, a superficial burn (first-degree burn). However, a wound that has edges that are well-approximated (i.e., they can be pulled together to meet neatly), such as a surgical incision, also heals through primary intention. Because there's no loss of tissue and little risk of infection, the healing process is predictable. These wounds usually heal in 4 to 14 days and result in minimal scarring (McNichol et al., 2022).

Secondary intention

A wound that involves some degree of tissue loss heals by secondary intention. The edges of these wounds can't be easily approximated, and the wound itself is described as *partial thickness* or *full thickness*, depending on its depth:
- Partial-thickness wounds extend through the epidermis and into, but not through, the dermis.

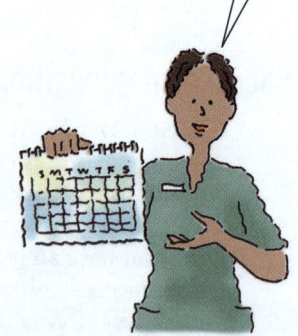

Wounds that heal by primary intention usually do so within 4 to 14 days.

- Full-thickness wounds extend through the epidermis and dermis and may involve subcutaneous tissue, muscle, and possibly bone (Bowers & Franco, 2020).

Getting under the skin

During healing, wounds that heal by secondary intention fill with granulation tissue, a scar forms, and reepithelialization occurs, primarily from the wound edges. Pressure injuries, burns, dehisced surgical wounds, and traumatic injuries are examples of this type of wound. These wounds also take longer to heal, result in scarring, and have a higher rate of complications, such as the development of an infection, than wounds that heal by primary intention (Sandy-Hodgetts et al., 2020).

Tertiary intention

When a wound is intentionally kept open to allow edema or infection to resolve or to permit removal of exudate, the wound heals by tertiary intention or *delayed primary intention*. These wounds result in more scarring than wounds that heal by primary intention but less scarring than wounds that heal by secondary intention.

Phases of wound healing

The healing process is the same for all wounds, whether the cause is mechanical, chemical, or thermal.

Four phases

The process of wound healing occurs in the following phases:
- hemostasis
- inflammation
- proliferation
- maturation

Although this categorization is useful, it's important to remember that healing rarely occurs in this strict order. Typically, the phases of wound healing overlap. (See *How wounds heal.*)

Hemostasis

Immediately after an injury, the body releases chemical mediators and intercellular messengers called *growth factors* that begin the process of cleaning and healing the wound.

Come on, guys! It's time to start the process of healing the wound!

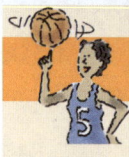

How wounds heal

The healing process begins at the instant of injury and proceeds through a repair "cascade," as outlined here.

1. When tissue is damaged, serotonin, histamine, prostaglandins, and blood from the injured vessels fill the area. Blood platelets form a clot, and fibrin in the clot binds the wound edges together.

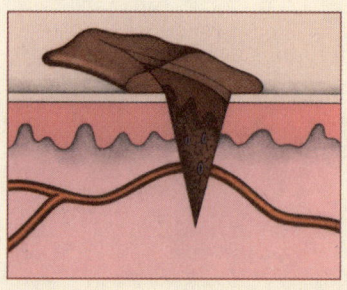

2. Lymphocytes initiate the inflammatory response, increasing capillary permeability. Wound edges swell; white blood cells from surrounding vessels move in and ingest bacteria and cellular debris, demolishing the clot. Redness, warmth, swelling, pain, and loss of function may occur.

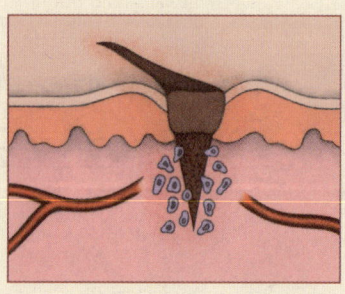

3. Adjacent healthy tissue supplies blood, nutrients, fibroblasts, proteins, and other building materials needed to form soft, pink, and highly vascular granulation tissue, which begins to bridge the area. Inflammation may decrease, or signs and symptoms of infection (increased swelling, increased pain, fever, and pus-filled discharge) may develop.

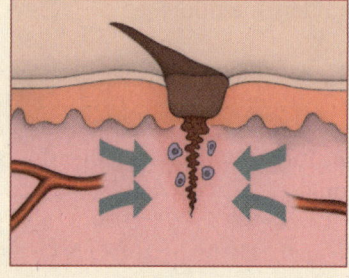

4. Fibroblasts in the granulation tissue secrete collagen, a gluelike substance. Collagen fibers crisscross the area, forming scar tissue.

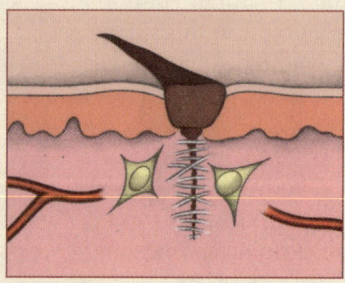

5. Meanwhile, epithelial cells at the wound edge multiply and migrate toward the wound center. A new layer of surface cells replaces the layer that was destroyed. New, healthy tissue or granulation tissue (if the blood supply is inadequate) appears.

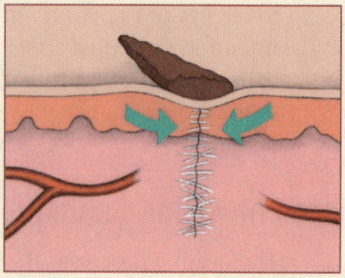

6. Damaged tissue (including lymphatics, blood vessels, and stromal matrices) regenerates. Collagen fibers shorten, and the scar diminishes in size. Scar size may decrease and normal function return, or the scar may hypertrophy, leading to the formation of a keloid and the development of contractures.

Slow that flow!

When blood vessels are damaged, the small muscles in the walls of the vessels contract (vasoconstriction), reducing the flow of blood to the injury and minimizing blood loss. Vasoconstriction can last as long as 30 minutes.

Next, blood leaking from the inflamed, dilated, or broken vessels begins to coagulate. Collagen fibers in the wall of the damaged blood vessels activate the platelets in the blood in the wound. Aided by the action of prostaglandins, the platelets enlarge and stick together to form a temporary plug in the blood vessel, which helps prevent further bleeding. The platelets also release additional vasoconstrictors, such as serotonin, which help prevent further blood loss. Thrombin forms in a cascade of events stimulated by the platelets, and a clot forms to close the small vessels and stop the bleeding (Bowers & Franco, 2020).

This initial phase of wound healing occurs almost immediately after the injury occurs and works quickly (within minutes) in small wounds but is less effective in stopping the bleeding in larger wounds.

Inflammation

The inflammatory phase is a defense mechanism that is a crucial component of the healing process. (See *Understanding the inflammatory response*.) During this phase, the wound is cleaned, and the process of rebuilding begins. This phase is marked by swelling, redness, pain, and heat at the wound site.

During the inflammatory phase, vascular permeability increases, permitting serous fluid carrying small amounts of cell and plasma protein to accumulate in the tissue around the wound (edema) (Norris, 2025). The accumulation of fluid causes the damaged tissue to appear swollen, red, and warm to the touch.

Seek and destroy

During the early phase of the inflammatory process, neutrophils (one type of white blood cell [WBC]) enter the wound. The primary role of neutrophils is *phagocytosis,* which is the removal and destruction of bacteria and other contaminants.

As neutrophil infiltration slows, monocytes appear. Monocytes are converted into activated macrophages and continue the job of cleaning the wound. The macrophages play a key role early in the process of granulation and reepithelialization by producing growth factors and by attracting the cells needed for the formation of new blood vessels and collagen (Norris, 2025).

Telling time

The inflammatory phase of healing is important in preventing wound infection. The process is negatively influenced if the patient

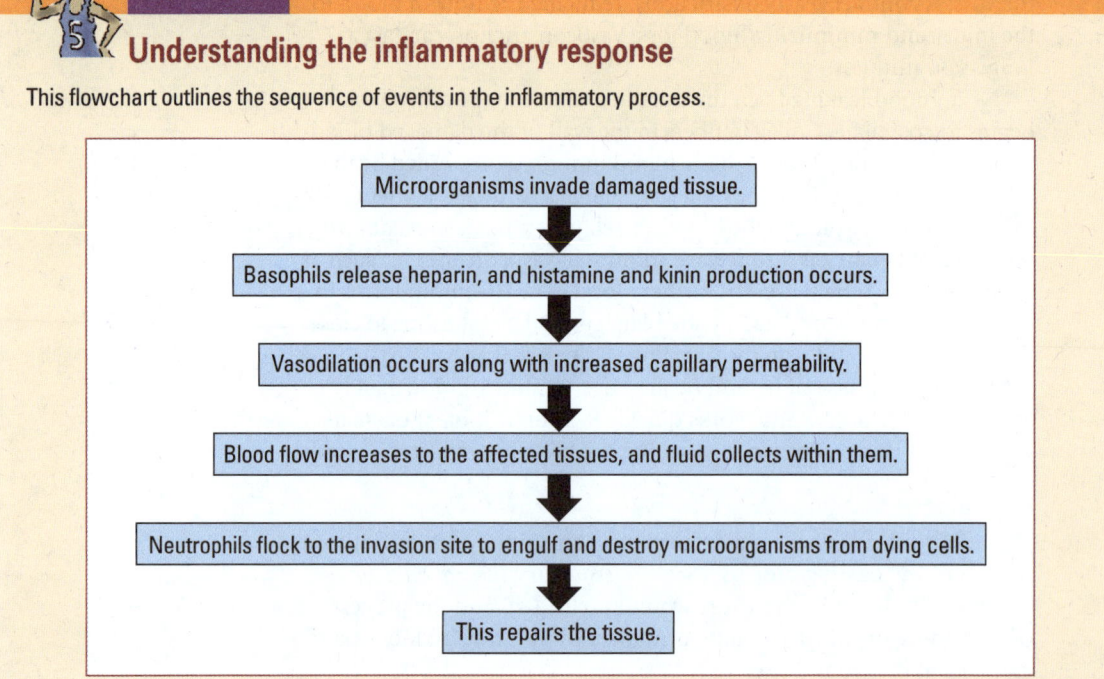

Understanding the inflammatory response

This flowchart outlines the sequence of events in the inflammatory process.

Microorganisms invade damaged tissue.

↓

Basophils release heparin, and histamine and kinin production occurs.

↓

Vasodilation occurs along with increased capillary permeability.

↓

Blood flow increases to the affected tissues, and fluid collects within them.

↓

Neutrophils flock to the invasion site to engulf and destroy microorganisms from dying cells.

↓

This repairs the tissue.

has a systemic condition that suppresses their immune system or if they're undergoing immunosuppressive therapy. In clean wounds, the inflammatory response lasts from 3 to 6 days. In dirty or infected wounds, the response can last much longer (Bennett et al., 2020).

Proliferation

During the proliferation phase of the healing process, the body:

- fills the wound with connective tissue (granulation)
- contracts the wound edges (contraction)
- covers the wound with epithelium (epithelialization)

Presto change–o!

The proliferation phase, which begins on day 3 and lasts until about day 21, takes much longer in wounds with extensive tissue loss. Although phases overlap, wound granulation generally starts when the inflammatory response is complete. As the inflammatory phase subsides, the wound drainage (exudate) begins to decrease (Bowers & Franco, 2020; World Union of Wound Healing Societies [WUWHS], 2018).

The proliferation phase involves the regeneration of blood vessels (angiogenesis) and the formation of connective or granulation tissue, which is fragile and can bleed easily. The development of granulation tissue requires an adequate supply of blood and nutrients. Endothelial cells in blood vessels in surrounding tissue reconstruct damaged or destroyed vessels by first migrating and then proliferating to form new capillary beds. As the beds form, this area of the wound takes on a red, granular appearance (Beeckman et al., 2020). This tissue is a good defense against contaminants, but it's also quite fragile and bleeds easily.

The rebuilding process

During the proliferation phase, growth factors prompt fibroblasts to migrate to the wound. Fibroblasts are the most common cell in connective tissue. They're responsible for making the *extracellular matrix*, a network of connective tissue that provides support to cells. At first, fibroblasts populate just the margins of the wound, but later they spread over the entire wound surface.

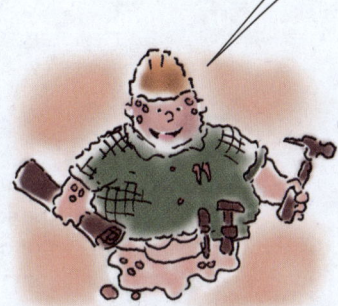

I'm your local fibroblast, and I'm here to build support for these cells.

Fibroblasts have the important task of synthesizing collagen fibers that, in turn, produce keratinocyte, a growth factor needed for reepithelialization. This process necessitates a delicate balance of collagen synthesis (making new) and lysis (removing old). If the process yields too much collagen, increased scarring results. If the process yields too little collagen, scar tissue is weak and easily ruptured. Because fibroblasts require a supply of oxygen to perform their important role, capillary bed regeneration is crucial to the process (Yousef et al., 2023).

Pulling it all together

As healing progresses, myofibroblasts and the newly formed collagen fibers contract, pulling the wound edges toward each other. Contraction reduces the amount of granulation tissue needed to fill the wound, thereby speeding the healing process. (See *Contraction versus contracture*.)

Complete healing occurs only after epithelial cells have completely covered the surface of the wound. As this occurs, keratinocytes switch from a migrating mode to a differentiating mode. The epidermis thickens and becomes differentiated, and the wound is closed. Any remaining scab comes off, and the new epidermis is toughened by the production of keratin, which also returns the skin to its original color.

Maturation

The final phase of wound healing is maturation, which is marked by shrinking and strengthening of the scar. This is a gradual, transitional phase of healing that can continue for months or even years after the wound has closed.

Contraction versus contracture

Contraction and contracture occur during the wound healing process. Although they have mechanisms in common, it's important to understand how contraction and contracture differ.

Contraction

Contraction, a desirable process that takes place during healing, occurs when the edges of a wound pull toward the center of the wound to close it. Contraction continues to close the wound until tension in the surrounding skin causes it to slow and then stop.

Contracture

Contracture is an undesirable process and a common complication of burn scarring. Typically, contracture occurs after healing is complete. Contracture involves excessive pulling or shortening of tissue, resulting in an area of tissue with only limited ability to move. It's especially problematic over joints, which may be pulled to a flexed position. Stretching is the only way to overcome contracture, and patients typically require physical therapy.

During this phase, fibroblasts leave the site of the wound, vascularization is reduced, the scar shrinks and becomes pale, and the mature scar forms. If the wound involved extensive tissue destruction, the scarred area won't contain hair, sweat, or sebaceous glands.

The wound gradually gains tensile strength. In primary intention wounds, tissues will achieve approximately 30% to 50% of their original strength between days 1 and 14. When fully healed, the tissue will achieve, at best, approximately 80% of its original strength. Scar tissue will always be less elastic than the surrounding skin (McNichol et al., 2022).

Factors that affect wound healing

The healing process is affected by many factors. The most important influences include (Beeckman et al., 2020):

- nutrition
- oxygenation
- infection
- age
- chronic health conditions
- medications
- smoking

Nutrition

Proper nutrition is arguably the most important factor affecting wound healing. Unfortunately, malnutrition is a common finding among patients with wounds. For older adults, the problem is more pervasive.

Poor nutrition prolongs hospitalization and increases the risk of medical complications, with the severity of complications being directly related to the severity of the malnutrition. In older patients, malnutrition is known to increase the risk of pressure injuries and to delay wound healing. It may also contribute to poor tensile strength in healing wounds, with an associated increase in the risk of wound dehiscence (Beeckman et al., 2020).

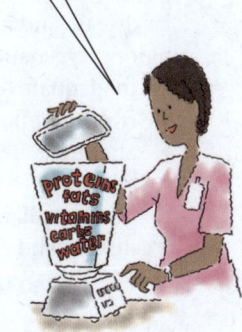

Good nutrition is key when it comes to getting well.

Protein is key

Protein is critical for wounds to heal properly. In fact, a person needs to double the recommended dietary allowance of protein (from 0.8 g/kg/day to 1.6 g/kg/day) before tissue begins to heal. If a significant amount of body weight has been lost in connection with the injury, as much as 50% of the lost weight must be regained before healing will begin. A patient who lacks protein reserves heals slowly, if at all, and a patient who's borderline malnourished can easily become malnourished under this increased demand.

The body needs protein to form collagen during the proliferation phase. Without adequate protein, collagen formation is reduced or delayed, and the healing process slows. Studies of malnourished patients indicate that they have lower levels of serum albumin, which results in slower oxygen diffusion and, in turn, a reduction in the ability of neutrophils to kill bacteria. Wound exudate alone can contain up to 100 g of protein per day (McNichol et al., 2022).

Other necessary nutrients

Fatty acids (lipids) are used in cell structures and play a role in the inflammatory process. Also, vitamins C, B complex, A, and E and the minerals iron, copper, zinc, and calcium are important in the healing process. A zinc deficiency adversely impacts the proliferation phase by slowing the rate of epithelialization and decreasing the strength of collagen produced, therefore decreasing the quality of healing.

In addition to protein and zinc, collagen synthesis requires supplies of carbohydrates and fat. Collagen cross-linking requires adequate amounts of vitamins A and C, iron, and copper. Vitamin C, iron, and zinc are important for developing tensile strength during the maturation phase of wound healing (McNichol et al., 2022).

Oxygenation

Healing depends on a consistent supply of oxygen. For example, oxygen is critical for leukocytes to destroy bacteria and fibroblasts to stimulate collagen synthesis. If the supply is hindered by poor blood flow to the wound or if the patient's oxygen intake is impaired, the result is the same: impaired healing (Beeckman et al., 2020).

Possible causes of inadequate blood flow to the area of the wound include pressure, arterial occlusion, or prolonged vasoconstriction, possibly associated with such medical conditions as peripheral vascular disease and atherosclerosis. Possible causes of lower than systemic blood oxygenation include:

- inadequate oxygen intake
- hypothermia or hyperthermia
- anemia
- alkalemia
- other medical conditions such as chronic obstructive pulmonary disease and congestive heart failure

Infection

An infection can affect wound healing or be a complication of the healing process. Infection can be systemic or localized in the wound. A systemic infection, such as pneumonia, increases the patient's metabolism and thus consumes the fluids, nutrients, and oxygen the body needs for healing (Bennett et al., 2020).

Keeping it local

A localized infection in the wound itself is more common. Any break in the skin allows bacteria to enter. The infection may occur as part of the injury or may develop later in the healing process. For example, when the inflammatory phase lingers, wound healing is delayed, and metabolic by-products of bacterial ingestion accumulate in the wound. This buildup interferes with the formation of new blood vessels and the synthesis of collagen. Infection can also occur in a wound that has been healing normally. This situation occurs particularly in larger wounds involving extensive tissue damage. New or increased pain, redness, heat, and drainage are signs of a new infection (Sandy-Hodgetts et al., 2020). In any case, healing cannot progress until the cause of the infection is addressed.

For patients living in long-term care facilities, infection may result from fecal contamination. Fecal incontinence affects 20% of long-term care patients and is associated with increased mortality (Frank et al., 2020). Typically, those impacted are patients with poorer overall health.

Age

Skin changes that occur with aging cause a prolonged healing time in older adult patients. Although delayed healing is partially due to physiologic changes, also it can be complicated by other problems

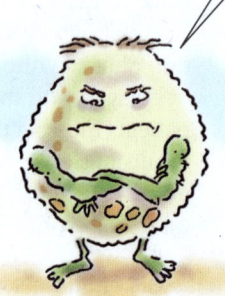

If there's a break in the skin, I'll be sure to find it. Infections are my specialty.

associated with aging, such as poor nutrition and hydration, the presence of a chronic condition, and the use of multiple medications (Beeckman et al., 2020). (See *Effects of aging on wound healing.*)

Chronic health conditions

Respiratory problems, atherosclerosis, diabetes, and malignancies can increase the risk of wounds and interfere with wound healing. These conditions can interfere with systemic and peripheral oxygenation and nutrition, which affect healing (Bowers & Franco, 2020).

Getting complicated

Impaired circulation, a common problem for patients with diabetes and other disorders, can cause tissue hypoxia (lack of oxygen). Neuropathy associated with diabetes reduces the ability to sense pressure. As a result, patients with diabetes may experience trauma, especially to the feet, without realizing it. Insulin dependency can impair leukocyte function, which adversely affects cell proliferation (Boulton et al., 2022).

Hemiplegia and quadriplegia involve the breakdown of muscle tissue and reduction in the padding around the large bones of the lower body. Because a patient with one of these conditions lacks sensation, they're at risk for developing chronic pressure injuries.

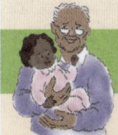

Ages and stages

Effects of aging on wound healing

These factors impede wound healing in older adults:
- slower turnover rate in epidermal cells
- poorer oxygenation at the wound due to increasingly fragile capillaries and a reduction in skin vascularization
- altered nutrition and fluid intake resulting from physical changes that can accompany aging, such as reduced saliva production, a declining sense of smell and taste, and decreased stomach motility
- altered nutrition and fluid intake attributable to troubling personal or social issues, such as loose-fitting dentures, financial concerns, eating alone after the death of a spouse, and problems preparing or obtaining food
- impaired function of the respiratory or immune systems
- reduced dermal and subcutaneous mass leading to an increased risk of chronic pressure injuries
- healed wounds that lack tensile strength and are prone to reinjury

Night and day shifts

Normally, a healthy person shifts position every 15 minutes or so, even during sleep. This shifting prevents tissue damage due to ischemia. Anything that impairs the ability to sense pressure, including spinal cord lesions, the use of pain medications, and cognitive impairment, puts the patient at risk (because the patient can't feel the growing discomfort of pressure and respond to it) (Avsar et al., 2021).

Medications

Any medication that reduces a patient's movement, circulation, or metabolic function, such as sedatives and tranquilizers, has the potential to inhibit the patient's ability to sense and respond to pressure. Additionally, because movement promotes adequate oxygenation, lack of motion means that peripheral blood delivers less oxygen to the extremities than it should. This decrease in oxygen is especially problematic for older adults. Remember, oxygen is important; without it, the healing process slows, and the potential for complications rises.

Interruptions!

Some medications, such as steroids and chemotherapeutic agents, reduce the body's ability to mount an appropriate inflammatory response. This reduction in response interrupts the inflammatory phase of healing and can dramatically lengthen healing time, especially in a patient with a compromised immune system. The use of antibiotics for long periods may place the patient at greater risk of developing an infection, which can affect wound healing (Bennett et al., 2020).

Smoking

Carbon monoxide, a component of cigarette smoke, binds to the hemoglobin in the blood in the place of oxygen. This binding significantly reduces the amount of oxygen circulating in the bloodstream, which can impede wound healing (Beeckman et al., 2020), and occurs to a lesser extent in people regularly exposed to secondhand smoke.

Complications of wound healing

The most common complications associated with wound healing are:
- hemorrhage
- dehiscence and evisceration
- infection
- fistula formation

Hemorrhage

Internal hemorrhage (bleeding) can result in the formation of a hematoma, which is a blood clot that solidifies to form a hard lump under the skin. Hematomas are commonly found around bruises.

External hemorrhage is visible bleeding from the wound. External bleeding during healing isn't unusual because the newly developed blood vessels are fragile and rupture easily (which is one reason a wound needs to be protected by a dressing). However, each time the new blood vessels suffer damage, healing is delayed while repairs are made.

Dehiscence and evisceration

Dehiscence is a separation of skin and tissue layers. It's most likely to occur 3 to 11 days after the injury was sustained and may follow surgery. Evisceration is similar but involves protrusion of underlying visceral organs as well. (See *Recognizing dehiscence and evisceration*.)

Dehiscence and evisceration may constitute a surgical emergency, especially if they involve an abdominal wound. If a wound opens without evisceration, it may need to heal by secondary intention (Sandy-Hodgetts et al., 2020). Poor nutrition and advanced age (typically, over age 65) are two factors that increase a patient's risk of dehiscence and evisceration.

Infection

Infection is a relatively common complication of wound healing that should be addressed promptly. Infection can lead to a bacterial infection that spreads to surrounding tissue. Signs that infection may be at work include:

- redness and warmth of the margins and tissue around the wound
- fever
- edema
- pain (or a sudden increase in pain)
- pus
- increase in exudate or a change in its color
- odor
- discoloration of granulation tissue
- further wound breakdown or lack of progress toward healing

Fistula formation

A fistula is an abnormal passage between two organs or between an organ and the skin. In a wound, it may appear as an undermining or a sinus tract (tunneling) in the skin around the wound. If a sinus tract is present, it's important to determine its extent and direction.

Recognizing dehiscence and evisceration

In wound dehiscence (top), the layers of a wound separate. In evisceration (bottom), the viscera (in this case, a bowel loop) protrude through the wound.

Wound dehiscence

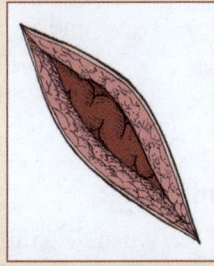

Evisceration of bowel loop

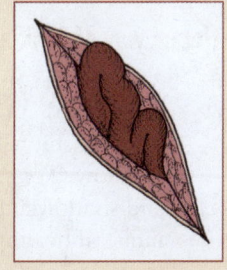

Wound classification

The words used to describe observations of a specific wound have to communicate the same meaning to other members of the health-care team, insurance companies, regulators, the patient's family, and, ultimately, the patient. This is a tall order when even wound care experts debate the descriptive phrases they use. (*Slough* or *eschar? Undermining* or *tunneling?* How much drainage is *moderate?* Is the color green or yellow? Does the drainage have an odor?)

The best way to classify wounds is to use the basic system described here, which focuses on three categories of funda-mental characteristics:

1. wound age
2. wound depth (extent of tissue loss)
3. wound color

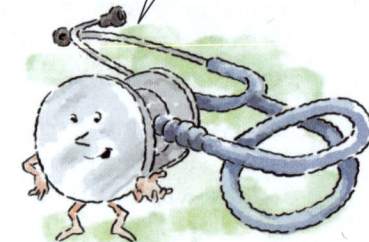

When it comes to classifying wounds, the magic number is 3—age, depth, and color.

Wound age

When determining the age of a wound, it must first be determined if the wound is acute or chronic. Wound experts generally agree that a wound that does not heal within 3 months is considered a chronic wound (Bowers & Franco, 2020).

A different way of thinking

A wound is considered to be acute if it's new or making progress as expected. A chronic wound is any wound that isn't healing in a timely fashion. The main idea is that, in a chronic wound, healing has slowed or stopped, and the wound is no longer getting smaller and shallower. Even if the wound bed appears healthy, red, and moist, if healing fails to progress, it should be considered a chronic wound.

More bad than good

Chronic wounds don't heal as simply as acute wounds. The drain-age in chronic wounds contains a greater amount of destructive enzymes, and fibroblasts (the cells that function as the architects in wound healing) seem to lose their "oomph." Cells in this type of wound are less effective at producing collagen, divide less often, and send fewer signals to other cells telling them to divide and fill the wound. In other words, the wound changes from one that's vigorous and ready to heal to one that's downright lazy (Bowers & Franco, 2020)!

Wound depth

Wound depth is another fundamental characteristic used to classify wounds. During wound assessment, record wound depth as partial thickness or full thickness. (See *Classifying wound depth*.)

Partial thickness

Partial-thickness wounds usually heal very quickly because they involve only the epidermal layer of the skin or extend through the epidermis into (but not through) the dermis. The dermis remains at least partially intact to generate the new epidermis needed to close the wound. Partial-thickness wounds are also less susceptible to infection because part of the body's first level of defense (the skin) is still intact. These wounds tend to be painful, however, and need protection from the air to reduce pain and to decrease the risk of infection (McNichol et al., 2022).

Full thickness

Full-thickness wounds penetrate completely through the skin into underlying tissues. The wound may expose adipose tissue (fat), muscle, tendon, or bone. In the abdomen, adipose tissue or omentum (the covering of the bowel) may be seen. If the omentum is penetrated, the bowel may protrude through the wound (evisceration). Granulation tissue may be visible if the wound has started to heal.

Classifying wound depth

Wounds are classified as partial thickness or full thickness according to the depth of the wound. Partial-thickness wounds involve only the epidermis or extend into the dermis but not through it. Full-thickness wounds extend through the dermis into tissues beneath and may expose adipose tissue, muscle, or bone. These diagrams illustrate the relative depth of both classifications.

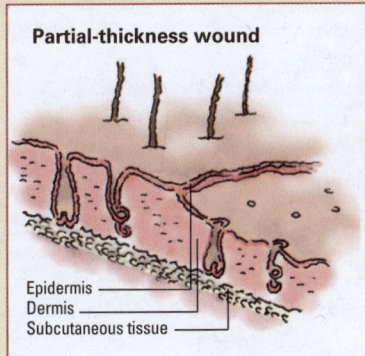

Partial-thickness wound

Epidermis
Dermis
Subcutaneous tissue

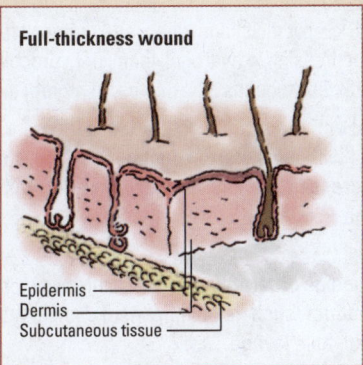

Full-thickness wound

Epidermis
Dermis
Subcutaneous tissue

Full-thickness wounds heal by granulation and contraction, which require more body resources and more time than the healing of partial-thickness wounds. When assessing a full-thickness wound, record its depth as well as the length and width.

The added pressure of pressure injuries

In the case of pressure injuries, wound depth helps to stage the pressure injury according to the classification system developed by the National Pressure Injury Advisory Panel (NPIAP) (2019). This classification system is described in the "Staging pressure injuries" section later in this chapter.

Wound color

Wounds are also classified by the color of the wound bed. Wound color helps the wound care team determine whether debridement is appropriate. (See *Tailoring wound care to wound color*.)

Be picky about wound bed color! Only red will do, and the best shade is red, not pale pink or grayish red. There are thousands of words to describe colors; however, assessment can be simplified by sticking to the red–yellow–black classification system. This system is a useful tool for developing effective wound care management plans.

Tailoring wound care to wound color

With any wound, healing can be stimulated by keeping the wound moist, clean, and free from debris. For open wounds, using wound color can guide the specific management approach to aid healing. Keep in mind that with varying skin colors, these colors may appear in different shades.

Wound color	Management technique
Red	• Cover the wound, keep it moist and clean, and protect it from trauma. • Use a transparent dressing, a hydrogel, foam, or hydrocolloid dressing over partial-thickness wounds to insulate and protect the wound.
Yellow	• Clean the wound and remove the yellow layer. • Cover the wound with a moisture-retentive dressing, such as a hydrogel or foam dressing, or a moist gauze dressing with or without a debriding enzyme. • Consider pulsatile lavage.
Black	• Debride the wound as ordered unless ischemia is suspected. Use an enzyme product (such as collagenase), conservative sharp debridement, or pulsatile lavage. • For wounds with inadequate blood supply and noninfected heel ulcers, do not debride. Keep them clean and dry.

Red means ahead

If the wound bed is red (the color of healthy granulation tissue), the wound is healthy, and normal healing is underway. When a wound begins to heal, a layer of pale pink granulation tissue covers the wound bed. As this layer thickens, it becomes red.

Mellow yellow

If the wound bed is yellow, beware! A yellow color in the wound bed may be a film of fibrin on the tissue. Fibrin is a sticky substance that normally acts as glue in tissue rebuilding. However, if the wound is unhealthy or too dry, fibrin builds up into a layer that can't be rinsed off and may require debridement. Tissue that has recently died due to ischemia or infection may also be yellow and must be debrided. Necrotic tissue in a wound bed that has the following characteristics is usually identified as slough: It is yellow, gray, green, or tan; it is adherent to the wound bed; and it is dry or moist.

Black = debridement

If the wound bed is black, be alarmed. A black wound bed signals necrosis (tissue death). Eschar (dead, avascular tissue) covers the wound, slowing the healing process and providing microorganisms with a site in which to proliferate. When eschar covers a wound, accurate assessment of wound depth is difficult and should be deferred until eschar is removed.

Ischemia exceptions

Typically, debridement is indicated for black wounds; however, ulcers caused by ischemia (damage due to inadequate blood supply) and uninfected heel pressure injuries are exceptions. Ischemic wounds won't heal until the blood supply is improved, and they're less likely to become infected if kept dry. The wound can be debrided and kept moist after the blood supply is reestablished. (The body can then fend off infection and heal the wound.)

Wound assessment

Gathering information about a wound requires the use of the senses of touch, sight, and smell. Be sure to assess drainage, the wound bed, and patient pain (Beeckman et al., 2020). Assess the wound bed and the surrounding skin only after they've been cleaned. When completing an assessment, remember that it doesn't matter what method you use to record observations—it's just important to be consistent.

Components of a complete wound assessment

When a wound is being assessed, be sure to record information about:

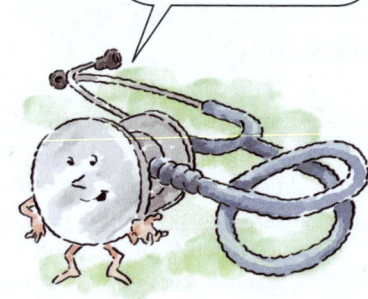

Record as much information about the wound as possible.

- Anatomic location
- Size
- Tunneling and undermining
- The wound bed
- Wound edges
- Periwound skin
- Drainage/exudates:
  - Amount
  - Consistency
  - Color
- Odor
- Extent of tissue loss (discussed previously)

Anatomic location

Identifying the location of the wound is important because location can assist in determining the etiology of the wound. Is it a pressure point, on the lower extremity, in the gluteal cleft, on the bottom of the foot? All of these locations suggest etiology.

Size

Record the length of the wound at the longest point in a head-to-toe direction, and record the width as the longest measurement perpendicular (at a right angle) to the length measurement. (See *Measuring a wound.*)

Get out the tape measure

The most common method of measuring wound dimensions is to use a tape measure. To prevent contamination and cross-contamination, make sure it's a disposable device.

Be sure to record any observed areas of discoloration of the intact skin around the wound opening separately, not as part of the wound bed. Record all measurements in centimeters.

Trace the wound

Another way to measure the wound is to use wound tracing (in which wound margins are traced on a sheet of clear plastic). Use tracing to calculate an approximate wound area. This method provides only a rough estimate but is simple and fairly quick.

Photography

Photography may be used to document wound progress; however, note that obtaining informed consent and maintaining safe storage of the photographs and digital content are required, per the Health Insurance

Measuring a wound

When measuring a wound, first determine the longest distance across the open area of the wound, in a head-to-toe direction. In this photograph, note the line used to illustrate this length.

A wound's width is simply the longest distance across the wound at a right angle to the length. Note the relationship between length and width in the photograph.

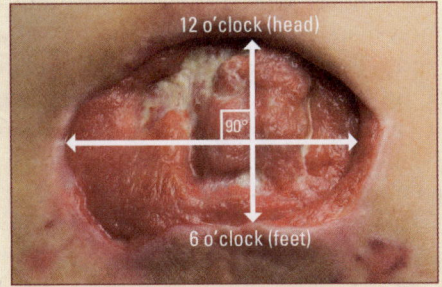

Photo credit: Shutterstock/Sergii Votit

Also, note the area of reddened, intact skin and white macerated skin. These areas would be measured and recorded as surrounding erythema and maceration, not as part of the wound itself. In this full-thickness ischial pressure injury, depth should be recorded and areas of tunneling or undermining noted.

Portability and Accountability Act (HIPAA) and the Health Information Technology for Economic and Clinical Health (HITECH) Act implications.

How deep

To measure the depth of the wound, gently insert the cotton-tipped swab into the deepest portion of the wound, and then carefully mark the probe where it meets the edge of the skin. Remove the applicator and measure the distance from the mark to the end to determine the depth.

Tunneling and undermining

It's also important to measure the following:
- Tunneling, also called *sinus tracts*, which are extensions of the wound bed into adjacent tissue
- Undermining (areas of the wound bed that extend under the skin)
These features are measured similarly to depth. Carefully insert a cotton-tipped swab to the bottom of the tunnel or to the end of the undermined area; next, mark the stick and measure the distance from the mark to the end of the swab. If a tunnel is large, palpate it with a gloved finger rather than a swab because the end of the tunnel can be sensed better with a finger.

The wound bed

The type of tissue in the ulcer base determines the potential for healing and the type of treatment. Know how to identify necrotic tissue, granulation tissue, and epithelial tissue.

Necrotic tissue (nonviable)

Necrotic tissue may appear as a moist yellow or gray area of tissue that's separating from viable tissue. When dry, necrotic tissue appears as thick, hard, and leathery black eschar. Slough tissue appears as yellow/tan/gray tissue and is dry or moist; also, it may be adherent or stringy in the base of the wound. Areas of necrotic or devitalized tissue may mask underlying abscesses and collections of fluid. Before the ulcer can begin to heal, necrotic tissue, drainage, and metabolic wastes must be removed from the wound (McNichol et al., 2022).

Granulation tissue

Granulation tissue appears as beefy red, bumpy, shiny tissue in the base of the ulcer. As a full-thickness ulcer heals, it develops more and more granulation tissue. Such factors as tissue oxygenation, tissue hydration, and nutrition can alter the color and quality of granulation tissue.

"Red Warning"

Usually, if a wound is red, it is healthy. However, looks can be deceiving; if a wound when touched bleeds easily (tissue is friable), this usually indicates excess bacteria (a bioburden) in the wound. Bioburden is not an "infection" but an overcolonization of bacteria in the wound bed and can often be treated with topical antiseptics (Bowers & Franco, 2020).

Epithelial tissue

Epithelialization is the regeneration of the epidermis across the ulcer surface. It appears as pale or dark pink skin, first becoming evident at ulcer borders in full-thickness wounds and as islands around hair follicles in partial-thickness wounds. Wound healing can be assessed and quantified by the percentage of surface covered by new epithelium.

Wound edges

Edges should be attached, moist, even, or flush with the wound base to enhance epithelialization (McNichol et al., 2022). When assessing wound edges, the skin should be smooth, not rolled, and tightly adherent to the wound bed. Premature "closure" of wound edges may be indicated by rolled edges (epibole) or dry and thickened edges. Rolled skin may indicate that the wound bed is too dry. Loose skin at the edges may indicate additional shearing injury (separation of skin layers), possibly due to a rough transfer or repositioning. In this case, to prevent recurrence, improve transfer and repositioning techniques.

Periwound skin

Be sure to assess the skin around the wound.

Rainbow connections

In the past, sailors used the color of the sky to predict danger at sea. In a similar fashion, the color of the skin around the wound can signal impending problems that can impede healing:

- White skin indicates maceration, or too much moisture, and the need for a protective barrier around the wound and a more absorbent dressing (and remember to keep the dressing in the wound and off the skin) (WUWHS, 2019b).
- Red skin can indicate inflammation, injury (e.g., tape burn, excessive pressure, or chemical exposure), or infection (Beeckman et al., 2020). Remember that inflammation is healthy only during the inflammatory phase of healing, not after!
- Purple skin can indicate bruising, a sign of trauma.

Finger tools

During the assessment of the area around a wound, the nurse's gloved fingers are an essential tool. For example, gentle probing of the tissue around the wound bed helps to determine if it's soft or hard (indurated). Indurated tissue, even in the absence of erythema (redness), is an indication of infection.

Similarly, if the patient has dark skin, it may be impossible to see color cues. This is when the sense of touch and fingers come in handy. Probe the area around the wound bed and compare the feel with the surrounding healthy skin. A tender area of skin that appears shiny and feels hard may indicate inflammation in such a patient.

Drainage/exudates

The wound bed should be moist but not overly moist. Moisture allows the cells and chemicals needed for healing to move about the wound surface.

To begin collecting information about wound drainage, inspect the dressing as you remove it and record answers to the following questions (WUWHS, 2019b):

- Is the drainage well contained, or is it oozing from the edges? If it's oozing, consider using a more absorbent dressing?
- In the case of an occlusive dressing, were the dressing edges well sealed? (A hydrocolloid in the gluteal cleft area becomes a greenhouse for bacteria if the edges are loose.) If the patient has fecal incontinence, it's even more important to note the seal status.
- Is the dressing saturated or dry?
- How much drainage is there: a scant, moderate, or large amount? Is there an odor?
- What are the color and consistency of the drainage? (See *Drainage descriptors*, page 448.)

Drainage descriptors

This chart provides terminology that can be used to describe the color and consistency of wound drainage.

Description	Color and consistency
Serous	• Clear or light yellow • Thin and watery
Sanguineous	• Red (with fresh blood) • Thin
Serosanguineous	• Pink to light red • Thin • Watery
Purulent	• Creamy yellow, green, white, or tan • Thick and opaque

Skipping the swab?

Furthermore, consider the texture of the drainage. If the drainage has a thick, creamy texture, the wound may contain an excessive amount of bacteria. However, this doesn't necessarily mean a clinically significant infection is present. Document the characteristics of the drainage. Drainage might be creamy because it contains WBCs that have killed bacteria. The drainage is also contaminated with surface bacteria that naturally live in moist environments on the human body.

Because of the possibility of bacterial contamination of the swab, swab cultures are not the best way to identify wound infections (Bowers & Franco, 2020). If a swab is used, the Levine method is suggested as the best method (McNichol et al., 2022):

- Cleanse the wound with normal saline solution (NSS) and blot dry with sterile gauze.
- Identify a healthy area of the wound, about 1 cm^2.
- Moisten the swab with nonpreserved NSS.
- Press on the wound area, rotating the swab (apply enough pressure to elicit tissue fluid).
- When the tip of the swab is saturated, break the tip (if needed) and insert it into a container using sterile technique.

Punch biopsy of tissue or needle aspiration of fluid may also be used. These methods require greater skill but are more likely to reveal accurate results.

Fish out of water

In dry wound beds, cells involved in healing, which normally exist in a fluid environment, are a bit like fish in a desert because they can't move. WBCs can't fight infection, enzymes like collagenase can't break down dead material, and macrophages can't carry away debris. The wound edges curl up to preserve moisture remaining in the edge, and epithelial cells (new skin cells) fail to grow over and cover the wound. Healing grinds to a halt, and necrotic tissue builds up.

Flood watch

Too much moisture poses a different problem. It floods the wound and spills out onto the skin, where the constant moisture causes the death of skin cells.

Odor

If kept clean, a noninfected wound usually produces little, if any, odor. (One exception is the odor normally present under a hydrocolloid dressing that develops as a by-product of the degradation process.) A newly detected odor might be a sign of infection; record such findings and report them to the healthcare provider. When documenting wound odor, it's important to include when the odor was noted and whether it went away with wound cleaning.

Odor eaters

If an odor develops, it can present an embarrassing or otherwise uncomfortable situation for the patient as well as their family, guests, and roommate. If an odor is noted, use an odor eliminator. Odor eliminators are compounds that bind with, and neutralize, the molecules responsible for the odor. (They differ from air fresheners, which are scents that mask odors.)

Pain

In addition to assessing wound characteristics, you must assess any pain related to the wound. It is important to note not only pain associated with the injury itself but also pain associated with healing and with therapies employed to promote healing. To fully understand the patient's pain, talk with them and ask about their level of pain on a scale of 0 to 10, with 10 being the worst pain they have ever experienced. Then watch to see how they respond to pain and the therapies provided. As always, remember to record the findings.

Listen and learn

If the patient is conscious and can communicate, have them rate their pain before and during each dressing change. If the patient says the dressing change itself is painful, you could consider administering pain medication before the procedure. Remember to document such pain and report it to the healthcare provider. Although there are less painful methods of removing dead tissue than wet-to-dry debridement, if the patient's pain isn't documented and communicated, wet-to-dry debridement orders may continue, and the patient may suffer unnecessary discomfort.

Useful tips for removing dressings

In general, when removing adherent dressings, it's less painful if the dressing is soaked off or if adhesive remover is used over intact skin. Also, keep the skin taut. Press down on the skin to release the dressing rather than just pulling the dressing off. Pull the dressing gently toward the wound using an index finger to gently release the skin from the adhesive.

Treatment for wounds

Treating impaired skin integrity involves a range of procedures, from basic wound care and wound irrigation to surgical wound management and closed-wound drain management.

Basic wound care

Basic wound care focuses on cleaning and dressing the wound. Because open wounds are colonized (or contaminated) with bacteria, practice clean technique using clean, nonsterile gloves during wound care unless sterile dressing changes are specified. Always follow standard precautions.

The goal of wound cleaning is to remove debris and contaminants from the wound without damaging healthy tissue (McNichol et al., 2022). The wound should be cleaned initially; repeat cleaning as needed, and always before a new dressing is applied.

The basic purpose of a wound dressing, which is to provide an optimal environment for the body to heal itself, should be considered before one is selected. Functions of a dressing include the following (WUWHS, 2022):

- protecting the wound from contamination and trauma
- providing compression if bleeding or swelling is anticipated
- applying medications
- absorbing drainage or debrided necrotic tissue from the wound bed
- filling the "dead space" in the wound
- protecting the skin surrounding the wound

The cardinal rule is to keep moist tissue moist and the surrounding skin dry. Ideally, a dressing should keep the wound moist, absorb drainage or debris, conform to the wound, and be adhesive to surrounding skin yet be easily removable

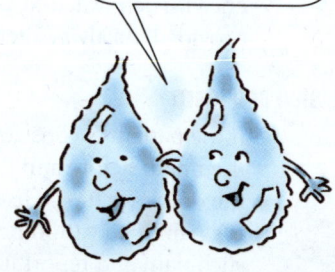

The cardinal rule of wound care is to keep moist tissue moist and dry tissue dry.

(WUWHS, 2019b). It should also be user-friendly, require minimal changes, decrease the need for a secondary dressing layer, and be cost-effective and comfortable for the patient.

Supplies

- hypoallergenic tape or elastic netting
- overbed table
- piston-type irrigating system
- two pairs of gloves
- cleaning solution (such as NSS) as ordered
- sterile 4 × 4-inch gauze pads
- selected topical dressing
- linen-saver pads
- impervious plastic trash bag
- disposable wound-measuring device

Getting ready

- Assemble the equipment at the patient's bedside. Use clean or sterile technique, depending on facility policy and wound care orders.
- Cut the tape into strips for securing dressings. Loosen lids on cleaning solutions and medications for easy removal.
- Attach an impervious plastic trash bag to the overbed table to hold used dressings and refuse.
- Before any dressing change, wash your hands and review the principles of standard precautions.
- Provide privacy, and explain the procedure to the patient to allay fears and promote cooperation.

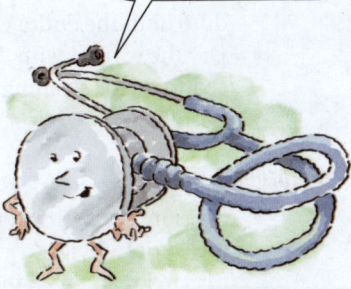

Be sure to wash your hands before and after each dressing change.

How it's done

- Position the patient in a way that maximizes comfort while allowing easy access to the wound site.
- Cover bed linens with a linen-saver pad to prevent soiling.

Cleaning the wound

- Open the cleaning solution container and carefully pour cleaning solution onto the opened plastic package of 4 × 4-inch gauze pads or into a bowl to avoid splashing. (The bowl may be clean or sterile, depending on facility policy.)
- Open other supplies as needed.
- Put on gloves.
- Gently roll or lift an edge of the soiled dressing to obtain a starting point. Support adjacent skin while gently releasing the soiled dressing from the skin. When possible, remove the dressing in the direction of hair growth. Assess the existing dressing for drainage, color, amount, and odor.

- Discard the soiled dressing and the contaminated gloves in the impervious plastic trash bag to avoid contaminating the clean or sterile field.
- Put on a clean pair of gloves (sterile or nonsterile, depending on facility policy or the wound care order).
- Inspect the wound. Note the color, amount, and odor of drainage and necrotic debris.
- Fold a sterile 4 × 4-inch gauze pad into quarters and grasp it. Make sure the folded edge faces outward.
- Alternatively, use a wound cleanser in a spray gun bottle.

Circles on the skin

- When cleaning, be sure to move from the least contaminated area to the most contaminated area. For a linear-shaped wound, such as an incision, gently wipe from top to bottom in one motion, starting directly over the wound and moving outward. For an open wound, such as a pressure injury, gently wipe in concentric circles, again starting directly over the wound and moving outward. Use a separate gauze pad each time the wound is cleaned.
- Discard the gauze pad in the plastic trash bag.
- Using a clean gauze pad for each wiping motion, repeat the procedure until the entire wound is cleaned.
- Dry the wound with 4 × 4-inch gauze pads, using the same procedure as for cleaning. Discard the used gauze pads in the plastic trash bag.

Don't forget to measure

- Measure the perimeter of the wound with a disposable wound-measuring device (e.g., a square, transparent card with concentric circles arranged in a bull's-eye fashion and bordered with a straight-edge ruler). Measure the longest length in a head-to-toe direction and the widest width.
- Measure the depth of a full-thickness wound.

Testing for tunneling

- Gently probe the wound bed and edges with a gloved finger or a flexible probe to assess for wound tunneling or undermining. Tunneling usually signals wound extension along fascial planes (Beeckman et al., 2020). Gauge tunnel depth by determining how far a gloved finger or the cotton-tipped applicator can be inserted.
- Next, reassess the condition of the skin and wound. Note the character of the clean wound bed and the surrounding skin.
- If adherent necrotic material is observed, notify a wound care specialist or a healthcare provider to ensure appropriate debridement.

Applying a dressing

- Prepare to apply the appropriate topical dressing if ordered. See *Choosing a wound dressing* for instructions for applying topical moist saline gauze, hydrocolloid, transparent, alginate, foam, and hydrogel dressings. For other dressings or topical agents, follow the facility's protocol or the manufacturer's instructions.

Choosing a wound dressing

The patient's needs and wound characteristics determine which type of dressing is used on a wound. As described in this box, different types of dressings maintain moisture, donate moisture, or absorb moisture.

Maintaining moisture

Gauze dressings

Made of absorptive cotton or synthetic fabric, gauze dressings are permeable to water, water vapor, and oxygen and may be impregnated with hydrogel or another agent. When uncertain about which dressing to use, you may apply a gauze dressing moistened in saline solution until a wound specialist recommends definitive treatment.

Hydrocolloid dressings

Hydrocolloid dressings are adhesive, moldable wafers made of a carbohydrate-based material and usually have waterproof backings. They're impermeable to oxygen, water, and water vapor, and most have some absorptive properties.

Transparent film dressings

Transparent film dressings are clear, adherent, and nonabsorptive. These polymer-based dressings are permeable to oxygen and water vapor but not to water. Their transparency allows visual inspection. Because they can't absorb drainage, they're used on partial-thickness wounds with minimal exudate.

Absorbing moisture

Alginate dressings

Made from seaweed, alginate dressings are nonwoven, absorptive dressings available as soft sterile pads or ropes. They absorb excessive exudate and may be used on infected wounds. As these dressings absorb exudate, many turn into a gel that keeps the wound bed moist and promotes healing. When exudate is no longer excessive, switch to another type of dressing.

Hydrofiber

These dressings are made of synthetic material and resemble alginates in shape, size, and absorbency. They absorb excessive exudate and may be used on infected wounds.

Foam dressings

Foam dressings are used when absorption is needed. They are spongelike polymer dressings that may be impregnated or coated with other materials. Foam dressings can be adhesive or nonadhesive, and they can be bordered or nonbordered.

Donating moisture

Hydrogel dressings

Most hydrogels are primarily water-based. They're available as a gel in a tube, as flexible sheets, gel impregnated gauze pads, and as saturated gauze packing strips. They may have a cooling effect, which eases pain, and are used when the wound needs moisture.

Semipermeable films

These films prevent evaporation from the wound bed, thus rehydrating the wound. Be careful; these dressings can sometimes cause skin tears when removed.

Source: World Union of Wound Healing Societies (WUWHS). (2022). Incision care and dressing selection in surgical wounds: Findings from a series of international meetings. *Wounds International.* https://woundsinternational.com/consensus-documents/incision-care-and-dressing-selection-surgical-wounds-findings-series-international-meetings/

Moist saline gauze dressing

- Moisten the gauze dressing with NSS. Wring out excess fluid.
- Open the gauze pad completely (often termed *fluffing*) and gently place the dressing into the wound. To separate surfaces within the wound, gently guide the gauze between opposing wound surfaces. To avoid damage to tissues, lightly fill the space—don't pack the gauze tightly.
- To protect the surrounding skin from moisture, apply a sealant or barrier.
- Change the dressing often enough to keep the wound moist.

Hydrocolloid dressing

- Choose a clean, dry, presized dressing, or cut one to overlap the wound by about 1 inch (2.5 cm). Remove the dressing from its package, pull the release paper from the adherent side of the dressing, and apply the dressing to the wound. Hold the dressing in place with your hand because the warmth of your hand will mold the dressing to the skin.

Smooth operator

- As you apply the dressing, carefully smooth out wrinkles and avoid stretching the dressing.
- If the dressing's edges need to be secured with tape, apply a skin sealant to the intact skin around the wound. After the area is dry, tape the dressing to the skin. The sealant protects the skin from tape burns and skin stripping and promotes tape adherence. Avoid using tension or pressure when applying the tape.
- Remove gloves and discard them in the impervious plastic trash bag. Dispose of refuse according to facility policy, and wash hands.
- Change a hydrocolloid dressing every 2 to 7 days as necessary; change it immediately if the patient complains of pain, the dressing no longer adheres, or leakage occurs. Remember, hydrocolloids are occlusive and provide a barrier when intact. If drainage is leaking out, then bacteria can go in!

Transparent dressing

- Clean and dry the wound as described earlier.
- Select a dressing to overlap the wound by 1 to 2 inches (2.5 to 5 cm).
- Gently lay the dressing over the wound; avoid wrinkling the dressing. To prevent shearing force, don't stretch the dressing over the wound. Press firmly on the edges of the dressing to promote adherence. Although this type of dressing is self-adhesive, the edges may have to be taped in place to prevent them from curling.
- Change the dressing every 3 to 5 days, depending on the amount of drainage. If the seal is no longer secure or if accumulated tissue

fluid extends beyond the edges of the wound and onto the surrounding skin, change the dressing. Occlusive dressings that are no longer secure or that are leaking onto the surrounding skin may cause a risk for infection or skin breakdown. The dressing should be monitored to be sure it is dry, secure, and intact.

Alginate/Hydrofiber dressing

- Apply the alginate or Hydrofiber dressing to the wound surface. Cover the area with a secondary dressing (such as gauze pads or transparent film) as ordered. Secure the dressing with tape or elastic netting.
- Change the dressing when strikethrough occurs (i.e., when the drainage outline can be seen on the secondary dressing). This means the alginate/Hydrofiber has absorbed the maximum amount. When the drainage stops or the wound bed looks dry, stop using alginate/Hydrofiber dressings.

Foam dressing

- Gently lay the foam dressing over the wound. Sometimes, if the wound is deep and dead space is not filled, foams become secondary dressings.
- Use tape, elastic netting, or gauze to hold the dressing in place if it is not bordered or adhesive.
- Change the dressing when the foam no longer absorbs the exudate, and there is strikethrough on the top or edges of the dressing.

Hydrogel dressing

- Apply gel to the wound bed to cover the bed with a layer of gel.
- Cover partial-thickness wounds with a secondary dressing (transparent film or a nonadherent dressing). For full-thickness wounds, use gel-impregnated gauze (4 × 4-inch gauze or strip). If this is unavailable, apply gel over the wound bed and fill the dead space with fluffed, NSS-moistened gauze.
- Change the dressing daily or as needed to keep the wound bed moist.
- If the hydrogel dressing you select comes in sheet form, cut the dressing to overlap the wound by 1 inch (2.5 cm); then apply in the same fashion as a hydrocolloid dressing. Don't forget to protect the periwound skin with skin prep!

Practice pointers

- Be aware that infection may cause foul-smelling drainage, persistent pain, severe erythema, induration, and elevated skin and body temperatures. Advancing infection or cellulitis can lead to septicemia.
- Severe erythema may signal worsening cellulitis, which means the offending organisms have invaded the tissue and are no longer localized.

Wound irrigation

Irrigation cleans tissues and flushes cell debris and drainage from an open wound. It also helps prevent premature surface healing over an abscess pocket or infected tract.

After irrigation, fill open wounds to absorb additional drainage. Always follow the standard precaution guidelines by the Centers for Disease Control and Prevention (CDC) (2017).

Supplies

- waterproof trash bag
- linen-saver pad
- emesis basin
- clean gloves
- sterile gloves
- goggles
- gown, if indicated
- sterile water or NSS
- soft rubber or plastic catheter
- sterile container
- materials as needed for wound care
- sterile irrigation and dressing set
- commercial wound cleaner
- 35-mL piston syringe with 19G needle or catheter
- skin protectant wipe (skin sealant) or other protective skin barriers

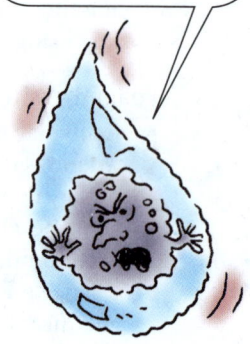

NO!!!!! I was so comfy living in that wound! Darn wound irrigation!

Getting ready

- Assemble equipment in the patient's room. Check the expiration date on each sterile package and inspect for tears.
- Don't use any nonpreserved solution that has been open longer than 24 hours. As needed, dilute the prescribed irrigant to the correct proportions with sterile water or NSS. Allow the solution to reach room temperature, or warm it to 90° to 95° F (32.2° to 35° C).
- Open the waterproof trash bag and place it near the patient's bed. Form a cuff by turning down the top of the trash bag.

How it's done

- Check the healthcare provider's order, assess the patient's condition, and identify allergies. Explain the procedure to the patient, provide privacy, and position the patient correctly for the procedure. Put the linen-saver pad under the patient and place the emesis basin below the wound so that the irrigating solution flows from the wound into the basin.
- Wash hands, and put on a gown and gloves.
- Remove the soiled dressing, and then discard the dressing and gloves in the trash bag.

- Establish a clean or sterile field with all the equipment and supplies needed for wound irrigation and dressing. Pour the prescribed amount of irrigating solution into a clean or sterile container. Put on sterile gloves and a gown and goggles, if indicated. (See *Irrigating a deep wound*.)

Irrigating a deep wound

When preparing to irrigate a wound, attach a 19G needle or catheter to a 35-mL piston syringe. This setup delivers an irrigation pressure of 8 psi, which is effective in cleaning the wound and reducing the risk of trauma and wound infection. To prevent tissue damage or, in an abdominal wound, intestinal perforation, avoid forcing the needle or catheter into the wound.

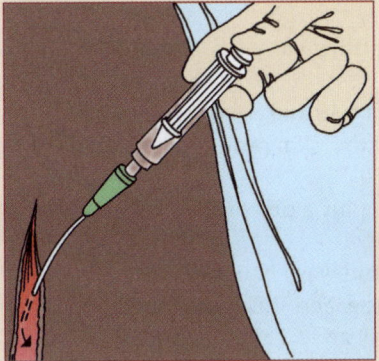

Irrigate the wound with gentle pressure until the prescribed amount has been administered and the solution returns clear. Allow the emesis basin to remain under the wound to collect any remaining drainage.

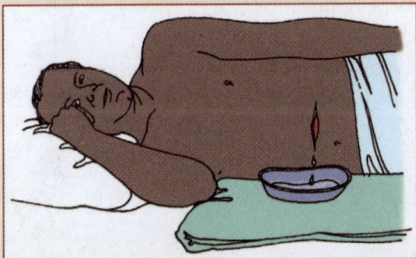

Syringe irrigation is another alternative. Where possible, direct the flow at a right angle to the wound and allow the fluid to drain by gravity. Doing so requires careful positioning of the patient, either in bed or on a chair. The patient may need an analgesic agent during the treatment.

If irrigation isn't possible, gently swab away exudate before using an antiseptic or saline solution to clean the wound (taking care not to push loose debris into the wound). If permitted by facility policy, use sharp, sterile scissors to snip off loose dead tissue—never pull it off.

From clean to dirty

- Fill the syringe with the irrigating solution and connect the catheter to the syringe. Gently instill a slow, steady stream of solution into the wound until the syringe empties. Make sure the solution flows from the clean to the dirty area of the wound to prevent contamination of clean tissue by exudate. Be sure the solution reaches all areas of the wound.
- Refill the syringe, reconnect it to the catheter, and repeat the irrigation. Continue to irrigate the wound until the prescribed amount of solution has been administered or until the solution returns clear. Note the amount of solution administered. Then remove and discard the catheter and syringe in the waterproof trash bag.

Positioned for success

- Keep the patient positioned to allow further wound drainage into the basin.
- Clean the area around the wound with NSS and pat dry with gauze; wipe intact surrounding skin with a skin protectant wipe and allow it to dry.
- Fill the wound lightly if ordered, and apply a dressing.
- Remove and discard gloves and gown.
- Make sure the patient is comfortable and wash hands.
- Dispose of drainage, solutions, trash bag, and soiled equipment and supplies according to facility policy and CDC guidelines.

Practice pointers

- Try to coordinate wound irrigation with the healthcare provider's visit so that they can inspect the wound.
- Irrigate with a bulb syringe if the wound is small or not particularly deep or if a piston syringe is unavailable. However, use a bulb syringe cautiously because this type of syringe *doesn't* deliver enough pressure to adequately clean the wound and may increase the risk of aspirating drainage.

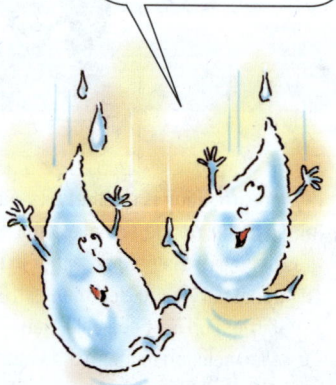

Infection-preventing procedures also allow you to monitor fluid and electrolyte imbalance.

Surgical wound management

When caring for a surgical wound, procedures that help prevent infection by stopping pathogens from entering the wound are carried out. In addition to promoting patient comfort, such procedures protect the skin's surface from maceration and excoriation caused by contact with irritating drainage. They also allow measurement of wound drainage to monitor fluid and electrolyte balance.

The primary method used to manage a draining surgical wound is a dressing, negative-pressure wound therapy, or a pouch. Usually, lightly seeping wounds with drains, and wounds with minimal purulent drainage, can be managed with dressings (WUWHS, 2022).

What a lovely dress

Dressing a surgical wound calls for sterile technique and sterile supplies to prevent contamination. The color of the wound may be used to help determine which type of dressing to apply. Be sure to change the dressing often enough to keep the skin dry. Always follow standard precautions according to CDC, APSIC, and WUWHS (2022) guidelines (CDC, 2017; Ling et al., 2019).

Supplies

- waterproof trash bag
- clean gloves
- sterile gloves
- gown and face shield or goggles, if indicated
- sterile 4 × 4-inch gauze pads
- selected primary dressing(s)
- sterile cotton-tipped applicators
- sterile dressing set
- topical medication, if ordered
- selected securing (adhesive or other tape, Montgomery straps, a fishnet tube elasticized dressing support, or a T-binder)
- skin protectant
- sterile NSS
- optional: forceps, nonadherent pads, collodion spray or acetone-free adhesive remover, graduated container

For a wound with a drain

- sterile scissors
- sterile 4 × 4-inch gauze pads without cotton lining
- ostomy pouch or another collection pouch
- sterile precut tracheostomy pads or drain dressings
- adhesive tape (paper or silk tape if the patient is hypersensitive)
- surgical mask

Getting ready

- Ask the patient about allergies to tapes and dressings. Assemble all equipment in the patient's room. Check the expiration date on each sterile package, and inspect for tears.
- Open the waterproof trash bag, and place it near the patient's bed. Position the bag to avoid reaching across the sterile field or the wound when disposing of soiled articles. Form a cuff by turning

down the top of the trash bag to provide a wide opening and to prevent contamination of instruments or gloves by touching the bag's edge.

How it's done

- Explain the procedure to the patient to allay fears and to ensure cooperation.

Removing the old dressing

- Check the healthcare provider's orders for specific wound care and medication instructions. Note the location of surgical drains to avoid dislodging them during the procedure.
- Assess the patient's condition.
- Provide privacy, and position the patient as necessary. To avoid chilling the patient, expose only the wound site.
- Wash hands. Put on a gown and a face shield, if necessary. Then put on clean gloves.

Go toward the wound

- Loosen the soiled dressing by holding the patient's skin and pulling the tape or dressing toward the wound to protect the newly formed tissue and to prevent stress on the incision. Moisten the tape with acetone-free adhesive remover, if necessary, to make the tape removal less painful (particularly if the skin is hairy). Don't apply solvents to the incision because they could contaminate the wound.
- Slowly remove the soiled dressing. If the gauze adheres to the wound, loosen the gauze by moistening it with sterile NSS.
- Observe the dressing for the amount, type, color, and odor of drainage.
- Discard the dressing and gloves in the waterproof trash bag.

Caring for the wound

- Wash hands. Establish a sterile field with all the equipment and supplies needed for suture line care and the dressing change. If the healthcare provider has ordered ointment or other topical medications, squeeze the needed amount onto the sterile field. If an antiseptic from an unsterile bottle is being used, pour the antiseptic cleaning agent into a sterile container so your gloves don't become contaminated. Then, put on sterile gloves.

No cotton balls, please!

- Saturate the sterile gauze pads with the prescribed cleaning agent. Avoid using cotton balls because they may shed fibers in the wound, causing irritation, infection, or adhesion.
- Proceed to clean the wound.
- Irrigate the wound, if ordered, using the specified solution.

- If ordered, obtain a wound culture after cleaning and irrigating the wound.
- Pick up the moistened gauze pad or swab, and squeeze out the excess solution.

From top to bottom

- Working from the top of the incision, wipe once to the bottom and then discard the gauze pad. With a second moistened pad, wipe from top to bottom in a vertical path next to the incision (as shown below).

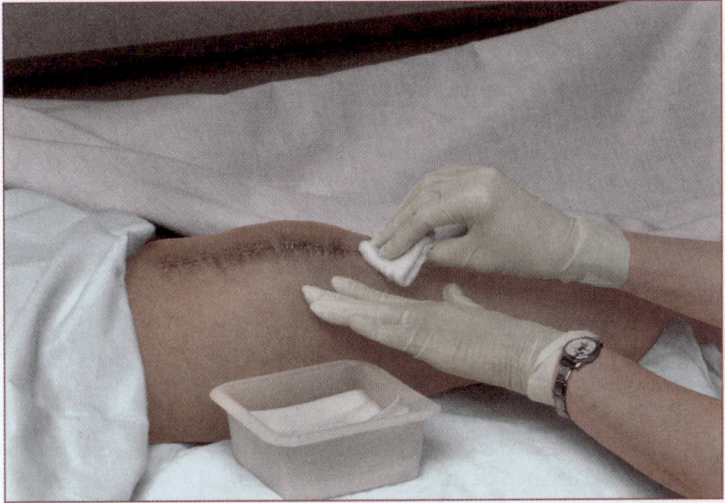

- Continue to work outward from the incision in lines running parallel to it. Always wipe from the clean area toward the less clean area. Use each gauze pad or swab for only one stroke to avoid tracking wound exudate and normal body flora from surrounding skin to the clean areas. Remember that the suture line is cleaner than the adjacent skin and the top of the suture line is usually cleaner than the bottom because more drainage collects at the bottom of the wound.
- Use sterile, cotton-tipped applicators for efficient cleaning of tight-fitting wire sutures, deep and narrow wounds, and wounds with pockets. Remember to wipe only once with each applicator.

Watch out for the drain!

- If the patient has a surgical drain, clean the drain's surface last. Because moist drainage promotes bacterial growth, the drain is considered the most contaminated area. Clean the skin around the drain by wiping in half or full circles from the drain site outward.

- Clean all areas of the wound to wash away debris, pus, blood, and necrotic material. Try not to disturb sutures or irritate the incision. Clean to at least 1 inch (2.5 cm) beyond the end of the new dressing. If you aren't applying a new dressing, clean to at least 2 inches (5 cm) beyond the incision.

Line them up . . .

- Check to make sure the edges of the incision are lined up properly, and check for signs of infection (heat, redness, swelling, induration, and odor), dehiscence, and evisceration. If these signs are observed or if the patient reports pain at the wound site, notify the healthcare provider.
- Wash the skin surrounding the wound with normal saline, and pat dry using a sterile 4 × 4-inch gauze pad. Avoid oil-based soap because it may interfere with pouch adherence.
- Apply any prescribed topical medication.
- Apply a skin protectant if needed.

. . . and then apply the dressing

Applying a new gauze dressing

- Gently place sterile 4 × 4-inch gauze pads at the center of the wound, and move progressively outward to the edges of the wound site. Extend the gauze at least 1 inch (2.5 cm) beyond the incision in each direction, and cover the wound evenly with enough sterile dressings (usually two or three layers) to absorb all drainage until the next dressing change, or apply a specific dressing ordered by the healthcare provider.
- If ordered, pack the wound with gauze pads or strips folded to fit, using sterile forceps. Avoid using cotton-lined gauze pads because cotton fibers can adhere to the wound surface and cause complications.
- Pack the wound, using the wet-to-damp method. Soak the packing material in solution and wring it out so that it's slightly moist to provide a moist wound environment that absorbs debris and drainage.
- Don't pack the wound tightly because doing so will exert pressure and may damage the wound. Use large absorbent dressings (abdominal pads, also known as *ABDs*) to form outer layers, if needed, to provide greater absorbency.
- Secure the dressing's edges to the patient's skin with strips of tape to maintain the sterility of the wound site (as shown). Alternatively, secure the dressing with a T-binder or hypoallergenic adhesive straps to prevent skin excoriation, which may occur with repeated tape removal necessitated by frequent dressing changes.

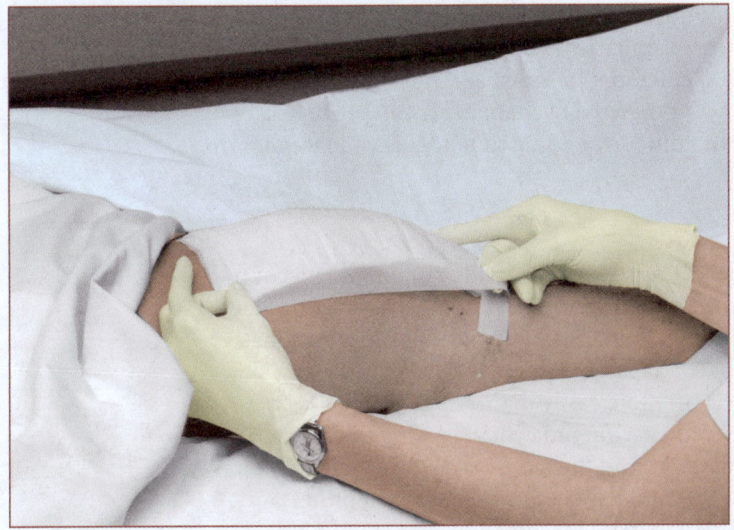

- Make sure the patient is comfortable.
- Properly dispose of the solutions and trash bag, and clean or discard soiled equipment and supplies according to the facility's policy.

Dressing a wound with a drain

- Use commercially precut gauze drain dressings or prepare a drain dressing by using sterile scissors to cut a slit in a sterile 4 × 4-inch gauze pad. Fold the pad in half, then cut inward from the center of the folded edge. Don't use a cotton-lined gauze pad, because cutting the gauze opens the lining and releases cotton fibers into the wound. Prepare a second pad the same way.
- Gently press one drain dressing close to the skin around the drain so that the tubing fits into the slit. Press the second drain dressing around the drain from the opposite direction so that the two dressings encircle the tubing.
- Layer two to four uncut sterile 4 × 4-inch gauze pads or large absorbent dressings around the tubing as needed to absorb expected drainage. Tape the dressing in place, or use a T-binder or hypoallergenic adhesive straps.

Practice pointers

- If the patient has two wounds in the same area, cover each wound separately with layers of sterile 4 × 4-inch gauze pads. Then cover each site with a large absorbent dressing secured to the patient's skin with tape. Don't use a single large absorbent dressing to cover both sites because drainage quickly saturates a pad, promoting cross-contamination.

- When filling a wound, don't fill it too tightly because doing so compresses adjacent capillaries and may prevent the wound edges from contracting. Remember to "open and fluff" gauze before placing it in the wound. Avoid overlapping damp gauze or any other dressing onto the surrounding skin because it macerates the intact tissue.

A time saver

- To save time when dressing a wound with a drain, use precut tracheostomy pads or drain dressings instead of custom-cut gauze pads to fit around the drain. If the patient is sensitive to adhesive tape, use paper or silk tape because it's less likely to cause a skin reaction and peels off more easily than adhesive tape. Use a surgical mask to cradle a chin or jawline dressing to provide a secure dressing and to avoid the need to shave the patient's hair.

- If ordered, use a collodion spray or similar topical protectant instead of a gauze dressing. This moisture- and contaminant-proof covering dries in a clear, impermeable film that leaves the wound visible for observation and avoids the friction caused by a dressing.

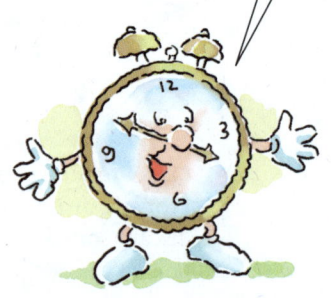

Using precut tracheostomy pads or drain dressings saves time.

- If a sump drain isn't adequately collecting wound secretions, reinforce it with an ostomy pouch or another collection bag. Use waterproof tape to strengthen a spot on the front of the pouch near the adhesive opening; then, cut a small x in the tape. Feed the drain catheter into the pouch through the x cut. Seal the cut around the tubing with more waterproof tape, then connect the tubing to the suction pump. This method frees the drainage port at the bottom of the pouch so the tubing doesn't have to be removed to empty the pouch. If more than one collection pouch is used for a wound or wounds, record drainage volume separately for each pouch. Avoid using waterproof material over the dressing because it reduces air circulation and promotes infection from accumulated heat and moisture.

Not the first time!!

- Because many healthcare providers prefer to change the first postoperative dressing themselves to check the incision, don't change the first dressing unless there are specific instructions to do so. If there aren't orders to change the dressing, and drainage comes through the dressing, reinforce the dressing with fresh sterile gauze. Request an order to change the dressing, or ask the healthcare provider to change it as soon as possible. A reinforced dressing shouldn't remain in place longer than 24 hours because it's an excellent medium for bacterial growth.

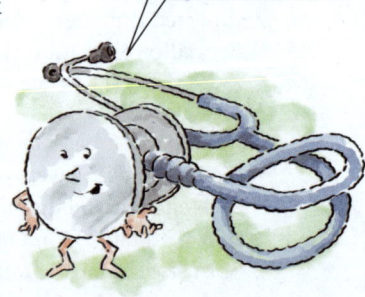

Don't perform the first dressing change unless you're given specific instructions to do so.

Check and recheck!

- For the recent postoperative patient or a patient with complications, check the dressing every 15 to 30 minutes or as ordered. For the patient with a healthy healing wound, check the dressing at least once every 8 hours.
- If the outside of the dressing becomes wet (e.g., from spilled drinking water), replace it as soon as possible to prevent wound contamination.
- If the patient will need wound care after discharge, provide appropriate teaching. If the patient will be doing self-care, stress the importance of using clean technique, and teach how to examine the wound for signs of infection and other complications. Also, demonstrate how to change dressings, and give written instructions for all procedures to be performed at home. If possible, have the patient do a return demonstration of the dressing change.

Closed-wound drain management

Typically inserted during surgery in anticipation of substantial postoperative drainage, a closed-wound drain promotes healing and prevents swelling by suctioning the serosanguineous fluid that accumulates at the wound site. By removing this fluid, the closed-wound drain helps reduce the risk of infection and skin breakdown, as well as the number of dressing changes.

Negative-pressure wound therapy (NPWT), also called *vacuum-assisted wound closure* (VAWC), is commonly used in deep surgical wounds or other larger wounds. Among other functions, it assists in healing by removing excess wound exudate, improves tissue perfusion and wound contraction, and reduces swelling (WUWHS, 2022). Other commonly used closed drainage systems include the Hemovac drain and the Jackson–Pratt drain.

A closed-wound drain consists of perforated tubing connected to a portable vacuum unit. The distal end of the tubing lies within the wound and usually leaves the body from a site other than the primary suture line to preserve the integrity of the surgical wound. The tubing exit site is treated as an additional surgical wound; the drain is usually sutured to the skin.

If the wound produces heavy drainage, the closed-wound drain may be left in place for longer than 1 week. Drainage must be emptied and measured frequently to maintain maximum suction and to prevent strain on the suture line.

Supplies
- graduated biohazard cylinder
- sterile laboratory container, if needed
- alcohol pads
- gloves
- gown
- face shield
- trash bag
- sterile gauze pads
- antiseptic cleaning agent
- prepackaged povidone–iodine swabs

Getting ready
- Check the healthcare provider's order, and assess the patient's condition.
- Explain the procedure to the patient, provide privacy, and wash hands.

How it's done
- Unclip the vacuum unit from the patient's bed or gown.
- Don clean gloves and, using clean technique, release the vacuum by removing the spout plug on the collection chamber. The container expands completely as it draws in air. (See *Using a closed-wound drainage system.*)
- Empty the unit's contents into a graduated biohazard cylinder, and note the amount and appearance of the drainage. If diagnostic

---

Using a closed-wound drainage system

The portable closed-wound drainage system draws drainage from a wound site, such as the chest wall postmastectomy (shown at left), by means of a Y-tube. To empty the drainage, remove the plug and empty it into a graduated cylinder. To reestablish suction, compress the drainage unit against a firm surface to expel air and, while holding it down, replace the plug with your other hand (as shown in the center). The same principle is used for the Jackson–Pratt bulb drain (shown at right).

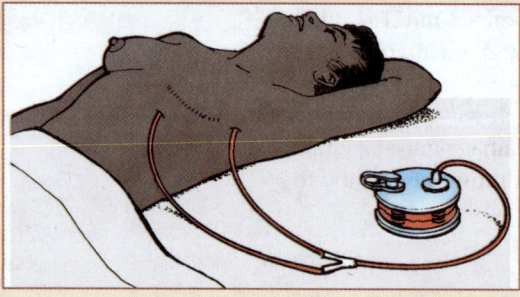
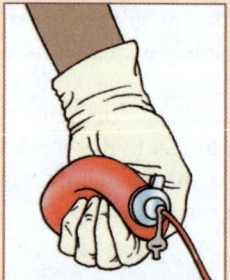
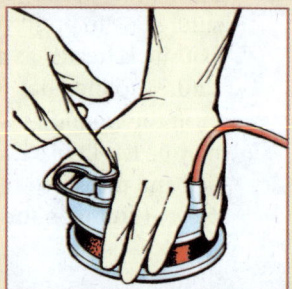

tests will be performed on the fluid specimen, pour the drainage directly into a sterile laboratory container, note the amount and appearance, and send it to the laboratory.
* Maintaining clean technique, use an alcohol pad to clean the unit's spout and plug.
* To reestablish the vacuum that creates the drain's suction power, fully compress the vacuum unit. With one hand holding the unit compressed to maintain the vacuum, replace the spout plug with your other hand.

No twist and shout!

* Check the patency of the equipment. Make sure the tubing is free from twists, kinks, and leaks because the drainage system must be airtight to work properly. The vacuum unit should remain compressed when manual pressure is released; rapid reinflation indicates an air leak. If reinflation occurs, recompress the unit and make sure the spout plug is secure.
* Secure the vacuum unit to the patient's gown. Fasten it below wound level to promote drainage. To avoid possible dislodgment, don't apply tension on drainage tubing when fastening the unit. Remove and discard gloves and wash hands thoroughly.

Be gentle

* Observe the sutures that secure the drain to the patient's skin; look for signs of pulling or tearing and for swelling or infection of surrounding skin. Gently clean the sutures with sterile gauze pads moistened with NSS or other solution as ordered.
* Properly dispose of drainage, solutions, and the trash bag, and clean or dispose of soiled equipment and supplies according to facility policy.

Practice pointers

* Empty the drain and measure its contents once during each shift if drainage has accumulated, more often if drainage is excessive. Removing excess drainage maintains maximum suction and avoids straining the drain's suture line.
* If the patient has more than one closed drain, number the drains so the drainage from each site can be clearly recorded.
* Document all care provided. (See *Documenting closed-wound drainage management.*)

Watch out!

* Note that the care of chest tubes with water seal drainage devices differs from the care of closed-wound drains. Be careful not to confuse the two, and never release the vacuum of a chest tube.

Take note!

Documenting closed-wound drainage management

Follow these tips when documenting the care of a closed-wound drainage unit. Record drainage color, consistency, type, and amount on the intake/output sheet. If the patient has more than one closed-wound drain, number the drains and record the information cited earlier separately for each drainage site.

Also, record:
* the date and time when the drain was emptied
* appearance of the drain site
* presence of swelling or signs of infection
* equipment malfunction and consequent nursing action
* the patient's tolerance of the treatment

A look at pressure injuries

Pressure injuries are a serious health problem. Although incidence figures vary widely because of differences in methodology, setting, and subjects, data gathered through 10 years of nationwide studies reveal that 10% to 15% of the general population suffers from chronic pressure injuries (Shi et al., 2021). Although this finding is significant in itself, prevalence in some groups—such as patients with spinal cord injuries, patients in intensive care units, and nursing home residents—can be as high as 50% (Chen et al., 2022).

At what cost?

Several types of costs are associated with pressure injuries: the cost in terms of suffering and diminished quality of life for patients, the cost to the healthcare industry in terms of resources consumed and manpower hours dedicated to managing the problem, and the monetary cost to individuals, health insurers, and government agencies (Shi et al., 2021). To encourage prevention, early intervention, and closer monitoring by the healthcare industry, many insurers and government agencies track outcomes to discern whether specific interventions help treat pressure injuries. Because pressure injuries are chronic conditions—that is, they're hard to heal and tend to recur frequently—prevention and early intervention are critical for more effective management.

Pressure injuries are costly—for the patient and for the healthcare industry.

OASIS

Data collected from Outcome and Assessment Information Set (OASIS) forms provide a basis for relating these costs to clinical outcomes. The OASIS-B1 form is currently used by home healthcare agencies, as mandated by the Centers for Medicare and Medicaid Services (CMS) (2023).

Close collaboration

Better disease management in pressure injury cases depends on closer collaboration among government agencies, insurers, and healthcare professionals. All involved are paying closer attention to prevention and the effectiveness of interventions, and they're finding better methods of quantifying and disseminating results. Starting in 2018, pressure injuries became a reportable condition for the CDC. In addition, current U.S. near-term healthcare objectives for the nation (Healthy People 2030) reflect an understanding of the problem's severity; one goal is to achieve by 2030 a reduction in pressure injuries–related hospitalization by 10% in patients older than 65 years of age (United States Department of Health and Human Services [USDHHS], 2023).

Causes

Chronic wounds are those that fail to heal in a timely manner, resist treatment, and tend to recur. Pressure injuries are chronic wounds resulting from tissue death due to prolonged, irreversible ischemia brought on by the compression of soft tissue (Bowers & Franco, 2020). In other words, pressure injuries are the clinical manifestation of localized tissue death due to a lack of blood flow in areas under pressure.

Simplify, simplify!

Time to simplify. First of all, different tissues have different tolerances for compression. Muscle and fat have comparatively low tolerances for pressure, whereas skin has a somewhat higher tolerance. All cells, regardless of tissue type, depend on blood circulation for the oxygen and nutrients they need. Tissue compression interferes with circulation, reducing or completely cutting off blood flow. The result, known as *ischemia*, is that cells fail to receive adequate supplies of oxygen and nutrients. Unless the pressure relents, cells eventually die. By the time inflammation signals impending necrosis on the surface of the skin, it's likely that necrosis has occurred in deeper tissues.

Location, location, location

Pressure injuries are most common in areas where pressure compresses soft tissue over a bony prominence in the body—that is, the tissue is pinched between the outer pressure and the hard underlying surface. The other three causal factors of skin breakdown are shear, friction, and moisture. Planning effective interventions for prevention and treatment requires a sound understanding of (1) the etiology of pressure injuries and (2) how to address the four causal factors.

Pressure

Capillaries are connected to arteries and veins through intermediary vessels called *arterioles* and *venules*. In healthy individuals, capillary filling pressure is approximately 32 mm Hg where arterioles connect to capillaries, and 12 mm Hg where capillaries connect to venules (Zaidi & Sharma, 2022). In frail or ill people, capillary filling pressures may be much lower. External pressure greater than capillary filling pressure can cause problems. External pressure that exceeds capillary perfusion pressure compresses blood vessels and causes ischemia in the tissues supplied by those vessels.

Tip of the iceberg

If the pressure continues long enough, capillaries collapse and thrombose, toxic metabolic by-products accumulate, and cells in nearby muscle and subcutaneous tissues begin to die. Muscle and fat are less tolerant of interruptions in blood flow than skin. Consequently, by the time signs of impending necrosis appear on the skin, underlying tissue has probably suffered substantial damage. Keep this "tip of the iceberg" effect in mind when assessing the size of a pressure injury. (See *Pressure points*.)

The pressure mounts

When external pressure exceeds venous capillary refill pressure (about 12 mm Hg), capillaries begin to leak. The resulting edema increases the amount of pressure on blood vessels, further impeding circulation. When interstitial pressure surpasses arterial intravascular pressure, blood is forced into nearby tissues (blanchable erythema). Continued capillary occlusion, lack of oxygen and nutrients, and buildup of toxic waste lead to necrosis of muscle, subcutaneous tissue, and, ultimately, the dermis and epidermis.

Spreading the load

The force associated with any given pressure increases as the amount of body surface exposed to the pressure decreases. For example, the force exerted on the buttocks of a person lying in bed is about 70 mm Hg. However, when the same person sits on a hard surface, the force exerted on the ischial tuberosities can exceed 100 mm Hg (Zaidi & Sharma, 2022). Consequently, bony prominences are particularly susceptible to

Pressure points

Pressure points are likely areas for pressure injury formation. These illustrations show the areas at highest risk for pressure injuries when the patient is in different positions.

Sitting

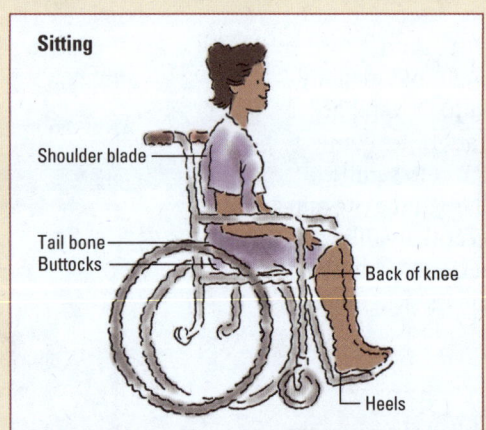

Shoulder blade

Tail bone
Buttocks

Back of knee

Heels

Lying

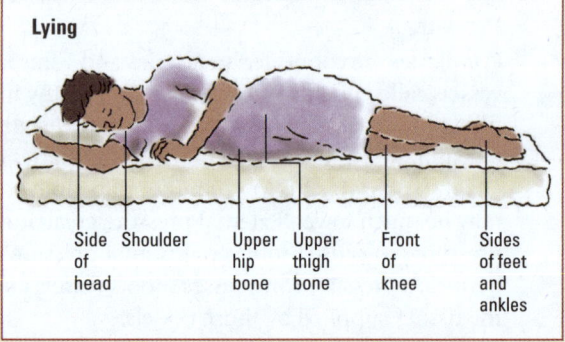

Side of head   Shoulder   Upper hip bone   Upper thigh bone   Front of knee   Sides of feet and ankles

pressure injuries. However, they aren't the only areas at risk. Pressure injuries can develop on any soft tissue subjected to prolonged pressure.

Between a bone and a hard place

When blood vessels, muscle, subcutaneous fat, and skin are compressed between a bone and an external surface such as a bed or chair, pressure is exerted on the tissues from the external surface and the bone. Essentially, the external surface produces pressure, and the bone produces counterpressure. These opposing forces create a cone-shaped pressure gradient. (See *Understanding the pressure gradient.*) Although the pressure impacts all tissues between these two points, tissues closest to the bony prominence suffer the greatest damage.

Long-term lows are losers

Over time, pressure causes a growing discomfort that prompts a person to change position before tissue ischemia occurs. In ulcer formation, an inverse relationship exists between time and pressure. Typically, low pressure for long periods is far more damaging than high pressure for short periods. For example, a pressure of 70 mm Hg sustained for 2 hours or longer almost always causes irreversible tissue damage, whereas a pressure of 240 mm Hg can be endured for a short time with little or no tissue damage. Furthermore, after the time–pressure threshold for damage passes, damage continues even after the pressure stops. Although pressure injuries can result from one period of sustained pressure, they're more likely to result from repeated ischemic events without adequate intervening time for recovery.

Understanding the pressure gradient

In this illustration, the V-shaped pressure gradient results from the upward force exerted by the supporting surface and the downward force of the bony prominence. Pressure is greatest on tissues at the apex of the gradient and lessens to the right and left of this point.

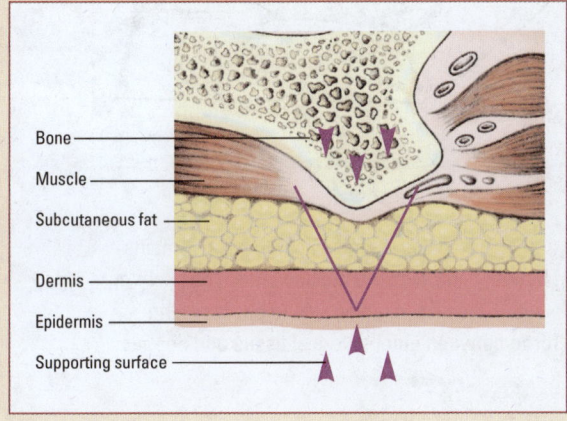

Bone
Muscle
Subcutaneous fat
Dermis
Epidermis
Supporting surface

Shear

Shearing force intensifies the pressure's destructive effects. Shear is a mechanical force that runs parallel, rather than perpendicular, to an area of skin; deep tissues feel the brunt of the force.

The shear truth of it

Shearing force is most likely to develop during repositioning or when a patient slides down after being placed in high-Fowler position. The force generated is enough to obstruct, tear, or stretch blood vessels. (See *Shearing force*.)

Shearing force reduces the length of time that tissue can endure a given pressure before ischemia or necrosis occurs. A sufficiently high level of shearing force can halve the amount of pressure needed to produce vascular occlusion. Research indicates that shearing force is responsible for the high incidence of triangular-shaped sacral ulcers and the large areas of tunneling or deep sinus tracts beneath these ulcers.

Shearing force

Shear is a mechanical force that is parallel, rather than perpendicular, to an area of tissue. As shown in this illustration, simply elevating the head of the bed increases shear and pressure in the sacral and coccygeal areas; gravity pulls the body down, but the skin on the back resists the motion because of friction between the

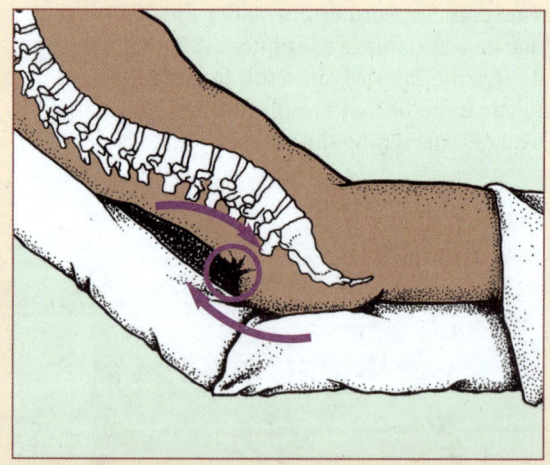

skin and the sheets. The skeleton and attached tissues move, but the skin remains stationary, held in place by friction between the skin and the bed linen. The skeleton and attached tissues actually slide within the skin, causing skin to pucker in the gluteal area, generating shearing force between outer layers of tissue and deeper layers.

Friction

Friction is another potentially damaging mechanical force. Friction develops as one surface moves across another surface—for example, the patient's skin sliding across the bedsheet. *Abrasions* are wounds created by friction.

Patients at particularly high risk for tissue damage due to friction include those who have uncontrollable movements or spastic conditions, patients who wear braces or appliances that rub against the skin, and older patients. Friction is also a problem for patients who have trouble lifting themselves during repositioning. Rubbing against the sheet can result in an abrasion, which increases the potential for deeper tissue damage. Elevating the head of the bed, as discussed earlier, generates friction between the patient's skin and the bed linen as gravity tugs the patient's body downward. As the skeleton moves inside the skin, friction and shearing force combine to increase the risk of tissue damage in the sacral area. Such dry lubricants as cornstarch and adherent dressings with slippery backings can help reduce the impact of friction.

Excessive moisture

Prolonged exposure to moisture can waterlog, or *macerate*, skin. Maceration contributes to pressure injury formation by softening the connective tissue. Macerated epidermis erodes more easily, degenerates, and eventually sloughs off. In addition, damp skin adheres to bed linen more readily, making friction's effects more profound. Consequently, moist skin is five times more likely to develop pressure injuries than dry skin. Excessive moisture can result from perspiration, wound drainage, bathing, or fecal or urinary incontinence.

Risk factors

Factors that increase the risk of developing pressure injuries include advancing age, immobility, incontinence, poor nutrition, and low blood pressure. High-risk patients, whether in an institution or at home, should be assessed regularly for pressure injuries.

Age

With advancing age, the skin becomes more fragile as epidermal turnover slows, vascularization decreases, and skin layers adhere less securely to one another. Older adults (those over 65 years of age) have less lean body mass and less subcutaneous tissue cushioning bony areas. Consequently, they're more likely to suffer tissue damage due to friction, shear, and pressure. (See *Aging and skin function*.)

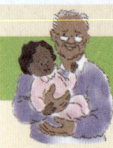

Ages and stages

Aging and skin function

Over time, skin loses its ability to function as efficiently or as effectively as it once did. As a result, the golden years of life place a person at greater risk for pressure injuries and tumors as well as various other skin conditions. This chart outlines the major changes that take place in the skin during the aging process and the implications of those changes for older adults.

Change	Implications
50% reduction in the cell turnover rate in the stratum corneum (outermost layer) and 20% reduction in dermal thickness	• Higher risk of infection because thinner skin is a less effective barrier to germs and allergens
Generalized reduction in dermal vascularization and an associated drop in blood flow to the skin	• Bruising more easily and increasing tendency of edema around wounds
Redistribution of subcutaneous tissue, which contains fewer fat cells in older adults, to the stomach and thighs	• Risk of hyperthermia or hypothermia • Higher incidence of ischemia (cell damage resulting from too little oxygen reaching cells) in compressed tissue of bony areas
Flattening of papillae in the dermoepidermal junction (meeting of the epidermis and dermis), which reduces adhesion between layers	• Much higher incidence of shear and tear injuries
Drop in the number of Langerhans cells (immune macrophages that attack invading germs) present in the skin	• Higher risk of infection • Slower sensitization response (redness, heat, discomfort), resulting in overuse of topical medications and more severe allergic reactions (because signs aren't evident early on)
50% decline in the number of fibroblasts and mast cells (cells that play a key role in the inflammatory response)	• Higher risk of infection
Marked reduction in the ability to sense pressure, heat, and cold, even though the same number of nerve endings in the skin are retained	• Higher incidence of pressure and thermal (hot and cold) damage to the skin • Higher incidence of ischemia (cell damage resulting from too little oxygen reaching cells) in compressed tissue • Higher incidence of skin tears
Significant decline in the number of sweat glands	• Difficulty with thermoregulation and increased risk of hyperthermia due to decreased production of sweat
Poorer absorption through the skin	• Risk of overdose of transdermal medications due to too frequent application
Reduction in the skin's ability to synthesize vitamin D	• Skin loses elasticity, and wrinkles develop

Source: Wang, Z., Man, M. Q., Li, T., Elias, P. M., & Mauro, T. M. (2020). Aging-associated alterations in epidermal function and their clinical significance. *Aging*, 12(6), 5551–5565. https://doi.org/10.18632/aging.102946

An older adult can experience altered pain perception, which can increase the risk of pressure injury development. Other common problems include poor nutrition, poor hydration, and impaired respiratory or immune systems.

Immobility

Immobility may be the greatest risk factor for pressure injury development. A risk assessment should always include the patient's ability to move in response to pressure sensations as well as the frequency with which their position is changed.

Incontinence

Incontinence increases a patient's exposure to moisture and, over time, increases their risk of skin breakdown. Urinary and fecal incontinences create problems as a result of excessive moisture and chemical irritation. Due to pathogens in stools, fecal incontinence can cause more skin damage than urinary incontinence. Feces contain both lipolytic and proteolytic enzymes, which are inactivated during passage through the gastrointestinal tract. When the feces come into contact with the urine, the urea in the urine is converted into ammonia. Ammonia causes a shift in the pH of the skin and feces to alkalinity, and this alkaline pH reactivates the enzymes in the feces.

Nutrition

Proper nutrition is vital to tissue integrity. A strong correlation exists between poor nutrition and pressure injuries, yet nutrition is all too commonly overlooked during treatment.

Albumin acumen

Increased protein is required for the body to heal itself. Albumin is one of the key proteins in the body. A patient's serum albumin level is an important indicator of their protein levels. A subnormal serum albumin level is a late manifestation of protein deficiency. Normal serum albumin levels range from 3.5 to 5.2 g/dL (Fischbach et al., 2022). Serum albumin deficits are ranked as:

- mild: greater than 3 to 3.5 g/dL
- moderate: 2.5 to 3 g/dL
- severe: less than 2.5 g/dL

Pressure injury occurrence and severity are linked to malnutrition. Multiple studies have established a direct correlation between pressure injury stage and degree of hypoalbuminemia (serum albumin level below 3.5 g/dL) (NPIAP, 2019). Monitor the serum albumin levels of a high-risk patient, and plan on nutritional intervention if they have hypoproteinemia.

Extra protein can help a patient's body heal itself.

Blood pressure

Low arterial blood pressure is clearly linked to tissue ischemia, particularly in vascular patients. When blood pressure is low, the body shunts blood away from the peripheral vascular system that serves the skin and toward vital organs to ensure their health. As perfusion drops, the skin is less tolerant of sustained external pressure, and the risk of damage due to ischemia rises.

Assessing risk factors

Several assessment tools are available to help determine a patient's risk of developing pressure injuries. The three most widely used scales are the Braden scale, the Norton scale, and the Waterlow scale (McNichol et al., 2022).

Common denominators

Most scales use the following factors to determine a patient's risk of developing pressure injuries:

- immobility
- inactivity
- incontinence
- malnutrition
- impaired mental status or sensation

Each category receives a value based on the patient's condition. The sum of these values determines the patient's score and level of risk. Scores for each category as well as the assessment as a whole guide the care team to develop appropriate interventions. Most healthcare facilities require an assessment score for all admitted patients.

The Braden scale

The Braden Pressure Sore Risk Assessment Scale is the most widely used scale. This tool scores etiologic factors that contribute to prolonged pressure as well as factors that contribute to diminished tissue tolerance for pressure. Factors scored in this assessment include sensory perception, moisture, activity, mobility, nutrition, and friction and shear. Each factor receives a score of 1 to 4, with the exception of friction and shear, which receives a score of 1 to 3. The highest possible score is 23; the lower the score, the higher the patient's risk of pressure injury. A score of 18 or lower denotes a risk of pressure injury.

In nursing home populations, most pressure injuries develop during the 2 weeks immediately following admission, so early identification of at-risk patients is crucial. The Wound Ostomy & Continence Nurses Society (WOCN) Guidelines for Pressure Ulcer Prevention (2017) recommends that all healthcare settings establish the following cadence for conducting risk assessment to ensure accuracy of assessments between/among nurses:

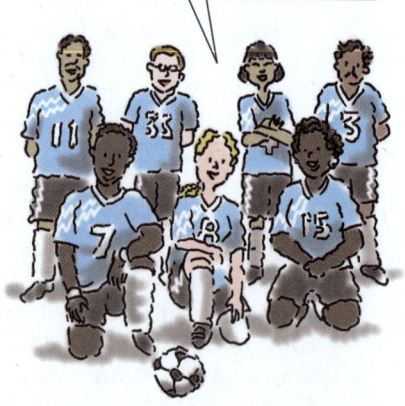

Overall assessment and scores for each category of pressure injury risk guide the medical team to develop appropriate interventions.

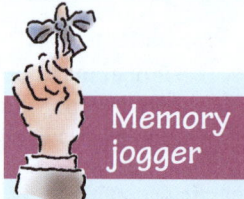

Memory jogger

To remember the five factors commonly used to determine a patient's risk of developing pressure injuries, think of the 5 I's:

Immobility

Inactivity

Incontinence

Improper nutrition (malnutrition)

Impaired mental status or sensation

- **Long-term care (LTC):** On admission and daily for a week—and then quarterly or follow the facility policy
- **Acute care:** On admission and daily on each shift
- **Long-term acute care (LTAC):** Daily for the first week, then weekly

Pressure injury prevention

Pressure injury prevention focuses on compensating for prevailing risk factors and addressing the underlying pathophysiology. When planning interventions, be sure to adopt a holistic approach and to consider all of the patient's needs.

Managing pressure

Managing the intensity and duration of pressure is a fundamental goal in prevention, especially for the patient with mobility limitations. Frequent, careful repositioning helps the patient avoid damaging repetitive pressure that can cause tissue ischemia and subsequent necrosis. When repositioning the patient, it's important to reduce the duration and intensity of pressure.

Positioning

Any time the patient is repositioned, look for telltale areas of reddened skin and make sure the new position doesn't place weight on these areas. Avoid the use of donut-shaped supports or ring cushions that encircle the ischemic area because these can reduce blood flow to an even wider expanse of tissue. If the affected area is on an extremity, use pillows to support the limb and reduce pressure. As noted earlier, avoid raising the head of the bed more than 30° to prevent tissue damage due to friction and shearing force.

Short stepping it

Inactivity increases a patient's risk of pressure injury development. To the degree that the patient is physically able, encourage activity. Start with a short step, such as helping them out of bed and into a chair. As tolerance improves, help them walk around the room and then down the hall.

Positioning a patient in bed

When the patient is on their side, never allow weight to rest directly on the greater trochanter of the femur. Instead, have the patient rest their weight on their buttock and use a pillow or foam wedge to maintain the position. This position ensures that no pressure is placed on the trochanter or sacrum. Also, a pillow placed between the knees or ankles minimizes the pressure exerted when one limb lies atop the other. (See *Repositioning a reclining patient.*)

Heel appeal

Heels present a particularly difficult challenge. Even with the aid of specially designed cushions, reducing the pressure on heels to below capillary refill pressure is almost impossible. Instead, suspend the patient's foot so the bony prominence on the heel is under no pressure. A pillow or foam cushion under the patient's calves can permit a comfortable position while suspending the foot. Take care to avoid knee contraction, however. Use a heel pressure redistribution device if the facility has this product.

Repositioning a reclining patient

When repositioning a reclining patient, use the Rule of 30, which is raising the head of the bed 30° (as shown top right). To prevent the buildup of shearing pressure, avoid raising the head of the bed more than 30°. When it must be raised more—at mealtimes, for instance—keep the periods brief.

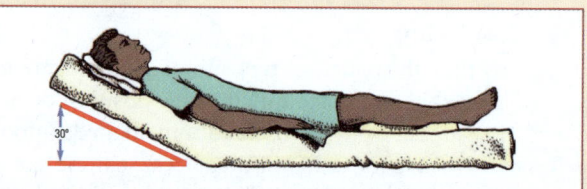

As the patient is repositioned from their left to their right side, make sure their weight rests on their buttock, not their hip bone. Resting weight on the buttock reduces pressure on the trochanter and sacrum. The angle between the bed and an imaginary lateral line through their hips should be about 30°. If needed, use pillows or a foam wedge to help the patient maintain the proper position (see illustration bottom right). Cushion pressure points, such as the knees and shoulders, with pillows as well.

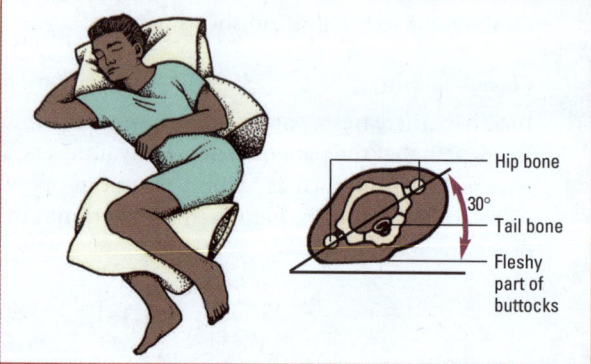

Positioning a seated patient

A patient is more likely to develop pressure injuries from sitting than from reclining. Sitting tends to focus all of the patient's weight on the relatively small surface areas of the buttocks, thighs, and soles. Much of this weight is focused on the small area of tissue covering the ischial tuberosities. Proper posture and alignment help ensure that the weight of the patient's body is distributed as evenly as possible.

Posture perfect

Proper posture alone can significantly reduce the patient's risk of pressure injuries at the ankles, elbows, forearms, wrists, and knees. Explain proper posture to the patient, if necessary, as described here:

- Sit with back erect and against the back of the chair, thighs parallel to the floor, knees comfortably parted, and arms horizontal and supported by the arms of the chair. This posture distributes weight evenly over the available body surface area.
- Keep feet flat on the floor to protect the heels from focused pressure and distribute the weight of the legs over the largest available surface area, which is the soles.
- Avoid slouching, which causes shearing force and friction and places undue pressure on the sacrum and coccyx.
- Keep the thighs and arms parallel to ensure that weight is evenly distributed all along the thighs and forearms, instead of being focused on the ischial tuberosities and elbows, respectively.
- Part the knees to keep knees and ankles from rubbing together.

The comforts of home

If the patient likes to use an ottoman or footstool, check to see if their knees end up above the level of their hips. If so, it means that their weight has shifted from the back of their thighs to the ischial tuberosities, and that they need to find a different footstool. The same problem—knees above hips—can occur if the chair itself is too short for the patient.

Patients at risk should reposition themselves every 15 minutes while sitting, if they can. Patients with spinal cord injuries can perform wheelchair pushups to intermittently relieve pressure on the buttocks and sacrum. This requires a fair amount of upper body strength, however, and some patients might not have the strength. Others may have injuries that preclude using this technique.

Pillows may be the most enduring support tools on the planet, but they're no longer the only options available. Today, people can choose from a vast array of support surfaces and cushioning aids. Special beds, mattresses, and seating options that employ foams, gels, water, and air as cushioning agents make it possible to tailor a comprehensive and personal system of supports for the patient.

Effective care depends on knowledge of the classes and types of products. Take time to learn about these products. (See *Pressure redistribution devices*.)

False security

Be informed, but be cautious as well. Using these devices can instill a false sense of security. It's important to remember that as helpful as these devices may be, they aren't substitutes for attentive care. Patients require individual turning schedules, regardless of the equipment used, and this schedule depends on an assessment of the patient's tolerance for pressure.

Beds and mattresses

When horizontal support surfaces are referred to, this most often means beds, mattresses, and mattress overlays. These products employ foams, gels, water, and air to minimize the pressure a patient experiences while lying in bed.

Pressure redistribution devices

Here are some special pads, mattresses, and beds that help redistribute pressure when a patient is confined to one position for long periods:
• Gel pads disperse pressure over a wide surface area.
• Water mattress or pads produce a wave effect that provides even distribution of body weight.
• Alternating-pressure air mattress involves alternating deflation and inflation of mattress tubes that changes areas of pressure.
• Foam mattress or pads, which must be a high-density foam, at least 3 to 4 inches (7.5 to 10 cm) thick, cushion skin, minimizing pressure. Solid foam is more effective than convoluted foam.

• Low-air-loss bed has a surface that consists of inflated air cushions. Each section is adjusted for optimal pressure relief for the patient's body size.
• Air-fluidized bed contains beads that move under an airflow to support the patient, thus reducing shearing force and friction and assisting in redistributing pressure.
• Mechanical lifting device, including lift sheets and other devices, prevents shearing by lifting the patient rather than dragging them across the bed.
• Padding, including pillows, towels, and soft blankets, can reduce pressure in body hollows.
• Foot cradle lifts the bed linens to remove pressure over the feet.

Beds

Some specialty beds and mattresses have low shear surfaces, provide some air circulation, and have pressure redistribution properties. Beds that have the "turn assist" feature help to *assist* nurses with turning the patient. These beds *do not* turn the patient enough to provide pressure redistribution. There are other beds that do 30° to 60° turns, and these beds are for pulmonary patients, *not* for pressure redistribution.

Mattresses

If the patient's weight completely compresses a mattress overlay, the overlay isn't helping. To make sure the patient isn't bottoming out, hand-check whenever a new overlay is put into service or if overlay breakdown is suspected. To hand-check an overlay, slide one hand, palm up and fingers outstretched, between the mattress overlay and the mattress. If the patient's body can be felt through the overlay, replace the overlay with a thicker one or add more air to the mattress.

Support aids for sitting

Products designed to help prevent pressure injuries while sitting fall into two broad categories: products that redistribute pressure and products that ease repositioning.

Redistributing pressure

Ambulatory and wheelchair-dependent patients should use seat cushions to distribute weight over the largest possible surface area. Wheelchair-dependent patients require an especially rugged seat cushion that can stand up to the rigors of daily use. In most instances, a good foam cushion of 3 to 4 inches (7.5 to 10 cm) thick suffices. However, many wheelchair-seating clinics now use computers to create custom seating systems tailored to fit the physiology and needs of each patient. For patients with spinal cord injuries, the selection of wheelchair seating is based on pressure evaluation, lifestyle, postural stability, continence, and cost. Custom seats and cushions are more expensive; however, the added expense is justifiable. Encourage wheelchair patients to replace their seat cushion as soon as their current one begins to deteriorate.

A position on repositioning

Repositioning is just as important when the patient is sitting as when they're reclining. For a patient requiring assistance in repositioning, devices such as overhead frames, trapezes, walkers, and canes are available. Healthcare personnel can help maneuver IV poles and other support equipment.

Managing skin integrity

An effective skin integrity management plan includes regular inspections for tissue breakdown, routine cleaning and moisturizing, and steps to protect the skin from incontinence, if this is an issue.

Inspecting the skin

The patient's skin should be routinely inspected for pressure areas, depending on the patient's assessed risk and their ability to tolerate pressure. Check for pallor and areas of redness, which are both signs of ischemia. Be aware that redness that occurs after the pressure is removed (called *reactive hyperemia*) is commonly the first external sign of ischemia due to pressure.

Cleaning the skin

Cleaning with a gentle soap and warm water usually suffices for daily skin hygiene. Use a soft cloth to pat, rather than rub, the skin dry. Avoid scrubbing or the use of harsh cleaning agents.

Moisturizing the skin

Skin becomes dry, flaky, and less pliable when it loses moisture. Dry skin is more susceptible to ulceration. Avoid powder, especially for older adult patients, because it can cause further drying of the skin. The number of skin moisturizing products available is truly staggering, so it shouldn't be hard to find one that the patient likes. The three categories of skin moisturizers are lotions, creams, and ointments.

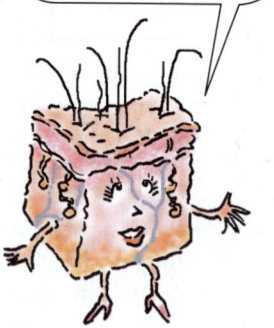

Effective management of skin integrity requires regular inspections as well as routine cleaning and moisturizing, and protecting the skin from incontinence.

Lotion notion

Lotions are dissolved powder crystals held in suspension by surfactants. Lotions have the highest water content and evaporate faster than any other type of moisturizer. Consequently, lotions must be applied more often than creams and ointments. The high water content is why lotions feel cool as they're applied.

Cream regime

Creams are preparations of oil and water or water in oil. Water-in-oil creams are more moisturizing because they provide an oily barrier that reduces water loss from the stratum corneum, the outermost layer of the skin. Creams don't have to be applied as often as lotions; three or four applications per day should do the trick.

Ointment appointment

Ointments are preparations of oil in water (typically lanolin or petrolatum) and are the best for skin protection against moisture. They're occlusive, meaning that they create a barrier over the skin that traps moisture and prevents water loss.

Protecting the skin

Although some moisture is good, too much is a problem. Waterlogged skin is easily eroded by friction and is more susceptible to irritants and bacteria colonization than dry skin. Close monitoring helps to head off problems before they escalate.

Skin protection is particularly important if the patient is incontinent. Urine and feces introduce chemical irritants and bacteria as well as moisture, which can speed skin breakdown. To effectively manage incontinence, determine the cause, and then plan interventions that protect skin integrity while addressing the underlying problem.

In older adults, don't assume that incontinence is a normal part of aging. It isn't. Instead, consider factors that can precipitate incontinence, such as:

- fecal impaction and tube feeding (can cause diarrhea)
- reaction to a medication (can cause urinary incontinence)
- urinary tract infection
- mobility problems (can keep the patient from reaching the bathroom in time)
- confusion or embarrassment (can keep the patient from asking for a bedpan or help to get to the bathroom)

Lend a helping hand

Whether the underlying cause is reversible or not, encourage the patient to ask for help when they need a bedpan or to go to the bathroom. Use incontinence collectors, adult briefs or under pads that wick and gel, and skin barriers, as appropriate, to minimize skin damage. Step up the frequency of inspections, cleaning, and moisturizing for these patients.

Assessing for pressure injuries

Pressure injuries can occur even with the best preventive measures. Effective treatment depends on a thorough assessment of the developing wound. Meaningful pressure injury assessment requires a systematic, objective approach. In addition to the wound assessment parameters described at the beginning of the chapter, also document the pressure injury history, including etiology, duration, and prior treatment.

On the border

Pressure injury borders can provide clues to healing potential. As discussed earlier, assess the skin around the pressure injury for:

- redness
- warmth

- induration or hardness
- swelling
- signs of infection

Before you examine the pressure injury, assess the patient's pain. In most cases, pressure injuries cause some degree of pain; in some cases, pain is severe. Have the patient rate their pain on a verbal or visual analog scale of 0 to 10, with 0 representing no pain and 10 representing severe pain. Similarly, ask the patient whether the pain interferes with their ability to function normally and, if so, to what degree.

Location

Common locations for pressure injuries include:

- sacrum
- coccyx
- ischial tuberosities
- greater trochanters
- elbows
- heels
- scapulae
- occipital bone
- sternum
- ribs
- iliac crests
- patellae
- lateral malleoli
- medial malleoli

Bottoming out

Pressure injuries are more common on the lower half of the body because it has more major bony prominences and more body weight than the upper half of the body. Two-thirds of pressure injuries occur within the pelvic girdle.

Characteristics

Tissue involvement ranges from blanchable erythema to the deep destruction of tissue associated with a full-thickness wound. Pressure against tissue interrupts blood flow and causes pallor due to tissue ischemia. If prolonged, ischemia causes irreversible and extensive tissue damage.

Reactive hyperemia

Usually, reactive hyperemia is the first visible sign of ischemia. When the pressure causing ischemia is released, the skin flushes red as blood rushes back into the tissue. This reddening is called *reactive hyperemia*, and it's due to a protective mechanism in the body that dilates vessels in the affected area to increase blood flow and speed oxygen to starved tissues. Reactive hyperemia first appears as a bright flush that lasts about one-half or three-quarters as long as the ischemic period. If the applied pressure is too high for too long, reactive hyperemia fails to meet the demand for blood, and tissue damage occurs (McNichol et al., 2022).

Blanchable erythema

Blanchable erythema (redness) can signal imminent tissue damage. Erythema results from capillary dilation near the skin's surface. In the patient with pressure injuries, the redness results from the release of ischemia-causing pressure. Blanchable erythema is redness that blanches (turns white) when pressed with a fingertip, and then immediately turns red again when pressure is removed. Tissue exhibiting blanchable erythema usually resumes its normal color within 24 hours and suffers no long-term damage. However, the longer it takes for tissue to recover from finger pressure, the higher the patient's risk of developing pressure injuries.

In dark-skinned patients, erythema is hard to discern. Use a bright light and look for taut, shiny patches of skin with a purplish tinge. Also, assess carefully for localized heat, induration, or edema, which can be better indicators of ischemia than erythema.

Nonblanchable erythema

Nonblanchable erythema can be the first sign of tissue destruction. In high-risk patients, nonblanchable tissue can develop in as little as 2 hours. The redness associated with nonblanchable erythema is more intense and doesn't change when compressed with a finger. If recognized and treated early, nonblanchable erythema is reversible.

What is not seen

In many cases, the full extent of ulceration can't be determined by visual inspection because there may be extensive undermining along the fascial planes. For example, tunneling can connect pressure injuries over the sacrum to those over the trochanter of the femur or the ischial tuberosities. These cavities can contain extensive necrotic tissue.

Staging pressure injuries

The most widely used system for staging pressure injuries is the classification system developed by the NPIAP (2019); see the information on pages 486–487.

NPIAP STAGING FOR LIGHTLY PIGMENTED SKIN

NPIAP NATIONAL PRESSURE INJURY ADVISORY PANEL

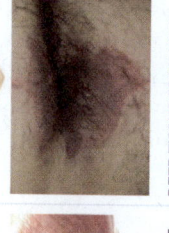

STAGE 1 PRESSURE INJURY: NON-BLANCHABLE ERYTHEMA OF INTACT SKIN

Intact skin with a localized area of non-blanchable erythema, which may appear differently in darkly pigmented skin. Presence of blanchable erythema or changes in sensation, temperature, or firmness may precede visual changes. Color changes do not include purple or maroon discoloration; these may indicate deep tissue pressure injury.

STAGE 2 PRESSURE INJURY: PARTIAL-THICKNESS SKIN LOSS WITH EXPOSED DERMIS

Partial-thickness skin loss with exposed dermis. The wound bed is viable, pink or red, moist, and may also present as an intact or ruptured serum-filled blister. Adipose (fat) is not visible and deeper tissues are not visible. Granulation tissue, slough and eschar are not present. These injuries commonly result from adverse microclimate and shear in the skin over the pelvis and shear in the heel.

STAGE 3 PRESSURE INJURY: FULL-THICKNESS SKIN LOSS

Full-thickness loss of skin, in which adipose (fat) is visible in the ulcer and granulation tissue and epibole (rolled wound edges) are often present. Slough and/or eschar may be visible. The depth of tissue damage varies by anatomical location; areas of significant adiposity can develop deep wounds. Undermining and tunneling may occur. Fascia, muscle, tendon, ligament, cartilage or bone is not exposed. If slough or eschar obscures the extent of tissue loss this is an Unstageable Pressure Injury.

STAGE 4 PRESSURE INJURY: FULL-THICKNESS LOSS OF SKIN AND TISSUE

Full-thickness skin and tissue loss with exposed or directly palpable fascia, muscle, tendon, ligament, cartilage or bone in the ulcer. Slough and/or eschar may be visible. Epibole (rolled edges), undermining and/or tunneling often occur. Depth varies by anatomical location. If slough or eschar obscures the extent of tissue loss this is an Unstageable Pressure Injury.

UNSTAGEABLE PRESSURE INJURY: OBSCURED FULL-THICKNESS SKIN AND TISSUE LOSS

Full-thickness skin and tissue loss in which the extent of tissue damage within the ulcer cannot be confirmed because it is obscured by slough or eschar. If slough or eschar is removed, a Stage 3 or Stage 4 pressure injury will be revealed. Stable eschar (i.e. dry, adherent, intact without erythema or fluctuance) on an ischemic limb or the heel(s) should not be softened or removed.

DEEP TISSUE PRESSURE INJURY: PERSISTENT NON-BLANCHABLE DEEP RED, MAROON OR PURPLE DISCOLORATION

Intact or non-intact skin with localized area of persistent non-blanchable deep red, maroon, purple discoloration or epidermal separation revealing a dark wound bed or blood-filled blister. Pain and temperature change often precede skin color changes. Discoloration may appear differently in darkly pigmented skin. This injury results from intense and/or prolonged pressure and shear forces at the bone-muscle interface.

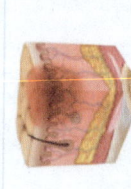
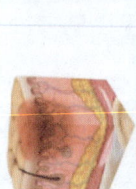
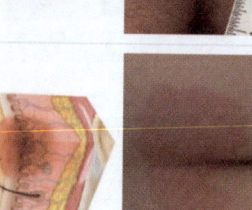
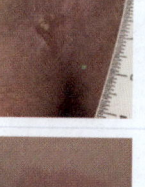
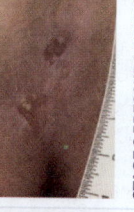
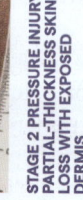
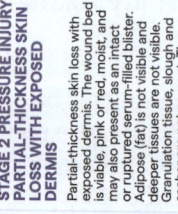
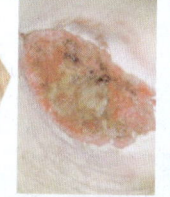

A pressure injury is localized damage to the skin and underlying soft tissue usually over a bony prominence or related to a medical or other device. The injury can present as intact skin or an open ulcer and may be painful. The injury occurs as a result of intense and/or prolonged pressure or pressure in combination with shear. The tolerance of soft tissue for pressure and shear may also be affected by microclimate, nutrition, perfusion, co-morbidities and condition of the soft tissue.

Hill•rom

(Reprinted with permission from NPIAP [https://npiap.com/page/PressureInjuryStages].)

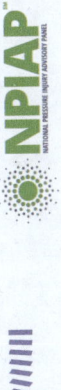

NPIAP STAGING FOR DARKLY PIGMENTED SKIN

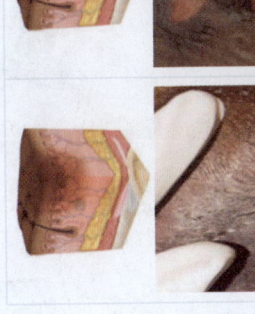
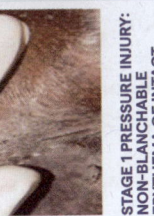
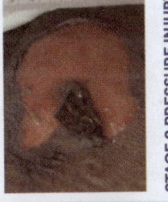
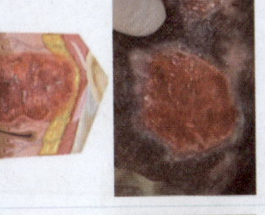

STAGE 1 PRESSURE INJURY: NON-BLANCHABLE ERYTHEMA OF INTACT SKIN

Intact skin with a localized area of non-blanchable erythema, which may appear differently in darkly pigmented skin. Presence of blanchable erythema or changes in sensation, temperature, or firmness may precede visual changes. Color changes do not include purple or maroon discoloration; these may indicate deep tissue pressure injury.

STAGE 2 PRESSURE INJURY: PARTIAL-THICKNESS SKIN LOSS WITH EXPOSED DERMIS

Partial-thickness skin loss with exposed dermis. The wound bed is viable, pink or red, moist, and may also present as an intact or ruptured serum-filled blister. Adipose (fat) is not visible and deeper tissues are not visible. Granulation tissue, slough and eschar are not present. These injuries commonly result from adverse microclimate and shear in the skin over the pelvis and shear in the heel.

STAGE 3 PRESSURE INJURY: FULL-THICKNESS SKIN LOSS

Full-thickness loss of skin, in which adipose (fat) is visible in the ulcer and granulation tissue and epibole (rolled wound edges) are often present. Slough and/or eschar may be visible. The depth of tissue damage varies by anatomical location; areas of significant adiposity can develop deep wounds. Undermining and tunneling may occur. Fascia, muscle, tendon, ligament, cartilage or bone is not exposed. If slough or eschar obscures the extent of tissue loss this is an Unstageable Pressure Injury.

STAGE 4 PRESSURE INJURY: FULL-THICKNESS LOSS OF SKIN AND TISSUE

Full-thickness skin and tissue loss with exposed or directly palpable fascia, muscle, tendon, ligament, cartilage or bone in the ulcer. Slough and/or eschar may be visible. Epibole (rolled edges), undermining and/or tunneling often occur. Depth varies by anatomical location. If slough or eschar obscures the extent of tissue loss this is an Unstageable Pressure Injury.

UNSTAGEABLE PRESSURE INJURY: OBSCURED FULL-THICKNESS SKIN AND TISSUE LOSS

Full-thickness skin and tissue loss in which the extent of tissue damage within the ulcer cannot be confirmed because it is obscured by slough or eschar. If slough or eschar is removed, a Stage 3 or Stage 4 pressure injury will be revealed. Stable eschar (i.e. dry, adherent, intact without erythema or fluctuance) on an ischemic limb or the heel(s) should not be softened or removed.

DEEP TISSUE PRESSURE INJURY: PERSISTENT NON-BLANCHABLE DEEP RED, MAROON OR PURPLE DISCOLORATION

Intact or non-intact skin with localized area of persistent non-blanchable deep red, maroon, purple discoloration or epidermal separation revealing a dark wound bed or blood-filled blister. Pain and temperature change often precede skin color changes. Discoloration may appear differently in darkly pigmented skin. This injury results from intense and/or prolonged pressure and shear forces at the bone-muscle interface.

TIPS FOR STAGING DARKLY PIGMENTED SKIN:

- Inspect for changes in pigmentation
- Palpate for edema
- Ask about pain in the area
- Moisten the skin
- Avoid direct light

Hillrom™

Educational materials produced by Hillrom in collaboration with NPIAP.
© 2020 NATIONAL PRESSURE INJURY ADVISORY PANEL | WWW.NPIAP.COM
APR41801 REV1 14-FEB-2020 ENG – US

(Reprinted with permission from NPIAP [https://npiap.com/page/PressureInjuryStages].)

Now appearing on stage

Pressure injury characteristics gained from the nurse's assessment can be used to stage the pressure injury. Staging reflects the anatomic depth of exposed tissue. Keep in mind that if the wound contains necrotic tissue, the stage can't be determined until the wound base can be seen.

Staging reflects the depth and extent of tissue involvement. Restaging isn't needed unless deeper layers of tissue are exposed by treatments such as debridement. Keep in mind that although staging is useful for classifying pressure injuries, it's only one part of a comprehensive assessment. Pressure injury characteristics and the condition of the surrounding skin provide equally important clues to the pressure injury's prognosis.

Mucosal pressure injuries

Pressure injuries that occur related to medical devices often form on mucosal tissue (lips, nares, urinary meatal opening, tongue, etc.) can't be staged with the pressure injury staging system. Mucous membranes do not have the same histologic structure as the skin. Classify these pressure injuries as partial or full thickness.

Reverse staging

When a pressure injury develops, and the tissue and structures are destroyed, they aren't replaced during the healing process. Therefore, a stage 4 pressure injury doesn't become a stage 3 as it becomes shallower, then a 2 and then a 1. This pressure injury is a healing stage 4 or a healed stage 4, period!

Treating pressure injuries

Treatment of pressure injuries follows the four basic steps common to all wound care (Beeckman et al., 2020; NPIAP, 2019):
1. Debride necrotic tissue and clean the wound to remove debris.
2. Provide a moist wound healing environment through the use of proper dressings.
3. Protect the wound from further injury.
   Provide nutrition that's essential to wound healing.

A key element in all pressure injury treatment plans is identifying and treating, when possible, the underlying pathophysiology. If the cause of the pressure injury remains, existing pressure injuries don't heal, and new pressure injuries develop.

That's so typical

Typically, wound care involves cleaning the wound, debriding necrotic tissue, and applying a dressing that keeps the wound bed moist. Topical agents are used to resolve various issues.

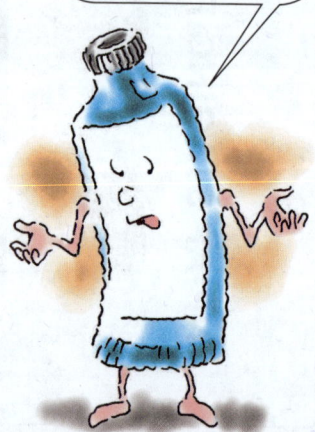

Topical agents can be used to treat some wound issues. Usually, cleaning, debriding, and dressings are part of treatment as well.

Pressure injury list of DO and DO NOT

With proper skin care and frequent position changes, patients and their caregivers can keep the patient's skin healthy, which a crucial element in pressure injury prevention. Here is some important information to pass along to patients:

DO...

• Change position at least once every 2 hours while reclining. Follow a schedule. Lie on the right side, then the left side, then the back, then the stomach (if possible). Use pillows and pads for support. Make small position changes between the 2-hour changes.

• Check your skin for signs of pressure injuries twice daily. Use a mirror to check areas you can't inspect directly, such as the shoulders, tailbone, hips, elbows, heels, and the back of the head. Report to the healthcare provider any breaks in the skin or changes in skin temperature.

• Follow the prescribed exercise program, including range-of-motion exercises every 8 hours or as recommended.

• Eat a well-balanced diet, drink lots of fluids, and strive to maintain the recommended weight.

DO NOT...

• Do not use commercial soaps or skin products that dry or irritate the skin. Instead, use oil-free lotions.

• Do not sleep on wrinkled bed sheets or tuck covers tightly into the foot of the bed.

Patient education

Remember that the goal of patient education is to improve the outcome. For any care plan to succeed after the patient leaves the hospital, the patient or caregiver must understand the care plan, be physically capable of carrying it out at home, and perceive value in the information and the outcomes. Therefore, education and goal establishment should take into consideration the preferences and lifestyles of the patient and their family whenever possible.

Teach the patient and their family how to prevent pressure injuries and what to do when they occur. (See *Pressure injury list of DO and DO NOT.*) Explain repositioning and show them what a 30° laterally inclined position looks like. If the patient needs assistance with repositioning, make sure they know the types of devices available and where to obtain them.

Mirror, mirror ...

Show the patient how they can inspect their back and other areas using a mirror. If the patient can't do this, a family member can help. Make sure they understand the importance of inspecting skin over bony prominences for pressure-related damage every day.

If the patient needs to apply dressings at home, make sure they know the proper way to apply and remove them. Tell them where to get supplies if they run low.

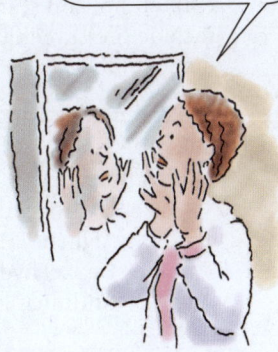

Teach the patient how to inspect their back and other areas using a mirror.

Ensuring proper nutrition can be difficult, but the patient and their family need to know how important proper nutrition is to the healing process. Provide materials on nutrition and maintaining an ideal weight, as appropriate. Show them how to create an easy-to-read chart of care reminders for a wall at home.

Pressure injuries should be reassessed weekly. Measure progress by the reduction in necrotic tissue and drainage and the increase in granulation tissue and epithelial growth. Clean, vascularized pressure injuries should show evidence of healing within 2 weeks. If they don't, and the patient has followed the guidelines for nutrition, repositioning, use of support surfaces, and wound care, it's time to reevaluate the care plan.

Quick quiz

1. The phases of wound healing are:
   A. hemostasis, inflammation, proliferation, and maturation.
   B. hemostasis, epithelialization, and scarring.
   C. epithelialization, inflammation, scarring, and maturation.
   D. chemical mediation, granulation, and maturation.

Answer: A. Though it rarely occurs in this order, the process of wound healing has four specific phases: hemostasis, inflammation, proliferation, and maturation.

2. A nurse is caring for a patient with a wound that is healing by secondary intention. Which description best describes this wound?
   A. A wound that is intentionally left open over a longer period of time to allow edema or infection to resolve or permit removal of exudate
   B. A full- or partial-thickness wound that is left open to fill with granulation tissue, followed by reepithelialization, then scar formation
   C. A superficial wound that heals through reepithelization
   D. A full-thickness wound that is surgically closed

Answer: B. Wounds that are left open to fill with granulation tissue, epithelium, and scar tissue heal by secondary intention. Examples include pressure injuries, burns, dehisced surgical wounds, and traumatic injuries.

3. A nurse is caring for a patient with a wound that needs to maintain moisture. Which of the following wound dressings are designed for this purpose?
   A. Hydrogel dressings
   B. Alginate, Hydrofiber, and foam dressings
   C. Gauze, hydrocolloid, and transparent film dressings
   D. Antimicrobial and foam dressings

Answer: C. Wound characteristics determine which type of dressing to use, and dressings are designed to either maintain, donate, or absorb moisture. Gauze, hydrocolloid, and foam dressings all maintain moisture in a wound.

4.   A pressure injury that is full-thickness with tissue damage or necrosis of subcutaneous tissue that can extend down to, but not through, underlying fasciae is which stage of a pressure injury?

    A.   Stage 1
    B.   Stage 2
    C.   Stage 3
    D.   Stage 4

Answer: C. Full thickness with destruction of but not through fasciae is a stage 3 pressure injury.

Scoring

 If you answered all four questions correctly, superb! You have a lot of integrity when it comes to knowledge of skin and wounds.

 If you answered three questions correctly, great! You're holding up well under the pressure.

    If you answered fewer than three questions correctly, relax! Just take a load off, review the chapter, and try again.

References

Avsar, P., Moore, Z., & Patton, D. (2021). Dressings for preventing pressure ulcers: How do thy work? *Journal of Wound Care, 30*(1), 33–39. https://doi.org/10.12968/jowc.2021.30.1.33

Beeckman, D. E., Campbell, K. E., LeBlanc, K., Campbell, J., Dunk, A. M., Harley, C., Holloway, S., Langemo, D., Romanelli, M., Tariq, G., & Vuagnat, H. (2020). Best practice recommendations for holistic strategies to promote and maintain skin integrity. *Wounds International*, 1–32. https://woundsinternational.com/best-prac-tice-statements/best-practice-recommendations-holistic-strategies-promote-and-maintain-skin-integrity/

Bennett, J., Dolin, R., & Blaser, M. (2020). *Principles and practice of infectious diseases* (9th ed.). Elsevier.

Boulton, A., Armstrong, D., Löndahl, M., Frykberg, R., Game, F., Edmonds, M., Orgill, D., Kramer, K., Gurtner, G., Januszyk, M., & Vileikyte, L. (2022). New evidence-based therapies for complex diabetic foot wounds. *American Diabetes Association Clinical Compendia, 2*, 1–23. https://doi.org/10.2337/db2022-02

Bowers, S., & Franco, E. (2020). Chronic wounds: Evaluation and management. *American Family Physician, 101*(3), 159–166.

Centers for Disease Control and Prevention (CDC). (2017). Guidelines for the prevention of surgical site infection. https://www.cdc.gov/infectioncontrol/guidelines/ssi/index.html

Centers for Medicare and Medicaid Services (CMS). (2023). Home health quality reporting program. https://www.cms.gov/medicare/quality-initiatives-patient-assessment-instruments/homehealthqualityinits

Chen, Z., Gleason, L. J. & Sanghavi, P. (2022). Accuracy of pressure ulcer events in U.S. nursing home ratings. *Medical Care, 60*(10), 775–783. https://doi.org/10.1097/MLR.0000000000001763

Fischbach, F., Fischbach, M. A., & Stout, K. (2022). *Fischbach's a manual of laboratory and diagnostic tests* (11th ed.). Wolters Kluwer.

Frank, C., Molnar, F., & Spencer, M. (2020). Fecal incontinence in older adults. *Canadian Family Physician, 66*(4), 264.

Ling, M. L., Apisarnthanarak, A., Abbas, A., Morikane, K., Lee, K. Y., Warrier, A., & Yamada, K. (2019). APSIC guidelines for the prevention of surgical site infections. *Antimicrobial Resistance and Infection Control, 8,* 174, https://doi.org/10.1186/s13756-019-0638-8

McNichol, L. L., Ratliff, C. R., & Yates, S. S. (2022). *Core curriculum: Wound management* (2nd ed.). Wolters Kluwer.

National Pressure Injury Advisory Panel (NPIAP). (2019). Prevention and treatment of pressure ulcers/injuries: Clinical practice guideline. https://npiap.com/page/Guidelines

Norris, T. L. (2025). *Porth's pathophysiology: Concepts of altered health states* (11th ed.). Wolters Kluwer.

Sandy-Hodgetts, K., Ousey, K., Conway, B., Nair, H., Serena, T., & Tariq, G. (2020). *International best practice recommendations for the early identification and prevention of surgical wound complications*. Wounds International. https://woundsinternational.com/best-practice-statements/international-best-practice-recommendations-early-indentification-and-prevention-surgical-wound-complications/

Shi, C., Dumville, J. C., Cullum, N., Rhodes, S., McInnes, E., Goh, E. L., & Norman, G. (2021). Beds, overlays, and mattresses for preventing and treating pressure ulcers: An overview of cochrane reviews and network meta-analysis. *Cochrane Database of Systematic Reviews, 8*(8), CD013761. https://doi.org/10.1002/14651858.CD013761.pub2

United States Department of Health and Human Services (USDHHS). (2023). Reduce the rate of pressure ulcer-related hospital admissions among older adults. *Healthy People 2030.* https://health.gov/healthypeople/objectives-and-data/browse-objectives/older-adults/reduce-rate-pressure-ulcer-related-hospital-admissions-among-older-adults-oa-04

Wang, Z., Man, M. Q., Li, T., Elias, P. M., & Mauro, T. M. (2020). Aging-associated alterations in epidermal function and their clinical significance. *Aging, 12*(6), 5551–5565. https://doi.org/10.18632/aging.102946

World Union of Wound Healing Societies (WUWHS). (2018). *Consensus round table meeting: Topical oxygen therapy for healing complex wounds*. Wounds International. https://woundsinternational.com/consensus-documents/consensus-round-table-meeting-portable-topical-oxygen-therapy-for-healing-complex-wounds/

World Union of Wound Healing Societies (WUWHS). (2019b). *Wound exudate: Effective assessment and management*. Wounds International. https://woundsinternational.com/world-union-resources/wuwhs-consensus-document-wound-exudate-effective-assessment-and-management/

World Union of Wound Healing Societies (WUWHS). (2022). *Incision care and dressing selection in surgical wounds: Findings from a series of international meetings*. Wounds International. https://woundsinternational.com/consensus-documents/incision-care-and-dressing-selection-surgical-wounds-findings-series-international-meetings/

Wound Ostomy and Continence Nurses Society-Wound Guidelines Task Force. (2017). WOCN 2016 guideline for prevention and management of pressure injuries (ulcers): An executive summary. *Journal of Wound Ostomy & Continence Nursing, 44*(3), 241–246. https://doi.org/10.1097/WON.0000000000000321

Yousef, H., Ajhajj, M., & Sharma, S. (2023). *Anatomy, skin (integument), epidermis.* StatPearls. https://www.ncbi.nlm.nih.gov/books/NBK470464/

Zaidi, S. & Sharma, S. (2022). *Pressure ulcer.* StatPearls. https://www.ncbi.nlm.nih.gov/books/NBK553107/

Chapter 16

Comfort, rest, and sleep

Just the facts

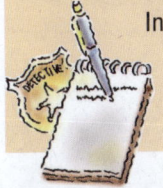

In this chapter, you'll learn:

◆ sleep stages and circadian rhythms

◆ types of sleep disorders and their causes.

Everyone needs comfort, rest, and sleep

Comfort, defined as the absence of pain (Cambridge Dictionary, 2023a), promotes rest, relaxation, and sleep. *Sleep* is a natural state of rest during which body activity and awareness of surroundings diminish (Cambridge Dictionary, 2023b). Sleep restores energy and well-being, enabling humans to function optimally.

Sleep is essential to quality of life and well-being. Every patient along the continuum of age from infancy to older adult needs restful sleep to enhance growth, healing, and general comfort. Not only do people feel better when they get enough sleep, but also during that time their bodies do many important tasks, such as processing new information.

Besides affecting the individual, sleep disturbances can have a direct impact on other family members' sleep patterns. For example, snoring may awaken the patient's spouse or prevent the spouse from falling asleep in the first place.

Primary or secondary

Sleep disorders may be primary or may arise secondary to a medical or psychiatric disorder, substance use, or environmental factors. Medical conditions such as Parkinson disease and thyroid disease can disrupt the body's sleep–wake cycles.

A vicious cycle

Psychiatric disorders such as depression or anxiety can cause chronic insomnia; in addition, chronic insomnia is a risk factor for depression and anxiety. High levels of stress may also contribute to sleep disorders, and lack of sleep may cause stress. Substances, including many that may be used to manage the effects of disordered sleep, may also disrupt sleep. These include alcohol, caffeine, and prescription medications—most notably, antihistamines, corticosteroids, and central nervous system drugs.

Sleep stages

Sleep occurs in four stages. With each stage, sleep becomes deeper, and brain waves grow progressively larger and slower, as shown on electroencephalogram (EEG).

Stage 1

The lightest stage of sleep, stage 1, occurs as a person falls asleep. The muscles relax, and brain waves are fast and irregular. Called *theta waves*, these spike-like waves have a low–medium amplitude and occur three to seven times per second. Stage 1 accounts for approximately 5% of an adult's total sleep time (Patel et al., 2022).

Stage 2

During stage 2, a deeper stage of sleep, theta waves continue but become interspersed with sleep spindles (sudden increases in wave frequency) and K complexes (sudden increases in wave amplitude). Stage 2 makes up about 45% of total sleep time (Patel et al., 2022).

Stage 3

Stage 3 is the deepest stage of sleep. Delta waves—large, slow waves of high amplitude and low frequency—appear on the EEG. In this stage, the body makes repairs and builds muscles, bones, and the immune system. Stage 3 makes up approximately 25% of total sleep time (Patel et al., 2022).

Stage 4

Stage 4 is a deep sleep called *rapid eye movement (REM) sleep*. During this stage, the sleeper shows darting eye movements, muscle twitching, and short, rapid brain waves resembling those seen during the waking state.

REM sleep usually begins about 90 minutes after sleep onset. Over the course of the night, REM periods lengthen. Overall, REM sleep accounts for approximately 25% of total sleep time (Patel et al., 2022).

(See *Sleep stages and brain waves.*)

Sleep stages and brain waves

Each sleep stage generates distinctive brain waves, as measured by EEG:
- During **stage 1,** which occurs as a person falls asleep, fast, irregular brain waves called *theta waves* appear on the EEG.
- During **stage 2,** theta waves are interspersed with wave phenomena called *sleep spindles* and *K complexes*.
- During **stage 3,** the EEG shows large, slow, high-amplitude waves, called *delta waves*.
- During **stage 4,** called *REM sleep*, short, rapid brain waves appear.

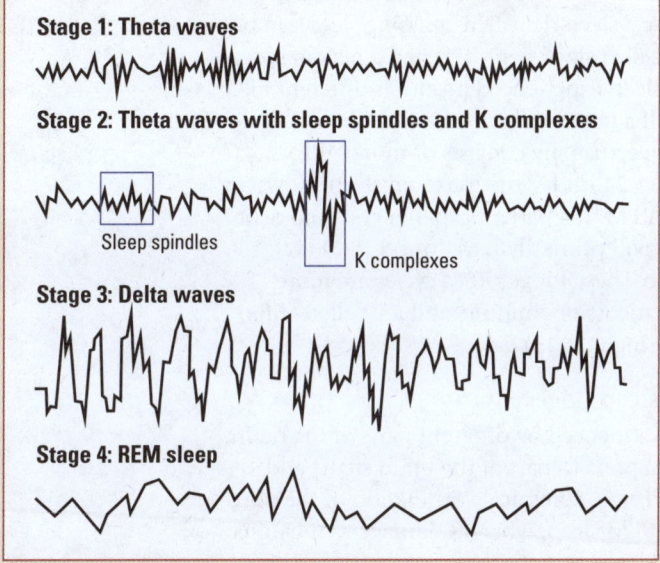

Stage 1: Theta waves

Stage 2: Theta waves with sleep spindles and K complexes

Sleep spindles

K complexes

Stage 3: Delta waves

Stage 4: REM sleep

To sleep, perchance to dream

Most story-like dreams take place during REM sleep. People awakened from REM sleep often report vivid dreams; in contrast, people awakened during stages 1 through 3 rarely do. Multiple research studies have shown that dreams are a compilation of random thoughts that the brain attempts to interpret as real.

Alternating sleep cycles

Throughout the night, REM (stage 4) and non-REM (NREM) (stages 1 through 3) sleep alternate in cycles of about 90 to 110 minutes each. The first cycle of REM (stage 4) is short and deep sleep (stage 3) is longer, but as the night

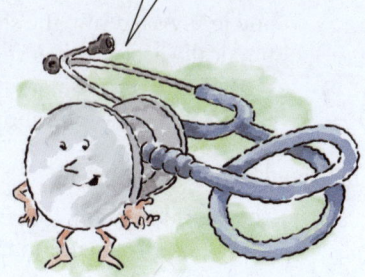

People awakened from REM sleep commonly report vivid story-like dreams.

wears on, periods of REM get longer, and less time is spent in deep sleep (Patel et al., 2022).

Functions of REM and NREM sleep

Scientists believe REM and NREM sleep serve different biological functions, although they don't know exactly what these functions are. NREM sleep is thought to stimulate brain growth, facilitate physical growth and recovery, or consolidate memory. REM sleep may support memory consolidation, but it also may help process information and emotions to prepare for wakefulness (Blumberg et al., 2020).

Lack of sleep impacts memory, cognitive function, and mood regulation, and it can even increase the risk of obesity, diabetes, and cardiovascular disease (Patel et al., 2022). A person with a disturbed night's sleep may have a sleep debt. This missing sleep can be recouped, usually during the next sleep period. When a person corrects sleep debt, the type of sleep experienced produces different EEG patterns than normal sleep. If a patient experiences less than 12 hours of sleep debt, the make-up sleep usually consists of more NREM sleep. If the sleep debt is 12 to 24 hours, the make-up sleep shows an increase in both NREM and REM. If a patient experiences sleep debt of more than 24 hours, they will primarily have longer REM cycles during the next sleep episode. These longer REM cycles are more intense, with more eye movements per minute, and are called "REM rebound effect" (Feriante & Singh, 2023).

Neurologic regulation of sleep stages

The various sleep stages are influenced by different parts of the brain. REM sleep is regulated by the pons (a part of the brain stem) and adjacent portions of the midbrain. Chemical stimulation of the pons may induce long periods of REM sleep, whereas damage to the pons may reduce or prevent REM sleep.

Paralysis and the pons

During REM sleep, neurons in the pons and midbrain that control muscle tone show various levels of activity: Some are active and others aren't. Reflecting this variable activity, certain body muscles remain inactive during REM sleep, especially those of the back, neck, arms, and legs. As a result, the sleeper is effectively paralyzed, so they can't physically act out whatever they're dreaming about. However, if these regulatory neurons malfunction, the sleeper may be more active during dreams, thrashing about or becoming violent.

Baths and the basal forebrain

The basal forebrain, located in front of the hypothalamus, controls NREM sleep. Damage to this region of the brain may cause difficulty falling asleep or staying asleep. Some neurons in the basal forebrain are activated by heat, which may explain the sleep-promoting benefits of taking a warm bath in the evening (Tai et al., 2021).

Factors that affect sleep

Factors affecting sleep quality and quantity include the patient's age, lifestyle, sleep environment, and medication use.

Age

Amounts and patterns of sleep differ at each major stage of the life cycle. Both REM and NREM sleep periods decrease with age. Older adults are also more likely to have trouble falling asleep and staying asleep.

Neonates, toddlers, and school age

Neonates sleep the most, averaging 17 to 18 hours a day, with REM accounting for roughly half of total sleep time. At first, a neonate sleeps in episodes of 3 to 4 hours. Although adult sleep begins with NREM, newborn sleep starts with REM. Gradually, as the infant sleeps longer at night, they develop circadian rhythms. It is recommended that neonates sleep 14 to 17 hours a day and infants sleep 12 to 15 hours a day, including naps. Toddlers, on the other hand, sleep 11 to 14 hours per day, including naps. Nap requirements vary, with some children taking naps up to age 5 years. By school age, children typically need 9 to 11 hours of sleep a day, with REM sleep accounting for about 20% of total sleep (Liu et al., 2022; Patel et al., 2022).

Tweens and teens

Preadolescents typically need about 8 to 10 hours of sleep. Due to hormonal changes with puberty, time spent in stage 2 of NREM and daytime sleepiness increase. Adolescent requirements aren't well defined. Many teenagers get too little sleep because of academic pressures and busy schedules.

Young adults

A typical young adult needs about 8 hours of sleep, although the requirement varies widely. Some young adults need as little as 6 or 7 hours, whereas others may need 9 or 10 hours to function optimally. Lifestyle choices such as increased screen time, school activities late in the day, and social obligations make this group vulnerable to sleep disturbances.

Middle-aged adults

In middle-aged adults, sleep requirements may remain unchanged from those of the young adult years. Typical sleep disturbances during middle age may stem from hormonal changes in people assigned female at birth, breathing-related disorders, and insomnia.

Older adults

Sleep problems are common among those over the age of 65 years; these include the following:

- Besides taking longer to fall asleep, they spend less time in deep NREM sleep, so their sleep is more easily interrupted or fragmented. (See *Sleep requirements of older adults.*)
- Early awakening is common in older adults and may result from an earlier rise in body temperature.
- Many seniors have trouble falling back to sleep after awakening to urinate. Patients who wake in the night to urinate should be encouraged to use night lights or have a lamp within easy reach to prevent falls. The path to the bathroom should also be unencumbered (National Institute on Aging, 2020).

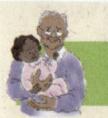

Ages and stages

Sleep requirements of older adults

It's a common misconception that older adults need much less sleep than younger adults. On the contrary, sleep requirements increase in older people because they tend to get decreased amounts of deep sleep and suffer frequent sleep interruptions.

Lifestyle

Travel, shift work, stress, and anxiety can greatly influence sleep. A person who travels through different time zones may experience jet lag, which is worse when traveling from west to east.

Environment

Sleep environment can greatly affect sleep quality. Negative environmental influences on sleep include noise, bright lights or sunlight, excessive activity, and an uncomfortable room temperature. When these influences are prominent, sleep can be difficult even for someone who's sleepy. Removing such stimuli produces an environment more conducive to sleeping (National Institute for Occupational Safety and Health, 2020).

The top physical factors related to sleepless nights are as follows:

- Bodily discomfort
- Noise
- Room temperature
- Light levels.

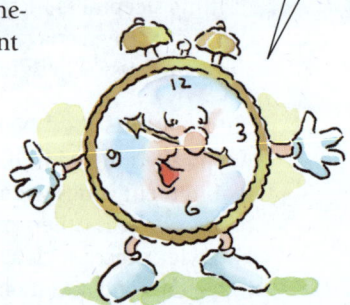

Travel, shift work, stress, and anxiety can greatly influence sleep. A person who travels through different time zones may suffer jet lag.

Hospital blues

Hospitalized patients commonly have trouble sleeping because of the following factors:

- They aren't in their own bed, and the noises of everyday hospital routines can be disruptive.
- If they're in a special care unit, such as intensive and cardiac care, the bells and whistles of equipment can disturb sleep or prevent a patient from getting to sleep.
- The stress of hospitalization and the fear of a bad prognosis or new procedures can impact routine sleeping patterns.
- The routines of regular vital signs measurement, doctor visits, and medication regimens can disrupt sleep.

Medications and substances

Medications of any kind may alter sleep patterns. Prescription drugs may cause somnolence (drowsiness) at inappropriate times; some may cause insomnia. Illicit drugs and other substances may also disturb established sleep patterns.

Alcohol

The impact of alcohol on sleep varies with the amount and time of consumption. In people without alcohol dependence issues, alcohol may have a sedative effect, increasing the amount of slow-wave sleep for the first 4 hours after sleep onset. After alcohol's effects wear off, sleep may be disrupted, with an increased amount of REM sleep and anxiety-causing dreams. People who are dependent on alcohol may have trouble falling asleep and staying asleep. Many have REM sleep disturbances (Koob & Colrain, 2020).

Withdrawal woes

During alcohol withdrawal, sleep deprivation is common. When sleep occurs, it's usually fragmented and accompanied by nightmares and anxiety-causing dreams.

No night–night

The most significant symptoms of sleep disturbances are insomnia at night (the most common symptom) and sleepiness during waking hours. A thorough medical and psychological history should be obtained from a patient who complains of sleep problems. The family may also need to be interviewed because the patient may be unaware of their sleep behavior.

Sometimes a physical examination is also warranted. Because sleep disorders are commonly linked to mood disorders, psychological tests may be administered as well.

Common sleep disorders

Some of the most common sleep disorders include circadian rhythm disorders, breathing-related sleep disorders, narcolepsy, primary hypersomnia, and primary insomnia.

Circadian rhythm disorders

Circadian refers to biological rhythms with a cycle of about 24 hours. (*Circadian* comes from the Latin phrase "circa diem," meaning "about a day.") The circadian rhythm functions as the body's internal "clock," regulating the 24-hour sleep–awake cycle and other body functions, such as body temperature, hormones, and heart rate. (See *Tick tock, it's the body clock*.)

The body's internal clock can reset itself to help a person adjust to such disturbances as seasonal changes, transitions to or from daylight savings time, or the start of a new workweek. However, it can't always easily overcome longer-lasting disruptions resulting from shift work or jet lag.

Tick tock, it's the body clock

The human body has an internal "clock" that follows a 24-hour cycle of wakefulness and sleepiness. This clock runs on circadian rhythms, which are linked to nature's cycle of light and darkness.

Organ "clocks"
Critical organs, such as the heart, liver, and kidneys, have their own "clocks" that work in a coordinated fashion with the body's master clock. Researchers know, for example, that certain cardiac events, such as heart attacks and sudden cardiac death, occur more commonly during specific times of the circadian cycle.

Night-shift blues
Up to 20% of night-shift workers experience sleep problems resulting from disruption of the body's natural rhythms. A condition known as "shift work sleep disorder" is a circadian rhythm disorder that can cause distress, trouble concentrating, and an increased risk of accidents (D'Ettore, et al., 2020).

Lark versus owl
The body's clock keeps us alert during daylight hours and makes us sleepy when night falls. All physiologic functions are geared toward being active during the day and

resting at night. The desire to sleep is strongest between 12 and 6 a.m.

Nonetheless, individual patterns of alertness vary; some people are relatively more alert during the day ("larks") while others are more alert at night ("night owls").

Mighty melatonin
The body's internal clock is regulated by melatonin, a hormone that causes sleepiness. Melatonin is secreted by the pineal gland, a structure located in the roof of the brain's third ventricle. Influenced by light, the pineal gland slows melatonin production during daylight hours to promote alertness and increases production when darkness falls, causing sleepiness.

It's not surprising that many older adults suffer from sleep disorders, because the body produces less melatonin as it ages (Martín Giménez et al., 2022).

Breathing-related sleep disorders

Breathing-related sleep disorders are marked by abnormal breathing during sleep. Obstructive sleep apnea (OSA) syndrome is the most common breathing-related sleep disorder (Mayo Clinic, 2021). Other disorders in this category include central sleep apnea syndrome and hypoventilation syndrome.

Breathing blockade

In OSA syndrome, the upper airway becomes blocked during sleep, impeding airflow. With sleep apnea, reduced airway muscle tone and the pull of gravity in the supine position further limit airway size during sleep. As tissue collapse worsens, the airway may become completely obstructed.

With partial or complete airway obstruction, the patient struggles to breathe. Blockage of airflow lasts 10 seconds to 1 minute and arouses the patient from sleep as the brain responds to decreased blood oxygen levels. (However, arousal is commonly partial and goes unrecognized by the patient.)

Snoring, then silence

This pattern causes disturbed and fragmented sleep, with periods of loud snoring or gasping when the airway is partly open, alternating with silence when the airway is blocked. (However, not everyone who snores has OSA syndrome.) The most common risk factors for OSA are being a person assigned male at birth, being older than 65 years, and having obesity (Yeghiazarians et al., 2021).

With arousal, the muscle tone of the tongue and airway tissues increases, causing the patient to awaken just enough to tighten the upper airway muscles and open the trachea. However, when they fall back to sleep, the tongue and soft tissue relax and the cycle begins again. This cycle may be repeated hundreds of times each night.

Repetitive cycles of snoring, airway collapse, and arousal may lead to cardiovascular problems such as high blood pressure, arrhythmias, coronary artery disease, pulmonary hypertension, metabolic syndrome, or stroke (Yeghiazarians et al., 2021). In some high-risk patients, sleep apnea may lead to sudden death from respiratory arrest during sleep.

Drowsy, irritable, and indifferent

Frequent awakenings during the night leave the patient sleepy during the day and can cause irritability or depression. The patient may suffer morning headaches and decreased mental functioning.

How sleepy is sleepy?

The Epworth Sleepiness Scale (ESS) is a tool to assess for abnormal daytime sleepiness. Although most people experience daytime sleepiness from time to time, regular daytime sleepiness could indicate and help diagnose a sleep disorder like sleep apnea. The ESS is a questionnaire in which the user rates the likelihood of dozing off in various situations using a 4-point Likert scale.

> People with severe, untreated sleep apnea have two to three times the risk of motor vehicle accidents.

Narcolepsy

Narcolepsy is characterized by sudden, uncontrollable attacks of deep sleep lasting up to 20 minutes. These "sleep attacks" come on without warning and may be accompanied by paralysis and hallucinations. Although the brief sleep is refreshing, the urge to sleep soon returns.

Sleep paralysis and hallucinations typically occur during sleep onset (hypnagogic hallucinations) or during the transition from sleep to wakefulness (hypnopompic hallucinations) (Slowik et al., 2022). Mostly visual, these hallucinations are intense, dreamlike images commonly involving the immediate environment.

Confounding cataplexy

More than 50% of patients with narcolepsy experience attacks of cataplexy, which is the sudden loss of muscle tone and strength. About 30% of patients with narcolepsy experience more subtle forms of cataplexy, in which the patient's head may drop or their jaw may slacken (Karna et al., 2023).

Cataplexy is commonly triggered by emotions. For example, the knees may buckle after the patient laughs, gets angry, or feels elated or surprised. Cataplexy typically lasts just a few seconds, and the patient remains alert during the episode. However, in severe cases, the patient falls and becomes completely paralyzed for up to several minutes. Narcoleptic sleep attacks may occur at any time of the day including during activities that call for undivided attention, such as driving.

Image problems

Besides causing car accidents, narcolepsy can be disabling, impairing work performance and disrupting leisure activities and interpersonal relationships. In children, narcolepsy impairs school performance and social relationships and invites ridicule from peers.

Primary hypersomnia

Primary hypersomnia is a condition of excessive sleepiness characterized by prolonged sleep periods at night or daytime sleep episodes occurring nearly every day. During long periods of drowsiness, the patient may exhibit automatic behavior, acting in a semi-controlled fashion. They may have trouble meeting morning obligations, commonly arriving late.

Symptomatic categories

Primary hypersomnia can present in the following ways:

- The patient may have isolated excessive daytime sleepiness unrelated to abnormal nocturnal awakenings.
- The patient may have abnormally long nighttime sleep and signs of sleep "drunkenness" (difficulty awakening completely, confusion, disorientation, poor motor coordination, and slowness) on awakening. Usually, the patient falls asleep easily at night and can stay asleep but seems out of sorts or even combative on awakening in the morning.

Primary insomnia

Insomnia is difficulty falling asleep and/or remaining asleep for a sufficient period of time. Although the exact causes are unknown, insomnia can be precipitated by stress, worry, environment, or any number of factors. (See *Factors contributing to insomnia*.)

Obsessing over insomnia

Insomnia can be acute or chronic. With chronic insomnia, the person may become preoccupied with getting enough sleep. The more the person tries to sleep, the greater their sense of frustration and distress, and the more elusive sleep becomes.

Insomnia commonly leads to daytime drowsiness that causes poor concentration, memory impairments, difficulty coping with minor problems, and reduced ability to enjoy family and social relationships.

Those with insomnia are more than twice as likely as the general population to have a fatigue-related motor vehicle accident. Those who sleep fewer than 5 hours per night may have a higher risk of multimorbidity of chronic disease (Sabia et al., 2022).

The Insomnia Severity Index (ISI) is the most accepted assessment tool for insomnia. The ISI determines the severity of insomnia by asking the patient to rate their experience with seven facets of insomnia

Factors contributing to insomnia

- reduced physical activity
- chronic conditions
- medications
- neurologic diseases such as Alzheimer disease
- stress and lifestyle changes

using a 5-point Likert scale. The questions relate to specific insomnia symptoms as well as how they impact daily life.

Another helpful tool to record sleep patterns is a sleep diary. When the provider asks a patient to keep a sleep diary over a set period of time, the patient uses this tool to keep track of when they fell asleep, how long it takes to fall asleep, when they woke up during the night, and when they arose in the morning. They can also use it to track any naps. Once the timeframe is complete, the patient shares the diary with their provider.

Treatments for sleep disturbances

Various therapies can be used to treat sleep disorders, depending on the source of the disorder. Asking the patient key questions in the assessment of sleep disorders may aid in treatment choices and possible referrals. (See *Key questions to ask about insomnia*.)

Breathing-related disorders

Treatments for breathing-related disorders such as OSA syndrome include lifestyle changes, continuous positive airway pressure (CPAP), and dental devices.

Lifestyle changes

Lifestyle changes, especially weight loss, are used to treat OSA syndrome. Weight loss reduces the amount of excess tissue in and around

---

Key questions to ask about insomnia

When a patient complains of insomnia, ask the following questions:
- When did the problem begin?
- Do you have a medical or mental illness that might affect your ability to sleep?
- What is your sleep environment like? Is it dark? Quiet? Bright? Noisy? Does it have a comfortable room temperature?
- What time do you usually go to bed?
- What time do you usually get up in the morning on weekdays? On weekends?

- Do you drink alcohol or smoke? Are you taking prescribed medications? Nonprescription preparations? Street drugs?
- What's your typical work schedule?
- How do you feel the day after a poor night's sleep?

Family inquiries

If possible, ask the patient's spouse or other family members if the patient snores or has unusual limb movements when they sleep.

the airway. Decreasing the body mass index to 30 or less significantly reduces the frequency of obstructive sleep episodes. However, even small weight reductions can improve the patient's condition.

Supine isn't sublime

Sleeping on the side rather than in a supine (back-lying) position may reduce apneic episodes. Avoiding alcohol and sleeping pills can decrease the number and duration of these episodes.

Continuous positive airway pressure

CPAP therapy during sleep is the most common and effective treatment for OSA syndrome. Positive pressure splints the airway open, preventing its collapse. The desired level of pressure varies with the type of CPAP device used. The patient wears either a full facial mask or a nasal mask.

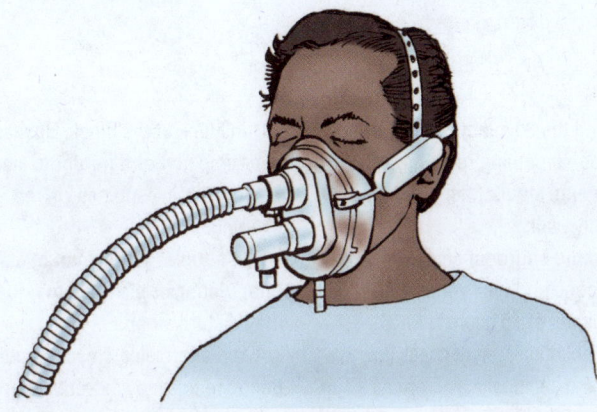

Dental devices

Oral appliances worn during sleep may help to relieve airway obstruction. However, they may be uncomfortable for some patients and may cause excessive salivation.

Insomnia

Treatments for insomnia include relaxation, sleep hygiene, behavioral interventions, cognitive therapy, alternative and complementary therapies, and medications.

Relaxation techniques

Because many people who experience insomnia display high levels of physiologic and cognitive arousal (both at night and during the day), relaxation-based interventions may provide relief. Techniques that help deactivate the arousal system include progressive muscle relaxation, abdominal or deep breathing, biofeedback, and imagery training.

Sleep hygiene

For some patients, insomnia can be decreased by simple lifestyle changes, sometimes called *sleep hygiene*. Such changes include going to bed at the same time every night, optimizing sleeping conditions, and avoiding naps during the day. (See *Getting hygienic about sleep*.)

Behavioral interventions

Behavioral interventions aim to change maladaptive sleep habits, reduce autonomic arousal, and alter dysfunctional beliefs and attitudes. A range of behavioral techniques may be used to treat chronic primary insomnia.

Getting hygienic about sleep

For most patients with insomnia, simple lifestyle measures, termed *sleep hygiene*, are the first line of treatment. When teaching patients about sleep hygiene, cover the following basics of sleep hygiene.

Sleep-promoting measures
- Use the bed only for sleep and sex, not for reading, watching television, or working.
- Establish a regular bedtime and a regular time for getting up in the morning. Stick to these times even on weekends and on vacations.
- Exercise in the evening. Energy levels bottom out a few hours after exercise, promoting sleep at that time.
- Take a hot bath 90 minutes to 2 hours before bedtime to decrease the core body temperature; this will help with falling asleep.

- During the 30 minutes before bedtime, do something relaxing, such as reading, meditating, or taking a leisurely walk.
- Keep the bedroom quiet, dark, relatively cool, and well ventilated.
- Eat dinner 4 to 5 hours before bedtime. At bedtime, a light snack (low in sugar and calories) may promote sleep.
- Spend 30 minutes in the sun each day. (However, be sure to use sunscreen and to take precautions against overexposure.)
- If sleep does not occur after 15 or 20 minutes, get up and go into another room. Read or perform a quiet activity, using dim lighting, until sleepiness occurs.

What not to do
- Don't use the bedroom for work, reading, or watching television.
- Avoid large meals before bedtime.

- Don't look at the clock. Obsessing over time makes it harder to sleep.
- Avoid naps, especially in the evening.
- Don't drink a large amount of fluid after dinner, or the need to urinate may disturb sleep.
- Avoid exercising close to bedtime because this may increase alertness.
- Avoid alcohol and caffeine in the evening.
- Don't engage in highly stimulating activities before bed, such as watching a frightening movie or playing competitive computer games.
- Quit smoking, because nicotine's effects may contribute to sleep loss.
- Avoid tossing and turning in bed. Instead, get up and read or listen to relaxing music. However, don't watch television because it emits bright, simulating light.

Source: Albakri, U., Drotos, E., & Meertens, R. (2021). Sleep health promotion interventions and their effectiveness: An umbrella review. *Int J Environ Res Public Health, 18*(11), 5533. https://doi.org/10.3390/ijerph18115533.

Stimulus control

Stimulus control centers on the theory that insomnia represents a learned response to bedtime and bedroom cues. This cognitive behavioral approach to impact sleep issues focuses on establishing a consistent sleep routine by recognizing the body's natural cues for sleep and wakefulness (MacDowell, 2022).

Biofeedback

In biofeedback, the patient is connected to a device that measures brain waves and other body functions. The patient is taught to read and understand the machine's feedback so they can learn to recognize certain states of tension or presleep stages and either avoid or repeat these states voluntarily.

Sleep restriction

The patient using this technique limits the amount of time spent in bed to increase the percentage of time in bed that is spent asleep. Sleep restriction creates a mild state of sleep deprivation, which may promote more rapid sleep onset and more "efficient" sleep.

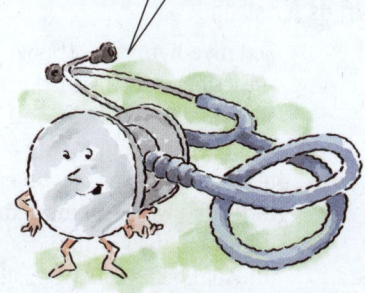

Unless the patient is an older adult, sleep restriction means just saying "No!" to naps!

To maintain a consistent sleep–awake pattern, the patient usually alters their bedtime rather than their rising time. Note that time in bed shouldn't be reduced to fewer than 5 hours per day. Naps aren't allowed (except for older adults).

Cognitive therapy

Cognitive therapy helps patients to identify their dysfunctional beliefs and attitudes about sleep (such as "I'll never fall asleep") and replace them with positive ones. Changing beliefs and attitudes can decrease the anticipatory anxiety that interferes with sleep. Cognitive therapy also focuses on actions intended to change behavior.

Alternative and complementary therapies

Alternative and complementary therapies that may be used to treat insomnia include acupressure, acupuncture, aromatherapy, massage, chiropractic, homeopathy, light and dark therapy, meditation, reflexology, visualization, tai chi, and yoga.

Supplements to sleep by

Some patients use herbal preparations (such as valerian, lavender, St. John's wort, and chamomile), nutritional substances, and other nonprescription preparations to treat insomnia. However, not all such products have been demonstrated to be consistently safe and effective (Suni, 2023b).

Dietary supplements sometimes recommended for insomnia relief include vitamins B_6, B_{12}, and D. Some practitioners also recommend calcium and magnesium. Tryptophan may relieve insomnia in some patients, but the patient must be monitored for possible adverse effects. Melatonin may increase sleepiness but should only be used on a short-term basis in small doses (Suni, 2023a).

Pharmacologic options

If insomnia persists despite other measures, the doctor may recommend drug therapy. The most commonly prescribed drugs are short-acting sedative-hypnotics (primarily benzodiazepines), non-benzodiazepine hypnotics (Z-drugs), melatonin receptor agonists, orexin receptor agonists, antidepressants, and antihistamines. (See *Pharmacologic therapy for sleep disorders*.)

Drugs for sleep

Sedative-hypnotics (benzodiazepines and Z-drugs) are commonly prescribed for the short-term management of insomnia. They work by slowing brain activity and making the patient feel sleepy. These drugs aid the patient in falling asleep, and some have the added benefit of helping them to stay asleep. Alcohol and other sedatives are contraindicated when taking sedative-hypnotic sleep aids, because taking other sedatives with sedative-hypnotic sleep aids increases the risk of unusual behaviors (e.g., sleepwalking, sleep eating, and talking) during sleep.

Drugs that may be prescribed for the long-term management of insomnia include the following:

- **Orexin receptor antagonists:** These drugs impact the sleep–wake cycle by decreasing the production of orexin, which causes alertness.
- **Melatonin receptor agonists:** These drugs make it easier for the patient to fall asleep by increasing the amount of melatonin in the body.

Antihistamines may be used for trouble falling or staying asleep in the short term but are not recommended for the long-term management of insomnia. Antihistamines work by causing a sedative effect, which helps induce sleep.

Antidepressants may be given in low dosages to combat insomnia, especially if the patient has a related psychiatric disorder or a history of substance misuse. However, because some antidepressants can exacerbate other disorders, such as mania and restless leg syndrome, the patient should be monitored closely.

Older adults or anyone who is at an increased risk for falls should be cautious when using any type of sleep aid due to the

Pharmacologic therapy for sleep disorders

This chart highlights the primary drug classes used to treat sleep disorders.

Drug class	Drug names	Patient teaching
Sedative-hypnotic benzodiazepine	• Temazepam • Flurazepam • Triazolam • Estazolam • Quazepam	• Daytime drowsiness, cognitive impairment, and abnormal behavior are common side effects • High potential for misuse and/or dependence as well as withdrawal symptoms • Because of the risk of breathing problems, should not be given to patients with sleep apnea or those who are also taking opioids
Nonbenzodiazepine hypnotic or Z-drug	• Zolpidem • Zaleplon • Eszopiclone	• Daytime drowsiness, cognitive impairment, and abnormal behaviors are possible side effects. Lesser risk of side effects than benzodiazepines • Potential for dependence
Melatonin receptor agonists	Ramelteon	• Dizziness, fatigue, and nausea are common side effects • Unlikely potential for misuse or dependence
Orexin receptor antagonists	• Suvorexant • Lemborexant • Daridorexant	• Daytime drowsiness is common, and cognitive impairment and abnormal behavior are possible side effects • May worsen depression • Potential for dependence and withdrawal symptoms
Antidepressants	• Doxepin	• Cognitive impairment and abnormal behavior are common side effects. An increase in suicidal thoughts is a possible serious side effect • Blurred vision • Contraindicated for older adults due to possible cardiovascular affects
Antihistamine with a sedating effect	• Doxylamine • Diphenhydramine	• Daytime drowsiness, cognitive impairment, dry mouth, and chest congestion are common side effects • Consistent use may lead to tolerance and dependence as well as withdrawal symptoms

Source: Martin, J. L., & Neubauer, D. N. (2022). Patient education: Insomnia treatments (Beyond the basics). *UpToDate*. https://www.uptodate.com/contents/insomnia-treatments-beyond-the-basics#H3748436209; Vallerand, A. H., & Sanoski, C. A. (2021). Davis's drug guide for nurses (17th ed.). F.A. Davis

risk of dizziness and altered cognition. During pregnancy and breastfeeding, benzodiazepines and Z-drugs are contraindicated, antihistamines can be used safely, and all other sleep aids should be used with caution and under the advice and care of a health care provider.

Quick quiz

1. A nurse is caring for a patient who has been diagnosed with a secondary sleep disorder. The nurse knows secondary sleep disorders **(Select all that apply):**

- A. Are multifaceted and complex.
- B. Require an interdisciplinary team approach.
- C. Are easy to understand and diagnose.
- D. Utilize multiple modalities.

Answer: A, B, and D. A secondary sleep disorder is a sleep problem that occurs because of a medical or psychiatric disorder, substance use, or environmental factors. Because secondary sleep disorders are complex, an interdisciplinary approach utilizing multiple modalities is essential.

2. Which statement is true regarding sleep and the older adult? These patients:

- A. sleep fewer hours at night because their sleep requirement is reduced with age.
- B. sleep more hours at night due to a higher need for restorative function.
- C. sleep fewer hours at night due to frequent sleep interruptions.
- D. sleep more deeply than younger adults.

Answer: C. Although the need for sleep doesn't decrease with age, older adults generally sleep fewer hours at night due to frequent interruptions such as trips to the bathroom and chronic pain.

3. When teaching a patient about sleep hygiene, the following recommendations should be included **(Select all that apply):**

- A. Use the bed only for sleep or sex.
- B. Install lights to fully illuminate the room.
- C. Avoid large meals right before bedtime.
- D. Go to bed at the same time every day.
- E. Exercise 30 minutes before bed.
- F. Increase the room temperature to make the room cozy.

Answer: A, C, and D. Sleep hygiene is a collection of recommendations that support healthy sleep patterns. The recommendations include establishing the bed to be used for sleep and sex only, setting regular sleep and wake times, avoiding heavy meals right before bed, exercising no later than 2 hours before bed, and creating a setting for sleep that is dark, cool, and quiet.

4. A nurse is caring for a 53-year-old person assigned male at birth with a body mass index (BMI) of 31 who lives alone. The patient reports headaches in the morning and difficulty concentrating at work. They say they use sleep hygiene practices and sleep approximately 7 hours every night. The patient's Epworth Sleepiness Scale (ESS) score indicates excessive daytime sleepiness. Which disorder description best fits this patient?

    A.   Narcolepsy.

    B.   Shift work sleep disorder.

    C.   Secondary insomnia due to anxiety.

    D.   Obstructive sleep apnea (OSA) syndrome.

Answer: D. This patient exhibits risk factors for, as well as symptoms of, OSA syndrome. These include being a person assigned male at birth, being over 65 years, having obesity, having excessive daytime sleepiness, and reporting adequate sleep time but not feeling rested.

Scoring

⭐⭐⭐ If you answered all four questions correctly, way to go! You're no slouch when it comes to sleeping.

  ⭐⭐ If you answered three questions correctly, good job! You're waking up to good sleep habits.

    ⭐ If you answered fewer than three questions correctly, don't lose sleep over it! Take a nap, review the chapter, and try again.

References

Albakri, U., Drotos, E., & Meertens, R. (2021). Sleep health promotion interventions and their effectiveness: An umbrella review. *International Journal of Environmental Research and Public Health, 18*(11), 5533. https://doi.org/10.3390/ijerph18115533

American Academy of Sleep Medicine. (2020). *Healthy sleep habits*. Sleep Education. https://sleepeducation.org/healthy-sleep/healthy-sleep-habits/

Blumberg, M. S., Lesku, J. A., Libourel, P. A., Schmidt, M. H., & Rattenborg, N. C. (2020). What is REM sleep? *Current Biology, 30*(1), R38–R49. https://doi.org/10.1016/j.cub.2019.11.045

Cambridge Dictionary. (2023a). *Comfort*. https://dictionary.cambridge.org/dictionary/english/comfort

Cambridge Dictionary. (2023b). *Sleep*. https://dictionary.cambridge.org/us/dictionary/english/sleep

D'Ettorre, G., Pellicani, V., Caroli, A., & Greco, M. (2020). Shift work sleep disorder and job stress in shift nurses: Implications for preventive interventions. *La Medicina del Lavoro, 111*(3), 195–202. https://doi.org/10.23749/mdl.v111i3.9197

Feriante, J., & Singh, S. (2023). *REM rebound effect*. StatPearls. StatPearls Publishing. https://pubmed.ncbi.nlm.nih.gov/32809548/

Karna, B., Sankari, A., & Tatikonda, G. (2023). *Sleep disorder*. StatPearls. StatPearls Publishing. https://www.ncbi.nlm.nih.gov/books/NBK560720/

Koob, G. F., & Colrain, I. M. (2020). Alcohol use disorder and sleep disturbances: A feed-forward allostatic framework. *Neuropsychopharmacology, 45*(1), 141–165. https://doi.org/10.1038/s41386-019-0446-0

Liu, J., Ji, X., Rovit, E., Pitt, S., & Lipman, T. (2022). Childhood sleep: Assessments, risk factors, and potential mechanisms. *World J Pediatrics,* 1–17. Published online. https://doi.org/10.1007/s12519-022-00628-z

MacDowell, R. (2022). *Stimulus control therapy.* Sleepopolis. https://sleepopolis.com/education/stimulus-control-therapy/

Martín Giménez, V. M., de Las Heras, N., Lahera, V., Tresguerres, J. A. F., Reiter, R. J., & Manucha, W. (2022). Melatonin as an anti-aging therapy for age-related cardiovascular and neurodegenerative diseases. *Frontiers in Aging Neuroscience, 14,* 888292. https://doi.org/10.3389/fnagi.2022.888292

Martin, J. L., & Neubauer, D. N. (2022). *Patient education: Insomnia treatments (Beyond the basics). UpToDate.* https://www.uptodate.com/contents/insomnia-treatments-beyond-the-basics#H3748436209

Mayo Clinic. (2021). *Obstructive sleep apnea.* https://www.mayoclinic.org/diseases-conditions/obstructive-sleep-apnea/symptoms-causes/syc-20352090

National Institute on Aging. (2020). *A good night's sleep.* https://www.nia.nih.gov/health/good-nights-sleep

National Institute for Occupational Safety and Health. (2020). *Creating a good sleep environment.* Centers for Disease Control and Prevention. https://www.cdc.gov/niosh/emres/longhourstraining/environment.html

Patel, A. K., Reddy, V., Shumway, K. R., & Araujo, J. F. (2022). *Physiology, sleep stages. StatPearls.* StatPearls Publishing. https://pubmed.ncbi.nlm.nih.gov/30252388/

Sabia, S., Dugravot, A., Léger, D., Ben Hassen, C., Kivimaki, M., & Singh-Manoux, A. (2022). Association of sleep duration at age 50, 60, and 70 years with risk of multimorbidity in the UK: 25-year follow-up of the Whitehall II cohort study. *PLoS Medicine, 19*(10), e1004109. https://doi.org/10.1371/journal.pmed.1004109

Slowik, J. M., Collen, J. F., & Yow, A. G. (2022). *Narcolepsy. StatPearls.* StatPearls Publishing.

Suni, E. (2023a). *Compare sleep aids.* Sleep Foundation. https://www.sleepfoundation.org/sleep-aids/compare-sleep-medications

Suni, E. (2023b). *Natural sleep aids.* Sleep Foundation. https://www.sleepfoundation.org/sleep-aids/natural-sleep-aids

Tai, Y., Obayashi, K., Yamagami, Y., Yoshimoto, K., Kurumatani, N., Nishio, K., & Saeki, K. (2021). Hot-water bathing before bedtime and shorter sleep onset latency are accompanied by a higher distal-proximal skin temperature gradient in older adults. *Journal of Clinical Sleep Medicine, 17*(6), 1257–1266. https://doi.org/10.5664/jcsm.9180

Vallerand, A. H., & Sanoski, C. A. (2021). *Davis's drug guide for nurses* (17th ed.). F.A. Davis.

Yeghiazarians, Y., Jneid, H., Tietjens, J. R., Redline, S., Brown, D. L., El-Sherif, N., Mehra, R., Bozkurt, B., Ndumele, C. E., & Somers, V. K. (2021). Obstructive sleep apnea and cardiovascular disease: A scientific statement from the American Heart Association. *Circulation, 144*(3), e56–e67. https://doi.org/10.1161/CIR.0000000000000988

Chapter 17

Pain management

Just the facts

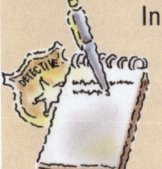

In this chapter, you'll learn:

♦ types and theories of pain

♦ effective ways to document pain assessment findings

♦ history and examination techniques for the patient with pain

♦ psychological characteristics of pain

♦ specific uses of pain medications

♦ physical therapies used in pain management

♦ roles of alternative and complementary therapies in relieving pain.

A look at pain

Pain is a perception that is complex in nature and helps to alert the body that a potential or real tissue damage is occurring. To put it succinctly, pain is whatever the patient says it is and it occurs whenever the patient says it does. When developing a plan for pain management with the patient, it is important that the nurse assess not only the physical manifestations of pain but also the subjective reports of pain as well.

Each patient reacts to pain differently because pain thresholds and tolerances vary from person to person. *Pain threshold* is a physiologic attribute that denotes the intensity of the stimulus needed to sense pain. *Pain tolerance* is a physiologic attribute that describes the amount of stimulus (duration and intensity) that the patient can endure before stating that they are in pain.

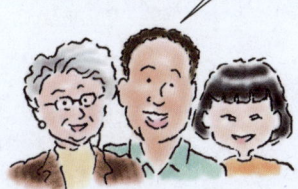

Reactions to pain vary from person to person and even within the same person at different times.

Beliefs about pain

Patients' attitudes, beliefs, expectations of themselves, coping resources, and beliefs about the health care system affect the entire spectrum of their pain behaviors.

Behavior and emotions are influenced by the interpretation as well as the facts of an event. This partly explains why patients may differ greatly in their beliefs about pain. Beliefs about pain are individualized; each patient has had different painful experiences and therefore has different expectations about pain and painful experiences. Coping with pain is specific to each patient within each event of pain in that patient's life.

Coping

The ability to cope is influenced by personal beliefs, judgments, and expectations about the consequences of the event. Personal beliefs, judgments, and expectations can influence mood directly and alter coping ability.

For example, if a person with low back pain fails to comply with prescribed exercises, this may be because the last time they did exercises for their low back they experienced pain, so they now foster a negative view of their abilities and an expectation of increased pain during exercise. These beliefs form a rationale for avoiding exercise.

Can you cope with these concepts?

Type of coping strategies include:

- **Overt or covert:**
  - *Overt* coping strategies include rest, drug therapy, and use of relaxation techniques.
  - *Covert* coping strategies include distraction, reassuring oneself that the pain will diminish, seeking information, and solving problems.
- Active and passive:
  - *Active* coping strategies—efforts to function despite pain or to distract oneself from pain—lead to adaptive functioning.
  - *Passive* coping strategies—restricting one's activities and depending on others for help in pain control—lead to greater pain and depression.

(See *Encouraging active pain-coping strategies*, page 515.)

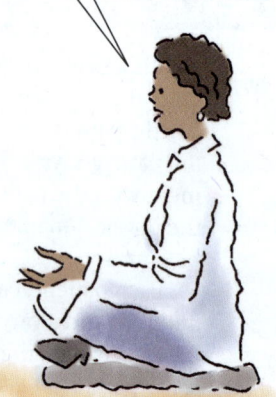

Rest and relaxation techniques can help patients cope with their pain.

Attention

Pain can change the way the patient processes pain-related and other information by focusing the patient's attention on bodily signals. As these signals change, the patient may assume these changes mean that the underlying disease is getting worse and, as a result, may report increased pain.

In contrast, a patient who doesn't attribute symptoms to worsening disease tends to report less pain, even if their disease actually is progressing.

Encouraging active pain-coping strategies

The patient's strategy for coping with pain may be active or passive. *Active* strategies include attempts to function despite pain. *Passive* strategies include relying on others for help in pain control.

If possible, steer the patient toward active coping strategies. A patient who uses active coping strategies tends to experience less pain and increased pain tolerance than one who uses passive strategies.

One strategy doesn't fit all

Keep in mind that one active coping strategy isn't necessarily better than another. A given strategy may be helpful in one situation, or for one patient, but not helpful in a different situation or for another patient.

Likewise, certain strategies may help at one time but prove ineffective in other situations or for different types of pain.

Out-of-control thoughts

The most detrimental feature of poor coping seems to be "catastrophizing"—thinking extremely negative thoughts about one's plight. If the patient falls into this trap, teach them that imagining more positive outcomes may help reduce their pain.

Too little feedback

Beliefs and expectations about a disease are hard to change. Patients tend to behave consistently with their beliefs and avoid experiences that might invalidate their beliefs. Often, health professionals refrain from challenging a patient who has irrational beliefs or a patient who excessively restricts their own activities due to their beliefs about pain. In doing so, health professionals fail to give patients valuable corrective feedback.

Physical links to pain

Just as physical factors can affect a patient's psychological condition, psychological factors can affect their mood, coping ability, and nociception (the sensation of pain).

Cognitive interpretations and affective arousal may influence physiology by increasing autonomic sympathetic nervous system (SNS) arousal and promoting endogenous opioid (endorphin) production.

Autonomic arousal

Thinking about pain and stress can increase muscle tension, especially in already painful areas. Chronic and excessive SNS arousal is a precursor to increased skeletal muscle tone. It may set the stage for hyperactive and persistent muscle contractions, which promote muscle spasms and pain.

Arousing sympathy

Patients who exaggerate the significance of their problems or ruminate on them too closely may cause arousal of the SNS, which predisposes them to further injury and can complicate recovery in other ways.

How thoughts affect endorphins

Studies show that thoughts can influence the concentration of endorphins available to control pain. Research results indicate that:

- a patient's feelings of self-efficacy predicted their pain tolerance; those with high self-efficacy had greater levels of endorphins (See *Psychological treatments and arthritis pain.*)
- naloxone, an opioid antagonist, blocked the pain-relieving effects of cognitive coping (which demonstrates how thoughts can directly affect endorphins and that self-efficacy may influence pain perception at least partially through endogenous opioids)
- lower concentrations of endorphins were associated with learned helplessness.

Pain assessment

Because pain is subjective, a thorough and accurate pain assessment must be done to ensure the patient receives effective pain relief.

Pain is influenced not just by physical pathology but also by cultural and social factors, expectations, mood, and perceptions of control. Expectations about pain and ways of expressing pain can dramatically influence pain thresholds and tolerance. Often, a person's first coping mechanism for the pain may be to try to ignore the pain; this patient may report moderate pain when asked but laugh with visitors or appear to not have pain. Not all patients cry out or shed tears with pain. Some patients may be quiet and reserved, wanting no visitors; others may be coping by trying to focus on something else. Even in the absence of visible injury the nurse must not question the presence of pain.

The patient knows best

Pain is *always* what the person says it is. When assessing pain, keep in mind the first principle of pain assessment: Pain is whatever the

---

Psychological treatments and arthritis pain

Research suggests that psychological treatments in patients with rheumatoid arthritis (RA) helps decrease pain and improve quality of life. RA is an autoimmune disorder that may result from impaired suppressor T-cell functioning and that causes inflammation of synovial membranes, joint pain, and stiffness. Psychological interventions decrease stress and pain and improve mood, feelings of self-efficacy, and quality of life. One study indicated that integration of psychological interventions is effective in reducing pain and improving mood in patients with RA. Therefore, a multidisciplinary approach that includes psychological interventions is recommended for effective treatment of patients with RA (Nagy et al., 2023).

patient says it is, occurring whenever they say it does. The patient's self-report of the presence and severity of pain is the most accurate, reliable means of pain assessment.

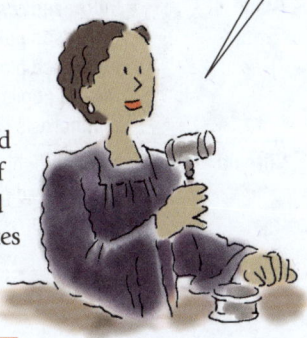

A nurse should never judge a patient's level of pain—pain is always what the person says it is.

Pain threshold and tolerance

Pain threshold refers to the intensity of the stimulus a person needs to sense pain. *Pain tolerance* is the duration and intensity of pain that a person tolerates before openly expressing pain. Tolerance has a strong psychological component. Remember that pain threshold and tolerance vary widely among patients. Identifying pain threshold and tolerance are crucial to pain assessment and the development of a pain management plan. Even so, keep in mind that pain threshold and tolerance may even fluctuate in the same patient as circumstances change.

Differentiating types of pain

Pain falls into three broad categories—acute pain, chronic nonmalignant pain (also called *chronic persistent pain*), and cancer pain.

Acute pain

Acute pain comes on suddenly—for instance, after trauma, surgery, or an acute disease—and lasts from a few days to a few weeks. Typically, it's described as sharp, intense, and easily localized to one area. It causes a withdrawal reflex and may trigger involuntary bodily reactions, such as sweating, fast heart and respiratory rates, and elevated blood pressure. (See *Acute pain: A sympathetic response.*)

Acute pain: A sympathetic response

In acute pain, certain involuntary (autonomic) reflexes may occur. Acute pain causes the sympathetic branch of the autonomic nervous system (ANS) to trigger the release of epinephrine and other catecholamines. These substances, in turn, cause physiologic reactions such as those seen in the fight-or-flight response.

It will get your attention
Sympathetic activation directs immediate attention to the injury site. This attention promotes reflexive withdrawal and fosters other actions that prevent further damage and enhance healing. For example, if you place your hand on a hot stove, the ANS immediately generates a reflex withdrawal that jerks your hand away and minimizes tissue damage.

Differentiating acute and chronic pain

Acute pain may cause certain physiologic and behavioral changes that may not be observed in a patient with chronic pain.

Type of pain	Physiologic evidence	Behavioral evidence
Acute	• Increased respirations • Increased pulse • Increased blood pressure • Dilated pupils • Diaphoresis	• Restlessness • Distraction • Worry • Distress
Chronic	• Normal respirations, pulse, blood pressure, and pupil size • No diaphoresis	• Reduced or absent physical activity • Despair, depression • Hopelessness

---

Acute pain may be constant (as in a burn), intermittent (as in a muscle strain that hurts only with activity), or both (as in an abdominal incision that hurts a little at rest and a lot with movement or coughing). It can also be prolonged or recurrent. (See *Differentiating acute and chronic pain*.)

So long now

Prolonged acute pain can last days to weeks. Usually, it results from tissue injury and inflammation (as from a sprain or surgery) and subsides gradually.

At the injury site, release or synthesis of chemicals heightens sensitivity in nearby tissues. This hypersensitivity, called *hyperalgesia*, is normal. In fact, tenderness and tissue hypersensitivity help protect the injury site and prevent further damage.

Over and over again

Recurrent acute pain refers to brief painful episodes that recur at variable intervals. Examples include pain related to sickle cell vascular occlusion crisis and migraine headache.

In migraine headache and some other recurrent conditions, pain serves no apparent useful purpose—no protective action can be taken, and tissue damage can't be prevented. However, in others, such as sickle cell disease, acute pain encourages the person to seek medical treatment.

Chronic nonmalignant pain

Pain is considered chronic when it lasts beyond the usual time expected for an injury to heal or an illness to resolve. Many experts define chronic nonmalignant pain as pain lasting 3 months or longer; such episodes of pain may recur during the patient's lifetime. Although it sometimes begins as acute pain, more typically it starts slowly and builds gradually. Unlike acute pain, chronic pain isn't protective and doesn't warn of significant tissue damage. Chronic pain is especially common in older adults, with management that can be complicated by multiple chronic health conditions, polypharmacy, and decreasing ability to metabolize medications (Rochon, 2022).

Chronic nonmalignant pain is unrelated to cancer. This type of pain is prevalent in one of five adults in the United States (Kunzmann, 2023). It is estimated that noncancer chronic pain accounts for 57% of all health care encounters (Gebke et al., 2023).

Causes of chronic pain include nerve damage such as in brain injury or unexplained and abnormal responses to tissue injury by the central nervous system (CNS). Chronic pain can be associated with serious disability (as in arthritis or avascular necrosis), or it may be related to poorly understood disorders such as fibromyalgia and complex regional pain syndrome. Neuropathic is another type of chronic pain. (See *Understanding neuropathic pain*.)

> Many experts define chronic nonmalignant pain as pain episodes lasting 3 months or longer that may recur during the patient's lifetime.

Understanding neuropathic pain

Commonly described as tingling, burning, or shooting, neuropathic pain is a puzzling type of chronic pain generated by the nerves. It commonly has no apparent cause and responds poorly to standard pain treatment.

We don't know the precise mechanism of neuropathic pain. Possibly, the peripheral nervous system has experienced damage that injures sensory neurons, causing continuous depolarization and pain transmission. Alternatively, it could result from repeated noxious stimuli that cause hypersensitivity and excitement in the spinal cord that results in chronic neuropathy in which a normally harmless stimuli causes pain.

The limb is gone, but the pain remains

Phantom pain syndrome is one example of neuropathic pain. This condition occurs when an arm or a leg has been removed but the brain still gets pain messages from the nerves that originally carried the limb's impulses. The nerves seem to misfire, causing pain.

Types of neuropathic pain

Neuropathic pain can involve peripheral or central pain.

Peripheral pain can occur as:

• *polyneuropathy*, which is pain felt along the peripheral nerves, as in diabetic neuropathy

• *mononeuropathy*, which is pain associated with an established injury and felt along the nerve, as in trigeminal neuralgia.

Central neuropathic pain can also be categorized as follows:

• *sympathetic pain*, which results from dysfunction of the ANS

• *deafferentation pain*, which is marked by elimination of sensory (afferent) impulses, as from damage to the central or peripheral nervous system (as in phantom pain).

High cost of chronic pain

Chronic pain may be so severe that it limits a patient's ability and desire to participate in career, family life, and even activities of daily living. If the pain is severe or intractable, the patient may experience decreased function, depression, opioid dependence, "doctor shopping" (see the *Shopping around* section on page 17), or suicide.

Assessment obstacles

Pain assessment may be especially difficult in a patient with chronic pain. Over time, the ANS adapts to pain, so the patient may lack typical autonomic responses, such as dilated pupils, increased blood pressure, and fast heart and respiratory rates. Also, their facial expression may not suggest pain. They may sleep periodically and shift their attention away from the pain. Regardless, a lack of outward signs of pain shouldn't influence the pain assessment.

Cancer pain

By the year 2030, the number of living cancer survivors in the United States is expected to reach 22.2 million (Pugh et al., 2021). Cancer pain is a complex problem. It may result from the disease itself or from treatment. Recent studies demonstrate that 56% of patients with cancer experience moderate to severe pain monthly (Pugh et al., 2021). Sometimes, pain results from the pressure of a tumor impinging on organs, bones, nerves, or blood vessels. In other cases, limitations in activities of daily living may lead to muscle aches. Although cancer pain can be treated with oral medications, including opioids, only one-third of patients with cancer pain achieve satisfactory relief. In addition to the presence of pain, suffering and quality of life should be assessed.

Treatments may cause pain

These cancer treatments may cause pain:
- chemotherapy, radiation, or drugs used to offset the impact of these therapies on blood counts and infection risk (such as mouth sores; peripheral neuropathy; and abdominal, bone, or joint pain from chemotherapy agents)
- surgery
- biopsies
- blood withdrawal
- lumbar punctures.

The Joint Commission on pain management standards

The Joint Commission (TJC) has issued standards for pain assessment, management, and documentation. These standards require health care workers to ask patients about pain when they're admitted.

Any patient who reports pain must be assessed further by licensed personnel. Facility policies must identify standardized pain screening tools to be used for pain assessments on all patients.

Policies and procedures should be reviewed for information on which screening tools are to be used, frequency of pain assessment, and when further assessment and actions are to be taken. For example, in many facilities a pain level of 4 or higher on a scale of 0 to 10 requires intervention.

Pain assessment scores must be monitored and recorded regularly—and at least as vigilantly—as vital signs. To meet TJC standards, pain assessment data should be recorded in a way that promotes reassessment. Most electronic medical record systems in the hospital systems include fields for entering information related to pain reassessment after medication administration.

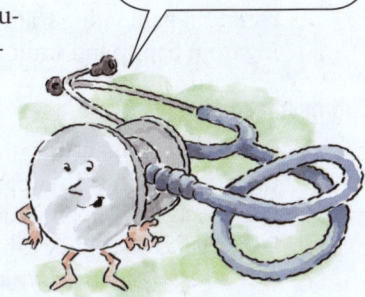

> According to TJC, good clinical practice dictates that any patient who reports pain must be assessed further by licensed personnel.

TJC standards also mandate that health care facilities plan and support activities and resources that assure pain recognition and use of appropriate interventions. These activities include:

- initial pain assessment
- regular reassessment of pain
- education of health care workers about pain assessment and management
- development of quality improvement plans that address pain assessment and reassessment.

Pain assessment tools

When a patient is admitted, ask them if they currently are in pain or have ongoing problems with pain. If they have ongoing pain, find out if they have an effective treatment plan. If so, continue with this plan if possible. If they do not have such a plan, use an assessment tool, such as a pain rating scale, to further assess the pain.

Pain rating scales

Pain rating scales quantify pain intensity—one of pain's most subjective aspects. These scales offer several advantages over semistructured and unstructured patient interviews:

- They're easier to administer.
- They take less time.
- They can uncover concerns that warrant a more thorough investigation.
- When used before and after a pain control intervention, they can help determine if the intervention was effective.

All shapes and sizes

Pain rating scales come in many varieties. When choosing an appropriate scale for your patient, consider their visual acuity, age, reading ability, and level of understanding.

Pain intensity rating scale

Pain can be evaluated in a nonverbal manner for pediatric patients 3 years and older or for adult patients with language difficulties. One common pain rating scale consists of six faces with expressions ranging from happy and smiling to sad and teary.

Putting a face on pain

To use a pain intensity rating scale, tell the patient that each face represents a person with progressively worse pain. Ask them to choose the face that best represents how they feel. Explain that, although the last face has tears, they can choose this face even if they are not crying. (See *Using a pain intensity rating scale.*)

Visual analog scale

The visual analog scale is a horizontal line, 10 cm (3⅝") long, with word descriptors at each end: "no pain" on one end and "pain as bad as it can be" on the other. The scale may also be used vertically.

Drawing the line on pain

Ask the patient to place a mark along the line to indicate the intensity of the pain. Then measure the line in millimeters up to the mark. This measurement represents the patient's pain rating. Be aware that this scale may be too abstract for some patients to use. (See *Visual analog scale.*)

Using a pain intensity rating scale

A pediatric patient or an adult patient with language difficulties may not be able to express the pain they are feeling. In such instances, use the pain intensity scale below. Ask your patient to choose the face that best represents the severity of their pain, on a scale from 0 to 5.

0

1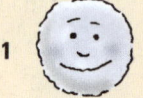

2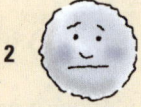

3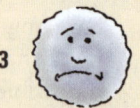

4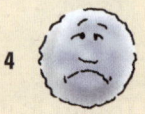

5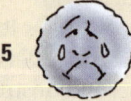

Visual analog scale

To use the visual analog scale, ask the patient to place a line across the scale to indicate their current level of pain. The pain rating is determined by measuring the distance, in millimeters, from "no pain" to their marking.

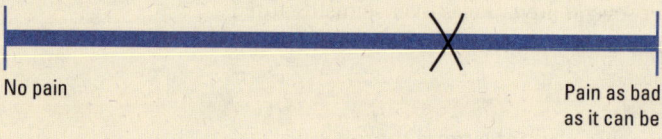

No pain | Pain as bad as it can be

Numerical rating scale

The numerical rating scale (NRS) is perhaps the most used pain rating scale. Simply ask the patient to rate their pain on a scale from 0 to 10, with 0 representing no pain and 10 representing the worst pain imaginable. Instead of giving a verbal rating, the patient can use a horizontal or vertical line consisting of descriptive words and numbers.

Although most patients find the NRS quick and easy to use, it may be too abstract for some patients. The NRS may also be frustrating to the patient who hurts, but their pain is not unbearable. Many patients have the belief that, to request pain medication, they have to be suffering. If the patient is in pain, the nurse should assess and offer pain medication on a regular basis, as stated in their facility's policies and procedures. The number should be used to assess pain management and not to judge whether a person needs to be medicated. (See *Using the numerical rating scale*.)

Verbal descriptor scale

With the verbal descriptor scale, the patient chooses a description of their pain from a list of adjectives, such as "none," "annoying," "uncomfortable," "dreadful," "horrible," and "agonizing."

Using the numerical rating scale

An NRS can help the patient quantify their pain. Have them choose a number from 0 (indicating no pain) to 10 (indicating the worst pain imaginable) to reflect their current pain level. The patient can either circle the number on the scale itself or verbally state the number that best describes the pain.

No pain   **0   1   2   3   4   5   6   7   8   9   10**   Pain as bad as it can be

Not as simple as it sounds

To be on the safe side, don't assume that the patient knows how to use the scale. Provide teaching and then verify that they understand what was taught. Be sure to document teaching and the method of evaluating their understanding.

Work toward a comfort goal

Help the patient establish a comfort goal—a numerical pain level that will enable them to perform self-care activities, such as ambulation, coughing, and deep breathing. Usually, a level of 3 or less on a 0-to-10 scale is an adequate comfort level.

If the patient chooses a comfort goal of four or higher, teach them that unrelieved pain can damage their health. Discuss concerns they may have about using analgesics, and clear up misconceptions such as those related to developing dependence on a drug.

When to evaluate the pain management plan

If the patient rates the pain as 10, they're experiencing severe pain—a sign that the pain management plan is ineffective. Consult with the health care provider about increasing the analgesic dose or adding another analgesic.

When to use a vertical scale instead

Like some children, many adults who speak languages that are read from right to left (or vertically) may have trouble with the NRS because it's horizontal. They may find a vertical scale easier to use. When using a vertical scale, place 0 at the bottom of the scale and 10 at the top.

Like the NRS, the verbal descriptor scale is quick and easy, but it does have drawbacks:
- The patient's choices are limited.
- Patients tend to choose moderate rather than extreme descriptors.
- Some patients may not understand all the adjectives.

Overall pain assessment tools

Overall pain assessment tools evaluate pain in multiple dimensions, providing a wider range of information. These tools are time consuming and may be more practical for outpatient use. However, an overall pain assessment may be useful for a hospitalized patient with hard-to-control chronic pain. Be sure to document the patient's pain according to your facility's policy. (See *Documenting pain assessment findings.*)

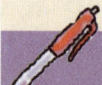

Take note!

Documenting pain assessment findings

Be sure to document baseline pain assessment findings so that all team members can refer to the information for later comparison. Standardized documentation forms may be used as a guide for pain assessment.

If the patient has unrelieved pain, frequent pain assessments are necessary. To make pain assessment findings more visible, consider using a graphic sheet that documents pain severity next to vital signs.

Pain assessment flow sheet

A pain assessment flow sheet provides a convenient way to track the patient's pain level and responses to interventions over time. On a typical flow sheet, record information about the patient's pain severity rating, therapeutic interventions, effects of each intervention, and adverse effects of treatments (such as nausea and sedation).

A pain assessment flow sheet is useful inside and outside the hospital. After discharge, the patient and their family may want to use the flow sheet along with a pain diary in which the patient records their activities, pain intensity, and pain interventions. The diary can reveal the extent to which pain management measures and activities affect the pain level.

Analgesic infusion flow sheet

If the patient is receiving an analgesic infusion, use an analgesic infusion flow sheet to speed documentation and track their progress. Information to record on the flow sheet includes:

- medication name and dosage
- date and time of each dose
- concentration of dose
- volume infused and volume remaining.

Oral medication flow sheet

An oral medication flow sheet can be a valuable tool for:
- patients who will receive analgesics after discharge
- home care patients with pain caused by progressive illness
- patients with chronic nonmalignant pain.

Common side effects to opioid pain medications include drowsiness, constipation, confusion, and respiratory depression.

History and physical examination

Accurate pain assessment yields information that serves as the basis for an individualized pain management plan. For a patient with acute pain, a brief assessment may be adequate to formulate an appropriate plan.

However, a patient with chronic pain may require a thorough assessment that evaluates physical and psychosocial factors. Still, even the best history and examination techniques may not produce the definitive findings needed to make a precise diagnosis and to clearly identify the origin of chronic pain. Usually, history and physical findings help the health care provider interpret the results of diagnostic tests.

Patient history

Assessment begins with the patient interview. If they have acute pain from a traumatic injury, the interview may last for mere seconds. If they have chronic pain, it may be lengthy.

When interviewing a patient with chronic pain, try to elicit information that sheds light on their thoughts, feelings, behaviors, and physiologic responses to pain. Also find out about the environmental stimuli that can alter their response to pain. With a patient who is experiencing chronic pain, their lifestyle most likely has been affected by the pain. Find out if there are any activities that the person used to enjoy doing that are now impossible because of the pain.

Questions to ask

During the interview, assess the cognitive, affective, and behavioral components of the patient's pain experience. Doing so can help later when working with the patient to develop pain management goals. Also ask questions to determine how the pain affects their mental state, relationships, and work performance.

Pain characteristics
Question the patient about these characteristics of their pain:
- *onset and duration*—when did the pain begin? Did it come on suddenly or gradually? Is it intermittent or continuous? How often does it occur? How long does it last? Is it prolonged or recurrent?
- *location*—ask the patient to point to the painful parts of the body or to mark these areas on a diagram. Be sure to assess each pain site separately.
- *intensity*—using a pain rating scale, ask the patient to quantify the intensity of the pain at its worst and at its best.

- *quality*—ask the patient what the pain feels like, in their own words. Does it have a burning quality? Is it knifelike? Do they feel pressure? Throbbing? Soreness?
- *relieving factors*—does anything help relieve the pain, such as a certain position or heat or cold applications? Besides helping to pinpoint the cause of the pain, the answers may aid in developing a pain management plan.
- *aggravating factors*—what seems to trigger the pain? What makes it worse? Does it get worse when the patient moves or changes position?

The assessment technique of onset, provoke, quality, radiate, severity, and time (OPQRST) may be valuable when assessing pain. Each letter stands for a crucial aspect of pain to explore.

Medical and surgical history

The patient's medical history may offer clues to the source of pain or a condition that may exacerbate it. Ask them to list all of their past medical conditions, even those that have been resolved. Also question them about previous surgeries.

Past experience with pain

Explore the patient's experiences with pain. If they experienced significant pain in the past, they may have anticipatory fear of future pain—especially if they received inadequate pain relief.

Play "20 Questions"

Ask the patient which previous treatments—pharmacologic and otherwise—they tried, and find out which treatments helped and which didn't help. Keep in mind that nonpharmacologic treatments include physical and occupational therapy, acupuncture, hypnosis, meditation, biofeedback, heat and cold therapy, transcutaneous nerve stimulation, and psychological counseling.

Drug history

Obtain a complete list of the patient's medications. (Many medications can alter the effectiveness of analgesics.) Besides prescribed drugs, ask if they take over-the-counter preparations, vitamins, nutritional supplements, or herbal or homemade remedies. Record the name, dose, frequency, administration route, and adverse effects of each agent used. Also ask about drug allergies.

Find out if the patient currently takes or has previously taken medications to control pain and whether they were effective. If the patient currently receives analgesics, have the patient describe exactly how they take them. If the patient hasn't been taking medications according to instructions, they may need additional teaching on proper administration. If a particular analgesic agent or regimen didn't work for them in the past, the regimen and dose may need to be tailored to be effective.

Satisfaction survey

Ask the patient if they're satisfied with the level of pain relief the current medications bring. Find out how long these drugs take to work and whether the pain returns before the next dose is due.

Question the patient about adverse effects, such as nausea, constipation, and drowsiness. If they're taking opioids for pain relief, note any worries they have about becoming drug dependent. Listen carefully for concerns they may have about any medication.

Social history

Thorough pain assessment includes a social history. Many social factors can influence the patient's perception and reports of pain and vice versa. This information also helps guide interventions.

Find out how the patient feels about themselves, their place in society, and their relationships with others. Ask about marital status; occupation; support systems; financial status; hobbies; exercise and sleep patterns; responsibilities; and religious, spiritual, and cultural beliefs. Determine patterns of alcohol use, smoking, and illicit drug use.

Chronic pain can have wide-ranging effects on a person's life. If the patient has chronic pain, explore the impact it has on moods, emotions, expectations, coping efforts, and resources. Also ask how their family responds to their condition.

The individualized meaning of pain

To provide culturally sensitive care, determine the meaning of pain for each patient—particularly in the context of culture and religion. Determine how cultural background and religious beliefs may affect pain experience. In some cultures, pain is openly expressed. Other cultures value stoicism and denial of pain. A patient who comes from a culture that values stoicism may lead you to believe that they are not in pain.

Be sure not to stereotype the patient. Keep in mind that, within each culture, the response to pain may vary from person to person. Also recognize personal values, biases, and cultural beliefs. Personal awareness can help keep personal beliefs from impacting the evaluation of the patient's pain response.

Physical examination

Start the physical examination by observing the patient. They may display a broad range of behaviors to convey pain, distress, and suffering. Some behaviors are controllable. Others, such as heavy perspiration or pupil dilation, are involuntary.

Observe the patient before and during the physical examination, and note and document behaviors. (See *Pain behavior checklist.*) Use these observations to help quantify the pain.

Overt means observable

These overt behaviors may indicate that the patient is experiencing pain:
- verbal reports of pain
- vocalizations, such as sighs and moans
- altered motor activities (frequent position changes, guarded positioning, slow movements, and rigidity)
- limping
- grimacing and other expressions
- functional limitations, including reclining for long periods
- actions to reduce pain such as taking medication.

If acute, think "autonomic"

Next, measure the patient's blood pressure, heart and respiratory rates, and pupil size. Acute pain may raise their blood pressure, speed their heart and respiratory rates, and dilate their pupils.

Pain behavior checklist

A pain behavior is something a patient uses to communicate pain, distress, or suffering. Place a check in the box next to each behavior observed while talking to the patient.

- Asking such questions as, "Why did this happen to me?"
- Asking to be relieved from tasks or activities
- Avoiding physical activity
- Being irritable
- Clenching teeth
- Frequently shifting posture or position
- Grimacing
- Holding or supporting the painful body area
- Limping
- Lying down during the day
- Moaning
- Moving in a guarded or protective manner
- Moving very slowly
- Requesting help with walking
- Sighing
- Sitting rigidly
- Stopping frequently while walking
- Taking medication
- Using a cane, cervical collar, or other prosthetic device
- Walking with an abnormal gait

Remember, however, that these autonomic responses may be absent in a patient with chronic pain because the body gradually adapts to pain. Don't assume lack of autonomic responses means lack of pain.

To complete the examination, use a systematic technique to perform palpation, percussion, and auscultation. If the patient is in severe pain, the examination may need to be shortened and completed later, when the pain has decreased.

Psychological characteristics of pain

If diagnostic tests don't find a physical basis for the patient's pain, some health care providers may label the pain *psychogenic*. Psychogenic pain refers to pain associated with psychological factors. A patient with psychogenic pain may have organic pathology, or a psychological disorder may be the predominant influence on pain intensity.

Common psychogenic pain syndromes include chronic headache, muscle pain, back pain, and stomach or pelvic pain of unknown cause.

Keep it real

Keep in mind that psychogenic pain is *real* pain and doesn't mean the patient is malingering. Remember, too, that, although pain can cause emotional distress, such distress isn't necessarily the cause of the psychogenic pain.

If objective physical findings don't substantiate the patient's complaints or if their pain severity rating seems excessive considering their physical findings, consider referring them to a psychologist or psychiatrist who specializes in evaluating chronic pain.

Shopping around

Many patients with chronic pain go from provider to provider and undergo exhausting procedures seeking a diagnosis and effective treatment. If their pain doesn't respond to treatment, they may feel health care providers, employers, and family are blaming—or doubting—them. In time, pain may become the central focus of their lives. They may withdraw from society, lose their jobs, and alienate family and friends.

Not surprisingly, many patients with chronic pain feel anxious, depressed, demoralized, helpless, hopeless, frustrated, angry, and isolated. They may suffer from insomnia, disruption of usual activities, drug misuse and dependence, anger, and violence. Some even attempt suicide.

Road to success

For health care providers, assessment and management of patients with pain—especially chronic pain—can be equally frustrating. However, through careful assessment and regular reevaluation, the odds for successful pain management can increase—even in patients with seemingly intractable or chronic pain.

Treating pain successfully

When caring for a patient experiencing pain, there are three overall goals:
* to reduce pain intensity
* to improve the patient's ability to function
* to improve the patient's quality of life.

To accomplish these goals, the nurse must work with the patient to agree on goals that are mutually desirable, realistic, measurable, and achievable. In addition, focus on the nociceptive and emotional aspects of pain. A patient responds to a painful physical condition based, in part, on their subjective interpretation of illness and symptoms. The patient's beliefs about the meaning of pain and their ability to function despite discomfort are important aspects of coping ability.

Harmful beliefs

Maladaptive responses to pain are more likely in a patient who believes that:
* they have a serious debilitating condition
* disability is a necessary aspect of pain
* activity is dangerous
* pain is an acceptable reason to reduce one's responsibilities.

Sometimes it pays to be a control freak

Many factors can promote or disrupt a patient's sense of control over the pain experience. These factors include:
* personal beliefs and expectations about pain
* coping ability
* social supports
* specific disorder that is causing the pain
* response of employers.

These factors also influence a patient's investment in treatment, acceptance of responsibility, perceptions of disability, adherence to treatment, and support from significant others. To start the patient on the road to successful pain management, consider physical, psychosocial, and behavioral factors—and the changes that occur in these relationships over time.

Interdisciplinary pain management team

An interdisciplinary team approach promotes effective pain management. Team members typically include a health care provider, a nurse, a pharmacist, a social worker, a spiritual advisor, a psychologist, physical and occupational therapists, an anesthesiologist or a certified registered nurse anesthetist, a pain management specialist and, of course, the patient and their family.

Treating types of pain

In addition to the three overall goals of treating pain, consider ways to treat specific types of pain.

Treating acute pain

The cause of acute pain can be diagnosed and treated, and the pain resolves when the cause is treated or analgesics are given. Drug regimens and invasive procedures that aren't reasonable for extended periods can be used more freely in acute pain. With acute pain, it's important to stay ahead of the pain. Many health care providers order pain medication around the clock to be given to the patient.

Treating chronic nonmalignant pain

Medical treatment for chronic nonmalignant pain must be based on the patient's long-term benefit, not just the current complaint of pain. Drug therapy and surgery, which typically provide only partial and temporary relief, should be individualized.

Drug treatment alone almost never effectively relieves chronic nonmalignant pain; the patient must receive a combination of treatments. These may include drugs, nondrug therapies, temporary or permanent invasive therapies (such as nerve blocks or surgery), cognitive-behavioral therapy, alternative and complementary therapies, and self-management techniques.

It pains me to say this

Even with medical management, however, chronic nonmalignant pain can be lifelong. Therefore, treatments that carry significant risks or those that aren't likely to prove effective over the long term may be inappropriate.

Rehab rewards

In many cases, treatment of chronic nonmalignant pain must focus on rehabilitation rather than a cure. Rehabilitation aims to:

- maximize physical and psychological functional abilities
- minimize pain experienced during rehabilitation and for the rest of the patient's life
- teach the patient how to manage residual pain and how to handle pain exacerbation caused by increased activity or unexplained reasons.

Treating cancer pain

Whether pain results from cancer or its treatment, it may cause the patient to lose hope—especially if they think the pain means illness is progressing. They're then likely to suffer additional feelings of help-lessness, anxiety, and depression.

However, most types of cancer pain can be managed effectively, diminishing physical and mental suffering.

Unwise to undertreat

Unfortunately, cancer pain commonly goes undertreated because of:

- inadequate knowledge of—or attention to—pain control by health care professionals
- failure of health care professionals to properly assess pain
- reluctance of patients to report their pain
- reluctance of patients and health care providers to use morphine and other opioids due to fear of developing dependence on a drug.

Undertreated cancer pain diminishes the patient's activity level, appetite, and sleep. It may prevent the patient from working produc-tively, enjoying leisure activities, or participating in family or social situations.

Go for the goal

The success of a pain management plan hinges on having the patient choose an appropriate goal—a pain intensity rating that will reduce their discomfort to a tolerable level and let them engage comfortably in self-care activities. Team members should work together to choose a rating scale for measuring the patient's pain intensity and to develop appropriate pain management goals.

Thorough documentation and pain assessment tools communi-cate vital patient information to all team members. If the patient has chronic pain, periodic team meetings may also be crucial.

Pharmacologic pain management

Pain management can be pharmacologic or nonpharmacologic. Pharmacologic pain management includes nonopioid analgesics, opioids, and adjuvant analgesics. In addition, nonpharmacologic pain management can include alternative and complementary therapies.

Nonopioid analgesics

Nonopioid (nonnarcotic) analgesics are used to treat pain that's *nociceptive* (caused by stimulation of injury-sensing receptors) or *neuropathic* (arising from nerves). These drugs are particularly effective against the somatic component of nociceptive pain such as joint and muscle pain. In addition to controlling pain, nonopioid analgesics reduce inflammation and fever.

Drug types in this category include:
- acetaminophen
- nonsteroidal anti-inflammatory drugs (NSAIDs)
- salicylates such as aspirin.

Solo or combo

When used alone, acetaminophen and NSAIDs provide relief from mild pain. NSAIDs can also relieve moderate pain; in high doses, they may help relieve severe pain. Given in combination with opioids, nonopioid analgesics provide additional analgesia, allowing a lower opioid dose and, thus, a lower risk of adverse effects.

Opioids

Opioids (narcotics) include derivatives of the opium (poppy) plant and synthetic drugs that imitate natural opioids. Unlike NSAIDs, which act peripherally, opioids produce their primary effects in the CNS. Opioids include opioid agonists, opioid antagonists, and mixed agonist–antagonists.

Opioid agonists

Opioid agonists are used to treat moderate to severe pain without causing loss of consciousness. Opioid agonists include:
- codeine
- fentanyl
- hydromorphone
- methadone
- morphine (including sustained-release tablets and intensified oral solution)
- oxycodone.

Opioid antagonists

Opioid antagonists aren't pain medications but block the effects of opioid agonists. They're used to reverse adverse drug reactions, such as respiratory and CNS depression produced by opioid agonists. Unfortunately, by reversing analgesic effects, they may cause the patient's pain to recur.

Attached but not stimulating

Opioid antagonists attach to opiate receptors but don't stimulate them. As a result, they prevent other opioids, enkephalins, and endorphins from producing their effects. Opioid antagonists include naloxone and naltrexone.

Mixed opioid agonist–antagonists

As their name implies, mixed opioid agonist–antagonists have agonist and antagonist properties. The *agonist component* relieves pain, and the *antagonist component* reduces the risk of toxicity and drug dependence. These agents also decrease the risk of respiratory depression and drug misuse. These agents include:
- buprenorphine
- butorphanol
- nalbuphine
- pentazocine hydrochloride (combined with pentazocine lactate, naloxone, aspirin, or acetaminophen).

Potent potential

Originally, mixed agonist–antagonists seemed to have less potential for developing dependence than pure opioid agonists. However, butorphanol and pentazocine reportedly have caused dependence.

Adjuvant analgesics

Adjuvant analgesics are drugs that have other primary indications but are used as analgesics in some circumstances. Adjuvants may be given in combination with opioids or used alone to treat chronic pain. Patients receiving adjuvant analgesics should be reevaluated periodically to monitor their pain level and to check for adverse reactions.

Adjuvant combinations

Drugs used as adjuvant analgesics include certain anticonvulsants, local and topical anesthetics, muscle relaxants, tricyclic antidepressants, serotonin 5-hydroxytryptamine agonists, selective serotonin reuptake inhibitors, ergotamine alkaloids, benzodiazepines, psych stimulants, cholinergic blockers, and corticosteroids.

Nonpharmacologic pain management

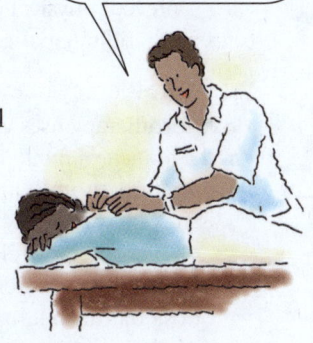

Nonpharmacologic approaches include whirlpools, hot packs, massage, and yoga.

Nonpharmacologic therapies can also help manage pain. Many people are concerned about the overuse of drugs for conventional pain management, and some people simply prefer to self-manage their health issues.

Something for everyone

Collectively speaking, nonpharmacologic approaches offer something for nearly everyone. They range from the relatively conventional (whirlpools, hot packs) to the electrifying (vibration, electrical nerve stimulation), sensual (aromatherapy, massage), serene (meditation, yoga), and high-tech (biofeedback).

Nonpharmacological therapies fall into three main categories:
- physical therapies
- alternative and complementary therapies
- cognitive and behavioral therapies.

In addition to being used alone, some nonpharmacological therapies can be combined with drug therapy. A combination approach may improve pain relief by enhancing drug effects and allowing lower dosages.

Plenty of perks

Nonpharmacologic approaches have other benefits in addition to pain management. For example, they help reduce stress, improve mood, promote sleep, and give the patient a sense of control over pain.

Opt for more options

The techniques discussed in this chapter can be effective for a wide range of patients. Additional options may help with pain relief. Some options may require an order from a health care provider.

Physical therapies

Physical therapies use physical agents and methods to aid rehabilitation and restore normal functioning after an illness or injury. These therapies are relatively cheap and easy to use. With appropriate teaching, patients and their families can use them on their own, which helps them participate in pain management.

Physical therapies include:
- hydrotherapy
- thermotherapy
- cryotherapy
- vibration
- transcutaneous electrical nerve stimulation (TENS).

Therapeutic goals

In addition to easing pain, physical therapies reduce inflammation, ease muscle spasms, and promote relaxation. The goals of physical therapies are to:

- promote health
- prevent physical disability
- rehabilitate patients disabled by pain, disease, or injury.

Hydrotherapy

Hydrotherapy uses water to treat pain and disease. Sometimes called the *ultimate natural pain reliever*, water comforts and soothes while providing support and buoyancy. Depending on the patient's medical issue, the water can be hot or cold, and liquid, solid (ice), or steam.

Hydrotherapy relaxes muscles, raises or lowers tissue temperature (depending on water temperature), and eases joint stiffness (as in RA or osteoarthritis). In pain management, hydrotherapy is most commonly used to treat acute pain—for instance, from muscle sprains or strains.

Jet set

Whirlpool baths—bathtubs with jets that force water to circulate—aid in rehabilitating injured muscles and joints. Depending on the desired effect, the water can be hot or cold. The water jets act to massage soothing muscles. (See *Pools that ease pain*.)

Pools that ease pain

Hydrotherapy commonly takes the form of a whirlpool bath, which uses water jets to help ease pain.

Pool tips
• When administering whirlpool therapy, keep water temperature between 52° and 109° F (11.1° and 42.8° C), depending on the body surface area being treated and the patient's physical condition.
• Use a hydraulic chair to help the patient get into and out of the whirlpool tub.

This illustration shows a patient whose leg injury is being treated in a whirlpool.

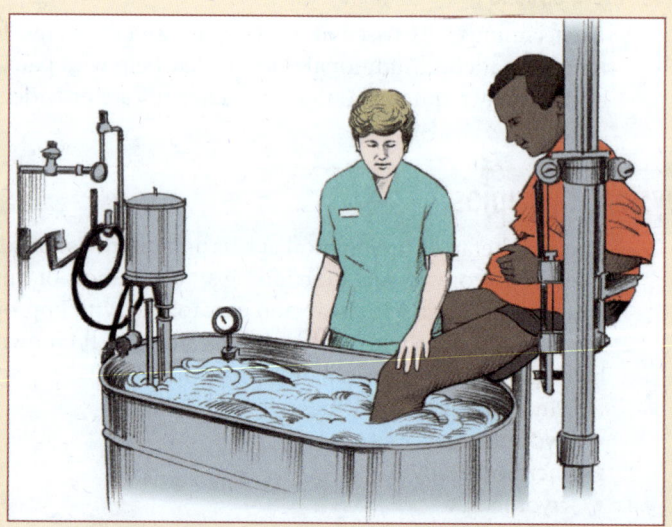

Whirlpools and certain other hydrotherapy treatments can be done at home. However, the more intensive forms are best done in a supervised clinical setting where the treatment and the patient's response can be monitored.

Secrets revealed

Hydrotherapy's pain-relieving properties are related to the physics and mechanics of water and its effect on the human body. When a body is immersed in water, the resulting weightlessness reduces stress on joints, muscles, and other connective tissues. This buoyancy may relieve some types of pain instantly.

Hot water hydrotherapy eases pain through a sequence of events triggered by increased skin temperature. As skin temperature rises, blood vessels widen and skin circulation increases. As resistance to blood flow through veins and capillaries drops, blood pressure decreases. The heart rate then rises to maintain blood pressure. The result is a significant drop in pain and an increase in comfort.

Some restrictions apply

As with any treatment, be aware of these potential hazards of hydrotherapy:

- Hydrotherapy may cause burns, falls, or light-headedness.
- Stop the treatment session if the patient feels light-headed, dizzy, or faint.
- Don't keep the patient in a heated whirlpool for more than 20 minutes.
- Instruct the patient to wipe their face frequently with a cool washcloth so they avoid getting overheated.
- Know that hydrotherapy isn't recommended for pregnant people; children; older adult patients; or patients with diabetes, hypertension, hypotension, or multiple sclerosis.

Thermotherapy

Thermotherapy refers to application of dry or moist heat to decrease pain, relieve stiff joints, ease muscle aches and spasms, improve circulation, and increase the pain threshold. Dry heat can be applied with a K-pad or an electric heating pad. Moist heat can be applied with a hot pack, a warm compress, or a special heating pad. Dry and moist heat involves conductive heating—heat transfer that occurs when the skin directly contacts a warm object.

Uses of thermotherapy

Thermotherapy is used to treat pain caused by:

- headache
- muscle aches and spasms

- earache
- menstrual cramps
- temporomandibular joint disease
- fibromyalgia (syndrome of chronic pain in the muscles and soft tissues surrounding joints).

Benefits of thermotherapy

Thermotherapy enhances blood flow, increases tissue metabolism, and decreases vasomotor tone. Analgesic effects are produced by suppressing free nerve endings. It also may reduce the perception of pain in the cerebral cortex.

Regional heating—heat therapy of selected body areas—can bring immediate temporary pain relief. This method may have a systemic effect, too, resulting from autonomic reflex responses to localized heat application. The reflex-mediated responses may raise body temperature, enhance blood flow, and cause other physiologic changes in areas distant from the heat application site. (See *Thermo thoughts* for considerations when using heat therapy.)

Cryotherapy

Cryotherapy involves applying cold to a specific body area. In addition to reducing fever, this technique can provide immediate pain relief and help reduce or prevent edema and swelling.

Thermo thoughts

Before administering thermotherapy, take these considerations into account:
- Determine the patient's awareness level and ability to communicate their response to the treatment.
- Measure the temperature of the heating agent before applying it. It should be 104° to 113° F (40° to 45° C) when it contacts the skin.
- Be aware that some patients may prefer a slightly lower (or higher) temperature. Keep the heating agent at a temperature that's comfortable for the patient.
- Wrap the heating agent so it doesn't directly contact the patient's skin.
- Regularly assess skin at the heat application site for irritation and redness.
- Frequently evaluate the patient's response to treatment and their pain level.
- Stop the treatment if the patient's pain increases.
- Don't apply heat to an area that's infected, bleeding, or receiving radiation therapy or where oil or menthol has been applied.
- Know that thermotherapy is contraindicated in patients with vascular insufficiency, neuropathy, skin desensitization, or neoplasms.

Cryotherapy methods include cold packs and ice bags for pain relief measures. These measures should only be used for 20 minutes. Ice is used in acute injury along with rest, compression, and elevation (RICE).

Quite a contrast

In another cryotherapy technique, known as *contrast therapy*, cold and heat application are applied alternately during the same session. Contrast therapy may benefit patients with RA and certain other conditions.

Typically, the session begins by immersing the patient's feet and hands in warm water for 10 minutes. Next come four cycles of cold soaks (each lasting 1 to 4 minutes) alternating with warm soaks (each lasting 4 to 6 minutes).

Freezing out pain

Cryotherapy is commonly used for acute pain—especially when caused by a sports injury (such as a muscle sprain). It may also be indicated for pain resulting from:
- acute trauma
- joint disorders such as RA
- headache such as migraine
- muscle aches and spasms
- incisions
- surgery.

Constrict and reduce

Cryotherapy constricts blood vessels at the injury site, reducing blood flow to the site. This, in turn, thickens the blood, resulting in decreased bleeding and increased blood clotting.

Cold application also slows edema development, prevents further tissue damage, and minimizes bruising.

In addition, cryotherapy decreases sensitivity to pain by cooling nerve endings. It eases muscle spasms by cooling muscle spindles—the part of the muscle tissue responsible for the stretch reflex. (See *Applying cold to a muscle sprain*, page 540.) Contrast therapy is thought to stimulate endocrine function, reduce inflammation, decrease congestion, and improve organ function.

Remember this

When administering cryotherapy, remember these points:
- As appropriate, encourage the patient to try cold application. Many patients aren't aware that cold relieves pain.
- Before applying cold, assess the injury site and the patient's pain level. Evaluate them for impaired circulation (such as from

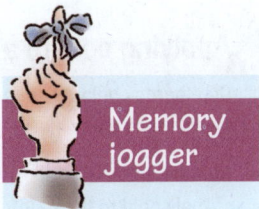

Memory jogger

RICE Therapy

For an acute injury, remember RICE:

Rest

Ice

Compression

Elevation

Applying cold to a muscle sprain

Cryotherapy helps reduce pain and edema when used during the first 24 to 72 hours after an injury. For best results, follow these guidelines.

Method and materials
• Apply cold to the painful area four times daily for 20 minutes each time.
• Use enough crushed ice to cover the area.
• Place the ice in a plastic bag, and place the bag inside a pillowcase or a large piece of cloth, as shown here. Then apply the bag over the painful area for the specified treatment time.

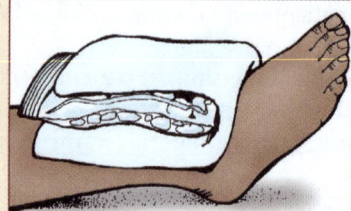

The old switcheroo
• After 24 to 72 hours, when swelling has subsided, switch to thermotherapy.

Wise words
• Inform the patient that ice eases pain in a joint that has begun to stiffen—but caution them not to let the analgesic effect lull them into overusing the joint.

Raynaud disease), inability to sense temperature (such as from neuropathy), extreme skin sensitivity, and inability to report the response to treatment (for instance, a young child or a confused patient).
• Measure the temperature of the cooling agent. It should be no colder than 59° F (15° C).
• When administering moist cold, keep in mind that moisture intensifies cold.
• Wrap cold packs so they don't directly contact the patient's skin. Keep them at a comfortable temperature.
• Stop the treatment if the patient's skin becomes numb.
• Use caution when applying ice to the elbow, wrist, or outer part of the knee. These sites are more susceptible to cold-induced nerve injury.
• Be aware that refreezable gel packs and chemical packs may be colder than ice and may leak.
• Regularly assess the patient for adverse effects such as skin irritation, joint stiffness, numbness, frostbite, and nerve injury.
• Don't apply cold to areas that have poor circulation or have received radiation.

Vibration

Vibration therapy eases pain by inducing numbness in the treated area. This technique, which works like an electric massage, may be effective for disorders such as:
• muscle aches
• headache
• chronic nonmalignant pain

- cancer pain
- fractures
- neuropathic pain.

Hospitalized patients need an order from the health care provider to use a vibrating device. Outpatients may choose from various devices available without a prescription.

Good vibrations

A vibrating device can be stationary or handheld. Stationary devices range from vibrating cushions to full beds and recliners. The patient lies or sits on the device and receives the treatment passively.

The patient or caregiver moves a handheld vibrator (also known as a massage gun or a muscle gun) above or below the painful area. Some handheld vibrators are battery operated; others plug into a wall outlet.

Points to remember

Remember these points when administering vibration therapy:
- Before using vibration therapy, teach the patient about this method, including how it works and when it should and shouldn't be used.
- Tell the patient they may feel a warm sensation initially.
- Apply the vibrator to an area above or below the pain site.
- For more effective pain relief, use the highest vibration speed the patient can tolerate.
- Apply the vibrating device for 1 to 15 minutes at a time, two to four times daily, or as ordered.
- Determine the length of treatment needed to achieve adequate pain relief. Continue to assess the patient's response to treatment.
- Stop the treatment if the patient experiences discomfort, pain, or excessive skin redness or irritation.
- Don't use vibration therapy if the patient has thrombophlebitis or bruises easily.
- Don't apply the vibrator over burns, cuts, or incision sites.
- If the patient will self-administer this therapy, provide appropriate teaching. Advise them to assess their pain level before the session, immediately afterward, and later to assess how long pain relief lasts. Doing so helps determine the optimal length of treatment. (Usually, the longer the session, the longer the duration of pain relief.)

Transcutaneous electrical nerve stimulation

In TENS therapy, a portable, battery-powered device transmits painless alternating electric current to peripheral nerves or directly to a painful area. Used postoperatively and for patients with chronic pain, TENS reduces the need for analgesic drugs and helps the patient resume normal activities. TENS therapy must be prescribed by a health care provider.

The patient usually wears the TENS unit on a belt. Units have several channels and lead placements. The settings allow adjustment of wave frequency, duration, and intensity. (See *Positioning TENS electrodes*, page 543.)

Typically, a course of TENS therapy lasts 3 to 5 days. Some conditions (such as phantom pain) may require continuous simulation. Others, such as a painful arthritic joint, call for shorter treatment periods—perhaps 3 to 4 hours.

Top TENS list

TENS can provide temporary relief of acute pain (such as postoperative pain) and ongoing relief of chronic pain (such as in sciatica). Specific pain problems that have responded to TENS include:
- chronic nonmalignant pain
- cancer pain
- bone fracture pain
- low back pain
- sports injuries
- myofascial pain
- neurogenic pain (as in neuralgia and neuropathy)
- phantom pain
- arthritis pain
- menstrual pain.

Still a mystery

Although TENS has existed for over 30 years, experts still aren't sure exactly how it relieves pain. Some believe that it works according to the gate-control theory, which proposes that painful impulses pass through a "gate" in the brain. According to this theory, TENS alters the patient's perception of pain by closing the gate to painful stimuli.

TENS to-do list

Consider these points when administering TENS therapy:
- To ensure that the patient is a willing and active participant in TENS therapy, provide complete instructions on using and caring for the TENS unit as well as expected results of treatment.
- Before TENS therapy begins, assess the patient's pain level and evaluate for skin irritation at the sites where electrodes will be placed.
- Be aware that the safety of TENS during pregnancy hasn't been established.

Positioning TENS electrodes

In TENS, electrodes placed around peripheral nerves or incision sites transmit mild electrical impulses, which are believed to block pain messages.

Perfect placement

Electrode placement usually varies, even for patients with similar complaints. Electrodes can be placed in several ways:
• to cover or surround the painful area, as for muscle tenderness or spasm, or for painful joints
• to capture the painful area between electrodes, as for incisional pain.

These illustrations show combinations of electrode placement (red squares) and areas of nerve stimulation (shaded light red strips) for low back and leg pain.

Placement tips

• If the patient has peripheral nerve injury, place electrodes proximal to the injury (between the brain and the injury site) to avoid increasing their pain.
• If a site lacks sensation, place electrodes on adjacent dermatomes (areas of skin innervated by sensory fibers from a single spinal nerve).

• Don't place electrodes in a hypersensitive area. Doing so can increase pain.

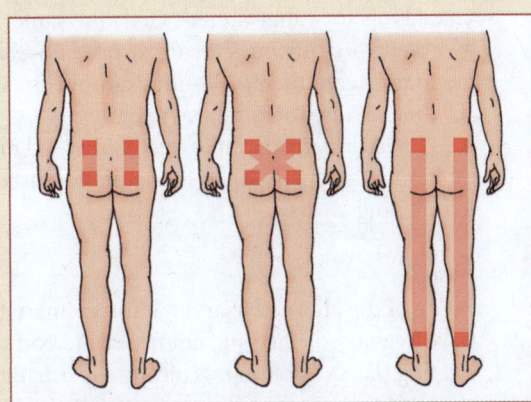

TENS taboos

- Don't use TENS if the patient has undiagnosed pain, uses a pacemaker, or has a history of heart arrhythmias.
- Don't apply a TENS unit over the carotid sinus, an open wound, or anesthetized skin.
- Don't place the unit on the head or neck of a patient who has a vascular disorder or seizure disorder.

Alternative and complementary therapies

Alternative and complementary therapies greatly expand the range of therapeutic choices for patients suffering pain. Today, patients are increasingly seeking these therapies—not just to treat pain but also to address many other common health conditions. Various theories have been offered to explain the increased interest in alternative and complementary therapies. (See *Understanding the alternative trend*, page 544.)

Wholly holistic

Regardless of the problem for which they're used, alternative and complementary therapies address the whole person—body, mind, and spirit—rather than just signs and symptoms.

Defining the terms

Although alternative and complementary therapies are usually discussed together, they aren't exactly the same:

- *Alternative* therapies are those used *instead* of conventional or mainstream therapies—for example, the use of acupuncture rather than analgesics to relieve pain.
- *Complementary* therapies are those used *in conjunction with* conventional therapies—such as meditation used as an adjunct to analgesic drugs.

East meets west

Some of the alternative and complementary therapies practiced today have been used since ancient times and come from the traditional healing practices of many cultures—particularly in the Eastern part of the world.

Understanding the alternative trend

Why are more people turning to alternative and complementary therapies to treat health problems? One reason is that most therapies are noninvasive and cause few adverse reactions.

People with certain chronic conditions may be drawn to these therapies because conventional medicine has few, if any, effective treatments for them. Also, people are encouraged by reports that document their effectiveness, although some reports may not be reliable or legitimate.

Focus on the whole

Conventional medicine tends to treat only signs and symptoms, whereas alternative and complementary therapies focus on the whole person (i.e., holism).

Time—and more time

Many people also value the extra time alternative practitioners spend with the patient and the attention they pay to the patient's temperament, behavioral patterns, and perceived needs. In an increasingly stressful world, people are searching for someone who will take the time to listen to them and to treat them as people, not just bodies displaying signs and symptoms.

Spiritual hunger

Some people view modern society as spiritually malnourished and are hungry for meaning. These patients view alternative practitioners as more responsive to this need than those who practice conventional medicine.

Cultural connections

Lastly, in a culturally diverse country such as the United States, a wide variety of traditional healing practices and beliefs exist. Some are based on the same principles that underlie alternative and complementary therapies.

Many mainstream Western health care providers have become more open-minded about these therapies—in fact, some health care providers even administer them. However, other providers object to them on the grounds that they aren't based solely on empirical science.

Pain relief prospects

Alternative and complementary therapies commonly relieve some types of pain that don't respond to Western techniques. They may prove especially valuable when a precise cause evades Western medicine, such as typically occurs in chronic low back pain.

Cognitive and behavioral approaches

Cognitive approaches to pain management focus on influencing the patient's interpretation of the pain experience. *Behavioral* approaches help the patient develop skills for managing pain and changing their reaction to it.

Cognitive and behavioral approaches to managing pain include meditation, biofeedback, and hypnosis. These techniques improve the patient's sense of control over pain and allow them to participate actively in pain management.

Meditation

Meditation is thought to relieve stress and reduce pain through an effect called the *relaxation response*—a natural protective mechanism against overstress. Learning to activate the relaxation response through meditation may offset some of the negative physiologic effects of stress.

Biofeedback

Biofeedback uses electronic monitors to teach patients how to exert conscious control over autonomic functions. By watching the fluctuations of various body functions on a monitor, patients learn how to change a particular body function by adjusting thoughts, breathing pattern, posture, or muscle tension.

As they modify vital functions, patients may develop the ability to control pain without using conventional treatments.

Hypnosis

Hypnosis harnesses the power of suggestion and altered levels of consciousness to produce positive behavior changes and treat various conditions. Under hypnosis, a patient typically relaxes and experiences changes in respiration, which may lead to a positive shift in behavior and a greater sense of well-being.

Quick quiz

1. Which of the following can influence pain perception? (*Select all that apply*).
   A. Beliefs
   B. Past experience
   C. Coping ability
   D. Judgments
   E. Gender

   Answer: A, B, C, D. Pain perception is influenced by beliefs, judgments, past experiences with pain, and coping ability.

2. What are the three types of pain?
   A. Acute, nonacute, and surgical
   B. Acute, chronic, and cancer
   C. Acute, subacute, and mild
   D. Acute, referred, and terminal

   Answer: B. The three types of pain are acute, chronic, and cancer pain.

3. Which type of pain responds to opioid medication?
   A. Acute pain
   B. Chronic pain
   C. Cancer pain
   D. All of the above

   Answer: D. All of the different types of pain can be treated with opioids.

4. Which are common side effects of opioids?
   A. Constipation, respiratory depression, nausea
   B. Confusion, insomnia, altered taste
   C. Depression, fatigue, weight loss
   D. Low blood pressure, thirst, restlessness

   Answer: A. Constipation, respiratory depression, and nausea are common side effects of opioids.

Scoring

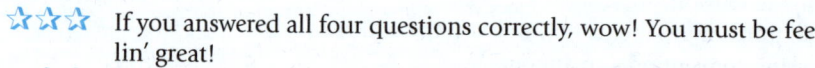

⭐⭐⭐ If you answered all four questions correctly, wow! You must be feelin' great!

⭐⭐ If you answered three questions correctly, good job! Your strategy is working!

⭐ If you answered two or fewer questions correctly, feel no pain! Review the chapter and try again.

References

Gebke, K., McCarberg, B., Shaw, E. Turk, D., Wright, W. & Semel, D. (2023). A practical guide to recognize, assess, treat and evaluate (RATE) primary care patients with chronic pain. *Postgraduate Medicine, 135*(3), 244–253. https://doi.org/10.1080/00325481.2021.2017201

Kunzmann, K. (2023, April 15). *Chronic pain prevalence remains among 1 in 5 US adults.* Retrieved from https://www.hcplive.com/view/chronic-pain-prevalence-remains-among-1-5-us-adults

Nagy, Z., Szigedi, E., Takács, S., & Császár-Nagy, N. (2023). The effectiveness of psychological interventions for rheumatoid arthritis (RA): A systematic review and meta-analysis. *Life (Basel, Switzerland), 13*(3), 849. https://doi.org/10.3390/life13030849

Pugh, T., Squarize, F., & Kiser, A. (2021). A comprehensive strategy to pain management for cancer patients in an inpatient rehabilitation facility. *Frontiers in Pain Research, 2,* 688511.

Rochon, R. (2022). *Drug prescribing for older adults.* http://www.uptodate.com/drug-prescri.bing-for-older-adults

Chapter 18

Nutrition

Just the facts

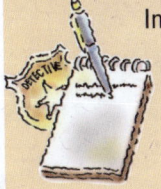

In this chapter, you'll learn:

◆ the role nutrients play in health promotion

◆ current nutrient standards for health promotion

◆ the purpose of digestion and absorption

◆ structures of the gastrointestinal (GI) tract wall, digestive organs, and accessory organs, as well as their functions in digestion and absorption

◆ ways to promote proper diet.

A look at nutrition

Nutrition refers to the processes by which a living organism ingests, digests, absorbs, transports, uses, and excretes *nutrients* (food and other nourishing material) (Academy of Nutrition and Dietetics, 2021). Nutrition as a science is primarily concerned with the properties of food that build healthy bodies and promote well-being.

More than just a pretty process

Because nutrition is essential to good health and disease prevention, any person involved in health care needs a thorough knowledge of nutrition and the body's nutritional requirements throughout the life span. Additionally, the study of nutrition should focus on health promotion.

Nutrients

There are two types of nutrients:

- *Nonessential nutrients* are nutrients that aren't needed in the diet because they're manufactured by the body.
- *Essential nutrients* are nutrients that must be acquired through food because the body can't produce them on its own in adequate quantities.

Certain and essential

For nutrition to be adequate, a person must receive certain essential nutrients, including carbohydrates, fats, proteins, vitamins, minerals, and water. These nutrients are required for proper growth and functioning. If the digestive system is not functioning properly, the body may struggle to make use of these nutrients.

Close relationships

Each nutrient has several specific metabolic functions, but no nutrient works alone. Close metabolic relationships exist among all of the basic nutrients as well as with their metabolic products.

Nutrient breakdown

Nutrients can be used by the body for its immediate needs, or they can be stored for later use. The body breaks down nutrients into simpler compounds for absorption in the stomach and intestines in two ways:
- mechanical breakdown, which begins in the gastrointestinal (GI) tract with chewing.
- chemical breakdown, which starts with salivary enzymes in the mouth and continues with acid and enzyme action through the rest of the GI tract.

Role of a lifeline

Nutrients play a vital role in maintaining health and wellness. They have several important functions:
- providing energy, which can be stored in the body or transformed for vital activities
- building and maintaining body tissue
- controlling metabolic processes, such as growth, cell activity, enzyme production, and temperature regulation.

Metabolism

Regulated mostly by hormones, metabolism is a combination of several processes by which energy is extracted from certain nutrients (carbohydrates, proteins, and fats) and then used by the body. Vitamins and minerals don't directly provide energy, but they're an important part of the metabolic process. Metabolism can be broken down into two parts:
- *Catabolism* is the breakdown of complex substances into simpler ones, resulting in the release of energy.
- *Anabolism* is the synthesis of simple substances into more complex substances. This process provides the energy necessary for tissue growth, maintenance, and repair.

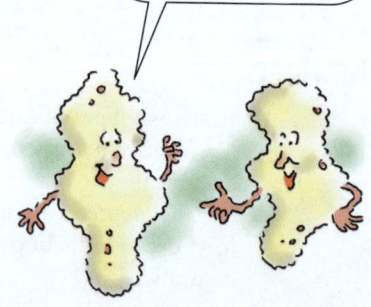

Metabolism, regulated mostly by hormones like us, is a combination of several processes by which energy is extracted from certain nutrients and then used by the body.

Energy

Energy, in the form of adenosine triphosphate, is produced as a by-product of carbohydrate, fat, and protein metabolism. The amount of energy in food products is measured in kilocalories (kcal), which are commonly referred to as *calories* (Sánchez López de Nava & Raja, 2022).

Through the processes of digestion and absorption, energy is released from food into the body. Small amounts of energy are stored within cells for immediate use. Larger amounts of energy are stored in glycogen and fat tissue to fuel long-duration activities.

Balancing act

In a healthy adult, the rate of anabolism equals the rate of catabolism, and energy balance is achieved. In other words, energy balance occurs when the caloric intake from food equals the number of calories expended. These calories may be used for voluntary activities (physical activity) or involuntary activities (basal metabolism).

Nutrition and health promotion

Many patients may consider themselves healthy because they don't feel sick. However, to provide the best care for patients, it's important to become familiar with the holistic meaning of the term *health*, which incorporates aspects of the patient's internal and external environments.

Health promotion considers all of a patient's needs, including physical, emotional, mental, and social. Only when these needs are met is a person considered to be healthy or well. Furthermore, wellness implies a state of balance between a person's activities and goals. Maintaining this balance allows the patient to maintain their energy and ability to function productively in society. A nutritious diet provides the basis for health promotion and disease prevention, making it an important part of caring for any patient.

Approaches to health promotion

There are two main approaches to health promotion:

- The *traditional approach* is reactive; it focuses on treating symptoms after they appear.
- The *preventive approach* involves identifying and eliminating risk factors to stop health problems from developing.

The current health and wellness movement in the United States is grounded in the preventive approach, with a focus on maintaining health and preventing illness and disease. Most Americans, however, don't get the recommended amount of physical activity, which can put them at greater risk for such disorders as heart disease, diabetes, cancer, and hypertension (Jurdana, 2021).

Healthy People 2030

The US national health goals, which were originally published in the US Department of Health and Human Services (USDHHS, 2020) *Healthy People 2000* and have been updated every 10 years since then, also reflect a preventive wellness philosophy. Prominent themes in the latest report, *Healthy People 2030*, include

- choosing a healthy diet, including increased amounts of fruits and vegetables
- maintaining weight control through physical exercise and diet
- decreasing foods high in sugar and saturated fat
- monitoring for and reducing high-risk factors for disease.

Not one, not two, but three!

Promoting health, establishing wellness, and preventing disease is a three-part process. (See *Three parts to prevention*.)

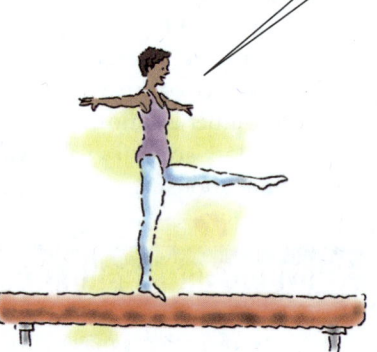

Wellness implies a state of balance between a person's activities and goals. Maintaining this balance allows the patient to maintain their energy and ability to function productively in society.

Three parts to prevention

Health promotion and disease prevention efforts can be categorized into three groups.

Primary prevention

Examples of primary prevention measures, which focus on health promotion, include
- conducting nutrition classes to promote healthy eating patterns
- modifying menus in restaurants and offering low-fat or low-sugar alternatives
- offering fresh fruit and vegetables in workplace cafeterias.

Secondary prevention

Secondary prevention, which focuses on risk reduction, may include such measures as
- screening for potential diseases (hypercholesterolemia, osteoporosis)
- nutritional counseling for people at risk for cardiovascular diseases and diabetes

Tertiary prevention

Examples of tertiary prevention measures, which focus on disease treatment and rehabilitation, include
- physical rehabilitation for a patient who has had a stoke
- cardiac rehabilitation for the patient who has had myocardial infarction
- diabetes education classes for the patient with newly diagnosed type 1 or type 2 diabetes.

Source: World Health Organization (WHO). (2023). Health promotion and disease prevention. https://www.emro.who.int/about-who/public-health-functions/health-promotion-disease-prevention.html

Nutrition and a balanced diet

The nurse is responsible for making sure the patient maintains optimal nutritional health, even though they may be combatting illness or recovering from surgery. It's essential to stress to the patient the importance of good nutrition in maintaining health and recovering from illness so that they can continue sound nutritional practices when they're discharged from the inpatient setting.

Nutritional status

Nurses use their knowledge of nutrition to promote health through education and counseling of sick and healthy patients. This counseling includes encouraging patients to consume appropriate types and amounts of food. It also means considering poor food habits as a contributing factor in a patient with chronic illness. Therefore, assessing nutritional status and identifying nutritional needs to meet the requirements of a balanced diet are primary activities in planning patient care.

Assessing nutritional status

A patient's nutritional status can influence the body's response to illness and treatment. Regardless of the patient's overall condition, evaluation of their nutritional health is an essential part of a nursing assessment. This process also includes determining nutritional risk factors and individual needs.

Good nutrition

Good nutrition, or *optimal nutrition*, is essential in promoting health, preventing illness, and restoring health after an injury or illness. To achieve optimal nutrition, one must eat a varied diet containing carbohydrates, proteins, fats, vitamins, minerals, water, and fiber in sufficient amounts. Although excesses of certain nutrients can be detrimental to a patient's health, intake of essential nutrients should be greater than the minimum requirements to allow for variations in health and disease and to provide stores for later use (Bhupathiraju & Hu, 2023).

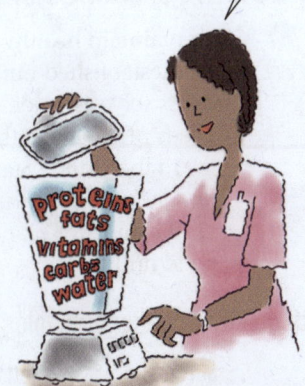

Optimal nutrition requires a varied diet of carbs, proteins, fats, vitamins, minerals, water, and fiber in sufficient amounts.

Poor nutrition

Undernutrition, or *malnutrition*, is a state of inadequate or excess nutritional intake. It's most common among people living in poverty, especially those with greater nutritional requirements, such as older adults, pregnant people, children, and infants. It can also occur in hospitals and long-term care facilities because the patients in these environments have illnesses that place added stress on their bodies, raising nutritional requirements (Morley, 2021).

Don't underestimate undernutrition

Undernutrition occurs when a patient consumes fewer daily nutrients than their body requires, resulting in a nutritional deficit. Typically, an undernourished patient is at greater risk for physical illnesses. They may also suffer from limitations in cognitive and physical status.

Undernutrition can result from

- inability to metabolize nutrients
- inability to obtain the appropriate nutrients from food
- accelerated excretion of nutrients from the body
- illness or disease that increases the body's need for nutrients.

Don't overdo it

In contrast, *overnutrition*, also a form of malnutrition, occurs when a patient consumes an excessive amount of nutrients. For example, overnutrition may occur in patients who self-prescribe mega-doses of vitamins and mineral supplements and in those who overeat. These practices can result in damage to body tissue or obesity.

Nutrient guidelines and standards

To maintain healthy populations, most resource-abundant countries have established nutrition standards for major nutrients. These standards serve as guidelines for nutrient intake based on the nutritional needs of most healthy population groups.

In the United States, the first nutrient standards, called *recommended dietary allowances (RDAs)*, were published during World War II as a guide for planning and acquiring food supplies and promoting good nutrition.

Understanding the terminology of US guidelines

Dietary reference intakes (DRIs) are the most recent version of the US nutrient standards. Because DRIs consider an individual's gender and age group and aren't limited to preventing nutrient-deficiency diseases, these standards are more comprehensive than RDAs in measuring a patient's nutritional status and long-term health (National Academy of Sciences, 2023). (See *Dietary reference intakes.*)

The published standards of other countries, such as Canada and Britain, are similar to US standards. In countries where quality of food and nutrition are lacking, standards are set by the Food and Agriculture Organization and the World Health Organization. No

Dietary reference intakes

DRIs consist of a set of four nutrient-based reference values developed by the Food and Nutrition Board (FNB) of the National Academy of Sciences (2023). These values have replaced and expanded on the familiar RDAs. DRIs can be used for planning and assessing diets. They include updated values for RDAs as well as values for estimated average requirement (EAR), adequate intake (AI), and tolerable upper intake level (UL).

Recommended dietary allowance

The RDA of a nutrient is the average daily dietary intake needed to meet the requirements of virtually all healthy people in a given life stage or gender group. Critics argue that RDAs merely prevent nutritional deficiencies rather than promote optimal health.

Estimated average requirement

The EAR of a nutrient is the average daily dietary intake needed to meet the requirements of half of all healthy people in a given life stage or gender group. Determination of this value isn't based solely on preventing nutritional deficiencies but also includes concepts related to risk reduction and bioavailability of a given nutrient.

Adequate intake

An AI value is assigned to a nutrient if the FNB lacks sufficient information to establish an RDA and an EAR. The AI value is a recommended daily intake level based on estimates of nutrient intake by a group of healthy people.

Tolerable upper intake level

The UL is the highest level of nutrient intake that doesn't pose an adverse health effect to almost all individuals in the general population.

Source: National Institutes of Health. (n.d.). *Nutrient recommendations and databases*. Office of Dietary Supplements. https://ods.od.nih.gov/HealthInformation/nutrientrecommendations.aspx

matter who sets forth the standards, the goal is the same: to promote good health and to prevent disease through sound nutrition.

Dietary Guidelines for Americans 2020-2025

The US Department of Agriculture and the Department of Health and Human Services released the first Dietary Guidelines and Food Guide Pyramid in 1980 to enable an individual to prepare a well-balanced diet through variety, balance, and moderation of choices. These guidelines have been revised several times, with the most recent Dietary Guidelines released in December 2020.

The US dietary guidelines recommend that people 2 years and older eat a healthy assortment of foods from the basic food groups. They also emphasize the importance of

- choosing foods that are low in added sugars, refined grains, sodium (salt), cholesterol, and saturated and trans fats
- eating more foods such as fruits, vegetables, whole grains, and fat-free and low-fat dairy products
- eating reasonable portions and balancing calories with physical activity to manage weight
- getting at least 30 minutes of moderate physical exercise on most days for adults. (The guidelines for children recommend at least 60 minutes of physical activity on most days of the week.)

All mine

Dietary Guidelines for Americans 2020-2025 uses an updated food pyramid called *MyPlate*. This infographic promotes an interactive and individualized approach to improving diet and lifestyle. MyPlate helps people transfer the principles of the *Dietary Guidelines* into healthy eating and lifestyle choices (United States Department of Agriculture [USDA], 2020). (See *Anatomy of MyPlate*.)

MyPlate features

MyPlate uses wedges of different widths and colors on a plate to represent the recommended amount of food a person should choose from a food group. Since its creation in 2010, MyPlate has become more interactive, with online resources, phone applications, and even integration with smartwatches and smart speakers.

Anatomy of MyPlate

The USDA's food guidance system—called MyPlate—symbolizes a personalized approach to healthy eating. Designed to be simple, the infographic reminds consumers to make healthy food choices and to be active every day. The five food groups are illustrated on a familiar family place setting. These five food groups are fruits, vegetables, grains, proteins, and dairy.

Key Behaviors:

Balancing Calories
- Enjoy your food, but eat less.
- Avoid oversized portions.

Foods to Increase
- Make half your plate fruits and vegetables.
- Make at least half your grains whole grains.
- Switch to fat-free or low-fat (1%) milk.

Foods to Reduce
- Compare sodium in foods like soup, bread, and frozen meals, and choose foods with lower amounts of sodium.
- Drink water instead of sugary drinks.

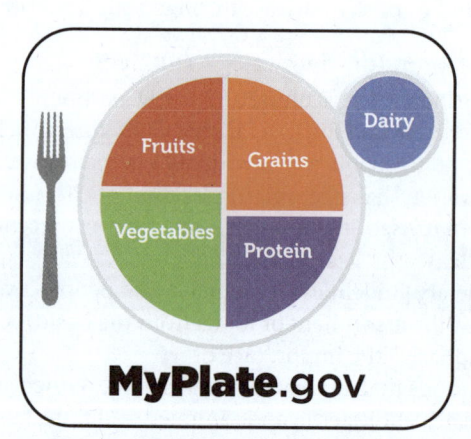

Source: USDA. (2020). What is MyPlate? https://www.myplate.gov/eat-healthy/what-is-myplate

The MyPlate website makes recommendations based on health needs for specific populations, such as children and adolescents, people of childbearing age, pregnant and breastfeeding individuals, people with hypertension, older adults, and overweight children and adults (USDA, 2020). (See *Daily Food Plans*, page 557.)

Food group recommendations

Each portion on the plate represents one of the five food groups: grains, vegetables, fruits, protein, and dairy. Each portion is designated in size in relation to the amount that is needed.

Daily Food Plans

To determine which food intake pattern to use for an individual, this chart gives an estimate of individual calorie needs. The calorie range is based on age, gender, height and weight, and physical activity level. Each Daily Food Plan is associated with a worksheet that is personally developed based on the above factors to give each individual a plan that is unique.

Age group (years)	Calorie range
Children	
2–3	1,000–1,400
*Females**	
4–8	1,200–1,600
9–13	1,400–2,000
14–18	1,800–2,000
19–30	2,000–2,200
31–50	1,800–2,000
51+	1,600–1,800
*Males**	
4–8	1,200–1,600
9–13	1,600–2,200
14–18	2,000–2,800
19–30	2,600–2,800
31–50	2,400–2,600
51+	2,200–2,400

*Note: In this box, "females" means people assigned female at birth, and "males" means people assigned male at birth.

Source: USDA. (2011). Estimated calorie needs per day table. https://www.fns.usda.gov/estimated-calorie-needs-day-age-gender-and-physical-activity-level

Grain group

Foods in the grain group are sources of complex carbohydrates, vitamins, minerals, and fiber. This group has two subgroups: *whole grains* and *refined grains*. Whole grains have not been processed to remove the entire grain kernel; refined grains have. This distinction is important when selecting grains for a healthy diet. To help the patient consume their recommended servings of foods from this food group, suggest that they

- consume what is recommended by the Daily Food Plan based on their age, gender, and physical activity level
- make sure that half of all grains consumed each day are whole grains
- be aware that 1 oz is approximately one slice of bread, one cup of breakfast cereal, or half cup of cooked rice, cereal, or pasta
- choose items made with little fat and sugar
- select several servings of food made from whole grains to add fiber
- avoid baked products that are high in fat and sugar, such as cakes and cookies

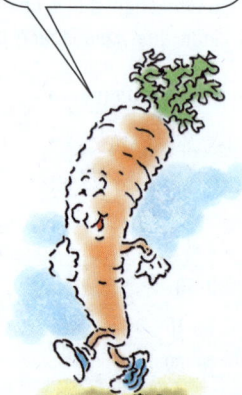

I know what I'm talking about! Eat your veggies!

Vegetable group

Vegetables provide sources of vitamin A, vitamin C, folate, iron, magnesium, and fiber. To help the patient select healthy food choices from the vegetable group, urge them to:

- Fill half of a dinner plate with vegetables and fruits.
- Consume plenty of dark green vegetables, such as broccoli; spinach; and other dark, leafy greens.
- Select orange vegetables, such as carrots and sweet potatoes.
- Eat dry beans and peas, such as pinto beans, kidney beans, and lentils.
- Vary the types of vegetables consumed, being sure to choose from all vegetable subgroups (dark green; red and orange; beans, peas, lentils; starchy vegetables; and other vegetables) several times per week.

Fruit group

The fruit group provides sources of vitamin A, vitamin C, and potassium. The foods in this group are naturally low in fat and sodium. To help with selections from the fruit group, suggest that the patient follow these recommendations:

- Fill at least half their plate with fruits and vegetables.
- Select a variety of fruits. Although fruits can be consumed in various forms, including fresh, frozen, canned, or dried fruits, the use of fruit juices should be limited.
- When drinking fruit juice, choose 100% fruit juice instead of fruit-flavored juices.
- When choosing canned fruits, choose fruits that are canned in their own juice, not in syrup.

Dairy group

Foods in this group provide protein, vitamins, and minerals. To help the patient with healthy choices from the milk group, encourage them to follow these recommendations:

- Eat or drink up to three cups a day based on their Daily Food Plan, which is specific to age and gender nutritional requirements.
- Pick low-fat or fat-free milk, yogurt, and other milk products.
- Choose lactose-free products or other calcium sources, such as fortified foods, if the patient doesn't like milk or is lactose intolerant.

Protein group

Foods in this group provide protein, vitamins, and minerals. To help the patient with healthy meat and bean food group choices, suggest that they follow these recommendations (USDA, 2020):

- Consume the required nutritional amount for their age and gender based on their Daily Food Plan.
- Consume low-fat or lean meats and poultry.
- Eat meats that are baked, broiled, or grilled.
- Vary selections among fish, beans, peas, nuts, and seeds.

Vegetarian diets

People may choose to follow vegetarian diets for religious, environmental, ethical, health, or other reasons. When compared with nonvegetarian diets, vegetarian diets are usually lower in saturated fat and cholesterol and higher in fiber, carbohydrates, magnesium, boron, folate, antioxidants, carotenoids, and phytochemicals. Those who follow a vegetarian diet have a lower risk of obesity, cancer, heart disease, hypertension, dementia, and type 2 diabetes mellitus (Hargreaves et al., 2021). On the other hand, vegetarians are at risk for protein, iron, and vitamin B_{12} deficiencies. If they avoid dairy products, they're also at risk for calcium and vitamin D deficiencies (Hargreaves et al., 2021).

There are three basic types of vegetarian diets, which vary according to the needs or beliefs of the person following the diet:

- **Lacto-ovo vegetarian** diets include dairy products and eggs.
- **Lactovegetarian** diets include no animal food sources except for dairy products.
- **Vegan** diets include no animal food sources. For patients on such a diet, the use of soybeans and its by-products, along with plant foods, can help provide a balanced diet.

Well-planned vegetarian diets can be nutritionally balanced for any patient, including a person who is pregnant or nursing. (See *Tips for the vegetarian.*)

Tips for the vegetarian

Strategies for meeting protein requirements
If the patient is a vegetarian or vegan, suggest these tips to help ensure that they're meeting their daily protein requirements:
• Eat a variety of foods from all included food groups, being sure to include all nutrients.
• Consume adequate calories; this will prevent the body from using amino acids for fuel.
• Use low-fat or nonfat products, and moderately consume nuts and seeds to maintain a low-fat diet.
• To increase fiber and iron content, select whole grains whenever possible.
• To aid iron absorption, include a vitamin C source at every meal.
• Use vitamin supplements, especially vitamin B_{12} (for strict vegans).

Strategies for meeting dietary guidelines
To help a vegetarian patient meet all the nutrition recommendations of *Dietary Guidelines for Americans 2020-2025* with the use of the MyPlate plan, offer the following suggestions (National Library of Medicine, 2022):

• Eat a variety of foods to meet caloric needs.
• Plan meals around sources of protein that are low in fat. This includes beans, lentils, and rice. Avoid using cheeses that are high in fat to replace meat.
• Increase calcium intake by using calcium-fortified, soy-based beverages, which are typically low in fat and cholesterol.
• Prepare food dishes that are usually made with meat or poultry, such as lasagna or pizza, as vegetarian dishes. Doing so increases the number of servings of vegetables while reducing saturated fat and cholesterol.
• Consider vegetarian products that look, and commonly taste, like meat dishes, such as soy-based sausages and "veggie burgers." These vegetable products are usually low in saturated fat and cholesterol-free.

A look at digestion and absorption

The basic purpose of digestion and absorption is to deliver essential nutrients to the cells in order to sustain life. To break food down into these essential nutrients, the body sends it through various mechanical and chemical processes in the GI tract or *alimentary canal*. Successful digestion and absorption depend on the coordinated function of the GI tract wall's muscles and nerves, the GI tract organs, and the accessory organs of digestion. (See *Structures of the GI system*, page 561.)

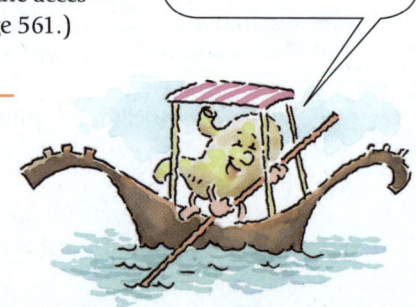

There's nothing like a trip down the alimentary canal after a good meal.

GI tract wall structures

The wall of the GI tract consists of four major layers:
• visceral peritoneum
• tunica muscularis
• submucosa
• mucosa.

Structures of the GI system

The GI system includes the alimentary canal (pharynx, esophagus, stomach, and small and large intestines) and the accessory organs (liver, biliary duct system, and pancreas).

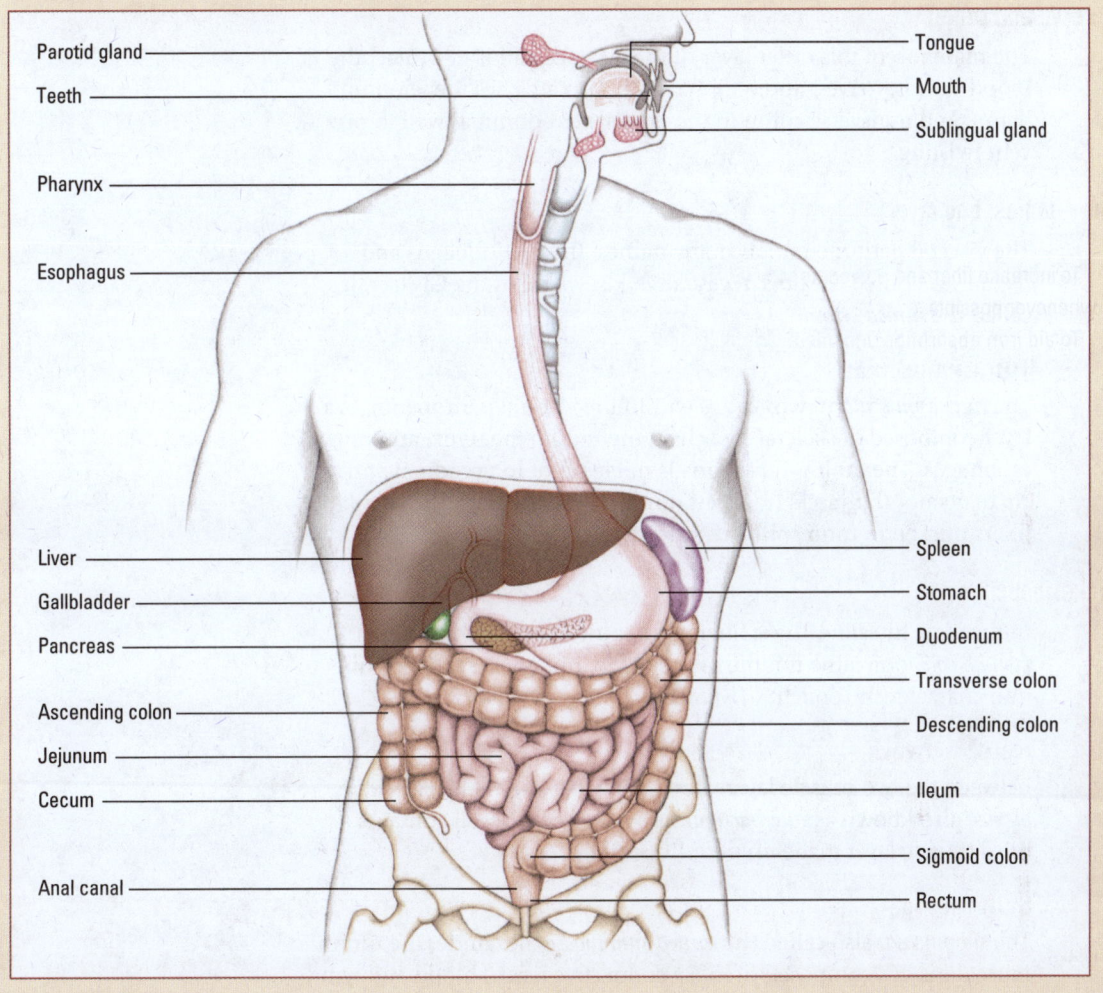

Parotid gland

Teeth

Pharynx

Esophagus

Liver

Gallbladder

Pancreas

Ascending colon

Jejunum

Cecum

Anal canal

Tongue

Mouth

Sublingual gland

Spleen

Stomach

Duodenum

Transverse colon

Descending colon

Ileum

Sigmoid colon

Rectum

Visceral peritoneum

The *visceral peritoneum* is the GI tract's outer covering. It covers most of the abdominal organs and lies next to an identical layer, the *parietal peritoneum*, which lines the abdominal cavity.

To serve and protect

The main job of this outer layer of the GI tract wall is to protect the blood vessels, nerves, and lymphatics. It also attaches the jejunum, ileum, and transverse colon to the posterior abdominal wall to prevent twisting.

Many names, one layer

The visceral peritoneum has many names. In the esophagus and rectum, it's called the *tunica adventitia*. Elsewhere in the GI tract, it's called the *tunica serosa*.

Tunica muscularis

The *tunica muscularis*, which lies within the visceral peritoneum, is a layer composed of skeletal muscle in the mouth, pharynx, and upper esophagus. The tunica muscularis is made up of longitudinal and circular smooth muscle fibers. At points along the tract, the circular fibers thicken to form sphincters.

Pucker pouches

In the large intestine, these fibers gather into three narrow bands *(teniae coli)* down the middle of the colon and pucker the intestine into characteristic pouches *(haustra)*.

Nerve network

Between the two muscle layers lies a nerve network—the *myenteric plexus*, also known as *Auerbach plexus*. The stomach wall contains a third muscle layer made up of oblique fibers.

Submucosa

The *submucosa*, also called the *tunica submucosa*, lies under the tunica muscularis. It's composed of loose connective tissue, blood and lymphatic vessels, and another nerve network called the *submucosal plexus* or *Meissner plexus*.

Mucosa

The *mucosa*, the innermost layer of the GI tract wall, is also called the *tunica mucosa*. This layer consists of epithelial and surface cells and loose connective tissue. Villi from surface cells secrete gastric and protective juices and absorb nutrients.

GI tract wall functions

The nerves and muscles of the GI tract wall work jointly to ensure that food moves spontaneously through the digestive system (motility). GI tract functions include innervation and secretion.

GI tract innervation

Distention of the submucosal plexus in the submucosa or myenteric plexus in the tunica muscularis stimulates the transmission of nerve signals to the smooth muscle, which initiates contraction and relaxation of these muscles, called *peristalsis*. During peristalsis, longitudinal fibers of the tunica muscularis shorten the lumen length and circular fibers reduce the lumen diameter (Tobias & Sadiq, 2022).

GI tract secretion

Five major substances secreted by the GI tract contribute to the chemical process of digestion:

- *Mucus* protects the lining of the GI tract and aids in motility.
- *Enzymes* are proteins that break down nutrients.
- *Acid (and various buffer ions)* contributes to the level of alkalinity or acidity (pH) needed to activate digestive enzymes.
- *Electrolytes (and water)* carry nutrients through the GI tract and aid in the absorption process.
- *Bile* emulsifies fat to promote intestinal absorption of fatty acids, cholesterol, and other lipids.

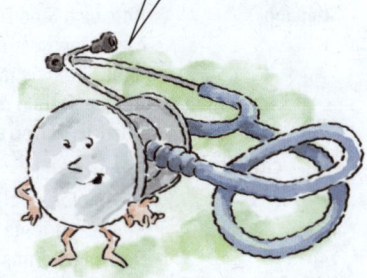

The nerves and muscles of the GI tract wall work together to ensure that food moves spontaneously through the digestive system (motility).

How digestion and absorption work

The organs of the GI tract play a major role in mechanical and chemical digestion and absorption of food and fluid. (See *Functions of the digestive system organs*, page 564.) Aided by the GI tract wall and accessory organs, the organs of the GI tract process nutrients in three phases of digestion:

- cephalic
- gastric
- intestinal.

Functions of the digestive system organs

This chart lists the digestive system organs and their primary functions.

Organ	Function
Mouth	• Breaks down food into smaller particles • Releases saliva to promote chewing and swallowing • Secretes amylase (ptyalin)
Esophagus	• Propels food downward into the stomach
Stomach	• Acts as a food reservoir • Mixes food with gastric secretions (hydrochloric acid, pepsin, mucus, intrinsic factor) • Begins protein digestion • Absorbs water, alcohol, and some drugs
Liver	• Produces bile • Metabolizes carbohydrates, protein, and fat • Stores nutrients • Detoxifies drugs and waste products
Gallbladder	• Concentrates and stores bile • Releases bile into the duodenum
Pancreas	• Produces and secretes insulin and glucagon • Produces and secretes digestive enzymes: proteases, lipase, and amylase
Small intestine	• Secretes hormones to stimulate the secretion of pancreatic juices, bile, and intestinal enzymes • Secretes digestive enzymes: peptidases, disaccharidases • Absorbs iron, magnesium, and calcium (duodenum) • Absorbs water-soluble vitamins and simple sugars (jejunum) • Absorbs amino acids, peptides, fat-soluble vitamins, fats, cholesterol, bile salts, and vitamin B_{12} (ileum)
Large intestine	• Absorbs water, sodium, potassium, and vitamin K formed by colonic bacteria • Eliminates solid waste

Cephalic phase

The cephalic phase of digestion uses the GI tract organs of the mouth, pharynx, and esophagus to begin the mechanical processes of digestion. Mechanical digestion breaks down food into smaller particles, which increases the surface area on which digestive enzymes can work.

Mouth

Digestion begins in the mouth (also called the *buccal cavity* or *oral cavity*). Ducts connect the mouth with the three major pairs of salivary glands:

- parotid
- submandibular
- sublingual.

These glands secrete the enzyme *ptyalin* (a salivary amylase) to moisten food during chewing (mastication) and begin breaking down starch into maltose. (See *Causes of dry mouth in older adults*.)

Pharynx

The *pharynx* is a cavity extending from the base of the skull to the esophagus. The pharynx aids swallowing by grasping food and propelling it toward the esophagus.

Esophagus

A muscular tube, the esophagus extends from the pharynx through the mediastinum to the stomach.

Down the hatch

When a person swallows, the cricopharyngeal sphincter in the upper esophagus relaxes, allowing food to enter the esophagus. In the esophagus, the glossopharyngeal nerve activates peristalsis, which moves the food bolus down toward the stomach.

One slippery bolus

As food passes through the esophagus, glands in the esophageal mucosal layer secrete mucus, which lubricates the bolus and protects the mucosal membrane from damage caused by poorly chewed foods.

Stomach express

Because food is only in the mouth for a short time, digestion of starch is limited. The salivary amylase that's swallowed continues to work for another 15 to 30 minutes in the stomach before its inactivated by gastric acids. By the time the food bolus is traveling toward the stomach, the stomach has begun secreting digestive juices (hydrochloric acid [HCl] and pepsin).

Gastric phase

When food enters the stomach, the gastric phase of digestion begins. (See *Sites and mechanisms of gastric secretion*, page 566.)

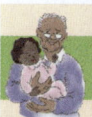

Ages and stages

Causes of dry mouth in older adults

As people age, salivation decreases, leading to dry mouth and a reduced sense of taste. Certain drugs (such as anticholinergics, antihistamines, tricyclic antidepressants, phenothiazines, clonidine, and opioid analgesics can also decrease salivation. Be sure to take a drug history for older adults. Other causes of dry mouth include facial nerve paralysis, salivary duct obstruction, Sjögren syndrome, and radiation of the mouth or face.

Sites and mechanisms of gastric secretion

The body of the stomach lies between the lower esophageal, or *cardiac*, sphincter and the pyloric sphincter. Between these sphincters lie the fundus, body, antrum, and pylorus. These areas have a rich variety of mucosal cells that help the stomach carry out its tasks.

Glands and gastric secretions

Cardiac glands, pyloric glands, and gastric glands secrete 2 to 3 L of gastric juice daily through the stomach's gastric pits.
- The *cardiac glands* (near the lower esophageal sphincter [LES]) and the *pyloric glands* (near the pylorus) secrete thin mucus.
- The *gastric glands* (in the body and fundus) secretes hydrochloric acid (HCl), pepsinogen, intrinsic factor, and mucus.

Protection from self-digestion

Specialized cells line the gastric glands, gastric pits, and surface epithelium. Mucous cells in the necks of the gastric glands produce thin mucus. Mucous cells in the surface epithelium produce alkaline mucus. Both substances lubricate food and protect the stomach from self-digestion by corrosive enzymes.

Other secretions

Argentaffin cells produce gastrin, which stimulates gastric secretion and motility. Chief cells produce pepsinogen, which breaks proteins down into polypeptides.

Large parietal cells scattered throughout the fundus secrete HCl and intrinsic factor. HCl degrades pepsinogen, maintains an acid environment, and inhibits excess bacterial growth. Intrinsic factor promotes vitamin B_{12} absorption in the small intestine.

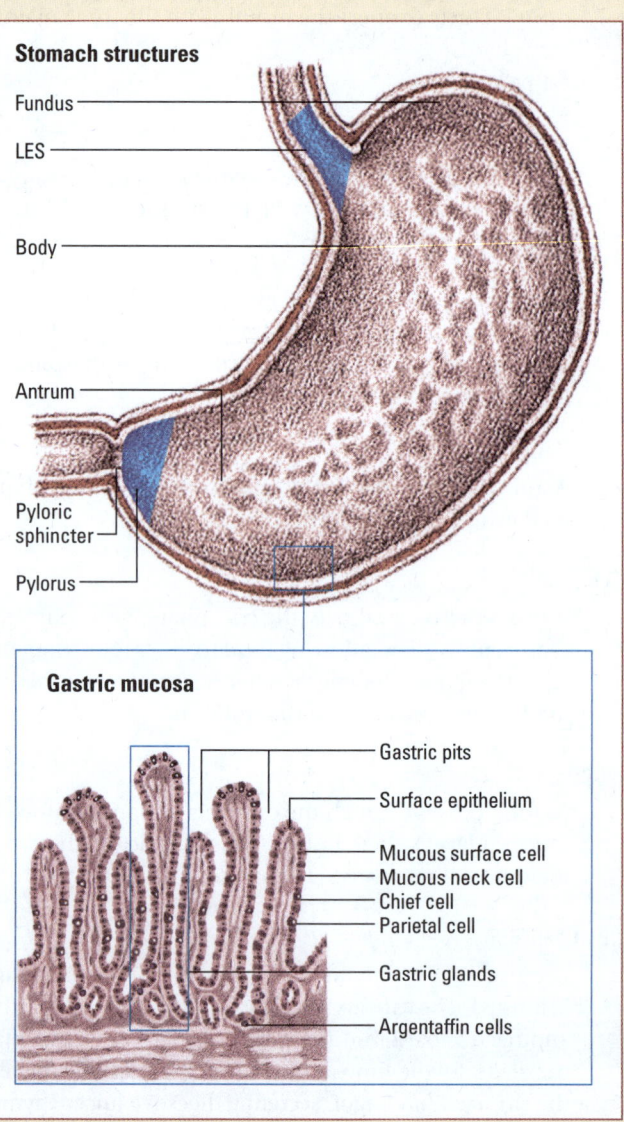

Stomach structures

Fundus
LES
Body
Antrum
Pyloric sphincter
Pylorus

Gastric mucosa

Gastric pits
Surface epithelium
Mucous surface cell
Mucous neck cell
Chief cell
Parietal cell
Gastric glands
Argentaffin cells

Source: Heda, R., Toro, F., & Tombazzi, C. R. (2023). Physiology, pepsin. *StatPearls*. https://www.ncbi.nlm.nih.gov/books/NBK537005/

Stomach

Chemical digestion, which occurs as food mixes with digestive enzymes, begins in the stomach. The stomach acts, in part, as a temporary storage area for food and has four main regions:

- cardia
- fundus
- body
- antrum.

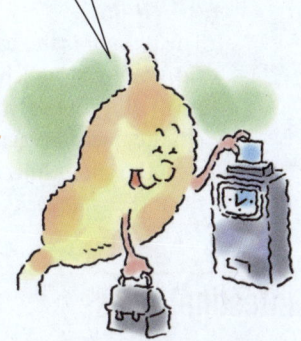

I punch the clock for chemical digestion. It all starts with me!

Cardia

The cardia lies near the junction of the stomach and esophagus. Relaxation of the cardiac sphincter in this region allows food to pass from the esophagus to the stomach.

Fundus

The *fundus* is an enlarged portion above and to the left of the esophageal opening into the stomach. Continued peristaltic activity in this region propels the intact food bolus toward the stomach body.

Body

The *body* is the middle portion of the stomach. In this region, distention of the stomach wall due to the food bolus stimulates secretion of gastrin.

Gassing up with gastrin

Gastrin, in turn, stimulates the stomach's motor functions and release of digestive secretions by the gastric glands. Highly acidic (pH of 0.9 to 1.5), these secretions consist mainly of HCl, intrinsic factor (which helps the body absorb vitamin B_{12}), and proteolytic enzymes (which help the body use proteins) (Hsu et al., 2022). (See *GI system changes in older adults*.)

HCl helps absorb calcium and iron and activates gastric enzymes that kill most food-borne bacteria. HCl is also needed to convert the enzyme pepsinogen into pepsin.

Enzyme with pep

Pepsin becomes the major protein-splitting enzyme and, in turn, activates the secretion of the gastric mucus that protects the gastric lining. The mucus also helps move the food bolus along the path to the small intestine.

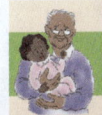

Ages and stages

GI system changes in older adults

Age-related changes in the GI system can lead to conditions that impact nutrition. Reduced gastric acid secretion in older adults can result in pernicious anemia, iron deficiency anemia, and reduced calcium absorption. Reduced production of bile acid, enlargement of the common bile duct, and increased output of cholecystokinin can lead to biliary stasis, cholelithiasis, and reduced appetite.

Nothing but alcohol

Normally, except for alcohol, little food absorption occurs in the stomach. Peristaltic contractions in the stomach body churn the food into tiny particles and mix it with gastric juices, forming chyme.

Antrum

The *antrum* is the lower portion of the stomach, lying near the junction of the stomach and the duodenum. Stronger peristaltic waves move the chyme from the stomach body into the antrum. Here, the chyme backs up against the pyloric sphincter before being released into the small intestine and triggering the intestinal phase of digestion. (See *Stomach emptying.*)

Intestinal phase

Most absorption occurs during the intestinal phase of digestion, which involves the small and large intestines.

Small intestine

The longest organ of the GI tract, the *small intestine* is a tube measuring about 20 ft (5 to 6 m) long. It performs most of the work of digestion and absorption. (See *Digestion and absorption in the small intestine.*)
  The small intestine has three major divisions:
- *duodenum:* the longest and most superior division
- *jejunum:* the middle portion and shortest segment
- *ileum:* the most inferior portion.

Break it down, please

In the small intestine, intestinal wall contractions and digestive enzymes break down carbohydrates, proteins, and fats so the intestinal mucosa can facilitate absorption of these nutrients into the bloodstream (along with water and electrolytes). These nutrients are then available for use by the body.

Stomach emptying

The rate of stomach emptying depends on several factors, including gastrin release, neural signals generated when the stomach wall distends, and the enterogastric reflex.

Enterogastric reflex

The *enterogastric reflex* is a response in which the duodenum releases secretin and gastric-inhibitory peptide and the jejunum secretes cholecystokinin. Both reactions decrease gastric motility.

Digestion and absorption in the small intestine

The small intestine performs most of the work of digestion and absorption. Here's a summary of the small intestine's major tasks.

Mechanical digestion

- Small muscles mix chyme.
- Peristaltic motions propel the food mass over the length of the intestine.
- Surface villi mix chyme at the intestinal wall, enhancing absorption.
- Long muscle moves the food mass in a circular motion, providing new surface sites for absorption.
- Segmentation rings from circular muscle mix the food into soft masses and then mix it with secretions.

Chemical digestion

- Lipase breaks fats into fatty acids and glycerides.
- Amylase converts starch to the disaccharides maltose and sucrose.
- Enterokinase activates trypsinogens, which become trypsin.
- Trypsin and chymotrypsin split protein molecules into small peptides and then into individual amino acids.

- Disaccharidases convert their respective disaccharides to monosaccharides.
- Bile from the liver helps to digest and absorb fat.
- Carbohydrate foods are changed into simple sugars.
- Fats are changed into fatty acids and glycerides.
- Proteins are changed into amino acids.
- Vitamins and minerals are also released.

Absorption

- Microvilli, villi, and mucus absorb essential nutrients.
- Absorption is controlled by diffusion—passive for the small materials and carrier-assisted for larger items.
- Digestive contents are mostly water soluble and can be absorbed directly into the circulation.
- Fatty contents aren't water soluble; they must pass through the villi, then into the lymph system, and finally into the bloodstream.

Source: Norris, T. L. (2025). *Porth's pathophysiology: Concepts of altered health status* (11th ed.). Wolters Kluwer.

The great intestinal wall

The intestinal wall has structural features that significantly increase its absorptive surface area. These features include

- *plicae circulares*: circular folds of the intestinal mucosa or mucous membrane lining
- *villi*: fingerlike projections on the mucosa
- *microvilli*: tiny cytoplasmic projections on the surface of epithelial cells.

Secretion police

The small intestine also releases hormones that help control the secretion of bile, pancreatic juice, and intestinal juice.

Large intestine

The main tasks of the large intestine are absorption of body water and elimination of digestive waste. In addition, the large intestine harbors the bacteria *Escherichia coli*, *Enterobacter aerogenes*, *Clostridium perfringens*, and *Lactobacillus bifidus*. All of these bacteria help synthesize vitamins, hormones, and lipids and break down cellulose into usable carbohydrates (Norris, 2025). Bacterial action also produces *flatus*, which helps propel stools toward the rectum.

Protection from bacterial action

The mucosa of the large intestine also produces alkaline secretions from tubular glands composed of goblet cells. This alkaline mucus lubricates the intestinal walls as food pushes through, protecting the mucosa from acidic bacterial action.

From start to finish

The large intestine extends from the ileocecal valve (the valve between the ileum of the small intestine and the first segment of the large intestine) to the anus. The large intestine has five segments:
- cecum
- ascending colon
- transverse colon
- descending and sigmoid colons
- rectum.

Cecum

The *cecum*, a saclike structure, makes up the first few inches of the large intestine. The cecum is connected to the ileum of the small intestine by the ileocecal pouch.

Ascending colon

The ascending colon rises on the right posterior abdominal wall and then turns under the liver at the hepatic flexure. By the time chyme passes through the ileocecal valve and enters the ascending colon of the large intestine, it has been reduced to mostly indigestible substances.

Transverse colon

The transverse colon is located above the small intestine, passing horizontally across the abdomen and below the liver, stomach, and spleen. It proceeds to turn downward at the left colic flexure. Through blood and lymph vessels, the large intestine has absorbed all but about 100 mL of water from the chyme by the time it leaves the transverse colon. It also absorbs large amounts of sodium and chloride.

Fiber makes it happen

Because dietary fiber isn't digested, it travels through the large intestine unabsorbed and contributes to the formation of feces.

Descending and sigmoid colons

The descending colon starts near the spleen and extends down the left side of the abdomen into the pelvic cavity. The sigmoid colon descends through the pelvic cavity, where it becomes the rectum. The descending and sigmoid colons are responsible for evacuation. Contents move slowly along the tract, enabling water and electrolytes to be absorbed.

Rectum

The *rectum*, the last few inches of the large intestine, terminates at the anus.

Mass movement

In the lower colon, long and relatively sluggish contractions cause propulsive waves or *mass movements*. Normally occurring several times per day, these movements propel intestinal contents into the rectum and produce the urge to defecate.

Accessory organs of digestion and absorption

Accessory organs of the digestive system—the liver, biliary duct system, and pancreas—contribute hormones, enzymes, and bile vital to digestion and absorption.

I don't mean to brag, but I'm the body's largest gland!

Liver

The body's largest gland, the highly vascular liver, is enclosed in a fibrous capsule in the right upper quadrant of the abdomen. The *lesser omentum*, a fold of the peritoneum, covers most of the liver and anchors it to the lesser curvature of the stomach. The *hepatic artery* and *hepatic portal vein,* as well as the common bile duct and hepatic veins, pass through the lesser omentum.

Functioning features

The liver's functional unit, the *lobule*, consists of a plate of hepatic cells, or *hepatocytes*, that encircle a central vein and radiate outward. Separating the hepatocyte plates from each other are *sinusoids*, the liver's capillary system. Reticuloendothelial macrophages (*Kupffer cells*) lining the sinusoids remove bacteria and toxins that have entered the blood through the intestinal capillaries (Norris, 2025).

Go with the blood flow

The sinusoids carry oxygenated blood from the hepatic artery and nutrient-rich blood from the portal vein. Unoxygenated blood leaves through the central vein and flows through hepatic veins to the inferior vena cava.

Many functions, one organ

The liver performs many important functions in the processes of digestion and absorption. The liver (Norris, 2025)

- aids in carbohydrate metabolism
- detoxifies various endogenous and exogenous toxins, such as drugs and alcohol
- synthesizes plasma proteins, nonessential amino acids, and vitamin A
- stores essential nutrients, such as vitamins K, D, B_{12}, and iron
- removes ammonia from body fluids, converting it to urea for excretion in urine
- converts glucose to glycogen and stores it as fuel for the muscles
- produces and secretes bile to aid in digestion
- stores fats and converts the excess sugars to fats to store in other parts of the body
- removes naturally occurring ammonia from body fluids, converting it to urea for excretion in the urine.

Biliary duct system

The biliary duct system consists of a network of ducts and includes the gallbladder.

Ducts

Think of ducts as a subway system transporting bile through the GI tract. *Bile* is a greenish liquid composed of water, cholesterol, bile salts, and phospholipids. From the liver, bile travels via the common bile duct to the small intestine, entering through the duodenum.

When bile salts are missing

When bile salts are absent from the intestinal tract, lipids are excreted and fat-soluble vitamins are absorbed poorly.

Report on bile production

The liver recycles about 80% of bile salts into bile, combining them with bile pigments (biliverdin and bilirubin, the breakdown products of red blood cells) and cholesterol (Norris, 2025). The liver secretes this alkaline bile continuously. Bile production may increase from stimulation of the vagus nerve, release of the hormone secretin, increased blood flow in the liver, and the presence of fat in the intestine. (See *GI hormones: Production and function*.)

Gallbladder

The *gallbladder* is a pear-shaped organ joined to the ventral surface of the liver by the cystic duct. The gallbladder
- stores and concentrates bile produced by the liver
- releases bile into the common bile duct for delivery to the duodenum in response to the contraction and relaxation of the sphincter of Oddi.

Cholecystokinin contraction

The secretion of the hormone cholecystokinin causes the gallbladder to contract. This contraction allows the release of bile into the common bile duct for delivery to the duodenum.

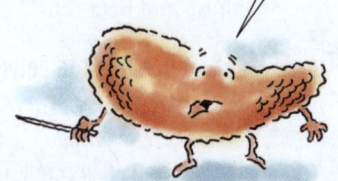

I may not be as large as the liver, but I perform important exocrine and endocrine functions.

Pancreas

The *pancreas* is a somewhat flat organ that lies behind the stomach. Its head and neck extend into the curve of the duodenum, and its tail lies against the spleen. The pancreas performs exocrine and endocrine functions.

GI hormones: Production and function

When stimulated, GI structures secrete four hormones. Each hormone plays a different part in digestion.

Hormone and production site	Stimulating factor or agent	Function
Gastrin Produced in pyloric antrum and duodenal mucosa	• Pyloric antrum distention • Vagal stimulation • Protein digestion products • Alcohol	Stimulates gastric secretion and motility
Gastric inhibitory peptides Produced in duodenal and jejunal mucosa	• Gastric acid • Fats • Fat digestion products	Inhibits gastric secretion and motility
Secretin Produced in duodenal and jejunal mucosa	• Gastric acid • Fat digestion products • Protein digestion products	Stimulates secretion of bile and alkaline pancreatic fluid
Cholecystokinin Produced in duodenal and jejunal mucosa	• Fat digestion products • Protein digestion products	Stimulates gallbladder contraction and secretion of enzyme-rich pancreatic fluid

Source: Norris, T. L. (2025). *Porth's pathophysiology: Concepts of altered health status* (11th ed.). Wolters Kluwer.

Exocrine function

The pancreas's exocrine function involves scattered cells that secrete between 1,000 and 4,000 mL of digestive enzymes every day (Karpińska & Czauderna, 2022). Lobules and lobes of the clusters *(acini)* of enzyme-producing cells release secretions into ducts that merge into the pancreatic duct. The pancreatic duct runs the length of the pancreas and joins the bile duct from the gallbladder before entering the duodenum. The vagus nerve stimulates the production and release of secretin and cholecystokinin, which are the two hormones responsible for regulating the rate and amount of pancreatic secretions (Morisset, 2020).

Endocrine function

The endocrine function of the pancreas involves the islets of Langerhans. Two types of cells formulate the islets of Langerhans: alpha and beta cells.

The ABCs of alpha and beta cells

Over 1 million of these alpha and beta cells are in the islets. Alpha cells secrete *glucagon*, a hormone that stimulates glycogenolysis in the liver; beta cells secrete *insulin* to promote carbohydrate metabolism. Both hormones flow directly into the blood. Their release is stimulated by blood glucose levels.

Pancreatic duct

Running the length of the pancreas, the *pancreatic duct* joins the bile duct from the gallbladder before entering the duodenum. Vagal stimulation and release of the hormones secretin and cholecystokinin control the rate and amount of pancreatic secretion.

A look at altered nutrition

Patients with nutritional problems may experience signs and symptoms, including excessive weight loss or gain, anorexia, or muscle wasting. Lifestyle habits, culture, and economic resources can also affect a person's nutritional status. Remember that nutritional deficiencies may exist for months or years before clinical signs appear. Also, be aware that patients hospitalized for more than 2 weeks risk developing a nutritional disorder. (See *Evaluation of nutritional findings.*)

> Remember that patients hospitalized for more than 2 weeks risk developing a nutritional disorder.

Evaluation of nutritional findings

This chart can be used to help interpret nutritional assessment findings.

Body system or region	Sign or symptom	Implications
General	• Weakness and fatigue • Weight loss	• Anemia or electrolyte imbalance • Decreased calorie intake, increased calorie use, or inadequate nutrient intake or absorption
Skin, hair, and nails	• Dry, flaky skin • Dry skin with poor turgor • Rough, scaly skin with bumps • Petechiae or ecchymoses • Sore that won't heal • Thinning, dry hair • Spoon-shaped, brittle, or ridged nails	• Vitamin A, vitamin B complex, or linoleic acid deficiency • Dehydration • Vitamin A or essential fatty acid deficiency • Vitamin C or K deficiency • Protein, vitamin C, or zinc deficiency • Protein or zinc deficiency • Iron, biotin, zinc, or protein deficiency.
Eyes	• Night blindness; corneal swelling, softening, or dryness; Bitot spots (gray triangular patches on the conjunctiva) • Red conjunctiva	• Vitamin A deficiency • Riboflavin deficiency
Throat and mouth	• Cracks at corner of mouth • Magenta tongue • Beefy, red tongue • Soft, spongy, bleeding gums • Swollen neck (goiter)	• Riboflavin or niacin deficiency • Riboflavin deficiency • Vitamin B_{12} deficiency • Vitamin C deficiency • Iodine deficiency
Cardiovascular	• Edema • Tachycardia and hypotension	• Protein deficiency • Fluid volume deficit
GI	• Ascites	• Protein deficiency
Musculoskeletal	• Bone pain and bow leg • Muscle wasting • Pain in calves and thighs	• Vitamin D or calcium deficiency • Protein, carbohydrate, and fat deficiency • Thiamine deficiency
Neurologic	• Altered mental state • Paresthesia	• Dehydration and thiamine or vitamin B_{12} deficiency • Vitamin B_{12}, pyridoxine, or thiamine deficiency

Source: Kesari, A., & Noel, J. Y. (2023). Nutritional assessment. *StatPearls*. https://www.ncbi.nlm.nih.gov/books/NBK580496/

Excessive weight loss

Patients with nutritional deficiencies frequently experience weight loss. Weight loss may result from decreased food intake, decreased food absorption, increased metabolic requirements, or a combination of all three. Other possible causes of weight loss include endocrine, neoplastic, GI, and psychiatric disorders; chronic disease; infection; and neurologic lesions that cause paralysis and dysphagia.

Consumption conundrums

Excessive weight loss may also occur if the patient has a condition that prevents them from consuming a sufficient amount of food, such as painful oral lesions, ill-fitting dentures, or a loss of teeth. In addition, poverty, fad diets, excessive exercise, or certain drugs may contribute to excessive weight loss.

Excessive weight gain

When a person consumes more calories than their body requires for energy, their body stores excess adipose tissue, resulting in weight gain. Emotional factors (such as anxiety, guilt, and depression), as well as social factors, can trigger overeating, resulting in excessive weight gain. Excessive weight gain is also a primary sign of many endocrine disorders. In addition, patients with conditions that limit activity, such as cardiovascular or respiratory disorders, may also experience excessive weight gain. (See *Overweight children*.)

Anorexia

Defined as a lack of appetite despite a physiologic need for food, *anorexia* commonly occurs with GI and endocrine disorders. It can also result from anxiety, chronic pain, poor oral hygiene, and changes in taste or smell that normally accompany aging. Short-term anorexia rarely jeopardizes health, but chronic anorexia can lead to life-threatening malnutrition. *Anorexia nervosa* is a psychological condition in which the patient severely restricts food intake, resulting in excessive weight loss.

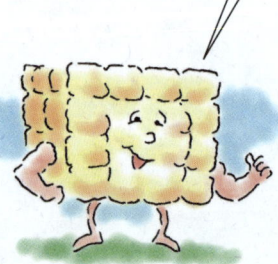

I'm an essential component to avoid atrophy, which can lead to lots of other unwanted conditions!

Muscle wasting

Commonly a result of chronic protein deficiency, muscle wasting, or *atrophy*, results when muscle fibers lose bulk and length. The muscles involved shrink and lose their normal contour, appearing

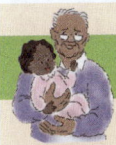

Ages and stages

Overweight children

Like adults, the number of children considered overweight has dramatically increased in recent years. Nearly 20% of children and teens are overweight (as determined by their body mass index) (Centers for Disease Control and Prevention [CDC], 2022). Being overweight as a child increases the risk of being overweight as an adult.

More weight, more risks
Children who are overweight are more likely to have high cholesterol and high blood pressure (risk factors for heart disease) as well as type 2 diabetes. They also are more likely to suffer from poor self-esteem and depression.

Counting causes
During the nutritional assessment, look for these common causes of excessive weight gain in children:

- lack of exercise
- sedentary lifestyle (involving an excessive amount of watching television, using computers, or playing video games)
- unhealthy eating habits.

Healthy habits
To prevent weight gain and to promote a healthy lifestyle, help the child develop an exercise plan and explain nutritious eating habits.

emaciated or even deformed. Associated signs and symptoms include chronic fatigue; apathy; anorexia; dry skin; peripheral edema; and dull, sparse, dry hair.

Lifestyle habits

Eating habits are developed in childhood and can vary greatly from one person to another. Peer pressure and gender role stereotypes can affect a person's eating patterns. Food fads can also interfere with a healthy eating pattern.

Fast-paced lives place families in tough situations when trying to provide well-balanced meals while maintaining busy schedules. The ready availability of prepackaged foods and fast-food options makes these unhealthy options appealing.

Culture and beliefs

Culture plays a large role in the type of food eaten and dietary habits and patterns. The nurse should be considerate of cultural preferences when caring for patients.

Religious beliefs also play a large role in dietary habits. For example, certain religions may restrict a particular food during a religious holiday, whereas others may encourage fasting. Still others restrict the kinds of foods that can be eaten in the same meal. The nurse should ask the patient if they have any dietary restrictions.

Economic resources

A person's economic resources or lack of resources can severely alter their eating patterns and food choices. Low-income families, especially older adults, may need to sacrifice their food money to buy much-needed prescriptions or to pay bills.

Preventing altered nutrition

The most important way a nurse can help prevent altered nutrition is to teach the patient about proper diet and health promotion. To accomplish this goal, try to increase the patient's understanding of what a healthy diet includes. Knowledge doesn't always guarantee that the patient will follow a healthy diet, but the odds are greater if they understand healthy food choices.

Promoting optimal intake

Illness greatly affects a person's eating habits and desire for food. Food should be served in an attractive, appetizing manner and be at the right temperature. The room should be pleasant and void of distractions. The patient's food preferences should be considered.

Pain and nausea medications should be timed to help the patient achieve optimal relief at mealtimes. Providing oral care before meals promotes taste and comfort. If possible and the patient's condition permits, the patient should receive meals sitting upright and out of bed in a chair. This position facilitates chewing and makes choking and reflux of stomach contents less likely.

Assisting an adult with feeding

Confusion, arm or hand immobility, injury, weakness, or restrictions on activities or positions may prevent a patient from eating independently. When this occurs, feeding the patient becomes a key nursing responsibility. An injured or debilitated patient may experience depression and subsequent anorexia. Meeting such a patient's nutritional needs requires determining food preferences; conducting the feeding in a friendly, unhurried manner; encouraging self-feeding to promote independence and dignity; and documenting intake and output.

Supplies
- meal tray
- overbed table
- linen-saver pad or towels
- clean linens
- flexible straws
- basin of water
- feeding syringe
- assistive feeding devices, if necessary

Getting ready
- Raise the head of the bed if the patient's condition allows. Fowler or semi-Fowler position makes swallowing easier and reduces the risk of aspiration and choking.
- Before the meal tray arrives, give the patient soap, a basin of water or a wet washcloth, and a hand towel *to clean their hands.*
- Wipe the overbed table with soap and water or sanitizing wipes.
- When the meal tray arrives, compare the name on the tray with the name on the patient's wristband. Check the tray to make sure it contains foods appropriate for the patient's condition. (See *Special diets.*)

How it's done
- Because many adults consider being fed demeaning, allow the patient some control over mealtime by letting them choose the pace of the meal or decide the order in which they eat various foods.
- Encourage the patient to feed themselves if they can. If they're restricted to the prone or the supine position but can use their arms and hands, encourage them to try foods they can pick up, such as sandwiches. If they can assume Fowler or semi-Fowler position but have limited use of their arms or hands, teach them how to use assistive feeding devices. (See *Using assistive feeding devices.*)
- If necessary, tuck a napkin or towel under their chin to protect their gown from spills. Use a linen-saver pad or towel to protect bed linens.
- To ensure comfort for both the nurse and the patient during feeding, position a chair next to the patient's bed.
- Set up the patient's tray, remove the plate from the tray warmer, and discard all plastic wrappings. Next, cut the food into bite-size pieces.

Special diets

Patients who are hospitalized may have different diets according to their diagnosis or reason for hospitalization. Also, dietary intake can vary to promote healing or to prevent complications such as a nothing-by-mouth (NPO) status before surgery. Always check the health care provider's orders before giving patients their meals to make sure that they're receiving the correct diet.

Nothing by mouth

The term *nothing by mouth,* or *NPO* (non per os), is actually the withholding of food or liquids. It may be indicated to
- clear the GI tract of contents before surgery or a diagnostic procedure
- prevent aspiration in high-risk patients
- treat severe nausea and vomiting
- prevent aspiration during surgery
- rest the GI tract to promote healing
- treat medical problems such as a bowel obstruction.

Clear liquid

A clear-liquid diet includes only liquids that don't contain residue. It includes juices without pulp (such as apple or cranberry), tea, gelatin, and clear broth. This type of diet is commonly used as the first diet ordered after surgery or before some diagnostic tests.

Full liquid

A full-liquid diet includes all fluids as well as foods that become a liquid at room temperature, such as ice cream or sherbet. It may also include strained cream-based soups, pudding, and milkshakes. This diet is commonly ordered for postoperative patients after a clear-liquid diet has been tolerated. It's also used for patients who can't chew properly, such as after a stroke.

Soft

A soft diet includes foods that are soft, with reduced fiber. They may be further chopped or pureed for patients who have difficulty chewing or have no teeth. This diet is most commonly used for patients after surgery when a full-liquid diet has been tolerated.

Diet as tolerated

As tolerated means that dietary preferences can change as the patient's tolerance changes. For instance, a postoperative patient may start out with clear liquids but may progress to a regular diet if they haven't experienced nausea or vomiting.

Restrictive diets

A restrictive diet is a diet based on the patient's disease or metabolic status that limits calorie content, certain foods, or a particular nutrient, such as sodium, potassium, and fat. For example, a patient who has obesity may be on a diet to limit calorie intake and a cardiac patient may need to limit sodium intake.

Peas at 12, corn at 3

- To help a blind or visually impaired patient feed themselves, describe the placement of various foods on their plate corresponding to the hours on a clock face. Maintain consistent placement for subsequent meals.
- Ask the patient which food they prefer to eat first to promote a sense of control over the meal. Some patients prefer to eat one food at a time, whereas others prefer to alternate foods.
- If the patient has difficulty swallowing, offer liquids carefully with a spoon or feeding syringe to help prevent aspiration. Pureed or soft foods, such as custard or flavored gelatin, may be easier to swallow than liquids. If the patient doesn't have difficulty swallowing, use a flexible straw to reduce the risk of spills.

Using assistive feeding devices

Various feeding devices, available through occupational therapy, can help the patient who has limited arm mobility, grasp, range of motion (ROM), or coordination. Before introducing the patient to an assistive feeding device, assess their ability to master it. Don't introduce a device they won't be able to manage. If their condition is progressively disabling, encourage them to use the device only until their mastery of it falters.

Introduce the assistive device before mealtime, with the patient seated in a natural position. Explain its purpose, show the patient how to use it, and encourage them to practice before the meal. After meals, wash the device thoroughly, and store it in the patient's bedside stand. Document the patient's progress, and share it with staff and family members to help reinforce the patient's independence. Specific devices are discussed here.

Plate guard

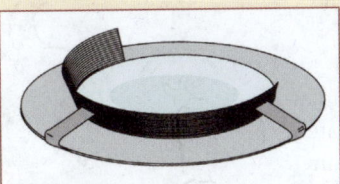

A plate guard blocks food from spilling off the plate. Attach the guard to the side of the plate opposite the hand the patient uses to feed themselves. Guiding the patient's hand, show them how to push food against the guard to secure it on the utensil. Then have them try again with food of a different consistency. If the patient tires, feed them the rest of the meal. At subsequent meals, encourage the patient to feed themselves for progressively longer periods until they can feed themselves an entire meal.

Universal cuffs

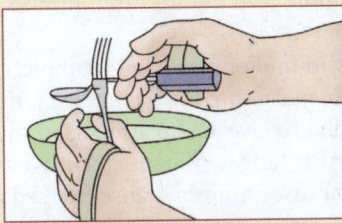

Universal cuffs are flexible bands that help the patient with flail hands or diminished grasp. Each cuff contains a slot that holds a fork or spoon. Attach the cuff to the hand the patient uses to feed themselves. Then place the fork or spoon in the cuff slot. Bend the utensil to facilitate feeding.

Swivel spoon

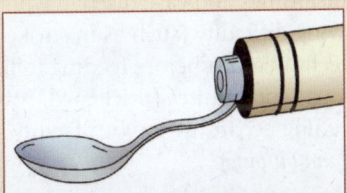

A swivel spoon helps the patient with limited ROM in their forearm or an intention tremor and will fit in universal cuffs. This device helps to keep the spoon level no matter the position of the patient's arm.

Long-handled utensils

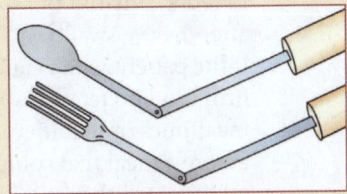

Long-handled utensils have jointed stems to help the patient with limited ROM in their elbow and shoulder.

Utensils with built-up handles

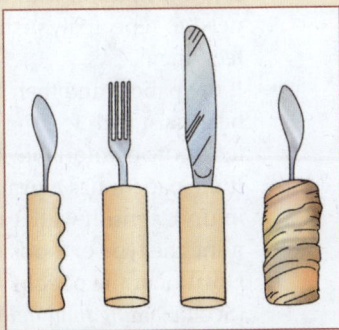

Utensils with built-up handles can help the patient with diminished grasp. They can be purchased or improvised by wrapping tape around the handles.

We now pause for a break

- Ask the patient to indicate when they're ready for another mouthful. Pause between courses and whenever the patient wants to rest. During the meal, wipe the patient's mouth and chin as needed.
- When the patient finishes eating, remove the tray. If necessary, clean up spills and change the linens. Provide mouth care.

Practice pointers

- Don't feed the patient too quickly, because this can upset them and impair digestion.
- If the patient is restricted to the supine position, provide foods that they can chew easily. If they're restricted to the prone position, to reduce the risk of aspiration, feed liquids carefully and only after they've swallowed their food.
- If the patient won't eat, try to find out why. For example, confirm food preferences. Also, make sure the patient isn't in pain at mealtimes or that they didn't receive any treatments immediately before a meal that could cause fatigue or nausea. Find out if any medications they're taking cause anorexia, nausea, or sedation. Be sure to clear the bedside of emesis basins, urinals, bedpans, and similar distractions at mealtimes.

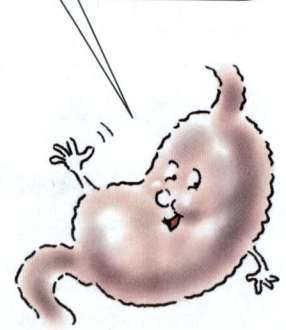

Feeding a patient too quickly can impair digestion.

A plausible pattern

- Establish a pattern and schedule for feeding the patient, and share this information with the rest of the staff so the patient doesn't need to repeatedly instruct staff members about the best way to feed them.
- If the patient and their family are willing, suggest that family members assist with feeding. Involving the family may make the patient feel more comfortable at mealtimes and ease discharge planning.
- If the patient has a swallowing difficulty (such as in stroke or head injury), consult with a speech therapist before feeding to best determine the type of foods the patient requires (thickened, soft, etc.).
- Document the patient's feeding according to your facility's policy. (See *Recording fluid intake and output.*)

Feeding tube insertion and removal

Inserting a feeding tube into the stomach or duodenum allows patients who can't or won't eat to receive nourishment. A feeding tube also permits the administration of supplemental feedings to patients who have high nutritional requirements, such as unconscious patients or those with extensive burns. The preferred feeding tube route is nasal, but the oral route may be used for patients with such conditions as a deviated septum or a head or nose injury.

Recording fluid intake and output

Accurate intake and output records help evaluate a patient's fluid and electrolyte balance, suggest various diagnoses, and influence the choice of fluid therapy. These records are mandatory for patients with burns, renal failure, electrolyte imbalance, recent surgical procedures, heart failure, or severe vomiting and diarrhea and for patients receiving diuretics or corticosteroids. Intake and output records are also significant in monitoring patients with nasogastric (NG) tubes or drainage collection devices and those receiving IV therapy.

Fluid intake consists of all fluid entering the patient's body, including beverages, fluids contained in solid foods taken by mouth, and foods that are liquid at room temperature, such as flavored gelatin, custard, ice cream, and some beverages.

Additional intake includes GI instillations, bladder irrigations, and IV fluids.

Fluid output consists of all fluid that leaves the patient's body, including urine, loose stools, vomitus, aspirated fluid loss, and drainage from surgical drains, NG tubes, and chest tubes.

When recording fluid intake and output, enlist the patient's help if possible. Record amount in cubic centimeters (cc) or milliliters (mL). Measure; don't estimate. For a small child, weigh diapers if appropriate. Monitor intake and output during each shift, and notify the health care provider if amounts differ significantly over a 24-hour period. Document findings in the appropriate location; describe any fluid restrictions and the patient's adherence.

Source: Simpson, D., & Mcintosh, R. (2021). Measuring and monitoring fluid balance. *British Journal of Nursing*, 30(12), 706–710. https://www.britishjournalofnursing.com/content/clinical/measuring-and-monitoring-fluid-balance/

Can't stomach this

The health care provider may order duodenal feeding when the patient can't tolerate gastric feeding or when they expect gastric feeding to produce aspiration. The absence of bowel sounds or possible intestinal obstruction are contraindications for the use of a feeding tube.

Keep it flexible

Feeding tubes are made of silicone, rubber, or polyurethane and have small diameters and great flexibility. To ease passage, some feeding tubes are weighted with tungsten, and some need a guide wire to keep them from curling in the back of the throat. These small-bore tubes usually have radiopaque markings and a water-activated coating, which provides a lubricated surface.

Supplies

For gastric feedings

- feeding formula
- graduated container
- 120 mL of water
- gavage bag with tubing and flow regulator clamp
- towel or linen-saver pad
- 60-mL syringe
- pH test strip
- optional: infusion controller and tubing set (for continuous administration), adapter to connect gavage tubing to feeding tube

For nasal and oral care

- cotton-tipped applicators
- water-soluble lubricant
- lemon glycerin swabs
- petroleum jelly

Bulbs, catheters, and pumps

A bulb syringe or large catheter-tip syringe may be substituted for a gavage bag after the patient demonstrates tolerance for a gravity drip infusion. The health care provider may order an infusion pump to ensure accurate delivery of the prescribed formula.

Getting ready

- Be sure to refrigerate formulas prepared in the dietary department or pharmacy. Refrigerate commercial formulas only after opening them.
- Check the date on all formula containers.
- Discard expired commercial formula.
- Use powdered formula within 24 hours of mixing.

Shake…

- Always shake the container well to mix the solution thoroughly.
- Allow the formula to warm to room temperature before administration. Cold formula can increase the chance of irritation and diarrhea.
- Never warm the formula over direct heat or in a microwave because heat may curdle it or change its chemical composition. Also, hot formula may injure the patient.

…and pour

- Pour 60 mL of water into the graduated container.
- After closing the flow clamp on the administration set, pour the appropriate amount of formula into the gavage bag.

- To prevent bacterial growth, hang no more than a 4- to 6-hour supply at one time.
- Open the flow clamp on the administration set to remove air from the lines and to prevent air from entering the patient's stomach, which would cause distention and discomfort.

How it's done

- Provide privacy and wash hands.
- Inform the patient that they'll receive nourishment through the tube, and explain the procedure to them. If possible, give them a schedule of subsequent feedings.
- If the patient has a nasal or oral tube, cover their chest with a towel or linen-saver pad to protect them and the bed linens from spills.
- Assess the patient's abdomen for bowel sounds and distention.

Delivering a gastric feeding

- Elevate the bed to semi-Fowler or high-Fowler position to prevent aspiration by gastroesophageal reflux and to promote digestion.
- Check placement of the feeding tube to make sure it hasn't slipped out since the last feeding.
- Never give a tube feeding until you're sure the tube is properly positioned in the patient's stomach. Administering a feeding through a misplaced tube can cause formula to enter the patient's lungs.
- To check tube patency and position, remove the cap or plug from the feeding tube and use the syringe to aspirate gastric secretions gently.

Checking the pH

- Examine the aspirate, and place a small amount on the pH test strip. Proper placement of the gastric tube is likely if the aspirate has a typical gastric fluid appearance (grassy-green, clear and colorless with mucous shreds, or brown) and the pH is 5.0 or less.
- To assess gastric emptying, complete an abdominal assessment. If distention or pain is present, hold the feeding.
- Once gastric emptying is confirmed, connect the gavage bag tubing to the feeding tube. Depending on the type of tube used, an adapter may be needed to connect the two.
- If you're using a bulb or catheter-tip syringe, remove the bulb or plunger and attach the syringe to the pinched-off feeding tube to prevent excess air from entering the patient's stomach, which would cause distention.
- If you're using an infusion controller, thread the tube from the formula container through the controller according to the manufacturer's directions.
- Purge the tubing of air, and attach it to the feeding tube.

- Open the regulator clamp on the gavage bag tubing, and adjust the flow rate appropriately.
- When using a bulb syringe, fill the syringe with formula and release the feeding tube to allow formula to flow through it. The height at which the syringe is held will determine flow rate. When the syringe is three-quarters empty, pour more formula into it.
- To prevent air from entering the tube and the patient's stomach, never allow the syringe to empty completely.
- If an infusion controller is being used, set the flow rate according to the manufacturer's directions.

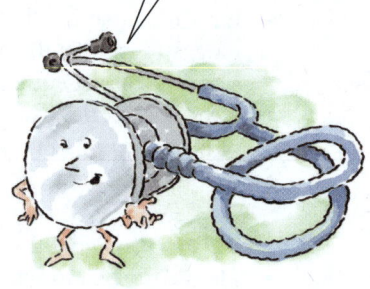

When using a bulb syringe, fill it with formula and release the feeding tube to allow formula to flow through it.

Slow and steady

- Always administer a tube feeding slowly—typically, 200 to 350 mL over 15 to 30 minutes, depending on the patient's tolerance and the health care provider's order—to prevent sudden stomach distention, which can cause nausea, vomiting, cramps, or diarrhea.
- After administering the appropriate amount of formula, flush the tubing by adding about 60 mL of water to the gavage bag or bulb syringe, or manually flush it using a barrel syringe. Flushing maintains the tube's patency by removing excess formula, which could occlude the tube.
- If a continuous feeding is being administered, flush the feeding tube every 4 hours to help prevent tube occlusion.

All done

- To discontinue gastric feeding (depending on the equipment being used), close the regulator clamp on the gavage bag tubing, disconnect the syringe from the feeding tube, or turn off the infusion controller.
- Cover the end of the feeding tube with its plug or cap to prevent leakage and contamination of the tube.
- Leave the patient in semi-Fowler or high-Fowler position for at least 30 minutes.
- Rinse all reusable equipment with warm water.
- Dry it and store it in a convenient place for the next feeding. Change equipment according to the facility's policy.

Practice pointers

- If the feeding solution doesn't initially flow through a bulb syringe, attach the bulb and squeeze it gently to start the flow. Then remove the bulb. Never use the bulb to force the formula through the tube.

- If the patient becomes nauseated or vomits, stop the feeding immediately. The patient may vomit if the stomach becomes distended from overfeeding or delayed gastric emptying.
- To reduce oropharyngeal discomfort from the tube, allow the patient to brush their teeth or care for their dentures regularly and encourage frequent gargling.
- If the patient is unconscious, administer oral care with wet sponge-tipped swabs every 4 hours. Use petroleum jelly on dry, cracked lips.

Parched

- Dry mucous membranes may indicate dehydration, which requires increased fluid intake.
- Clean the patient's nostrils with cotton-tipped applicators, apply lubricant along the mucosa, and assess the skin for signs of breakdown.
- During continuous feedings, assess the patient frequently for abdominal distention. Flush the tubing by adding about 50 mL of water to the gavage bag or bulb syringe. Flushing the tubing maintains the tube's patency by removing excess formula, which could occlude the tube.
- If the patient develops diarrhea, administer small, frequent, less concentrated feedings, or administer bolus feedings over a longer time.
- Make sure that the formula isn't cold and that proper storage and sanitation practices have been followed. The loose stools associated with tube feedings make additional perineal and skin care necessary. Changing to a formula that contains more fiber may eliminate liquid stools.

More fruits and veggies

- If the patient becomes constipated, the health care provider may increase the fruit, vegetable, or sugar content of the formula.
- Assess the patient's hydration status, because dehydration may produce constipation. Increase fluid intake as necessary. If the condition persists, administer an appropriate drug or enema, as ordered.
- Drugs can be administered through the feeding tube.
- Except for enteric-coated drugs or time-released medications, crush tablets or open and dilute capsules in water before administering them. Be sure to flush the tubing afterward to ensure full instillation of medication. Keep in mind that some drugs may change the osmolarity of the feeding formula and cause diarrhea. For more information regarding medication administration through a gastric tube, see Chapter 10.

Hold the wire

- Small-bore feeding tubes may kink, making instillation impossible. If this problem is suspected, try changing the patient's position or withdraw the tube a few inches and restart. Never use a guide wire to reposition the tube.
- Collect blood samples as ordered.
- Glycosuria, hyperglycemia, and diuresis can indicate an excessive carbohydrate level, leading to hyperosmotic dehydration, which may be fatal. Monitor blood glucose levels to assess glucose tolerance. Also, monitor serum electrolytes, blood urea nitrogen, serum glucose, serum osmolality, and other pertinent findings to determine the patient's response to therapy and assess their hydration status.

Check the flow

- Check the flow rate hourly to ensure correct infusion.
- For duodenal or jejunal feeding, most patients tolerate a continuous drip better than bolus feedings. Bolus feedings can cause such complications as hyperglycemia and diarrhea.
- Until the patient acquires a tolerance for the formula, it may need to be diluted to half or three-quarters strength to start and then the strength of the formula can be increased gradually.
- Patients under stress or who are receiving steroids may experience a pseudodiabetic state. Assess them frequently and consult with the health care provider about the need for insulin.
- Document the procedure and the feeding according to your facility's policy. (See *Documenting tube feedings.*)

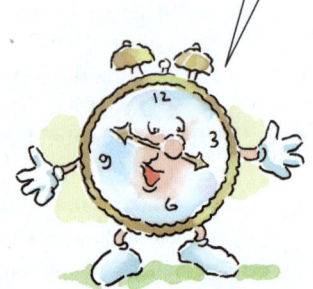

Check the flow rate hourly to ensure correct infusion.

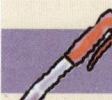

Take note!

Documenting tube feedings

When documenting tube feedings, be sure to include the details listed below:
- On the intake and output sheet, record the date, volume of formula, and volume of water.
- When charting, include abdominal assessment (including tube exit site, if appropriate); amount of residual gastric contents; verification of tube placement; amount, type, and time of feeding; and tube patency.
- Discuss the patient's tolerance of the feeding, including nausea, vomiting, cramping, diarrhea, and distention.
- Note the result of blood and urine tests, hydration status, and any drugs given through the tube.
- Include the date and time of administration set changes, oral and nasal hygiene, and results of specimen collections.

Quick quiz

1. The nurse is teaching the patient about preventing nutrition-related disease. Of the following interventions, which are considered primary prevention efforts? (**Select all that apply**)
    A. participation in a healthy cooking class
    B. making shopping lists that include fruits and vegetables
    C. screening for high cholesterol
    D. making a list of food swaps for high-sugar items
    E. teaching about meal planning

Answer: A, B, D, and E. Primary prevention efforts aim to prevent a disease or illness from occurring in the first place. Providing nutrition support and education helps the patient to make healthy nutrition choices on a daily basis in the hope of preventing nutrition-related diseases.

2. A patient is using the MyPlate dietary guidelines to help make healthy food choices. To meet their daily recommendations for grains, they must consume whole grains. Which of the following are considered whole grains? (**Select all that apply**)
    A. oatmeal
    B. brown rice
    C. white rice
    D. quinoa
    E. grits
    F. popcorn

Answer: A, B, D, and F. Oatmeal, brown rice, quinoa, and popcorn are all whole grains because they have not been processed to remove the grain kernel.

3. Which gastrointestinal (GI) hormone acts on both the gallbladder and the pancreas?
    A. gastric inhibitory peptides
    B. gastrin
    C. secretin
    D. cholecystokinin

Answer: D. Cholecystokinin stimulates the gallbladder to contract and release bile and encourages the release of enzyme-rich pancreatic fluid.

4. The nurse is caring for a patient who has an intention tremor and has trouble getting a spoon from the plate to their mouth without spilling. Which assistive feeding device would be the best choice to help with this issue?
    A.   universal cuff
    B.   swivel spoon
    C.   long-handled spoon
    D.   plate guard

Answer: B. A swivel spoon is the best choice for a patient with an intention tremor, because it keeps the spoon level even when jostling or shaking occurs.

Scoring

☆☆☆   If you answered all four questions correctly, gee whiz! Your nutritional knowledge is optimal.

☆☆   If you answered three questions correctly, great! Your ingestion of nutrition facts is quite sufficient.

☆   If you answered fewer than three questions correctly, no worries! Review the chapter, and absorb some more facts.

References

Academy of Nutrition and Dietetics. (2021). Definition of terms list. https://www.eatrightpro.org/practice/dietetics-resources/quality-management/definition-of-terms

Bhupathiraju, S. N., & Hu, F. (2023). *Overview of nutrition. Merck Manual Professional Version.* https://www.merckmanuals.com/professional/nutritional-disorders/nutrition-general-considerations/overview-of-nutrition

Centers for Disease Control and Prevention (CDC). (2022). Childhood obesity facts. https://www.cdc.gov/obesity/data/childhood.html

Faizan, U., & Rouster, A. S. (2023). *Nutrition and hydration requirements in children and adults. StatPearls.* https://www.ncbi.nlm.nih.gov/books/NBK562207/

Hargreaves, S. M., Raposo, A., Saraiva, A., & Zandonadi, R. P. (2021). Vegetarian diet: An overview through the perspective of quality of life domains. *International Journal of Environmental Research and Public Health, 18*(8), 4067. https://doi.org/10.3390/ijerph18084067

Heda, R., Toro, F., & Tombazzi, C. R. (2023). *Physiology, pepsin. StatPearls.* https://www.ncbi.nlm.nih.gov/books/NBK537005/

Hsu, M., Safadi, A. O., & Lui, F. (2022). *Physiology, stomach. StatPearls.* https://www.ncbi.nlm.nih.gov/books/NBK535425/

Jurdana, M. (2021). Physical activity and cancer risk. Actual knowledge and possible biological mechanisms. *Radiology and Oncology, 55*(1), 7–17. https://doi.org/10.2478/raon-2020-0063

Karpińska, M., & Czauderna, M. (2022). Pancreas: Its functions, disorders, and physiological impact on the mammals' organism. *Frontiers in Physiology, 13*, 807632. https://doi.org/10.3389/fphys.2022.807632

Kesari, A., & Noel, J. Y. (2023). *Nutritional assessment. StatPearls*. https://www.ncbi.nlm.nih.gov/books/NBK580496/

Morisset, J. (2020). Life with the pancreas: A personal experience. *Advances in Medical Sciences, 65*(1), 46-64. https://doi.org/10.1016/j.advms.2019.11.002

Morley, J. E. (2021). *Overview of undernutrition*. Merck Manual Professional Version. https://www.merckmanuals.com/professional/nutritional-disorders/undernutrition/overview-of-undernutrition

National Academy of Sciences. (2023). Dietary reference intakes for energy. https://nap.nationalacademies.org/catalog/26818/dietary-reference-intakes-for-energy

National Institutes of Health. (n.d.). *Nutrient recommendations and databases*. Office of Dietary Supplements. https://ods.od.nih.gov/HealthInformation/nutrientrecommendations.aspx

National Library of Medicine. (2022). *Vegetarian diet*. Medline Plus. https://medlineplus.gov/ency/article/002465.htm

Norris, T. L. (2025). *Porth's pathophysiology: Concepts of altered health status* (11th ed.). Wolters Kluwer.

Sánchez López de Nava, A., & Raja, A. (2022). *Physiology, metabolism. StatPearls*. https://www.ncbi.nlm.nih.gov/books/NBK546690/

Simpson, D., & Mcintosh, R. (2021). Measuring and monitoring fluid balance. *British Journal of Nursing, 30*(12), 706–710. https://www.britishjournalofnursing.com/content/clinical/measuring-and-monitoring-fluid-balance/

Tobias, A., & Sadiq, N. M. (2022). *Physiology, gastrointestinal nervous control. StatPearls*. https://www.ncbi.nlm.nih.gov/books/NBK545268/

United States Department of Health and Human Services (USDHHS). (2020). *Healthy people 2030*. https://health.gov/healthypeople

World Health Organization (WHO). (2023). Health promotion and disease prevention. https://www.emro.who.int/about-who/public-health-functions/health-promotion-disease-prevention.html

Chapter 19

Urinary elimination[*]

Just the facts

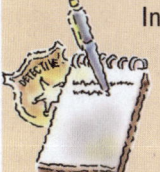

In this chapter, you'll learn:

♦ process of urine formation

♦ factors that affect urinary elimination

♦ common urinary abnormalities

♦ proper methods for obtaining urine specimens

♦ proper method for obtaining urine specific gravity

♦ steps for insertion, care, and removal of an indwelling urinary catheter

♦ proper method for applying a condom catheter.

A look at the urinary system

The urinary system consists of the kidneys, ureters, bladder, and urethra.

Kidneys

The essential functions of the urinary system—such as forming and excreting urine to maintain the proper balance of fluids and electrolytes, minerals, and organic substances for homeostasis—take place in the highly vascular kidneys. These bean-shaped organs are 4½ to 5 in (11.4 to 12.7 cm) long and 2½ in (6.4 cm) wide.

Located outside of the peritoneal cavity in the posterior upper abdomen on each side of the vertebral column, the two kidneys are protected by the contents of the abdomen. The right kidney extends slightly lower than the left kidney. The deep fissure called the *hilus* is where the blood vessels and nerves enter and leave the kidneys and connect the ureters to drain urine to the bladder. A layer of fat

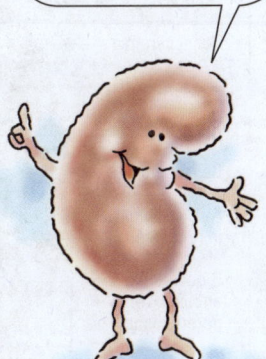

I'm essential to a well-balanced urinary system.

---

[*]Note: In this chapter, the term "male" refers to a person assigned male at birth, and the term "female" refers to a person assigned female at birth.

surrounds each kidney, offering further protection. Each kidney consists of three regions:

- renal cortex (outer region)
- renal medulla (middle region)
- renal pelvis (inner region) (See *A close look at the kidneys.*)

A close look at the kidneys

The kidneys are located in the lumbar area, with the right kidney situated slightly lower than the left to make room for the liver, which is just above it. The position of the kidneys shifts somewhat with changes in body position. Covering the kidneys are the fibrous capsule, perirenal fat, and renal fasciae.

Blood's cleansing journey

The kidneys receive waste-filled blood from the renal artery, which branches off the abdominal aorta. After passing through a complicated network of smaller blood vessels and nephrons, the filtered blood returns to circulation by way of the renal vein, which empties into the inferior vena cava.

Continuing the cleanup

The kidneys excrete waste products that the nephrons remove from the blood. These excretions combine with other waste fluids (such as urea, creatinine, phosphates, and sulfates) to form urine. An action called *peristalsis* (the circular contraction and relaxation of a tube-shaped structure) passes the urine through the ureters and into the urinary bladder. When the bladder has filled, nerves in the bladder wall relax the sphincter. In conjunction with a voluntary stimulus, this relaxation causes urine to pass into the urethra for elimination from the body.

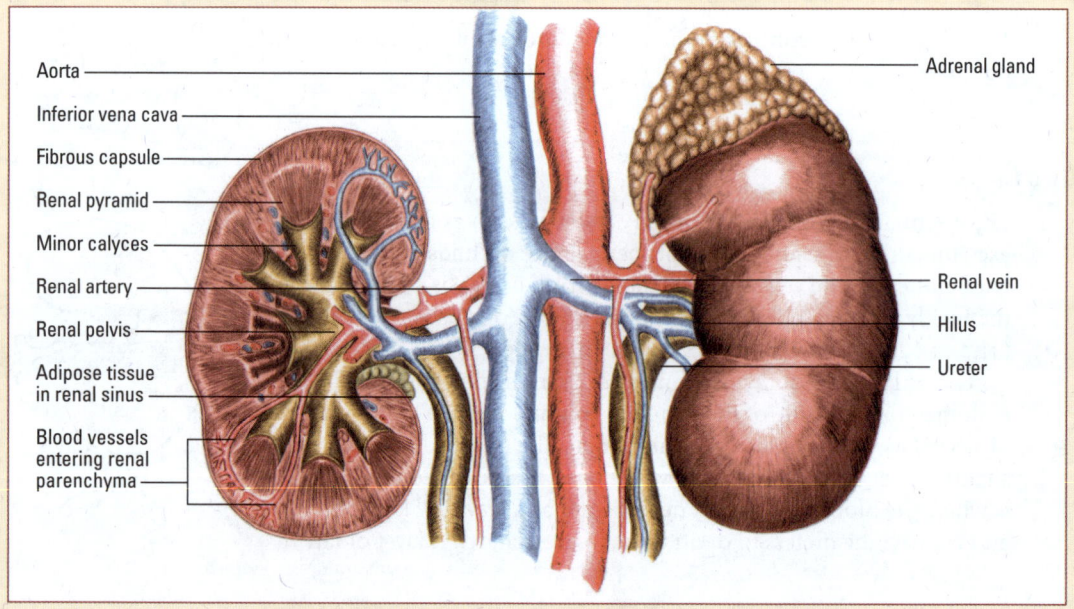

Aorta

Inferior vena cava

Fibrous capsule

Renal pyramid

Minor calyces

Renal artery

Renal pelvis

Adipose tissue in renal sinus

Blood vessels entering renal parenchyma

Adrenal gland

Renal vein

Hilus

Ureter

Filtering station

The outer portion of the kidney is called the *renal cortex*. It holds *nephrons*, which contain the glomerulus that filters blood, and tubules that selectively reabsorb substances back into the blood or secrete unneeded substances into the filtrate that becomes urine.

Renal wonder

The *renal medulla* contains 8 to 12 renal pyramids, which are striated wedges composed mostly of tubular structures. Each pyramid forms a lobe of the kidney, and the apices of the pyramid form the papillae. The tapered portion of each pyramid empties into a cuplike calyx that channels formed urine from the pyramids into the renal pelvis. The renal pelvis receives urine through the major calyces, and then urine moves into the ureters and finally to the bladder.

All in a day's work

Kidney functions include:

- elimination of wastes and excess ions (in the form of urine)
- blood filtration (by regulating chemical composition and blood volume)
- maintenance of fluid–electrolyte and acid–base balances
- production and release of renin to promote angiotensin II activation and aldosterone production in the adrenal gland
- promotion of erythropoietin (a hormone that stimulates red blood cell production and such enzymes as renin, which governs blood pressure and kidney function)
- conversion of vitamin D to a more active form

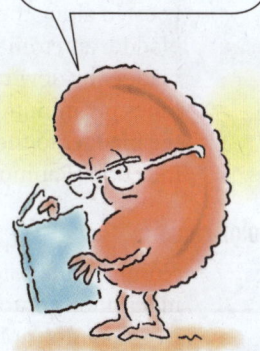

Hmm . . . It appears that I'm responsible for several important functions.

Making urine

The nephron is the functional unit of the kidneys. Each kidney contains roughly one million nephrons. Nephrons each consist of capillary structures, a proximal convoluted tubule, a loop of Henle, a distal convoluted tubule, and a collecting duct. Blood is filtered in the glomerulus, and the other structures reabsorb water, electrolytes, and substances needed to maintain constancy of the internal environment. Unneeded substances are secreted in the tubular filtrate for elimination. Urine gathers in the collecting tubules and ducts of the nephrons and then drains into the ureters, down into the bladder, and out through the urethra.

A wealth of minerals

Formed urine consists of water, sodium, chloride, potassium, calcium, magnesium, sulfates, phosphates, bicarbonates, uric acid, ammonium ions, creatinine, and urobilinogen (a derivative of bilirubin).

Go with the flow

Urine is produced in small or large amounts and can be dilute or concentrated. Urine is normally sterile; it contains fluid, salts, and waste products, but not bacteria, fungi, or protozoa (Taylor et al., 2023). Approximately 250 to 400 mL of urine is expressed when someone voids. Because the kidneys continue to fill the bladder even as it empties, it is normal for 5 to 10 mL of urine to remain in the bladder after urination. Daily urine output averages 720 to 2,400 mL, varying with fluid intake and environment.

Ureters

The ureters are a pair of muscular tubes that extend 10 to 12 in (25.5 to 30.5 cm) from the kidneys to the bladder. The left ureter is slightly longer than the right because of the left kidney's higher position. The diameter of each ureter varies from ⅛ to ¼ in (3 to 6 mm), with the narrowest part at the ureteropelvic junction.

Where the action is

Located along the posterior abdominal wall, the ureters enter the bladder anteromedially. They carry urine from the kidneys to the bladder by downward peristaltic contractions that occur one to five times per minute. If urine is retained in the kidneys or backflows from the bladder to the kidneys, this increases the patient's susceptibility to infection (Rabinowitz & Cubillos, 2022).

Color clues .

Normal urine color ranges from straw yellow to dark yellow. Certain medications or foods and reduced or increased fluid intake can alter its color. Amitriptyline can turn urine blue-green, and phenazopyridine may produce bright orange urine. Beets and blackberries may turn the urine pink. Very dilute urine is almost colorless, and concentrated urine can be dark amber or orange-brown.

Clear is cool

Freshly voided urine should appear clear with no sediment. Urine collected from an indwelling urinary catheter bag may contain mucus shreds, but urine in the tubing should still be clear.

Odor alert

The more dilute the urine, the fainter the odor. Concentrated urine has a strong odor, and collected urine that's long-standing may develop a strong ammonia smell. Certain infections may also cause urine to have a foul or offensive odor.

Bladder

Located in the pelvis, the bladder is a hollow, muscular organ that serves as a temporary storage reservoir for urine collection. The bladder lies on the pelvic floor behind the symphysis pubis; when it's full, it becomes displaced under the peritoneal cavity. Bladder capacity ranges from 500 to 1,000 mL in healthy adults and is lower in children and older adults. Micturition, the passing of urine, is controlled by the detrusor muscle and the external sphincter. The external sphincter stops micturition and maintains continence against high bladder pressure (Sam et al., 2022).

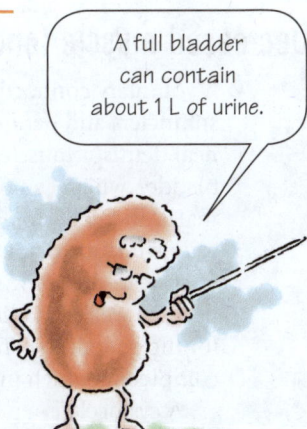

A full bladder can contain about 1 L of urine.

Urethra

The urethra is a small duct that carries urine from the bladder and out of the body. A female's urethra is only 1 to 2 in (3 to 4 cm) long and is anterior to the vaginal opening. Because a male's urethra must pass through the erectile tissue of the penis, it's about 7 to 8 in (18 to 20 cm) long. It has three main segments: prostatic, membranous, and penile (Stoddard & Leslie, 2023). The urethra is part of the reproductive system as well as the urinary system because it also transports semen.

Factors affecting urinary elimination

Several factors impact how urine is eliminated. These include body position, decreased muscle tone, fluid intake, hypotension, infection, loss of body fluid, medications, neurologic injury, nutrition, obstruction of urinary flow, psychological problems, and surgery.

Body position

The ability to empty the bladder during each voiding is dependent on proper body positioning, which is normally standing for males and sitting for females. If a patient is using a bedpan, it's best to position them in a sitting position on the bedpan for bladder emptying, if their condition allows. Offering a urinal to a male patient lying flat in bed will affect the patient's ability to initiate a urine stream and empty the bladder completely. Similarly, placing a female patient on a bedpan while lying flat in bed will affect the patient's ability to urinate and empty the bladder completely. To facilitate urination and complete bladder emptying, sitting up as one would on a commode is the most accommodating position.

Decreased muscle tone

A voluntary contraction and relaxation of the internal and external sphincters and perineal muscles controls urination. Weakened perineal detrusor muscles can result from chronic overdistention of the bladder, which can occur due to benign prostatic hypertrophy in males and pelvic organ prolapse in females (Sam et al., 2022). Other causes include diabetes mellitus, nerve damage, spinal cord injury, fracture of the spine, herniated disc, or infections. When these muscles become weak, muscle tone is decreased, so it becomes more difficult for the patient to control the urge to void or to empty the bladder completely, which may result in incontinence.

A cystocele is a protrusion of the bladder into the vaginal canal that occurs when the vaginal wall musculature weakens as a result of muscle straining. This type of straining can occur during childbirth or heavy lifting. It can cause stress incontinence, dribbling, frequency, an inability to empty the bladder completely, and an increased rate of infections (Makajeva et al., 2022).

Stretch and tone

A patient who has had a long-standing indwelling urinary catheter may have trouble regaining bladder control when the catheter is removed. The continuous drainage caused by the indwelling catheter doesn't allow the bladder to fill or stretch to capacity. Because the bladder wall doesn't stretch, atrophy can develop. Dribbling after the catheter is removed is usually temporary until bladder tone returns.

Fluid intake

A patient's fluid intake is directly related to urinary volume and frequency. Urine output decreases if fluid intake decreases. Similarly, urine output increases if fluid intake increases. If fluid intake increases significantly, the frequency of urination also increases.

The correlation of intake affecting output is regulated by several hormones, such as angiotensin I and II, aldosterone, erythropoietin, and antidiuretic hormone (ADH). The most important hormone is ADH, which regulates the amount of reabsorption that occurs in the nephrons of the kidney and conserves body water by reducing urine output. ADH is released when fluid intake is decreased. The kidney then reabsorbs more water and produces more highly concentrated urine. When fluid intake increases, the release of ADH is suppressed (Cuzzo et al., 2022).

Hypotension

Hypotension (low arterial blood pressure) reduces blood flow to the kidneys. Adequate blood flow to the kidneys is necessary for urine production. Thus, hypotension prevents filtration from occurring. Surgery, trauma, or severe fluid loss from vomiting or diarrhea can cause hypotension, which results in a decrease in circulating blood volume and decreased filtration and urinary excretion.

Infection

The urinary tract is sterile, except at the urinary meatus, and microorganisms there usually get washed away during urination. *Urinary tract infections* (UTIs) occur when microorganisms from the perineal or anal area come in contact with the urinary meatus and ascend into the urethra. UTIs are most common in females because of the shorter urethra and its close proximity to the anus. Symptoms of uncomplicated UTIs include urgency, frequency, and dysuria.

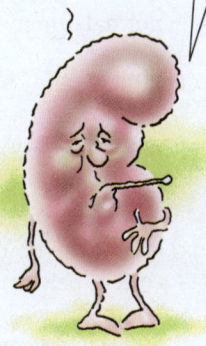

Females are particularly susceptible to UTIs.

Infection protection

UTIs can occur anywhere along the urinary tract, including the urethra, bladder, ureter, or kidney. Lower UTIs are more common and occur in the urethra or bladder. Upper UTIs occur in the ureters, kidneys, pelvis, or renal tubule system; they're more serious and can lead to kidney damage and renal failure. If left untreated, however, lower UTIs can progress to the kidneys and result in renal damage and renal failure (and become upper UTIs).

Loss of body fluid

Loss of body fluid can result from excessive diuresis caused by fever, exercise, vomiting, diarrhea, and excessive wound drainage or blood loss from surgery or trauma (Brinkman et al., 2022). The kidneys respond to this loss by increasing water absorption to conserve water, causing a decrease in urine output.

Medications

Diuretics are used to promote the excretion of water and electrolytes by the kidneys. Commonly used diuretics include furosemide, chlorothiazide, triamterene, hydrochlorothiazide, and spironolactone (Arumugham & Shahin, 2022).

Cholinergic medications, such as bethanechol (Urecholine), may be prescribed because they stimulate the contraction of the detrusor muscle, which promotes voiding. Urinary frequency or urgency may be treated with oxybutynin because of its antispasmodic effect on the detrusor muscle (Mayo Clinic, 2022).

Other medications can also impact urinary output. Opioids can decrease the glomerular filtration rate and the sensation of a full bladder. Phenothiazines, belladonna alkaloids, tricyclic antidepressants, and antihistamines have anticholinergic effects and can increase urine retention.

Neurologic injury

The frontal lobe of the brain controls voluntary urination. Hemorrhage, trauma, or a tumor in this lobe can result in urinary incontinence. A spinal cord injury or a stroke also can interfere with normal urinary elimination.

Reflex control

Injury to the sacral area of the spinal cord, which controls the urination reflex, can change urinary elimination patterns. When the bladder becomes full and stretched to capacity, it contracts, and urination occurs. This is called *reflex neurogenic bladder*. An *autonomous neurogenic bladder* can occur as a result of neurologic injury of the sacral spinal cord or pelvic nerves; it results in complete disruption of both motor and sensory nervous system control over the bladder (Leslie et al., 2022). Urine retention causing the bladder to fill without the bladder stretch mechanism in place can result in increased infections.

Nutrition

A diet consisting of foods high in water content such as soups, gelatin desserts, vegetables, and fruits increases urine output. Salty foods can decrease urine output, especially if water intake doesn't increase. Food and drinks containing caffeine (chocolate, coffee, tea, and cola), which is a diuretic, and alcohol can increase urine output.

Obstruction of urine flow

Obstruction of urine flow can lead to decreased urinary elimination. Structural abnormalities in the urinary system, including urinary tumors, renal stones, and an enlarged prostate gland, can cause obstructions. Obstruction can also result from clogs or kinks in an indwelling catheter. Unrelieved obstruction causes increased resistance to urine flow and can lead to hydronephrosis (distention of the renal pelvis).

An infection connection

Prolonged obstruction can lead to urinary stasis, a condition that provides a breeding ground for microorganisms and resulting UTIs.

Psychological factors

Urination is a voluntary function that's affected by internal and external factors. Stress and anxiety can cause a patient to contract their muscles involuntarily, making urination impossible or making the urge to urinate overwhelming. In addition, asking a patient for a urine sample or to urinate "on demand" can make them unable to urinate. The sound or feel of running water can intensify the need to urinate. If a patient has difficulty voiding, try pouring warm water over their inner thigh or perineal area to initiate urination. Though this technique can be effective, always consider a patient's need for privacy, especially when a bedpan or urinal must be used. Ensuring privacy may allow the patient to relax and be able to void.

Surgery

Most patients should be able to urinate within 6 to 8 hours after surgery. If a patient can't urinate following surgery, the cause may be depleted fluid volume due to limited fluid intake and blood loss during surgery. The stress that accompanies surgery can cause the release of ADH, which also decreases urinary output. Urine retention is also an adverse effect of some pain medications, such as opioids. Urinary, intestinal, or reproductive surgery also predisposes a patient to postoperative urinary retention. Trauma to the tissues causes edema and can obstruct urinary flow. The need for intervention should be assessed carefully.

How dry am I?

Medications used for spinal anesthesia or regional blocks can cause temporary urinary problems because they impair sensory and motor impulses that control urination. When the anesthetic wears off, the patient should be able to resume their normal voiding pattern. If not, position changes, walking when possible, privacy, and the sound of running water may facilitate voiding.

Common urinary abnormalities

Dysuria, hematuria, nocturia, polyuria, urinary frequency, urgency, and hesitancy and urinary incontinence are common abnormalities in the urinary system.

Dysuria

Pain during urination, or *dysuria*, commonly signals a lower UTI. The onset of the pain signifies the cause. Pain immediately before urination indicates bladder irritation or distention, whereas pain at the onset usually signals a bladder outlet obstruction (Mehta et al., 2022). Bladder spasms can cause pain at the end of the stream. Pain throughout urination may indicate pyelonephritis, especially when accompanied by fever, chills, hematuria, and flank pain.

Hematuria

Brown or bright red urine is a sign of hematuria or blood in the urine (National Institute of Diabetes and Digestive and Kidney Diseases (NIDDK), 2022). When the bleeding occurs during elimination, it can indicate the location of the underlying problem. For example, a urethral disorder will cause bleeding at the onset of urination. Bleeding at the end of the stream suggests a disorder of the bladder neck or prostate gland. When bleeding occurs throughout urination, it indicates a disorder located above the bladder neck. Hematuria can also be caused by gastrointestinal, vaginal, or some coagulation disorders or cancer. In addition, males may experience hematuria temporarily following urinary tract or prostate surgery or after a urethral catheterization.

Nocturia

Excessive urination at night, known as *nocturia*, is a common sign of kidney or lower urinary tract disorders. It can result from a disruption of normal urine patterns or overstimulation of the nerves and muscles that control urination. The following can also produce nocturia: cardiovascular, endocrine, or metabolic disorders; diuretics; and increased fluid intake.

In males, nocturia can result from benign prostatic hyperplasia (BPH), when significant urethral obstruction develops, or from prostate cancer.

Polyuria

Polyuria is the production and excretion of more than 2,500 mL of urine per day. This fairly common condition is usually a result of diabetes insipidus, diabetes mellitus, or diuretic use. Other causes of polyuria include urologic disorders, such as pyelonephritis and postobstructive uropathy, and some psychological, neurologic, and renal disorders. Patients with polyuria are at risk for developing hypovolemia.

Urinary frequency, urgency, and hesitancy

Urinary frequency commonly results from decreased bladder capacity and is a classic symptom of a UTI. Frequency also occurs with urethral stricture, neurologic disorders, pregnancy, and uterine tumors. For males, urinary frequency may emerge with BPH, urethral stricture, or a prostate tumor, all of which can put pressure on the bladder.

Pain picture

The sudden urge to urinate, or *urinary urgency*, when accompanied by bladder pain, is another symptom of a UTI. Even small amounts of urine in the bladder can cause pain because inflammation decreases bladder capacity. Urgency without pain may be a symptom of an upper motor neuron lesion.

Ready, set, go?

Difficulty starting a urine stream, or *urinary hesitancy*, can occur with a UTI, partial obstruction of the lower urinary tract, neuromuscular disorders, or the use of certain drugs.

Stalling

Urinary hesitancy is most common in male patients over the age of 50 with an enlarged prostate gland, which can cause partial obstruction of the urethra.

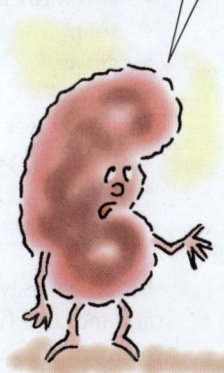

What to do, what to do? I can't decide if I want to go or not.

Urinary incontinence

Urinary incontinence is a common condition that may be transient or permanent with a minimal or significant release of urine. Possible causes include stress incontinence, tumor, bladder cancer and calculi, and such neurologic disorders as Guillain-Barré syndrome, multiple sclerosis, and spinal cord injury. In males, urinary incontinence may also be a symptom of BPH, prostate infection, or prostate cancer.

Intervening for issues with urinary elimination

When caring for a patient with altered urinary elimination, interventions may include bedpan and urinal use; collecting urine specimens; obtaining urine specific gravity; applying a condom catheter or male incontinence device; and insertion, care, and removal of an indwelling urinary catheter.

Bedpan and urinal use

Bedpans and urinals permit elimination by a patient who is bedfast and provide a way to accurately observe and measure urine and stool. A female patient can use a bedpan for urination and defecation. A male patient normally uses a urinal for urination and a bedpan for defecation. Be sure to offer these devices frequently—before meals, visiting hours, morning and evening care, and treatments or procedures. Always allow the patient privacy.

Supplies
- fracture or regular bedpan or urinal with cover
- toilet tissue
- two washcloths
- soap
- gloves
- towel
- linen-saver pad
- bath blanket
- pillow

Big and little

Bedpans are available in adult and pediatric sizes and disposable and reusable (must be sterilized) models. The fracture pan, a type of bedpan, is used when spinal injuries, body or leg casts, or other conditions prohibit or restrict turning the patient.

Getting ready
- Obtain the appropriate bedpan or urinal.
- If a metal bed pan is being used, warm it under running water to avoid startling the patient and stimulating muscle contraction, which hinders elimination.
- Dry the bedpan thoroughly and test its temperature.
- For a thin patient, place a linen-saver pad at the edge of the bedpan, or use a fracture pan to minimize pressure on the coccyx.

How it's done

- Always provide privacy.
- Put on gloves to prevent contact with body fluids, and comply with standard precautions.

Placing a bedpan

- If the patient's condition allows, elevate the head of the bed slightly to prevent hyperextension of the spine when the patient raises their buttocks.
- Rest the bedpan on the edge of the bed. Then turn down the corner of the top linens and draw up the patient's gown. Ask the patient to raise the buttocks by flexing their knees and pushing down on their heels. While supporting the patient's lower back with one hand, center the curved, smooth edge of the bedpan beneath the buttocks.
- If the patient can't raise their buttocks, lower the head of the bed to the horizontal position and help the patient roll onto one side with the buttocks facing you. Position the bedpan properly against the buttocks, and then help the patient roll back onto the bedpan. When the patient is positioned comfortably, raise the head of the bed if the patient's condition allows.

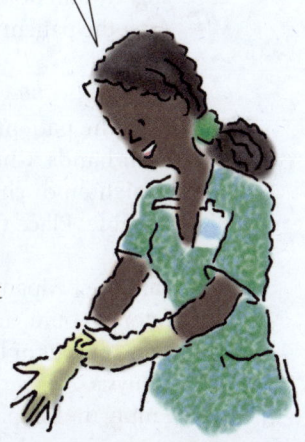

> Be sure to put on gloves before performing a procedure where there's a risk of contact with body fluids.

Position is everything

- After positioning the bedpan, if the patient's condition allows, elevate the head of the bed further, until the patient is sitting erect. This position aids in defecation and urination.
- If elevation of the head of the bed is contraindicated, tuck a small pillow or folded bath blanket under the patient's back to cushion the sacrum against the edge of the bedpan and support the lumbar region.
- Place the bed in a low position and raise the side rails to ensure their safety. Place toilet tissue and the call button within the patient's reach, and instruct them to push the button after elimination. If the patient is weak or disoriented, remain with them.
- Before removing the bedpan, lower the head of the bed slightly. Then ask the patient to raise the buttocks off the bed. Support the lower back with one hand, and gently remove the bedpan with the other to avoid skin injury caused by friction. If the patient can't raise their buttocks, ask them to roll off the pan while assisting with one hand. Hold the pan firmly with the other hand to avoid spills. Cover the bedpan and place it on the chair.
- Help clean the anal and perineal area, as necessary, to prevent irritation and infection. Turn the patient onto their side, wipe carefully with toilet tissue, clean the area with a damp washcloth and

soap, and dry with a towel. Clean a female patient from front to back to avoid introducing rectal contaminants into the vaginal or urethral openings.

Placing a urinal

- Lift the corner of the top linens, hand the urinal to the patient, and allow them to position it.
- If the patient can't position the urinal themselves, spread the legs slightly and hold the urinal in place to prevent spills.
- After the patient voids, carefully withdraw the urinal.

After use of a bedpan or urinal

- Give the patient a clean, damp, warm, soapy washcloth for their hands. Check the bed linens for wetness or soiling, and straighten or change them, if needed. Make the patient comfortable. Place the bed in the lowest position and raise the side rails.
- Take the bedpan or urinal to the bathroom. Observe the color, odor, amount, and consistency of its contents. If ordered, measure urine output or liquid stool, or obtain a specimen for laboratory analysis.
- Empty the bedpan or urinal into the toilet or hopper. Rinse with cold water and clean the bedpan thoroughly, using a disinfectant solution. Dry and return it to the patient's bedside stand.
- Use an air freshener, if necessary, to eliminate offensive odors and minimize embarrassment.
- Remove and discard gloves, and wash hands.

Practice pointers

- Explain to the patient that drug treatment and changes in environment, diet, and activities may disrupt the usual elimination schedule. Try to anticipate elimination needs, and offer the bedpan or urinal frequently to help reduce embarrassment and minimize incontinence.
- Avoid placing a bedpan or urinal on top of the bedside stand or overbed table to avoid contamination of clean equipment and food trays. Similarly, avoid placing it on the floor to prevent the spread of microorganisms from the floor to the patient's bed linens when the device is used.
- If the patient experiences pain or discomfort on a standard bedpan, use a fracture pan. The fracture pan is slipped under the buttocks from the front rather than the side. It's also shallower than a standard bedpan, so the patient may only need to move slightly to position it. If the patient has obesity or is otherwise difficult to lift, help from a coworker may be required.

- If the patient has an indwelling urinary catheter, carefully position and remove the bedpan to avoid tension on the catheter, which could dislodge it or irritate the urethra. After the patient defecates, wipe, clean, and dry the anal region, taking care to avoid catheter contamination. If necessary, clean the urinary meatus with soap and water or chlorhexidine. Always follow facility guidelines (Taylor et al., 2023).
- Avoid leaving the urinal, fracture pan, or bedpan in place for extended periods to prevent skin breakdown.

Collecting a random urine specimen

A random urine specimen is collected as part of the physical examination or at various times during hospitalization. It permits laboratory screening for urinary and systemic disorders as well as drug screening.

Supplies
- bedpan, fracture pan, or urinal with cover
- toilet tissue
- two washcloths
- soap
- gloves
- towel
- linen-saver pad
- specimen container and cover
- specimen label

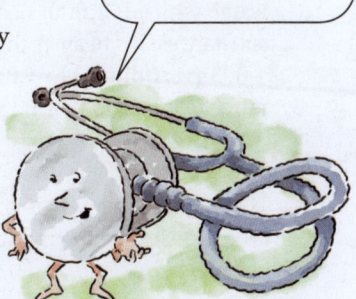

It's important to maintain a patient's dignity by providing as much privacy as the patient's condition allows.

Getting ready
- Tell the patient that a urine specimen is needed for laboratory analysis.
- Explain the procedure to the patient and their family, if necessary, to promote cooperation and prevent accidental disposal of specimens.

How it's done
- Provide privacy. Instruct the patient on bed rest to void into a clean bedpan or urinal, or ask the ambulatory patient to void into either one in the bathroom.

Pour, record, discard
- Put on gloves. Pour at least 120 mL of urine into the specimen container and cap it securely. If the patient's urine output must be measured and recorded, pour the remaining urine into the graduated container; otherwise, discard it. If urine is inadvertently spilled on the outside of the container, clean and dry it to prevent cross-contamination. Remove and discard gloves, and wash hands.

- Label the specimen container with the patient's name, room number, current date, and time of collection, according to the facility's guidelines. Attach the request form and send the specimen container immediately to the laboratory.

Clean and return

- Put on gloves. Clean the graduated container and urinal or bedpan, and return them to their proper storage area. Discard any gloves and disposable items.
- After gloves are removed, it's important to perform hand washing to prevent cross-contamination. Offer the patient a washcloth and soap and water to wash hands.
- Document the urine collection according to the facility's policy. (See *Documenting urine specimen collection.*)

Practice pointers

- Be sure to send the specimen to the laboratory immediately because delayed transport of the specimen may alter test results.
- If a patient is collecting a random urine specimen at home, provide the patient with an appropriate container to collect the specimen, and instruct them to keep it in the refrigerator (away from food items) for no more than 24 hours.

Take note!

Documenting urine specimen collection

Be sure to record the times of urine specimen collection and transport to the laboratory. Specify the test as well as the appearance, odor, color, and unusual characteristics of the specimen. If necessary, record urine volume in the intake and output record.

Obtaining urine specific gravity

Urine specific gravity is determined by comparing the weight of a urine specimen with the weight of an equivalent volume of distilled water, which is 1.000. Because urine contains dissolved salts and other substances, it's heavier than 1.000. Urine specific gravity ranges from 1.003 (very dilute) to 1.035 (highly concentrated); normal values range from 1.010 to 1.025.

The light does it

Urine specific gravity is commonly measured with a refractometer, which measures the refraction of light as it passes through a urine specimen.

High and low

Elevated specific gravity reflects an increased concentration of urine solutes, which occurs in conditions that cause renal hypoperfusion, and may indicate heart failure, dehydration, hepatic disorders, or nephrosis. Low specific gravity reflects a failure to reabsorb water and concentrate urine. It may indicate hypercalcemia, hypokalemia, alkalosis, acute renal failure, pyelonephritis, glomerulonephritis, or diabetes insipidus.

Controlled accuracy

Although urine specific gravity is commonly measured with a random urine specimen, a more accurate measurement is possible with a controlled specimen collected after withholding fluids for 12 to 24 hours.

Supplies
- refractometer
- gloves
- graduated specimen container

Getting ready
- Explain the procedure to the patient, including when the urine specimen is needed.
- To ensure patient cooperation, explain why fluids are being withheld and for how long.

How it's done
- Put on gloves, and collect a random or controlled urine specimen.
- Place a single drop of urine on the refractometer slide.
- Turn on the light and look through the eyepiece to see the specific gravity indicated on the scale. (Some instruments have a digital display.)
- Remove and discard gloves and disposable equipment, and wash hands.
- Document the procedure according to the facility's policy. (See *Documenting urine-specific gravity collection.*)

Practice pointers
- Follow the manufacturer's directors for calibrating the refractometer as appropriate.
- Replace the refractometer battery as needed.

Take note!

Documenting urine-specific gravity collection

Be sure to record the specific gravity, volume, color, odor, and appearance of the collected urine specimen.

Applying a condom catheter

Many patients don't require an indwelling urinary catheter to manage incontinence. For male patients, a condom catheter or male incontinence device reduces the risk of a UTI associated with catheterization. It also promotes bladder retraining when possible, helps prevent skin breakdown, and maintains the patient's self-image. A condom catheter is secured to the shaft of the penis and connected to a leg bag or drainage bag. It can cause skin irritation and edema.

Supplies
- condom catheter
- drainage bag

- extension tubing
- hypoallergenic tape or incontinence sheath holder
- commercial adhesive strip
- elastic adhesive or hook-and-loop fasteners, if needed
- gloves
- razor
- basin
- soap
- washcloth
- towel
- optional: solvent

Getting ready

- Explain the procedure to the patient.
- Fill the basin with lukewarm water.
- Bring the basin and other equipment to the bedside.

How it's done

- Wash hands, put on gloves, and provide privacy.

Applying the device

- If the patient is circumcised, wash the penis with soap and water, rinse well, and pat dry with a towel. If the patient isn't circumcised, gently retract the foreskin, and clean beneath it. Rinse well and dry. Replace the foreskin to avoid penile constriction.
- If necessary, shave the base and shaft of the penis to prevent the adhesive strip or skin-bond cement from pulling pubic hair.

Making it stick

- If a precut commercial adhesive strip is being used, insert the glans penis through its opening, and position the strip 1″ (2.5 cm) from the scrotal area. If an uncut adhesive is being used, cut a strip to fit around the shaft of the penis. Remove the protective covering from one side of the adhesive strip and press this side firmly to the penis to enhance adhesion. Remove the covering from the other side of the strip.

Positioning the catheter

- Position the rolled condom catheter at the tip of the penis, with its drainage opening at the urinary meatus. Allow 1″ to 2″ (2.5 to 5 cm) of space at the tip of the penis to prevent erosion and to allow for expansion when the patient voids.
- Unroll the catheter upward, past the adhesive strip on the shaft of the penis. Then gently press the sheath against the strip until it adheres. (See *How to apply a condom catheter.*)

How to apply a condom catheter

Apply an adhesive strip to the shaft of the penis about 1″ (2.5 cm) from the scrotal area.

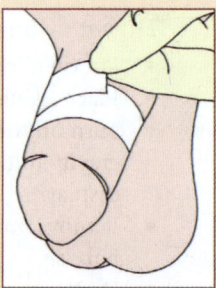

Then roll the condom catheter on to the penis past the adhesive strip, leaving about ½″ (1.3 cm) clearance at the end. Press the sheath gently against the strip until it adheres.

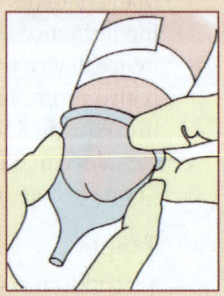

- After the condom catheter is in place, secure it with hypoallergenic tape or an incontinence sheath holder.
- Using extension tubing, connect the condom catheter to the leg bag or drainage bag. Remove and discard gloves, and wash hands.
- To protect the patient's skin and prevent UTIs, change the condom catheter at least every other day.

Removing the device

- Put on gloves. Simultaneously roll the condom catheter and adhesive strip off the penis and discard them. Remove and discard the hypoallergenic tape or incontinence sheath holder.
- Clean the penis with lukewarm water, rinse thoroughly, and dry. Check for swelling or signs of skin breakdown.
- Remove the leg bag by closing the drain clamp, unlatching the leg straps, and disconnecting the extension tubing at the top of the bag. Discard gloves and wash hands.

Practice pointers

- If hypoallergenic tape or an incontinence sheath holder isn't available, secure the condom with a strip of elastic adhesive or hook-and-loop fasteners. Apply the strip snugly; however, to avoid circulatory constriction, make sure that it isn't too tight.
- Inspect the condom catheter for twists and the extension tubing for kinks to prevent obstruction of urine flow, which could cause the condom to balloon and eventually displace. (See *Documenting use of a male incontinence device.*)

Take note!

Documenting use of a male incontinence device

Be sure to record the date and time that the incontinence device was applied and removed. Also, note skin condition and the patient's response to the device, including voiding pattern, to assist with bladder retraining.

Inserting an indwelling urinary catheter

An indwelling urinary catheter, also called a *Foley* or *retention catheter*, provides the patient with continuous urine drainage. It's inserted into the bladder, and a balloon is inflated at the catheter's distal end to prevent it from slipping out. To prevent injury and infection, insert the catheter with extreme care.

Supplies

- sterile indwelling catheter
  - latex or silicone #10 to #22 French (average adult size: #16 to #18 French)
- syringe filled with 5 to 8 mL of normal saline solution
- washcloth
- towel
- soap and water
- two linen-saver pads
- sterile gloves
- gloves

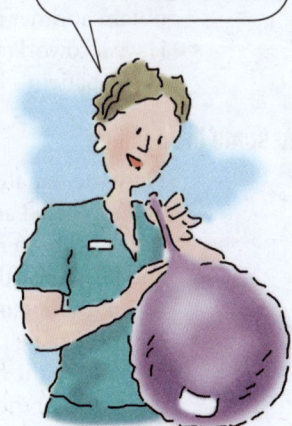

A Foley catheter has a balloon at the distal end to prevent it from slipping out. Now that's handy!

- sterile drape
- sterile fenestrated drape
- sterile cotton-tipped applicators (or cotton balls and plastic forceps)
- chlorhexidine or other antiseptic cleaning agents
- urine receptacle
- sterile water-soluble lubricant
- sterile drainage collection bag
- intake and output sheet
- optional: urine specimen container and laboratory request form, catheter securement device, gooseneck lamp or flashlight, pillows or rolled blankets or towels
  Note: Prepackaged, commercial, sterile disposable kits containing all necessary equipment are often available.

In case of contamination

Have an extra pair of sterile gloves and two appropriate-size catheters available at the bedside in case of contamination during insertion.

Getting ready
- Explain the procedure to the patient.
- Check the order on the patient's chart to determine if a catheter size or type has been specified.
- Verify the patient's identity using two patient identifiers.
- Wash hands.
- Select the appropriate equipment and assemble it at the patient's bedside.

How it's done
- Provide privacy. Check the patient's chart and ask when they voided last. Percuss and palpate the bladder to establish baseline data. Ask if the patient feels the urge to void. Make sure that the patient isn't allergic to chlorhexidine solution; if they're allergic, obtain another antiseptic cleaning agent.
- Have a coworker hold a flashlight or place a gooseneck lamp next to the patient's bed so the urinary meatus can be seen clearly.

Assume the position
- Place the female patient in the supine position, with knees flexed and separated and feet flat on the bed, about 2 feet (61 cm) apart. If this position is uncomfortable, ask the patient to flex one knee and keep the other leg flat on the bed. (See *Positioning the female patient with limited range of motion.*)
- Place the male patient in the supine position with legs extended and flat on the bed. Ask the patient to hold this position to give a clear view of the urinary meatus and to prevent contamination of the sterile field.

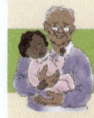

Ages and stages

Positioning the female patient with limited range of motion

The female patient with limited range of motion may need pillows or rolled towels or blankets for positioning support. If necessary, ask the patient to lie on the side with one knee drawn up to the chest during catheterization (as shown here).

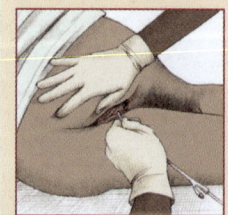

Sterile fieldwork

- Put on gloves. Clean the patient's genital area and perineum thoroughly with a prepackaged perineal cleansing cloth or soap and water, following the facility's guidelines. Dry the area with the towel. Remove gloves and wash hands.
- Place the linen-saver pads on the bed between the patient's legs and under the hips. To create the sterile field, open the prepackaged kit or equipment tray and place it between the female patient's legs or next to the male patient's hip. If the sterile gloves are on the top of the tray, put them on. Place the sterile drape under the patient's hips. Then drape the patient's lower abdomen with the sterile fenestrated drape so that only the genital area remains exposed. Take care not to contaminate the sterile gloves or sterile field.
- Open the rest of the kit or tray. Put on sterile gloves if you haven't already.
- Tear open the packet of chlorhexidine or other antiseptic cleaning agent, and saturate the sterile cotton balls or applicators.
- Open the packet of water-soluble lubricant and apply it to the catheter tip; attach the drainage bag to the other end of the catheter. (If a commercial kit is being used, the drainage bag may be attached.) Make sure that all tubing ends remain sterile and that the clamp at the emptying port of the drainage bag is closed to prevent urine leakage from the bag.

Female facts

- For the female patient, separate the labia majora and labia minora as widely as possible with the thumb, middle, and index fingers of your nondominant hand to have a full view of the urinary meatus. Keep the labia well separated throughout the procedure so they don't obscure the urinary meatus or contaminate the area when it's cleaned.

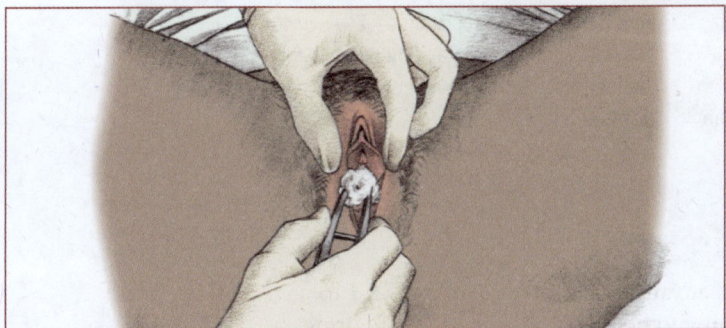

- With the dominant hand, use a sterile, cotton-tipped applicator (or pick up a sterile cotton ball with the plastic forceps) and wipe one side of the urinary meatus with a single downward motion (as shown here). Similarly, wipe the other side with another sterile applicator or cotton ball. Then wipe directly over the meatus with still another sterile applicator or cotton ball. After each wipe, dispose of the soiled cotton ball. During this process, it's important to practice sterile technique.

Male matters

- For the male patient, hold the penis with your nondominant hand. If the patient is uncircumcised, retract the foreskin. Then gently lift and stretch the penis to a 60° to 90° angle. Grasp the penis firmly, and hold the penis this way throughout the procedure to straighten the urethra and to maintain a sterile field.
- Use your dominant hand to clean the glans with a sterile cotton-tipped applicator or a sterile cotton ball held in the forceps. Clean in a circular motion, starting at the urinary meatus and working outward.
- Repeat the procedure, using another sterile applicator or cotton ball and taking care not to contaminate the sterile field or glove.
- Use the dominant hand to pick up the catheter and prepare to insert the lubricated tip into the urinary meatus. To facilitate insertion by relaxing the sphincter, ask the patient to cough as the catheter is inserted. Tell the patient to breathe deeply and slowly to further relax the sphincter and spasms. Hold the catheter close to its tip to ease insertion and control its direction. (See *Preventing indwelling catheter problems.*)

Preventing indwelling catheter problems

These precautions can help prevent problems with an indwelling urinary catheter:

• Never force the catheter during insertion. Instead, maneuver it gently as the patient bears down or coughs. If resistance is still met, stop and notify the healthcare provider. Sphincter spasms, strictures, misplacement in the vagina (in females), or an enlarged prostate (in males) may cause resistance.

• Establish urine flow, and then inflate the balloon to ensure that the catheter is in the bladder.

Advanced class

- For the female patient, advance the catheter 2 to 3 in (5.1 to 7.5 cm) while continuing to hold the labia apart—until urine begins to flow (as shown in this illustration). If the catheter is inadvertently inserted into the vagina, leave it there as a landmark. Then begin the procedure again using new supplies.

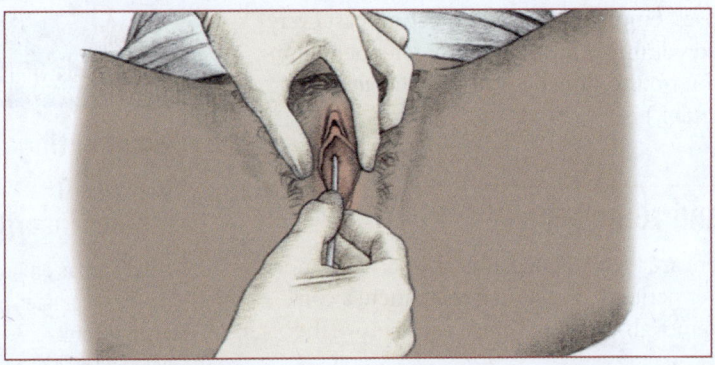

- For the male patient, advance the catheter to the bifurcation and check for urine flow (as shown below). If the foreskin was retracted, replace it to prevent compromised circulation and painful swelling.

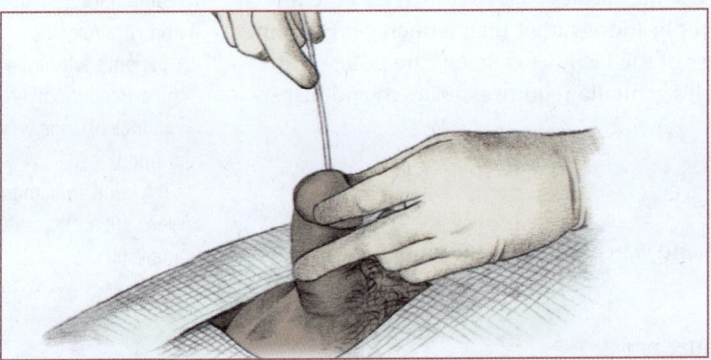

Inflate, hang, and secure

- When urine stops flowing, attach the saline-filled syringe to the Luer lock.
- Push the plunger and inflate the balloon to keep the catheter in place in the bladder.
- Hang the collection bag below the bladder level to prevent urine reflux into the bladder, which can cause infection, and to promote gravity drainage of the bladder. Make sure that the tubing doesn't get tangled in the bed's side rails.
- Secure the catheter to the patient's thigh per the facility's policy.
- Dispose of all used supplies properly, and wash hands.

Practice pointers

- The balloon size determines the amount of solution needed for inflation. The exact amount is usually printed on the distal extension of the catheter used for inflating the balloon.

- For monitoring purposes, empty the collection bag at least every 8 hours. Excessive fluid volume may require more frequent emptying to prevent traction on the catheter wall. (See *Documenting indwelling catheter insertion.*)

Indwelling catheter care and removal

When performed, catheter care is completed after the patient's morning bath, immediately after perineal care. When the patient's condition warrants catheter removal, the nurse must also remove the indwelling catheter.

Difference of opinion

Individual facility policy dictates whether a patient receives daily catheter care. There is currently much debate about the merits of daily catheter care because some studies suggest it increases the risk of infection and other complications rather than reducing it (Cowan, 2020). However, regardless of the facility's catheter care policy, the equipment and the patient's genitalia require assessment and inspection twice daily.

Supplies

For catheter care

- chlorhexidine or soap and water (or other antiseptic cleaning agent)
- sterile gloves
- eight sterile 4″ × 4″ gauze pads
- basin
- sterile absorbent cotton balls or cotton-tipped applicators
- leg bag
- collection bag
- adhesive tape
- optional: safety pin, rubber band, adhesive remover, antibiotic ointment, specimen container
  Note: Commercially prepared catheter care kits containing all necessary supplies are available.

For catheter removal

- absorbent cotton
- gloves
- alcohol pad
- 10-mL syringe with a Luer lock
- bedpan
- linen-saver pad
- optional: clamp for bladder retraining

Take note!

Documenting indwelling catheter insertion

If a patient has an indwelling catheter, be sure to record:
- date and time of catheter insertion
- size and type of catheter used
- amount, color, and other characteristics of urine drainage
- patient's tolerance of the procedure (if large volumes of urine were drained)
- if a urine specimen was sent for laboratory analysis

Getting ready
- Explain the procedure to the patient and provide privacy.
- Wash hands and bring all equipment to the patient's bedside.

How it's done
Catheter care
- Open the gauze pads, place several in the first basin, and pour chlorhexidine solution, soap and water, or other cleaning agents over them.

Avoid irritation
- Some facilities specify that, after wiping the urinary meatus with a cleaning solution, the nurse should wipe it off with wet, sterile gauze pads to prevent possible irritation from the cleaning solution. If this is the facility's policy, pour water into the second basin, and moisten three more gauze pads.
- Make sure that the lighting is adequate and the perineum and catheter tubing are clearly visible.
- Inspect the catheter for problems, and check the collected urine for mucus, blood clots, sediment, and turbidity. Then pinch the catheter between two fingers to determine if the lumen contains any material. If any of these conditions exist (or if the facility's policy requires it), obtain a urine specimen and notify the healthcare provider.
- Inspect the outside of the catheter where it enters the urinary meatus for encrusted material and suppurative drainage. Also, inspect the tissue around the meatus for irritation or swelling.

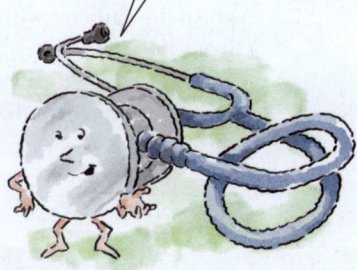

Adequate lighting is essential for indwelling catheter assessment and care.

Wipe away
- Put on sterile gloves. Use a saturated, sterile gauze pad or cotton-tipped applicator to clean the outside of the catheter and the tissue around the meatus. To avoid contaminating the urinary tract, always clean by wiping away from, never toward, the urinary meatus. Use a dry gauze pad to remove encrusted material.
- When cleaning the catheter, don't pull on it. Doing so can injure the urethra and the bladder wall. Moreover, it can expose a section of the catheter that was inside the urethra, and when the catheter is released, the newly contaminated section will reenter the urethra, introducing potentially infectious organisms.
- Remove gloves and wash hands.
- Use the plastic clamp on the tubing of the drainage bag to attach the bag to the sheet. If the bag doesn't have a clamp, wrap a rubber band around the drainage tubing, insert a safety pin through a loop of the rubber band, and pin the tubing to the sheet below the

bladder level. Then attach the collection bag, below the bladder level, to the bed frame.

Catheter removal

- Wash hands. Assemble the equipment at the patient's bedside. Explain the procedure to the patient and tell them that they may feel slight discomfort. Reassure the patient that the nursing staff will check them periodically during the first 6 to 24 hours after catheter removal to make sure that voiding resumes.
- Put on gloves. Attach the syringe to the Luer lock mechanism on the catheter. Place a linen-saver pad under the patient's buttocks.

Deflate the balloon

- Pull back on the plunger of the syringe to deflate the balloon by aspirating the injected fluid. The amount of fluid to be injected is usually indicated on the tip of the catheter's balloon lumen and on the patient's chart.
- Before removing the catheter, offer the patient a bedpan. Then grasp the catheter with the absorbent cotton and gently pull it from the urethra. Inspect the balloon to make sure that it's intact. If it isn't intact, notify the healthcare provider.
- Measure and record the amount of urine in the collection bag before discarding it. (See *Documenting indwelling catheter care and removal.*)

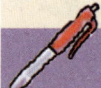

Take note!

Documenting indwelling catheter care and removal

When providing care for a patient with an indwelling catheter, be sure to record:
- the care performed
- care modifications required
- patient complaints
- condition of the perineum and urinary meatus
- characteristics of urine in the drainage bag
- whether a specimen was sent for laboratory analysis
- fluid intake and output (Usually, an hourly record is required for critically ill patients and hemodynamically unstable patients with renal insufficiency.)

Catheter removal
When removing a catheter, be sure to record:
- date and time of catheter removal
- patient's tolerance of the procedure
- when and how much the patient voided after removal (usually for the first 24 hours)
- any associated problems

Bladder retraining
For bladder retraining, be sure to record:
- date and time the catheter was clamped and released
- volume and appearance of urine

Practice pointers
- Some facilities may require the use of specific cleaning agents for catheter care, so check the policy manual before the procedure.

Stay low
- Avoid raising the drainage bag above the bladder level to prevent urine reflux, which may contain bacteria.
- If the patient will be discharged with an indwelling catheter, teach them how to use a leg bag.
- When changing catheters after long-term use (usually 30 days), a larger size catheter may be necessary because the meatus enlarges, causing urine to leak around the catheter.

Collecting urine from an indwelling catheter

Obtain an indwelling catheter specimen by clamping the drainage tube and emptying the accumulated urine into a container or by aspirating a specimen with a syringe. Both procedures require a sterile collection technique to prevent catheter contamination and a UTI. Clamping the drainage tube and emptying the urine into a container are contraindicated after genitourinary surgery.

Supplies
- gloves
- alcohol pad
- 10-mL syringe
- 21G or 22G 1½″ needle
- tube clamp
- sterile specimen container with a lid
- label
- laboratory request form

Getting ready
- About 30 minutes before collecting the specimen, clamp the drainage tube to allow urine to accumulate.

How it's done
- Wash hands and put on gloves. If the drainage tube has a built-in sampling port, wipe the port with an alcohol pad. Uncap the needle on the syringe and insert the needle into the sampling port at a 90-degree angle to the tubing. Aspirate the specimen into the syringe. (See *Aspirating a urine specimen.*)

Rubber made
- If the drainage tube doesn't have a sampling port and the catheter is made of rubber, obtain the specimen from the catheter. Other

Aspirating a urine specimen

To aspirate a urine specimen when the patient has an indwelling urinary catheter in place, clamp the tube distal to the aspiration port for about 30 minutes. Wipe the port with an alcohol pad, and insert a needle and a 10- or 20-mL syringe into the port perpendicular to the tube. Aspirate the required amount of urine, and expel it into the specimen container. Remove the clamp on the drainage tube.

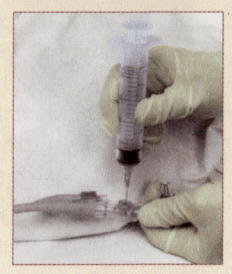

types of catheters leak after the needle is withdrawn. To withdraw the specimen from a rubber catheter, wipe it with an alcohol pad just above where it connects to the drainage tube. Insert the needle into the rubber catheter at a 45° angle and withdraw the specimen. *Never insert the needle into the shaft of the catheter because doing so may puncture the lumen leading to the catheter balloon.*

- Transfer the specimen to a sterile container, label it, and send it to the laboratory immediately or place it on ice. If a urine culture is ordered, include a list of current antibiotic therapy on the laboratory request form. Remove gloves and wash hands.

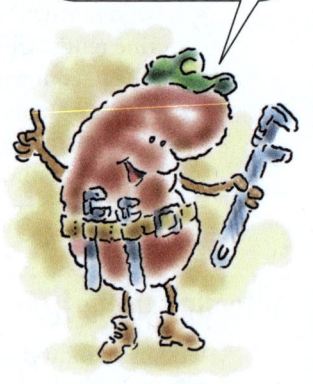

Don't forget to clamp the drainage tube before collecting urine.

Not rubber made

If the catheter isn't made of rubber or has no sampling port, wipe the area where the catheter joins the drainage tube with an alcohol pad. Disconnect the catheter, and allow urine to drain into the sterile specimen container. To prevent contamination, avoid touching the inside of the sterile container with the catheter, and don't touch anything with the catheter drainage tube. When the specimen has been collected, wipe both connection sites with an alcohol pad and join them. Cap the specimen container, label it, and send it to the laboratory immediately or place it on ice. Remove gloves and wash hands.

Needleless ports

If the catheter has a needleless sampling port, wipe the port with an alcohol pad. Insert the needleless syringe into the port and withdraw the specimen. Transfer the specimen to a sterile container, label it, and send it to the laboratory immediately or place it on ice. If a urine culture is ordered, include a list of current antibiotic therapy on the laboratory request form. Remove gloves and wash hands.

Practice pointers

- Be sure to unclamp the drainage tube after collecting the specimen to prevent urine backflow, which may cause bladder distention and infection.

Quick quiz

1. Which of the following is the main complication of benign prostatic hypertrophy (BPH)?
    A. Urethral obstruction
    B. Renal calculi
    C. Prostatitis
    D. Urinary tract infection (UTI)

Answer: A. A urethral obstruction is caused by BPH due to constriction of the urethra.

2. Which of the following is an abnormal constituent of urine?
    A. Urea
    B. Glucose
    C. Sodium chloride
    D. Hydrogen ions

Answer: B. Glucose is not normally found in urine and is not filtered by the kidneys.

3. A patient had surgery 8 hours ago and has not yet voided. Where should the nurse assess for bladder distention?
    A. Between ribs 11 and 12 and the umbilicus
    B. Over the costovertebral region of the flank
    C. In the left lower quadrant of the abdomen
    D. Between the symphysis pubis and the umbilicus

Answer: D. When the bladder becomes distended, it is palpable above the symphysis pubis.

4. A nurse is reviewing the lifestyle choices of a patient who complains of bladder urgency. Which of the following choices can increase bladder urgency?
    A. Exercise frequency
    B. Weight gain
    C. Caffeine intake
    D. Vitamin supplementation

Answer: C. Caffeine acts as a diuretic and can increase urinary frequency.

Scoring

☆☆☆ If you answered all four questions correctly, sensational! You are as smooth as a perfect indwelling catheter removal.

☆☆ If you answered three questions correctly, great! You've got a great capacity for knowledge.

☆ If you answered fewer than three questions correctly, don't worry. Review the chapter, and you'll begin to filter all the important facts!

References

Arumugham, V. B., & Shahin, M. H. (2022). *Therapeutic uses of diuretic agents*. In: *StatPearls*. StatPearls Publishing. https://www.ncbi.nlm.nih.gov/books/NBK557838/

Brinkman, J. E., Dorius, B., & Sharma, S. (2022). *Physiology, body fluids*. In: *StatPearls*. StatPearls Publishing. https://www.ncbi.nlm.nih.gov/books/NBK482447/

Cowan, H. (2020). Bridging the evidence gap in the care of indwelling urethral catheters. *Nursing Times, 116*(1), 56–58. https://www.nursingtimes.net/clinical-archive/infection-control/bridging-the-evidence-gap-in-the-care-of-indwelling-urethral-catheters-03-12-2019/

Cuzzo, B., Padal, S. A., & Lappin, S. L. (2022). *Physiology, vasopressin.* In: *StatPearls.* StatPearls Publishing. https://www.ncbi.nlm.nih.gov/books/NBK526069/

Leslie, S. W., Tadi, P., & Tayyeb, M. (2022). *Neurogenic bladder and neurogenic lower urinary tract dysfunction.* In: *StatPearls.* StatPearls Publishing. https://www.ncbi.nlm.nih.gov/books/NBK560617

Makajeva, J., Waters, C., & Safioleas, P. (2022). *Cystocele.* In: *StatPearls.* StatPearls Publishing. https://www.ncbi.nlm.nih.gov/books/NBK564303/

Mayo Clinic. (2022). Bladder control: Medications for urinary problems. https://www.mayoclinic.org/diseases-conditions/urinary-incontinence/in-depth/bladder-control-problems/art-20044220

Mehta, P., Leslie, S. W., & Reddivari, A. K. R. (2022). *Dysuria.* In: *StatPearls.* StatPearls Publishing. https://www.ncbi.nlm.nih.gov/books/NBK549918/

National Institute of Diabetes, and Digestive and Kidney Diseases (NIDDK). (2022). *Hematuria (blood in the urine).* U.S. Department of Health and Human Services. https://www.niddk.nih.gov/health-information/urologic-diseases/hematuria-blood-urine

Rabinowitz, R. & Cubillos, J. (2022). *Vesicoureteral reflux.* Merck Manual Professional Version. https://www.merckmanuals.com/professional/pediatrics/congenital-renal-and-genitourinary-anomalies/vesicoureteral-reflux-vur?query=Urinary%20Reflux

Sam, P., Nassereddin, A., & LaGrange, C. A. (2022). *Anatomy, abdomen and pelvis, bladder detrusor muscle.* In: *StatPearls.* StatPearls Publishing. https://www.ncbi.nlm.nih.gov/books/NBK482181/

Stoddard, N. & Leslie, S. (2023). *Histology, male urethra.* In: *StatPearls.* StatPearls Publishing. https://www.ncbi.nlm.nih.gov/books/NBK542238/

Taylor, C. R., Lynn, P., & Bartlett, J. (2023). *Fundamental of nursing: The art and science of person-centered care* (10th ed.). Wolters Kluwer.

Chapter 20

Bowel elimination

Just the facts

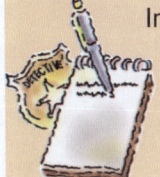

In this chapter, you'll learn:

♦ organs and structures that make up the GI system

♦ causes and characteristics of abnormalities in the GI system

♦ factors that affect bowel elimination

♦ abnormalities of bowel elimination

♦ methods for obtaining a stool specimen

♦ proper way to perform a test for occult blood

♦ proper way to administer an enema

♦ proper colostomy and ileostomy care.

A look at the GI system

The gastrointestinal (GI) system consists of two major divisions: the GI tract and the accessory organs.

GI tract

The GI tract, also called the *alimentary canal*, is a hollow tube that begins at the mouth and ends at the anus. It consists of smooth muscle alternating with blood vessels and nerve tissue. About 25′ (7.5 m) long, the GI tract includes the pharynx, esophagus, stomach, small intestine, and large intestine.

Open wide

Digestion begins in the mouth with chewing, salivating, and swallowing. Three pairs of glands (the parotid, submandibular, and sublingual) produce saliva. The tongue provides the sense of taste.

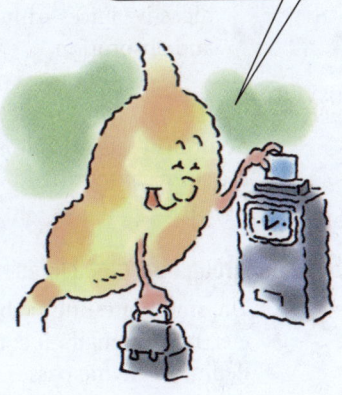

I couldn't do my job without my coworkers: the pharynx, the esophagus, and the small and large intestines.

Proceed to the pharynx

The pharynx, or throat, allows the passage of food from the mouth to the esophagus. It assists in swallowing and secretes mucus that aids in digestion. The epiglottis (a thin, leaf-shaped structure made of fibro-cartilage) is directly behind the root of the tongue. When food is swallowed, the epiglottis closes over the larynx and the soft palate lifts to block the nasal cavity, preventing food and fluid from aspirating into the airway.

Down the esophagus

The esophagus is a muscular, hollow tube about 10 in (25.5 cm) long that moves food from the pharynx to the stomach. When food is swallowed, the upper esophageal sphincter relaxes and the food moves into the esophagus. Specialized circular and longitudinal fibers contract, causing peristalsis, which propels food through the GI tract toward the stomach. The gastroesophageal sphincter at the lower end of the esophagus allows the contents to progress into the stomach and then remains closed to prevent the reflux of gastric contents.

Sitting in the stomach

The stomach is a dilated, saclike structure that serves as a reservoir for food. It lies obliquely in the left upper quadrant below the esophagus and diaphragm, to the right of the spleen, and partially under the liver. The stomach contains two important sphincters: the cardiac sphincter, which protects the entrance to the stomach, and the pyloric sphincter, which guards the exit.

The stomach has three major functions:

* stores food
* mixes food with gastric juices (hydrochloric acid [HCl])
* passes chyme—a watery mixture of partly digested food and digestive juices—into the small intestine for further digestion and absorption.

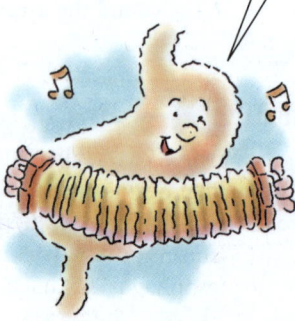

Large amounts of food are like music to my rugae!

Expands to size

Accordion-like folds in the stomach lining, called *rugae*, allow the stomach to expand when large amounts of food and fluid are ingested.

Slipping through the small intestine

The small intestine is about 20 ft (6.1 m) long. Named for its diameter, not its length, it consists of the duodenum, the jejunum, and the ileum. As chyme passes into the small intestine, the end products of digestion are absorbed through its thin mucous membrane lining into the bloodstream.

Leaping through the large intestine

The large intestine, or colon, is about 5 ft (1.5 m) long. Its main functions are

- absorbing excess water and electrolytes
- storing food residue
- eliminating waste products in the form of feces.

The large intestine includes, in the following order: the cecum; the ascending, transverse, descending, and sigmoid colons; the rectum; and the anus. The appendix, a fingerlike projection, is attached to the cecum. Bacteria in the colon produce gas, or flatus.

Accessory organs

Accessory GI organs include the liver, pancreas, gallbladder, and bile ducts. The abdominal aorta and the gastric and splenic veins also aid the GI system.

Spotting the liver

The liver is located in the right upper quadrant, under the diaphragm, and is the heaviest organ in the body, weighing about 3 lb (1.4 kg) in a healthy adult. It's divided into two major lobes by the falciform ligament.

The liver's functions include

- metabolizing carbohydrates, fats, and proteins
- detoxifying blood
- converting ammonia to urea for excretion
- synthesizing plasma proteins, nonessential amino acids, and clotting factors
- storage of vitamins A, D, E, K, and B_{12} and essential nutrients and minerals such as iron and copper.

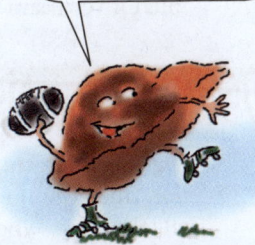

I'm a key player when it comes to digesting fats and absorbing fatty acids.

Believe in bile

The liver also secretes bile, a greenish fluid that helps digest fats and absorb fatty acids, cholesterol, and other lipids.

Gaping at the gallbladder

The gallbladder is a small, pear-shaped organ about 4 in (10 cm) long that lies halfway under the right lobe of the liver. Its main function is to store and concentrate bile. The small intestine initiates chemical impulses that cause the gallbladder to contract and empty bile into the duodenum.

Probing the pancreas

The pancreas, which measures 6 to 8 in (15 to 20.5 cm) in length, lies horizontally in the abdomen, behind the stomach. It consists of a head, a tail, and a body. The body of the pancreas is located in the right upper quadrant, and the tail is in the left upper quadrant, attached to the duodenum.

The pancreas releases insulin, glucagon, and other hormones and peptides into the bloodstream, and it produces pancreatic enzymes that are released into the duodenum for digestion.

Beholding the bile ducts

The bile ducts provide passageways for bile to travel from the liver to the intestines. Two hepatic ducts drain the liver, and the cystic duct drains the gallbladder. These ducts converge into the common bile duct, which then connects with the main pancreatic duct that empties the mixture of digestive enzymes and bile into the duodenum via the hepatopancreatic duct (also known as the ampulla of Vater) and the sphincter of Oddi (Hundt et al., 2022).

Visualizing the vascular structures

The abdominal aorta supplies blood to the GI tract. It enters the abdomen, separates into the left and right common iliac arteries, and then branches into many arteries that extend the length of the GI tract. The gastric and splenic veins drain absorbed nutrients and toxins into the portal vein of the liver. After entering the liver, the venous blood circulates and exits the liver through the hepatic vein, emptying into the inferior vena cava (Norris, 2025).

Digestion and elimination

Digestion starts in the oral cavity, where chewing (mastication), salivation (the beginning of starch digestion), and swallowing (deglutition) all take place. When a patient swallows, the hypopharyngeal sphincter in the upper esophagus relaxes, allowing food to enter the esophagus.

Long day's journey into the stomach

In the esophagus, the glossopharyngeal nerve activates peristalsis, which moves food down toward the stomach through wave-like muscular contractions. As food passes through the esophagus, glands in the esophageal mucosa layer secrete mucus, which lubricates the bolus and protects the mucosal membrane from damage caused by poorly chewed food.

Stomach emptying

Food can remain in the stomach for 3 to 4 hours. The rate of stomach emptying depends on gastrin release, neural signals generated when the stomach wall distends, and the enterogastric reflex. This reflex causes the duodenum to release secretin and cholecystokinin and the jejunum to secrete gastric-inhibitory peptide, both of which decrease gastric motility (Parikh & Thevenin, 2022).

Small intestine

Nearly all digestion and absorption take place in the small intestine. (See *Small intestine: How form affects absorption.*)

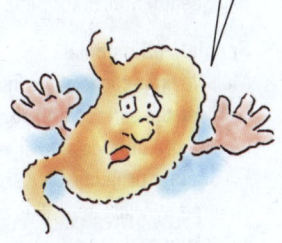

Fill and empty. Fill and empty. Do I ever get a break?

Small but mighty

In the small intestine, intestinal contractions and various digestive secretions break down carbohydrates, proteins, and fats. These actions enable the intestinal mucosa to absorb these nutrients into the bloodstream (along with water and electrolytes) for use by the body. Pancreatic enzymes, bile, and hormones from glands of the small intestine mix with chyme and aid in absorption and digestion.

By the time the chyme passes through the small intestine and enters the ascending colon of the large intestine, it's reduced to mostly indigestible substances.

Large intestine

The chyme bolus begins its journey through the large intestine, where the ileum and the cecum join with the ileocecal pouch. The bolus moves up the ascending colon and past the right abdominal cavity to the liver's lower border. It crosses horizontally below the liver and stomach, by way of the transverse colon, and descends the left abdominal cavity to the iliac fossa through the descending colon.

From there, the bolus travels through the sigmoid colon to the lower midline of the abdominal cavity, then to the rectum, and finally to the anal canal. The anus opens to the exterior through two sphincters. The internal sphincter contains thick, circular, smooth muscle under autonomic control; the external sphincter contains skeletal muscle under voluntary control.

Super absorption

The large intestine doesn't produce hormones or enzymes; however, it plays an important role in the production of B vitamins, especially biotin and vitamin K. It continues the absorption process through blood and lymph vessels in its submucosa. The proximal half of the large intestine absorbs all but about 100 mL of the remaining water in the colon. It also absorbs large amounts of sodium, potassium, and chloride (Azzouz & Sharma, 2022).

Small intestine: How form affects absorption

Nearly all digestion and absorption take place in the 20 ft (6.1 m) of the small intestine. The structure of the small intestine, as shown here, is key to digestion and absorption.

Specialized mucosa

Multiple projections of the intestinal mucosa increase the surface area for absorption by several hundredfold, as shown in the enlarged views.

Circular projections (Kerckring folds) are covered by villi. Each villus contains a lymphatic vessel (lacteal), a venule, capillaries, an arteriole, nerve fibers, and smooth muscle.

Each villus is densely fringed with about 2,000 microvilli, making it resemble a fine brush. The villi are lined with columnar epithelial cells, which dip into the lamina propria between the villi to form intestinal glands (crypts of Lieberkühn).

Types of epithelial cells

The type of epithelial cell dictates its function:
• Mucus-secreting *goblet cells* are found on and between the villi on the crypt mucosa.
• Specialized *Brunner glands* in the proximal duodenum also secrete large amounts of mucus to lubricate and protect the duodenum from potentially corrosive acidic chyme and gastric juices.
• Duodenal *argentaffin cells* produce the hormones secretin and cholecystokinin.
• *Undifferentiated cells* deep within the intestinal glands replace the epithelium.
• *Absorptive cells* consist of large numbers of tightly packed microvilli over a plasma membrane that contains transport mechanisms for absorption and produces enzymes for the final step in digestion.

Intestinal glands

The intestinal glands primarily secrete a watery fluid that bathes the villi with chyme particles. Fluid production results from local irritation of nerve cells and, possibly, from hormonal stimulation by secretin and cholecystokinin. The microvillous brush border secretes various hormones and digestive enzymes that catalyze final nutrient breakdown.

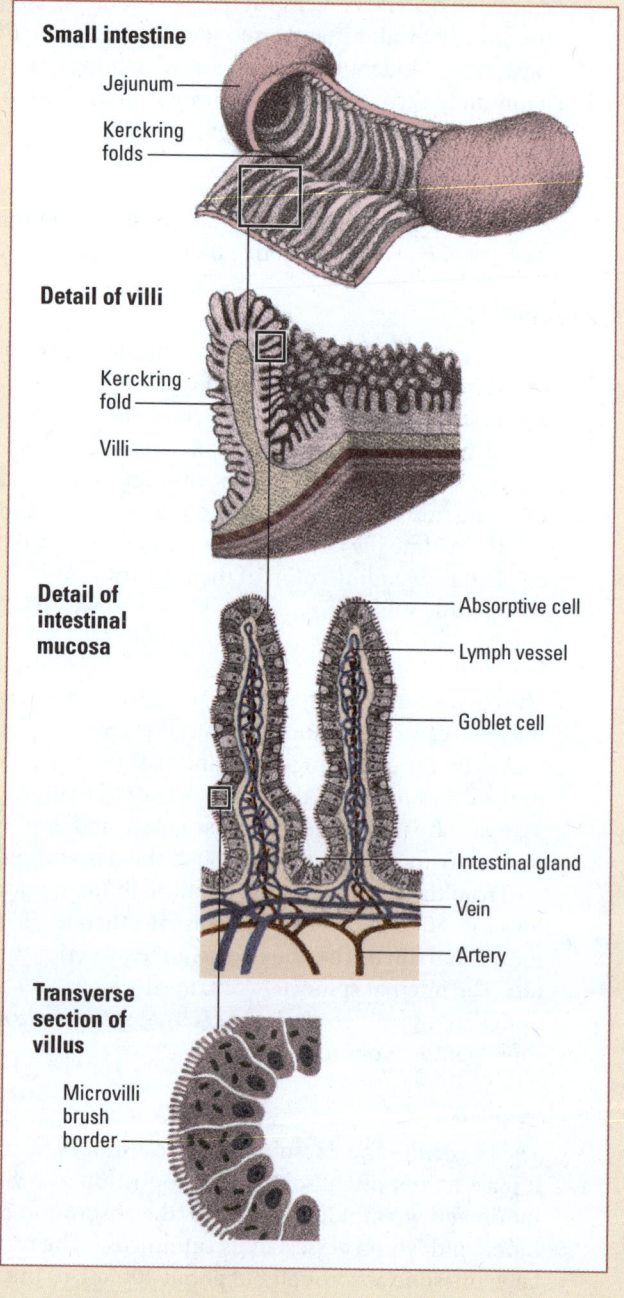

Small intestine
Jejunum
Kerckring folds

Detail of villi
Kerckring fold
Villi

Detail of intestinal mucosa
Absorptive cell
Lymph vessel
Goblet cell
Intestinal gland
Vein
Artery

Transverse section of villus
Microvilli brush border

Source: Norris, T. L. (2025). *Porth's pathophysiology: Concepts of altered health states* (11th ed.). Wolters Kluwer.

Bacteria in action

The large intestine harbors the bacteria *Escherichia coli, Enterobacter aerogenes, Clostridium perfringens,* and *Lactobacillus bifidus.* These bacteria help synthesize B vitamins and vitamin K and break down cellulose into usable carbohydrates. Bacterial action also produces flatus, which helps propel stool toward the rectum.

Mucosa on a mission

In addition, the mucosa of the large intestine produces alkaline secretions from tubular glands composed of goblet cells. This alkaline mucus lubricates the intestinal walls as food pushes through, protecting the mucosa from acidic bacterial action.

Mass movement

In the lower colon, long and relatively sluggish contractions cause propulsive waves or mass movements. These movements, which occur several times per day, propel intestinal contents into the rectum, producing the urge to defecate.

Defecation normally results from the defecation reflex, a sensory and parasympathetic nerve-mediated response, along with voluntary relaxation of the external anal sphincter. (See *GI changes with aging.*)

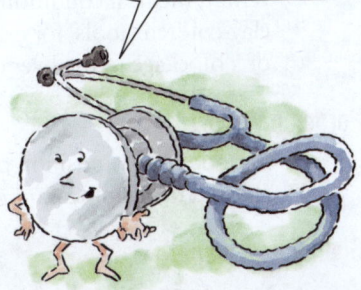

In the lower colon, long and relatively sluggish contractions cause propulsive waves or mass movements.

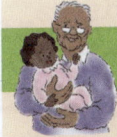

Ages and stages

GI changes with aging

Normal changes that typically impact those over the age of 65 years include diminished mucosal elasticity and reduced GI secretions that, in turn, modify some processes, such as digestion and absorption. GI tract motility, bowel wall and anal sphincter tone, and abdominal muscle strength may also decrease with age. Any of these changes may cause issues in an older patient ranging from loss of appetite to constipation.

Changes in the oral cavity also occur. Tooth enamel wears away, leaving the teeth prone to cavities. Periodontal disease increases, and the number of taste buds declines. Appetite loss can result from a diminishing sense of smell and a decrease in salivary gland secretion.

Liver changes

Normal physiologic changes in the liver include decreased liver weight, reduced regenerative capacity, and decreased blood flow to the liver. Because liver enzymes involved in oxidation and reduction markedly decline with age, the liver metabolizes drugs and detoxifies substances less efficiently.

Characteristics of normal stool

Stool is 25% solids and 75% water. The solids consist of bacteria, undigested fiber, fat, inorganic matter, and some protein.

Bili brown

The chemical conversion of bilirubin (a by-product of hemoglobin and other cellular breakdown) produces the brown color of stool. Other factors can alter the color of stool, such as diet and certain foods and medications. Diets high in fat and low in fiber may cause stool to be very light brown, beets turn stool to a reddish color, blueberries may darken the stool, and medications such as bismuth subsalicylate can turn stool black. Stool color can also be indicative of certain medical conditions such as GI bleeding or infections. White or clay-colored stools, for example, can signal a malabsorption disorder or a blockage in the liver or biliary system (Hopkins, 2023).

Pardon my odor!

Bacterial decomposition of protein in the solids produces stool's characteristic unpleasant odor.

Getting into shape

Stool normally has a soft consistency and a cylindrical form that mimics the shape of the rectum. Thin and ribbon-like stools may be a result of internal hemorrhoids or a warning sign of colorectal cancer.

Different strokes for different folks

Each patient's elimination pattern differs. The frequency of bowel movements can range from one or two bowel movements per day to one bowel movement every 2 or 3 days. If dietary fiber intake is reduced, fewer stools will be produced.

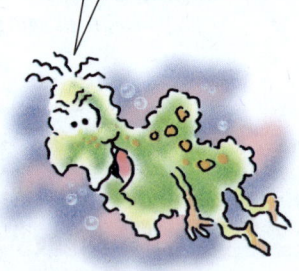

Stool's characteristic unpleasant odor is caused by decomposition of protein in the solids.

Factors affecting bowel elimination

Many factors affect bowel elimination including body position, exercise and activity, fecal diversion, fluid intake, ignoring the urge to defecate, lifestyle, medications, nutrition, and surgery.

Body position

Semisquatting or sitting is the most conducive position for having a bowel movement because it allows gravity to aid in stool movement. It also promotes contraction of the abdominal and pelvic muscles that are used during bowel elimination. A patient who uses a bedpan lying flat in bed may have difficulty having a bowel movement.

Exercise and activity

Good muscle tone and regular exercise facilitate peristalsis and aid in bowel elimination. Abdominal and pelvic muscles create the intra-abdominal pressure needed to have a bowel movement. Lack of or reduced physical activity can increase the chances of developing constipation. Also, loss of neurologic control due to illness or trauma may impair muscle tone.

Fecal diversion

Fecal diversion is the creation of an alternate route for bowel elimination. This procedure removes all or part of the colon, rectum, and anus. An alternative exit site, called a *stoma*, is created that redirects a portion of the remaining bowel through the abdominal wall to an incision on the abdomen. Fecal diversions may be temporary or permanent and are sometimes performed in a patient with bowel cancer or a bowel obstruction or to rest the bowel in inflammatory GI disorders such as Crohn disease.

All those ostomies

When a part of the small intestine is redirected through the abdominal wall, it's called an *ileostomy*. *Colostomy* refers to a fecal diversion that brings a portion of the large intestine or colon through the abdominal wall. (See *Reviewing types of ostomies*.)

Reviewing types of ostomies

The appropriate type of ostomy for a patient depends on the patient's condition. Temporary ostomies, such as a double-barrel or loop colostomy, help treat perforated sigmoid diverticulitis and other conditions in which intestinal healing is expected. Permanent colostomy or ileostomy accompanies extensive abdominal surgery such as the removal of a malignant tumor.

Double-barrel colostomy

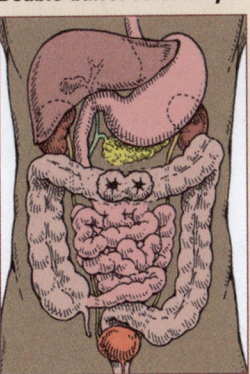

Loop colostomy

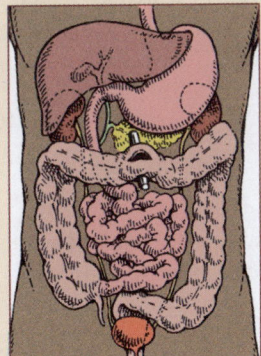

Permanent colostomy

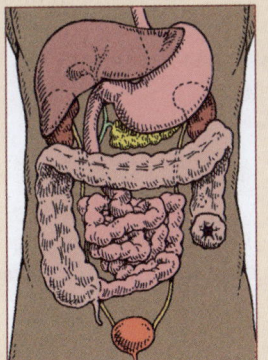

Ileostomy

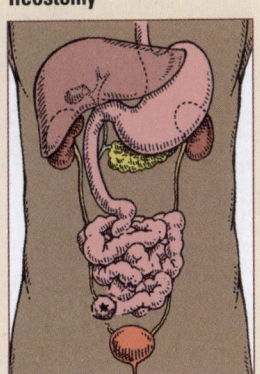

Fluid intake

As stated previously, stool is 75% water. If the body doesn't take in enough fluid, the bowel will conserve more water by absorbing it from the stool. Stools then become hard and difficult to pass.

A storage problem

The longer stool remains in the colon, the greater the amount of water absorbed, resulting in hard, dry stool. Conversely, stool that doesn't remain in the colon long enough for water to be absorbed will be loose and watery, resulting in fluid loss.

Ignoring the urge to defecate

If the initial reflex urge to defecate is ignored, it subsides in a few minutes. Stool remains in the rectum until another mass movement propels more stool into the rectum, creating another urge. A patient with a chronic condition, such as hemorrhoids, may ignore the urge because of painful bowel movements. Lack of privacy may also cause a patient to ignore the urge to defecate. Ignoring the urge to have a bowel movement can lead to constipation.

Lifestyle

Bowel elimination patterns are commonly part of patients' daily routines and are convenient for their lifestyle. Some patients may be used to waiting until they have the urge to defecate. An early riser may consistently have a bowel movement in the morning, whereas a patient who works the night shift may have their daily bowel movements in the late afternoon.

Here we go...or maybe not?

Vacation, changing jobs, and strong emotions such as anxiety, anger, fear, depression, or excitement can alter bowel habits. Hospitalization or a disruption in personal relationships can also be stressful enough to cause such a change.

Medications

Medications, such as opioids and iron preparations, can cause constipation. Antibiotics can cause diarrhea. Antacids can cause constipation or diarrhea.

To go or not to go

Stool softeners and laxatives are normally prescribed to increase stool consistency or bowel elimination. Other medications, such as antidiarrheals, are given to decrease stool frequency.

Nutrition

A high-fiber diet (20 to 30 g of dietary fiber per day) should produce enough bulk to assist in bowel elimination. Foods high in fiber include fruits, vegetables, and cereal grains.

Hard to tolerate

Certain patients may not be able to tolerate lactose (a sugar contained in milk products) or gluten (a protein found in barley, rye, buckwheat, and wheat) and should avoid foods containing these substances. If a lactose-intolerant patient eats or drinks milk products, it may cause abdominal distention, gas formation, abdominal cramping, and diarrhea. If a gluten-intolerant patient ingests foods containing gluten, it may result in bulky greasy stools, abdominal distention, and bloating.

Surgery

Surgery can significantly impact bowel elimination patterns. A patient who's scheduled for operative procedures is commonly required to restrict food and water intake preoperatively and postoperatively.

A surgical pause

Anesthesia slows GI motility for 1 to 2 days following surgery. GI or abdominal surgery may hinder a return of full bowel function for 3 to 4 days. Decreased bowel motility may also result from the bowel's exposure to air and handling during the surgical procedure.

A painless pause

Opioids used to manage pain postoperatively can reduce bowel motility. Fear of pain upon defecation, especially if the patient has an abdominal incision, can also inhibit normal bowel function.

Altered bowel function

Alterations in bowel function include constipation, diarrhea, distention, fecal impaction, fecal incontinence, and flatulence.

Constipation

Constipation is most common in patients over the age of 65 years. It can be caused by immobility, a sedentary lifestyle, and certain medications. A patient who's constipated may complain of a dull abdominal ache and a full feeling. Hyperactive bowel sounds, which may signal irritable bowel syndrome, are sometimes present. A patient with complete intestinal obstruction won't pass flatus or stool, with an absence of bowel sounds when listening past obstruction.

Diarrhea

Toxins, medications, or a GI condition such as Crohn disease can result in diarrhea. Typical symptoms include cramping, abdominal tenderness, anorexia, and hyperactive bowel sounds. Diarrhea accompanied by a fever suggests a toxin as the causative agent.

Distention

Distention may result from gas, a tumor, or a colon filled with stool. It can also suggest an incisional hernia, which may protrude when the patient lifts their head and shoulders.

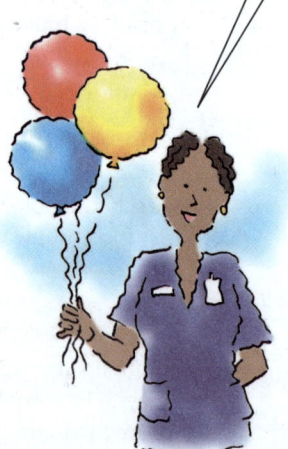

Do you sometimes feel like a balloon ready to pop?

Fecal impaction

Fecal impaction is a large, hard, dry mass of stool in the folds of the rectum or in the sigmoid colon. It's the result of prolonged retention and stool accumulation. Possible causes include poor bowel habits, inactivity, dehydration, improper diet (especially inadequate fluid intake), the use of constipation-inducing drugs, and incomplete bowel cleaning after a barium enema or barium swallow.

Fecal incontinence

Fecal incontinence is the involuntary elimination of feces from the bowel and may result from watery or loose stool. In patients over the age of 65 years, fecal incontinence commonly follows loss or impairment of anal sphincter control.

Flatulence

Flatus is the accumulation of gas in the GI tract resulting from swallowing air, diffusion in the blood, and bacterial action in the large intestine. Certain foods such as cabbage and onions, large amounts of carbonated beverages, smoking, and anxiety (which can cause excessive swallowing) can also produce flatus.

Nursing care for bowel elimination

Nursing care for bowel elimination includes stool specimen collection, testing the stool for occult blood, administering enemas, colostomy or ileostomy care, and irrigating a colostomy.

Stool specimen collection

Stool is collected to determine if blood, ova and parasites, bile, fat, pathogens, or ingested drugs are present. Stool characteristics such as color, consistency, and odor can reveal conditions including GI bleeding (indicated by dark, tarry, foul-smelling stool) and malabsorption (indicated by pale, greasy, foul-smelling stools called steatorrhea) (Perencevich & Saltzman, 2023).

Random or specific

Stool specimens are collected randomly or for specified periods such as for 72 hours. Proper collection requires careful instructions to the patient to ensure an uncontaminated specimen.

Supplies
- specimen container with lid
- gloves
- tongue blade
- paper towel or paper bag
- bedpan or portable commode
- three patient-care reminders (for timed specimens)
- laboratory request form

Getting ready
- Verify the patient's identity using two patient identifiers (not including the patient's room number).
- Inform the patient that a stool specimen is needed for laboratory analysis.
- Explain the procedure to the patient and their family, if possible, to ensure cooperation and to prevent the disposal of timed stool specimens.

How it's done
Collecting a random specimen

- The patient should be instructed to notify the nurse when they have the urge to defecate. Have the patient defecate into a clean, dry bedpan or portable commode. Instruct them to urinate and discard toilet tissue into an alternative basin so as not to contaminate the stool specimen because urine inhibits fecal bacterial growth and toilet tissue contains bismuth, which interferes with test results.
- Put on nonsterile gloves.

Stands out from the crowd

- Using a tongue blade, transfer a representative stool specimen from the bedpan to the specimen container, and cap the container. If the patient passes blood, mucus, or pus with the stool, include this with the specimen.
- Wrap the tongue blade in a paper towel or place it in a paper bag and discard it. Remove and discard gloves, and wash hands thoroughly to prevent cross-contamination.

Collecting a timed specimen

- Place a patient-care reminder stating SAVE ALL STOOL over the patient's bed, in the bathroom, and in the utility room.
- After putting on gloves, collect the first specimen, and include it in the total specimen.

Complete transfer

- Obtain the timed specimen by following the same steps as collecting a random specimen. Remember to transfer all stool to the specimen container.
- If stool must be obtained with an enema, use only tap water or normal saline solution.
- After labeling the container with the patient information, date, and time, send each specimen to the laboratory immediately with a laboratory request form. If unable to send the specimens immediately or as directed, refrigerate the specimens and send them all when collection is complete. Remove and discard gloves. Wash hands.
- Make sure the patient is comfortable after the procedure and has the opportunity to thoroughly perform hand and perianal hygiene. Offer assistance if help with perineal care is indicated.

Practice pointers

- Never place a stool specimen in a refrigerator that contains food or medication to prevent contamination. (See *Collecting a stool specimen.*)
- Notify the health care provider if the stool specimen looks unusual. (See *Documenting stool collection,* page 637.)

Education Corner

Collecting a stool specimen

If stool specimen collection at home is necessary, instruct the patient to collect it in a clean container with a tight-fitting lid, to put the container in a brown paper bag, and to keep it in the refrigerator (separate from food items) until it can be transported.

Assessing stool for occult blood

Fecal occult blood tests are valuable for detecting occult blood (hidden GI bleeding), which may be caused by a variety of conditions such as peptic ulcers, gastritis, inflammatory bowel disease, or colorectal cancer, and can distinguish between true melena and melena-like stools. Certain medications, such as iron supplements and bismuth compounds, can darken stools to resemble *melena*, which is black, tarry stool containing blood.

Look for blue

The Hemoccult slide (filter paper impregnated with guaiac) is a common occult blood screening test. This test produces a blue reaction in a fecal smear if occult blood loss exceeds 5 mL in 24 hours. A newer test, ColoCARE, requires no fecal smear (Helena Laboratories, 2023). (See *Home tests for fecal occult blood*.)

Repeat three times

To confirm a positive result, the test must be repeated at least three times while the patient follows a meatless, high-residue diet. A positive result doesn't necessarily confirm colorectal cancer, but it does

Documenting stool collection

When the stool collection is complete, be sure to record
- time of specimen collection and transport to the laboratory
- color, odor, and consistency of the stool
- unusual characteristics such as mucus or blood
- whether the patient had difficulty passing the stool.

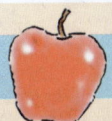

Education Corner

Home tests for fecal occult blood

Most fecal occult blood tests require the patient to collect a specimen of their stool and smear some of it on a slide. However, some newer tests don't require the patient to handle stool, making the procedure safer and simpler. One example is a test called *ColoCARE*. If a patient will be performing the ColoCARE test at home, include these instructions in the patient teaching:
- Tell them to avoid red meat, vitamin C supplements, and the use of laxatives for 2 days before the test and during the time of the collection(s).
- Advise the patient to check with their health care provider about the need for discontinuing medications before the test. Drugs that can interfere with test results include:
  – Antiplatelet medications such as aspirin
  – Nonsteroidal anti-inflammatory drugs such as indomethacin
  – Corticosteroids

- Tell the patient to flush the toilet twice just before performing the test to remove any toilet-cleaning chemicals from the tank.
- Instruct the patient to defecate into the toilet but to avoid throwing toilet paper into the bowl. Then, within 5 minutes, the patient should remove the test pad from its pouch and float it printed side up on the surface of the water.
- Tell the patient to watch the pad for 15 to 30 seconds to see if it changes to a blue or green color, and have them record the result on the reply card.
- Emphasize that the patient should perform this test with three consecutive bowel movements and then send the completed card to their provider. However, the patient should call their health care provider immediately if they note a color change in the first test (i.e., a positive test result).

Source: Helena Laboratories. (2023). *ColorCARE – instruction sheet*. ColorCARE Procedures 310Rev6. Helena.com/Procedures/310Rev6.pdf

indicate the need for further diagnostic studies. GI bleeding can result from conditions other than cancer, such as ulcers and diverticula. Fecal occult blood tests are easily performed on collected specimens or smears from a digital rectal examination.

Supplies
- test kit
- gloves
- glass or porcelain
- tongue blade or other wooden applicator

Getting ready
- Explain the procedure to the patient and their family, if possible, to ensure cooperation and prevent disposal of timed stool specimens.
- Provide privacy.
- Wash hands and bring all equipment to the patient's bedside.
- Verify the patient's identity using two patient identifiers (not including the patient's room number).

How it's done
- Put on gloves, and collect a stool specimen.

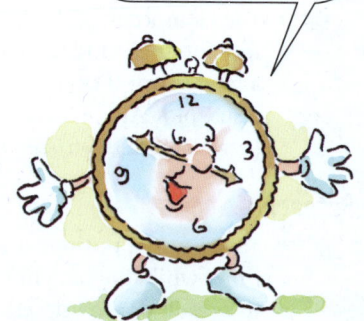

If a test is timed, be sure to read the results exactly when specified to ensure documentation of the correct result.

Hemoccult slide test
- Open the flap on the slide packet, and use a tongue blade or other wooden applicator to apply a thin smear of the stool specimen to the guaiac-impregnated filter paper exposed in box A, as shown in the first photo at the end of this section. Alternatively, after performing a digital rectal examination, wipe the finger used for the examination on a square of the filter paper.
- Apply a second smear from another part of the specimen to the filter paper exposed in box B because some parts of the specimen may not contain blood.
- Allow the specimens to dry for 3 to 5 minutes.
- Open the flap on the reverse side of the slide package, and place two drops of Hemoccult-developing solution on the paper over each smear, as shown in the second photo at the end of this section.

- If the test result is positive, a blue reaction will appear in 30 to 60 seconds.
- Record the results, and discard the slide package.
- Remove and discard gloves, and wash hands thoroughly.

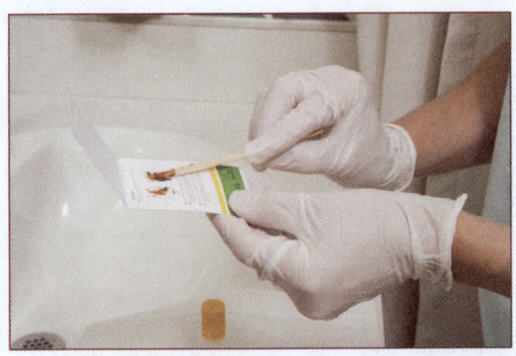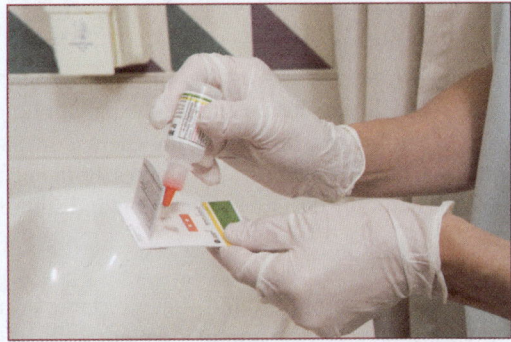

(Reprinted with permission from Henshaw, C. M., & Rassilyer-Bomers, R. (2025). *Craven & Hirnle's fundamentals of nursing: Concepts and competencies for practice* (10th ed., Figs. 1 and 3 in Procedure 35-1). Wolters Kluwer.)

Practice pointers

- Make sure stool specimens aren't contaminated with urine, soap solution, or toilet tissue, and test them as soon as possible after collection.
- Test samples from several portions of the same specimen because occult blood from the upper GI tract isn't always evenly dispersed throughout the formed stool. Blood from colorectal bleeding occurs mostly on the outer stool surface.

Repeat if positive

- If repeat testing is necessary after a positive result, explain the reason for the retest to the patient. Instruct them to maintain a high-fiber diet and to refrain from eating red meat, poultry, fish, turnips, and horseradish for 48 to 72 hours before the test and throughout the collection period because these substances may alter test results.
- As ordered, have the patient discontinue the use of iron preparations, bromides, iodides (such as antithyroid agents), indomethacin, colchicine, salicylates, potassium, bismuth compounds, steroids, and ascorbic acid for 48 to 72 hours before the test and during it to ensure accurate test results and to avoid possible bleeding. (See *Documenting a fecal occult blood test.*)

Take note!

Documenting a fecal occult blood test

Be sure to record the time and date of the test, the result, and any unusual characteristics of the stool tested. Report positive results to the health care provider.

Enema administration

Enema administration involves instilling a solution into the rectum and colon. In a retention enema, the patient holds the solution for 30 minutes to 1 hour. In an irrigating enema, the patient expels the solution almost completely within 15 minutes. Both enemas stimulate peristalsis by mechanically distending the colon and stimulating rectal wall nerves.

Enem-ies

Enemas are contraindicated after a recent colon or rectal surgery or a myocardial infarction and in a patient with an acute abdominal condition of unknown origin such as suspected appendicitis. They also should be administered cautiously to a patient with an arrhythmia.

Supplies

- prescribed solution
- bath (utility) thermometer
- enema administration bag with attached rectal tube and clamp
- IV pole
- gloves
- linen-saver pads
- bath blanket
- two bedpans with covers, or bedside commode
- water-soluble lubricant
- toilet tissue
- bulb syringe or funnel
- plastic bag for equipment
- water
- gown
- washcloth
- soap and water

Prep package

Prepackaged disposable enema sets are available, as are small-volume enema solutions in irrigating and retention types and pediatric sizes.

Getting ready

- Verify the patient's identity using two patient identifiers (not including the patient's room number).
- Explain the procedure to the patient and their family, if possible, to ensure cooperation.
- Provide privacy.
- Wash hands and bring all equipment to the patient's bedside.
- Prepare the prescribed type and amount of solution, as indicated. (See *Understanding types of enemas.*) The standard volume of an irrigating enema for an adult is 750 to 1,000 mL.
- Warm the solution to body temperature to reduce patient discomfort.

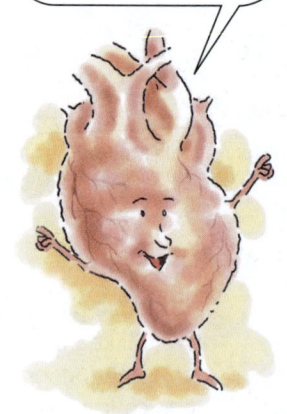

Enemas are contraindicated after a myocardial infarction, also known as a heart attack.

Understanding types of enemas

Enemas are used primarily for three purposes:
* cleaning
* lubricating (or emollient)
* and carminative (to promote expulsion of flatus).
  This chart outlines the preparation steps and purposes of common irrigating/evacuant and retention enemas.

Solution	Preparation	Purpose
Irrigating/Evacuant enemas		
Harris flush	Instill 1,000 mL of tap water.	Cleaning
Saline solution	If a commercially prepared solution isn't available, add two tsp of salt to 1,000 mL of tap water.	Cleaning
Soap and water	Add one packet of mild soap to 1,000 mL of tap water, and remove all bubbles before administering solution.	Cleaning
Retention enemas		
Oil	Instill 150 mL of mineral or arachis oil.	Cleaning and lubricating
1-2-3	Add 30 mL of 50% magnesium sulfate to 60 mL of glycerin. Add mixture to 90 mL of warm tap water.	Cleaning

Source: Taylor, C., Lynn, P., & Bartlett, J. (2023). *Fundamentals of nursing: The art and science of person-centered care* (10th ed.). Wolters Kluwer.

Working toward the right solution

* Clamp the tubing and fill the solution bag with the prescribed solution. Unclamp the tubing, flush the solution through the tubing, and then reclamp it. Flushing detects leaks and removes air that could cause discomfort if introduced into the colon.
* Hang the solution container on the IV pole and take supplies to the patient's room.

How it's done

* Check the health care provider's order and assess the patient's condition.
* Provide privacy. If administering an enema to a child, familiarize them with the equipment and allow a parent or another relative to remain with them during the procedure. (See *Giving an enema to a child*.)
* Instruct the patient to breathe through their mouth to relax the anal sphincter, which will ease catheter insertion.
* Wash hands and put on gloves. If clothing could become soiled, put on a gown.

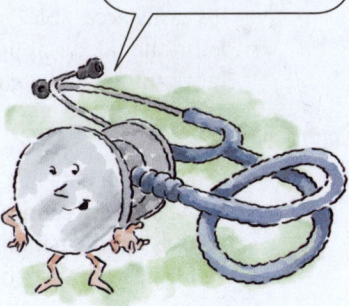

If administering an enema to a child, familiarize them with the equipment and allow a parent or another relative to remain with them during the procedure.

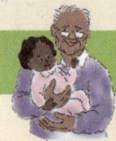

Ages and stages

Giving an enema to a child

Unless contraindicated, help the child into left lateral Sims position. After lubricating the end of the tube, separate the child's buttocks and push the tube gently into the anus, aiming it toward the umbilicus. Insertion depth varies based on the size of the child; if unsure, check with the health care provider.

Try this solution

To prevent rectal wall trauma, avoid forcing the tube. If the tube doesn't advance easily, let a little solution flow in to relax the inner sphincter enough to allow passage. If this doesn't work, stop the procedure and notify the provider.

Standard irrigating enema volumes for pediatric patients are 500 to 1,000 mL for a school-aged child, 250 to 500 mL for a toddler or preschooler, and 250 mL or less for an infant. Irrigating enema volumes should always be double-checked with the health care provider.

A matter of degree (and inches)

To avoid burning rectal tissues, don't administer an enema solution that's warmer than 100 °F (37.8 °C). Be sure not to raise the solution container higher than 12 in (30.5 cm) above bed level for a child or 6 to 8 in (15.2 to 20.3 cm) for an infant. Excessive pressure can force colonic bacteria into the small intestine or cause the colon to rupture.

- Assist the patient into left lateral Sims position to facilitate the flow of the solution into the descending colon. If contraindicated or if the patient reports discomfort, reposition them on their back or right side.

Prep procedures

- Place linen-saver pads under the patient's buttocks to prevent soiling the linens. Replace the top bed linens with a bath blanket.
- Have a bedpan or commode nearby and toilet tissue within the patient's reach. If the patient can use the bathroom, make sure that it's easily accessible.
- Lubricate the distal tip of the rectal catheter with water-soluble lubricant to facilitate rectal insertion and to reduce irritation.

Contraction reaction

- Separate the patient's buttocks and touch the anal sphincter with the rectal tube to stimulate contraction. Then, as the sphincter relaxes, tell the patient to breathe deeply through their mouth as you gently advance the tube.

- If the patient feels pain or if the tube meets continued resistance, notify the health care provider. This may signal an unknown stricture or abscess.

Go with the flow

- Hold the solution container slightly above bed level, and release the tubing clamp. Raise the container gradually to start the flow, usually at a rate of 75 to 100 mL/min for an irrigating enema. Use the slowest possible rate for a retention enema to avoid stimulating peristalsis and promote retention. Adjust the flow rate of an irrigating enema by raising or lowering the solution container according to the patient's retention ability and comfort. However, be sure not to raise it higher than 18 in (46 cm) above bed level for an adult.

> Use the slowest possible rate for a retention enema to avoid stimulating peristalsis and promote retention.

- Assess the patient's tolerance frequently during instillation. If they complain of discomfort, cramps, or the need to defecate, stop the flow by pinching or clamping the tubing. Instruct the patient to breathe slowly and deeply through the mouth to help relax the abdominal muscles and promote retention. Resume administration at a slower flow rate after a few minutes when discomfort passes. Stop the flow any time the patient complains of discomfort.

Sudden slowdown

- If the flow slows or stops, the catheter tip may be clogged with feces or pressed against the rectal wall. Gently turn the catheter slightly to free it without stimulating defecation. If the catheter tip remains clogged, withdraw the catheter, flush it with solution, and reinsert it.
- After administering most of the prescribed amount of solution, clamp the tubing. To avoid introducing air into the bowel, stop the flow before the container empties completely.
- To administer a commercially prepared, small-volume enema, first remove the cap from the rectal tube. Insert the rectal tube into the rectum and squeeze the bottle to deposit the contents in the rectum. Remove the rectal tube, replace the used enema unit in its original container, and discard.
- For a flush enema, stop the flow by lowering the solution container below bed level and allowing gravity to siphon the enema from the colon. Continue to raise and lower the container until gas bubbles cease or the patient feels more comfortable and abdominal distention subsides. Don't allow the solution container to empty completely before lowering it because this may introduce air into the bowel.

Time frame

- For an irrigating enema, instruct the patient to retain the solution for 15 minutes, if possible.
- For a retention enema, instruct the patient to avoid defecation for the prescribed time, or if a time is not prescribed, 30 minutes or longer for oil retention and 15 to 30 minutes for anthelmintic and emollient enemas.
- Position the patient on the bedpan with the call button within reach. If they will be using the bathroom or the commode, instruct them to call for help before attempting to get out of bed because the procedure may make the patient feel weak or faint. Also instruct them to call if they feel weak or in pain at any time.
- When the solution has remained in the colon for the recommended time or for as long as the patient can tolerate it, assist the patient onto a bedpan or to the commode or bathroom.

Wrapping it up

- Provide privacy. Instruct the patient not to flush the toilet.
- Assist the patient with cleaning, if necessary, and help them into bed. Place a clean linen-saver pad under them to absorb rectal drainage.
- Observe the contents of the toilet or bedpan. Carefully note fecal color, consistency, volume, and foreign matter such as blood, rectal tissue, worms, pus, mucus, or other unusual matter.
- Send specimens to the laboratory, if ordered.
- Rinse and wash the bedpan or commode.
- Properly dispose of the enema equipment. Store clean, reusable equipment. Discard gloves and gown, and wash hands.
- Document the procedure according to facility policy. (*See Documenting enema administration.*)

Practice pointers

- Schedule a retention enema before meals. A full stomach may stimulate peristalsis and make retention difficult. An oil retention enema may be followed by a soap and water enema 1 hour later to help expel the softened feces completely.
- If the patient has hemorrhoids, instruct them to bear down gently during tube insertion because bearing down causes the anus to open and facilitates insertion.

Take note!

Documenting enema administration

After an enema has been administered, be sure to record
- date and time of administration
- type and amount of solution administered
- special equipment used
- retention time
- approximate amount returned
- color, consistency, and amount of the return
- abnormalities within the return
- complications.

Colostomy and ileostomy care

A patient with a colostomy or an ileostomy must wear an external pouch to collect emerging fecal matter. The pouch also helps control odor and protect the stoma and peristomal skin. Most disposable pouching systems can be used for 2 to 7 days, although some models exceed 7 days.

Half-full

An external pouch must be emptied when it's one-third to half full. A patient with an ileostomy may need to empty the pouch more frequently, four or five times daily. A pouch should be changed immediately if a leak develops.

After meals

The best time to change a pouching system is when the bowel is least active, usually 2 to 4 hours after meals. After a few months, most patients can determine which time is best for them.

A protective seal

The type of pouch selected depends on the stoma's location and structure, availability of supplies, wear time, consistency of effluent, personal preference, and finances. The best adhesive seal and skin protection for the individual patient should also be considered.

Supplies

- pouching system
- stoma measuring guide
- stoma paste (if drainage is watery to pasty or stoma secretes excess mucus)
- plastic bag
- water
- washcloth and towel
- closure clamp
- toilet or bedpan
- water or pouch cleaning solution
- gloves
- facial tissues
- optional: paper tape, mild nonmoisturizing soap, skin shaving equipment, liquid skin sealant, pouch deodorant

Choices, choices, choices

Pouching systems may be drainable or closed-bottomed, disposable or reusable, adhesive-backed, and one-piece or two-piece. (See *Comparing ostomy pouching systems*, page 646.)

Getting ready

- Explain the procedure to the patient and family, if possible.
- Wash hands and bring all equipment to the patient's bedside.

How it's done

- Provide privacy and emotional support.

Comparing ostomy pouching systems

Available in many shapes and sizes, ostomy pouches are fashioned for comfort, safety, and easy application. A disposable closed-end pouch may meet the needs of a patient who irrigates, wants added security, or wants to discard the pouch after each bowel movement. Another patient may prefer a reusable, drainable pouch. Some commonly available pouches are described here.

One-piece disposable pouch

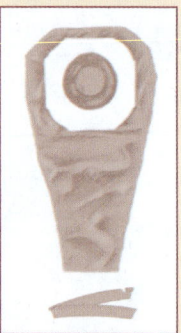

The patient who must empty the pouch often (because of diarrhea or a new colostomy or ileostomy) may prefer a one-piece, drainable, disposable pouch with a closure clamp attached to a skin barrier (see above).

This odor-proof, plastic pouch comes with an attached adhesive or Karaya seal. The bottom opening allows for easy draining. This pouch may be used permanently or temporarily, until stoma size stabilizes.

A one-piece closed-end pouch (above right) is also disposable and made of odor-proof plastic. It may come in a kit with an adhesive seal, a skin barrier, or a carbon filter for gas release. A patient with a regular bowel elimination pattern may choose this style.

Two-piece disposable pouch

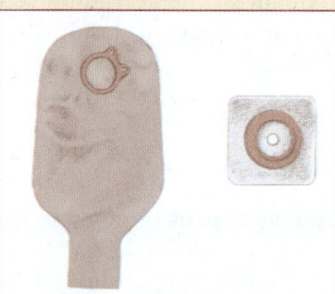

A two-piece disposable drainable pouch with a separate skin barrier (above) permits frequent changes and minimizes skin breakdown. Made of odor-proof plastic, this style comes with belt tabs and usually snaps to the skin barrier with a flange mechanism.

Reusable pouch

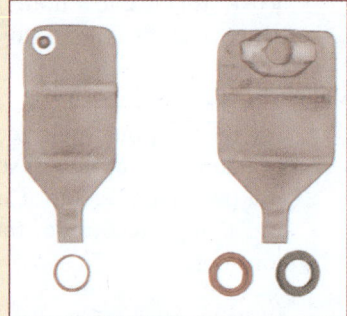

Typically made of sturdy, hypoallergenic plastic, the reusable pouch (above) comes with a separate custom-made faceplate and O-ring. Some reusable pouches have pressure valves for releasing gas. The device has a 1- to 2-month life span, depending on how frequently the patient empties the pouch.

Reusable equipment may benefit a patient who needs a firm faceplate or who wishes to minimize cost. However, many reusable ostomy pouches aren't odor-proof.

Source: United Ostomy Associations of America (UOAA). (2022). Colostomy and ileostomy pouches. https://www.ostomy.org/types-pouching-systems/

Fitting the pouch and skin barrier
- For a pouch with an attached skin barrier, measure the stoma using the stoma measuring guide. Select the opening size that matches the stoma.
- For an adhesive-backed pouch with a separate skin barrier, measure the stoma with the measuring guide and select the opening

that matches the stoma. Trace the selected size opening onto the
paper back of the skin barrier's adhesive side.

- Cut out the opening. (If the pouch has precut openings, which
  can be handy for a round stoma, select an opening that is 1/8 in
  [0.3 cm] larger than the stoma. If the pouch comes without an
  opening, cut the hole 1/8 in wider than the measured tracing.) The
  cut-to-fit system works best for an irregularly shaped stoma.
- For a two-piece pouching system with flanges, see *Applying a skin
  barrier and pouch.*

Can't feel a thing

- Avoid fitting the pouch too tightly; because the stoma has no pain
  receptors, a constrictive opening could injure the stoma or skin
  tissue without the patient feeling warning discomfort. Also, avoid

Applying a skin barrier and pouch

Fitting a skin barrier and ostomy pouch properly can be done in a few steps. Shown here is a commonly used two-piece pouching system with flanges.

STEP 1: Measure the stoma using a measuring guide.

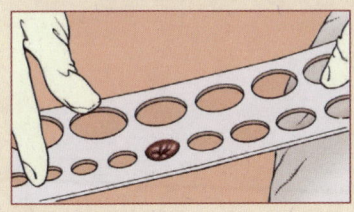

STEP 2: Trace the appropriate circle carefully on the back of the skin barrier.

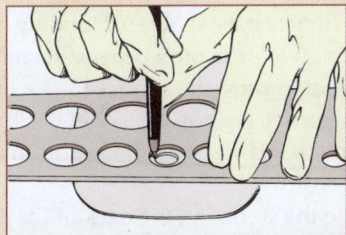

STEP 3: Cut the circular opening in the skin barrier. Bevel the edges to keep them from irritating the patient.

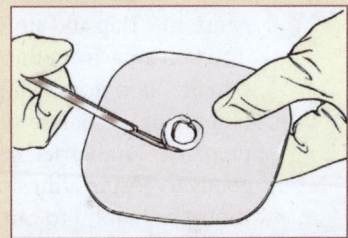

STEP 4: Remove the backing from the skin barrier and moisten it or apply barrier paste, as needed, along the edge of the circular opening.

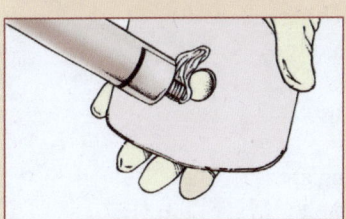

STEP 5: Center the skin barrier over the stoma, adhesive side down, and gently press it to the skin.

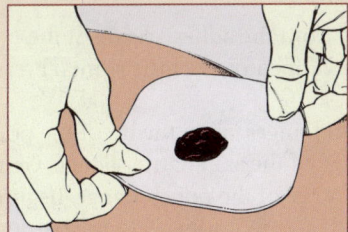

STEP 6: Gently press the pouch opening onto the ring until it snaps into place.

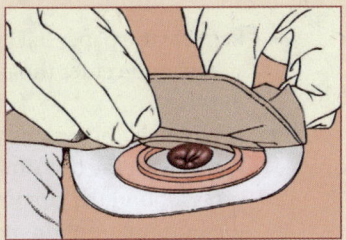

cutting the opening too big; this may expose the skin to fecal matter and moisture.

- If the patient has a descending or sigmoid colostomy, has formed stools, and has an ostomy that doesn't secrete much mucus, they may choose to wear only a pouch. In this case, make sure the pouch opening closely matches the stoma size.
- Between 6 weeks and 1 year after surgery, the stoma will shrink to its permanent size. At that point, pattern-making preparations will be unnecessary unless the patient gains weight, has additional surgery, or injures the stoma.

Explain each step to the patient so they understand the procedure and will have the tools to do it on their own eventually.

Applying or changing the pouch
- Collect all equipment.
- Wash hands and provide privacy.
- Explain the procedure to the patient because the patient will eventually perform the procedure themselves.
- Put on gloves.

Out with the old
- Remove and discard the old pouch in a plastic bag. Wipe the stoma and peristomal skin gently with a tissue.
- Carefully wash the peristomal skin with mild soap and water, and dry it by patting gently. Allow the skin to dry thoroughly. Inspect the peristomal skin and stoma. If necessary, shave surrounding hair (in a direction away from the stoma) to promote a better seal and to avoid skin irritation from hair pulling against the adhesive.
- If applying a separate skin barrier, peel off the paper backing of the prepared skin barrier, center the barrier over the stoma, and press gently to ensure adhesion.
- It may be helpful to outline the stoma on the back of the skin barrier (depending on the product) with a thin ring of stoma paste to provide extra skin protection. (Skip this step if the patient has a sigmoid or descending colostomy, formed stools, and little mucus.)

Peel and press
- Remove the paper backing from the adhesive side of the pouching system and center the pouch opening over the stoma. Press gently to secure.
- For a pouching system with flanges, align the lip of the pouch flange with the bottom edge of the skin barrier flange. Gently press around the circumference of the pouch flange, beginning at the bottom, until the pouch securely adheres to the barrier flange.

(The pouch will click into its secured position.) Holding the barrier against the skin, gently pull on the pouch to confirm the seal between the flanges.

Warm to the task

- Encourage the patient to stay quietly in position for about 5 minutes to improve adherence. The patient's body warmth also helps to improve adherence and to soften a rigid skin barrier.
- Attach an ostomy belt to further secure the pouch, if desired. (Some pouches have belt loops, and others have plastic adapters for belts.)
- Leave a bit of air in the pouch to allow drainage to fall to the bottom.
- Apply the closure clamp, if necessary.
- If desired, apply paper tape in a picture frame fashion to the pouch edges for additional security.

Emptying the pouch

- Put on gloves. Tilt the bottom of the pouch upward, and remove the closure clamp.
- Turn up a cuff on the lower end of the pouch and allow it to drain into the toilet or bedpan.
- Wipe the bottom of the pouch and reapply the closure clamp.
- If desired, the bottom portion of the pouch can be rinsed with cool tap water. Don't aim water up near the top of the pouch, because this may loosen the seal on the skin.
- A two-piece flanged system can also be emptied by unsnapping the pouch. Let the drainage flow into the toilet.

Gas release

- Release flatus through the gas release valve if the pouch has one. Otherwise, release flatus by tilting the pouch bottom upward, releasing the clamp, and expelling the flatus. To release flatus from a flanged system, loosen the seal between the flanges.
- Never release gas by making a pinhole in a pouch, because doing so destroys the odor-proof seal.

Practice pointers

- After performing and explaining the procedure to the patient, encourage self-care to promote independence.
- Use adhesive solvents and removers only after patch-testing the patient's skin. Some products may irritate the skin or produce hypersensitivity reactions. Consider using a liquid skin sealant, if available, to give skin tissue additional protection from drainage and adhesive irritants.

- Remove the pouching system if the patient reports burning or itching beneath it or if there's purulent drainage around the stoma. Notify the health care provider of skin irritation, skin breakdown, a rash, or an unusual appearance of the stoma or peristomal area.
- Use commercial pouch deodorants, if preferred. Most pouches are odor-free, and odor should be evident only when emptying the pouch or if it leaks. Instruct the patient to avoid odor-causing foods such as fish, eggs, onions, and garlic.
- If the patient wears a reusable pouching system, suggest they have two or more systems so one can be worn while one is being cleaned. Clean the pouching system with soap and water or a commercially prepared cleaning solution.
- Document the procedure according to facility policy. (See *Documenting colostomy and ileostomy care.*)

Colostomy irrigation

Irrigation of a colostomy serves two purposes: It allows a patient with a descending or sigmoid colostomy to regulate bowel function, and it cleans the large bowel before and after tests, surgery, or other procedures.

Colostomy irrigation may begin as soon as bowel function resumes after surgery. However, most clinicians recommend waiting until bowel movements are more predictable, which may take 4 to 6 weeks. Initially, the nurse or the patient irrigates the colostomy at the same time daily, recording the output and any spillage between irrigations.

Supplies

- colostomy irrigation set (contains an irrigation drain or sleeve, a water-soluble lubricant, a drainage pouch clamp, an irrigation bag with clamp, tubing, and a cone tip)
- 1,000 mL (1 quart) of tap water
- irrigant warmed to about 100 °F (37.8 °C)
- normal saline solution (for cleaning enemas)
- IV pole or wall hook
- washcloth and towel
- water
- ostomy pouching system
- linen-saver pad
- bedpan or chair
- mild nonmoisturizing soap rubber band or clip
- small dressing or bandage
- stoma cap
- gloves

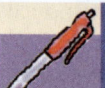

Take note!

Documenting colostomy and ileostomy care

When ostomy care is complete, be sure to record

- date and time of the pouching system change
- characteristics of drainage, including color, amount, type, and consistency
- appearance of the stoma and peristomal skin
- patient teaching
- patient's response to self-care and evaluation of their learning progress.

Getting ready

- Explain each step of the procedure to the patient to promote self-care.
- Provide privacy and wash hands.
- If the patient is in bed, place a linen-saver pad under them to protect the sheets from soiling.
- Put on gloves.
- Remove the ostomy pouch if the patient uses one.

How it's done

- Depending on the patient's condition, colostomy irrigation may be performed in bed using a bedpan or in the bathroom using a chair and the toilet.
- Set up the irrigation bag with the tubing and cone tip. If the patient remains in bed, place the bedpan beside the bed and elevate the head of the bed between 45° and 90°, if their condition allows. If irrigation occurs in the bathroom, have the patient sit on the toilet or on a chair facing the toilet, whichever offers more comfort.

Shoulder level

- Fill the irrigation bag with warmed tap water (or normal saline solution, if the irrigation is for bowel cleaning). Hang the bag on the IV pole or wall hook. The bottom of the bag should be at the patient's shoulder level to prevent the fluid from entering the bowel too quickly. Most irrigation sets also have a clamp that regulates the flow rate.
- Prime the tubing with irrigant to prevent air from entering the colon, which could possibly cause cramps and gas pains.
- Place the irrigation sleeve over the stoma. If the patient has a two-piece pouching system with flanges, snap off the pouch and save it. Snap on the irrigation sleeve.
- Place the open-ended bottom of the irrigation sleeve in the bedpan or toilet to promote drainage by gravity. If necessary, cut the sleeve so that it meets the water level inside the bedpan or toilet. Effluent may splash from a short sleeve or may not drain from a long sleeve.
- Lubricate a gloved finger with water-soluble lubricant and insert the finger into the stoma. If the patient is being taught to care for their own stoma, have them do this to determine the bowel angle at which to insert the cone safely. Expect the stoma to tighten when the finger enters the bowel and then to relax in a few seconds.
- Lubricate the cone with water-soluble lubricant to prevent it from irritating the mucosa.

- Insert the cone into the top opening of the irrigation sleeve and then into the stoma. Angle the cone to match the bowel angle. Insert it gently but snugly; never force it into place.

A slow flow

- Unclamp the irrigation tubing and allow the water to flow slowly. If there isn't a clamp to control the irrigant flow rate, pinch the tubing to control it. The water should enter the colon over 10 to 15 minutes. (If the patient reports cramping, slow or stop the flow, keep the cone in place, and tell the patient to take a few deep breaths until the cramping stops.) Cramping during irrigation may result from a bowel that's ready to empty, water that's too cold, a rapid flow rate, or air in the tubing.

Waiting to drain

- Have the patient remain stationary for 15 or 20 minutes so that the initial effluent can drain.
- If the patient is ambulatory, they can stay in the bathroom until all effluent empties, or they can clamp the bottom of the drainage sleeve with a rubber band or clip and return to bed. Explain that ambulation and activity stimulate elimination. Suggest to the nonambulatory patient that they lean forward or that they massage their abdomen to stimulate elimination.
- Wait about 45 minutes for the bowel to finish eliminating the irrigant and effluent. Then, remove the irrigation sleeve.

A clean machine

- If the irrigation was intended to clean the bowel, repeat the procedure with warmed normal saline solution until the return solution appears clear.
- Using a washcloth, mild soap, and water, gently clean the area around the stoma. Rinse and dry the area thoroughly with a clean towel.
- Inspect the skin and stoma for changes in appearance. Usually dark pink to red, the stoma color may change with the patient's status. Notify the provider of marked stoma color changes because a pale hue may result from anemia and substantial darkening suggests a change in blood flow to the stoma.
- Apply a clean pouch. If the patient has a regular bowel elimination pattern, they may prefer a small dressing, bandage, or commercial stoma cap.
- If the irrigation sleeve is disposable, discard it. If it is reusable, rinse it and hang it to dry along with the irrigation bag, tubing, and cone.

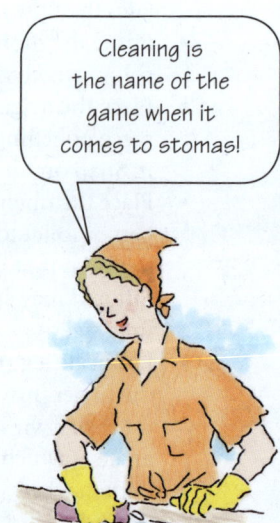

Cleaning is the name of the game when it comes to stomas!

Practice pointers

- Irrigating a colostomy to establish a regular bowel elimination pattern doesn't work for all patients. If the bowel continues to move between irrigations, try decreasing the volume of irrigant. Increasing the irrigant won't help, because that would stimulate peristalsis. Keep a record of results. Also, consider irrigating every other day.

Regulation station

- Irrigation may help to regulate bowel function in a patient with a descending or sigmoid colostomy. A patient with an ascending or transverse colostomy won't benefit from irrigation, and a patient with descending or sigmoid colostomy who's missing part of the ascending or transverse colon may not be able to irrigate successfully.

Diet and exercise

- If diarrhea develops, discontinue irrigations until stools regain form. Irrigation alone won't achieve regularity; the patient must also observe a nutritionally adequate diet and exercise regimen.
- If the patient has a stricture stoma that prohibits cone insertion, remove the cone from the irrigation tubing and replace it with a soft silicone catheter. Angle the catheter gently 2 to 4 in (5.1 to 10.2 cm) into the bowel to instill the irrigant. Don't force the catheter into the stoma, and don't insert it further than the recommended length, because it may perforate the bowel.
- Document the procedure according to your facility policy. (See *Documenting colostomy irrigation.*)

Take note!

Documenting colostomy irrigation

- Record the date and time of irrigation and the type and amount of irrigant.
- Note the stoma color and characteristics of drainage, including color, consistency, and amount.
- Record patient teaching.
- Describe teaching content and patient response to self-care instruction.
- Evaluate the patient's learning progress.

Quick quiz

1. A patient reports a burning sensation in the middle of their chest, rising from the stomach to their mouth. This occurs especially after eating large meals, drinking carbonated beverages, or lying down right after eating. These findings indicated dysfunction with which part of the gastrointestinal (GI) system?

   A. Epiglottis
   B. Upper esophageal sphincter
   C. Cardiac sphincter
   D. Pyloric sphincter

Answer: C. The cardiac (lower esophageal) sphincter is responsible for keeping acidic gastric contents in the stomach. When this sphincter fails, the acidic gastric contents regurgitate from the stomach back up into the esophagus. This can result in irritation and inflammation of the esophageal lining and subsequent burning.

2. A patient with a fecal diversion reports redness and dryness of the peristomal skin. What is an appropriate interpretation of these findings?

    A. These are normal peristomal skin findings and indicate that the ostomy fits the stoma and functions appropriately.

    B. This indicates that there is likely an issue with the maintenance of the ostomy site, and further assessment is necessary.

    C. These findings are evidence of a food allergy, and the nurse should assist the patient in documenting a 48-hour food diary.

    D. These are symptoms of an infection at the site of the ostomy surgical incision and need to be reported to the provider.

Answer: B. The skin around the ostomy is vulnerable to irritation if exposed to fecal contents. Irritation may be caused by various factors of ostomy management, including inadequate skin preparation, inappropriately sized ostomy equipment, or too-frequent pouch changes. Further assessment of an irritated site would be necessary.

3. The bacteria found in the large intestine are responsible for the synthesis of which of the following? (Select all that apply)

    A. Vitamin K

    B. Vitamin D

    C. Vitamin C

    D. Biotin

    E. Vitamin E

Answers: A, C, and D. The large intestine does not produce hormones or enzymes; however, it plays an important role in the production of vitamins K and B, especially biotin.

Scoring

⭐⭐⭐ If you answered all three questions correctly, super! You've really digested this chapter.

⭐⭐ If you answered two questions correctly, great! Your functions (brain, that is) are all in line.

⭐ If you answered fewer than two questions correctly, don't worry. Reread the chapter, and you'll soon swallow all the facts you need!

References

Azzouz, L., & Sharma, S. (2022). *Physiology, large intestine. StatPearls.* StatPearls Publishing. https://www.ncbi.nlm.nih.gov/books/NBK507857/

Helena Laboratories. (2023). *ColorCARE—instruction sheet.* ColorCARE Procedures 310Rev6. Helena.com/Procedures/310Rev6.pdf

Hopkins, J. (2023). What can your child's poop color tell you? https://www.hopkins-medicine.org/johns-hopkins-childrens-center/what-we-treat/specialties/gastroenterology-hepatology-nutrition/stool-color-overview.html

Hundt, M., Wu, C. Y., & Young, M. (2022). *Anatomy, abdomen and pelvis: Biliary ducts. StatPearls.* StatPearls Publishing. https://www.ncbi.nlm.nih.gov/books/NBK459246/

Norris, T. L. (2025). *Porth's pathophysiology: Concepts of altered health states* (11th ed.). Wolters Kluwer.

Parikh, A., & Thevenin, C. (2022). *Physiology, gastrointestinal hormonal control. StatPearls.* StatPearls Publishing. https://www.ncbi.nlm.nih.gov/books/NBK537284/

Perencevich, M., & Saltzman, J. R. (2023). Evaluation of occult gastrointestinal bleeding. In Lamont, J. T. & Travis, A. C. (Eds.), *UpToDate.* https://www.uptodate.com/contents/evaluation-of-occult-gastrointestinal-bleeding

Taylor, C., Lynn, P., & Bartlett, J. (2023). *Fundamentals of nursing: The art and science of person-centered care* (10th ed.). Wolters Kluwer.

United Ostomy Associations of America (UOAA). (2022). Colostomy and ileostomy pouches. https://www.ostomy.org/types-pouching-systems/

Appendices and index

Lippincott Advisor Problem–Based Care Plans Taxonomy

Activity intolerance

Acute anxiety

Acute confusion

Acute pain

ADL deficit

Altered body image perception

Altered breathing pattern

Altered health maintenance

Altered health seeking behavior

Altered skin integrity

Altered skin integrity risk

Altered tissue integrity risk

Altered tissue perfusion

Aspiration risk

Bathing/hygiene ADL deficit

Bleeding risk

Bowel incontinence

Caregiver fatigue

Chronic anxiety

Chronic confusion

Chronic low self-esteem

Chronic pain

Constipation

Constipation risk

Coping impairment

Corneal injury risk

Death anxiety

Deconditioning

Dehydration

Denial

Depression

Diarrhea

Discharge planning

Dressing ADL deficit

Electrolyte imbalance

Electrolyte imbalance risk

Fall risk

Fatigue

Fear

Fecal impaction

Feeding ADL deficit

Fluid overload

Fluid overload risk

Functional urinary incontinence

Grief

Hearing impairment

Hyperglycemia risk

Hypertension risk

Hypoglycemia risk

Hypotension

Hypotension risk

Hypovolemia

Impaired comfort

Impaired gas exchange

Impulsivity

Ineffective airway clearance

Ineffective airway clearance risk

Ineffective breastfeeding

Infection risk

Injury risk

Insomnia

Knowledge deficiency

Latex allergy reaction

Malnutrition risk

Memory impairment

Morbid obesity

Nausea

Nonadherence

Orthostatic hypotension

Overweight

Perioperative injury risk

Perioperative positioning injury

Polypharmacy

Pressure injury risk

Psychosocial/spiritual needs

Reflex urinary incontinence

Risky health behavior

Safety

Self-harm risk

Situational low self-esteem

Sleep deprivation

Suicide attempt risk

Surgical site infection risk

Thermal injury risk

Tobacco abuse

Toileting ADL deficit

Urinary retention

Venous thromboembolism risk

Ventilator failure to wean

Violence risk

Visual impairment

Vomiting

abduct: to move away from the midline of the body; the opposite of *adduct*

activities of daily living: activities performed every day, such as bathing, eating, and toileting

adduct: to move toward the midline of the body; the opposite of *abduct*

adjuvant medications: a group of medications used in combination to enhance the effects of pain medication and to treat concurrent symptoms or side effects

advance directive: written legal document that identifies a patient's wishes in advance about the types of health care they desire should the patient be unable to decide for themselves

aerobic: oxygen necessary for growth

affective: pertaining to emotions or feelings

agent: factor that by its presence or absence can lead to disease

agonist: drug that binds to a receptor to elicit a physiologic response

alveolus: in the lung, a small saclike dilation of the terminal bronchioles

American Nurses Association (ANA): professional organization for nurses made up of individual state nursing organizations with specialized units representing all nursing practice specialty areas

anaerobic: oxygen not required for growth

anion: ion with a negative electrical charge

anorexia: loss of appetite

antagonist: drug that binds to a receptor but doesn't produce a response or blocks the response at the receptor

antigen: foreign substance that causes antibody formation when introduced into the body

antiseptic: agent applied to living tissue to stop or slow the growth of microorganisms

apnea: cessation of breathing

asepsis: condition in which disease-producing microorganisms aren't present

assessment: the first step of the nursing process; involves data collection

atrophy: wasting away

auscultation: listening to body sounds using a stethoscope

autonomy: degree of independence of action

basal metabolic rate: amount of energy used by the body at absolute rest when in an awake state

base: substance with the ability to combine with hydrogen ions; alkali

binder: large bandage used to support a body part or keep a dressing in place

blood pressure: force exerted by the blood on the walls of the vessels; expressed in millimeters of mercury (mm Hg)

body image: feelings about one's body

body mechanics: use of body positioning or movement to prevent or correct problems related to activity or immobility

bone: dense, hard, connective tissue that composes the skeleton

bone marrow: soft tissue in the cancellous bone of the epiphyses; crucial for blood cell formation and maturation

bradycardia: abnormally slow heart rate; usually fewer than 60 beats/minute

bradypnea: abnormally slow respiratory rate; usually fewer than 10 breaths/minute

bronchiole: small branch of the bronchus

buccal: pertaining to the cheek

buffer: substance that helps to control pH through neutralization

bursa: fluid-filled sac lined with synovial membrane

calorie: unit of heat

capillary: microscopic blood vessel that links arterioles with venules

carpal: pertaining to the wrist

cartilage: connective supporting tissue occurring mainly in the joints, thorax, larynx, trachea, nose, and ear

case management: means of providing care that involves coordination of patient services

cation: positively charged ion

central nervous system: one of the two main divisions of the nervous system; consists of the brain and spinal cord

cilia: small, hairlike projections on the outer surfaces of some cells

colloid: fluid containing starches or proteins

communication: exchange of information

conceptual framework: formal explanation of how concepts are linked, with an emphasis on the relationship among them

confidentiality: maintenance of patient information as private

consciousness: state involving full awareness and ability to respond to stimuli

continuity of care: provision of services uninterrupted as the patient moves within the healthcare system

coping mechanism: method used to manage stress

coronary: pertaining to the heart or its arteries

cortex: outer part of an internal organ; the opposite of *medulla*

costal: pertaining to the ribs

crystalloid: a solution that's clear

critical thinking: process that's purposeful and disciplined and requires the use of reason and reflection to achieve insight and to determine conclusions

cultural diversity: wide-ranging ideas and opinions of persons that add to the fabric of society

culture: behavior and beliefs of a specific group; passed from one generation to the next

cutaneous: pertaining to the skin

cyanosis: bluish discoloration of the skin and mucous membranes

debridement: removal of dead tissue or foreign material from a wound

dehiscence: separation of a wound's edges

deltoid: shaped like a triangle (as in the deltoid muscle)

dermis: skin layer beneath the epidermis

diaphragm: membrane that separates one part from another; the muscular partition separating the thorax and abdomen

diarrhea: frequent elimination of watery stool

diffusion: movement of particles from an area of higher concentration to one of lower concentration

diagnosis/identification of patient needs: the second step of the nursing process; involves a determination of patient response to actual or potential health changes

discharge planning: coordination and arrangement of the patient's transition from one health care setting to another

disinfectant: solution used to kill microorganisms on inanimate objects

distal: far from the point of origin or attachment; the opposite of *proximal*

diuresis: formation and excretion of large amounts of urine

documentation: process of writing a record of patient information and care

dorsal: pertaining to the back or posterior; the opposite of *ventral* or *anterior*

duct: passage or canal

dyspnea: difficulty breathing or labored breathing

edema: accumulation of fluid in the interstitial space

empathy: the ability to understand and share the feelings of another

endocrine: pertaining to secretion into the blood or lymph rather than into a duct; the opposite of exocrine

epidermis: outermost layer of the skin; lacking vessels

ethics: professional standards of behavior that indicate right and wrong

evaluation: the last step of the nursing process; involves determining the effectiveness of nursing care

evidence-based care: approach that emphasizes decision making based on the best pertinent research-based evidence

evisceration: internal organ protrusion through an opening in a wound

exocrine: pertaining to secretion into a duct; the opposite of *endocrine*

extracellular fluid space: space outside of cells that contains fluid

febrile: state of temperature elevation

fistula: abnormal opening between organs or between an organ and body surface

flatus: gas or air in the GI tract

focused health assessment: data collection directly related to the patient's problems

fossa: hollow or cavity

functional health assessment: data collection focusing on the ability of the patient to perform activities of daily living

fundus: base of a hollow organ; the part farthest from the organ's outlet

gait: characteristics associated with walking

gastric lavage: instillation and removal of solution into the stomach

gland: organ that secretes or excretes substances

goal/plans: the third step in the nursing process; involves stating intended purpose (i.e., that which is to be achieved with the delivery of care)

health: optimal state of well-being

hematuria: blood in the urine

hemoglobin: protein found in red blood cells that contains iron

homeostasis: balance in the body

hormone: substance secreted by an endocrine gland that triggers or regulates the activity of an organ or cell group

host: person or thing that harbors a microorganism and allows it to grow

hypertension: elevated blood pressure

hypertonic: having a greater concentration than body fluid

hypotension: low blood pressure

hypotonic: having a lesser concentration than body fluid

hypoxemia: state in which the blood contains a lower than normal amount of oxygen

hypoxia: state in which the tissues have a decreased amount of oxygen

implementation: the fourth step of the nursing process, in which the plan of care is carried out

infarction: death of tissue due to ischemia

infiltration: seepage or leakage of fluid into the tissues

informed consent: legal document that a patient or legal guardian signs giving permission for a procedure after the patient or guardian has demonstrated an understanding of the procedure

inferior: lower; the opposite of *superior*

inspection: assessment technique that involves systematic observation

interstitial fluid: fluid contained between the cells

intracellular fluid compartment: fluid contained within the cells

intravascular fluid: fluid contained within the blood vessels and lymphatics

ion: charged particle that forms when an electrolyte separates in solution

ipsilateral: on the same side; the opposite of *contralateral*

ischemia: insufficient blood supply to a part

isotonic: having the same concentration as body fluid

joint: fibrous, cartilaginous, or synovial connection between bones

justice: treatment of all patients fairly and equally

Korotkoff sounds: sounds heard when auscultating blood pressure denoting systolic and diastolic pressures

laceration: wound caused by tearing of the tissues

laws: standards for human conduct and enforced by the government

lacrimal: pertaining to tears

lateral: pertaining to the side; the opposite of *medial*

leukocyte: white blood cell

ligament: band of white fibrous tissue that connects bones

living will: advance directive that states the medical care that a person would want or would refuse should the person be unable to give consent or refusal

lumbar: pertaining to the area of the back between the thorax and the pelvis

lymph: watery fluid in lymphatic vessels

maceration: tissue softening resulting from excessive moisture

malpractice: professional negligence

mammary: pertaining to the breast

meatus: opening or passageway

medial: pertaining to the middle; the opposite of *lateral*

medical asepsis: clean technique involving measures to reduce and control the number of microorganisms

membrane: thin layer or sheet

muscle: fibrous structure whose contraction initiates movement

National League for Nursing (NLN): a national nursing association that promotes excellence in nursing education and provides continuous development for nurse faculty and nursing education leaders

nerve: cordlike structure consisting of fibers that convey impulses from the central nervous system to the body

networking: process of interacting with colleagues who share common interests

neutropenia: decreased number of neutrophils

neutrophil: white blood cell that removes and destroys bacteria, cellular debris, and solid particles

noncompliance: inability to adhere to a prescribed regimen

normal flora: microorganisms that inhabit the body but usually cause no harm

nurse practice acts: state-established guidelines that govern the practice of nursing

nursing process: systematic method for delivering nursing care

objective data: information that's observable, measurable, and that can be verified and validated

oliguria: urine output of less than 400 mL in 24 hours, or less than 20 mL per hour

ophthalmic: pertaining to the eye

osmosis: movement of water through a semipermeable membrane from an area of higher water concentration (lower solute concentration) to an area of lower water concentration (higher solute concentration)

outcome: end product of nursing care; that which is hoped to be achieved

palpation: use of touch to determine size, shape, and consistency of underlying structures

parenteral nutrition: administration of nutrients by intravenous route

pathogen: organism capable of causing disease

percussion: use of tapping on a body surface with fingers to determine the density of the underlying structure or area

peristalsis: wavelike movement to progress contents through the intestines

phrenic: pertaining to the diaphragm

plantar: pertaining to the sole of the foot

plasma: colorless, watery fluid portion of lymph and blood

platelet: small, disk-shaped blood cell necessary for coagulation

pleura: thin serous membrane that encloses the lung

plexus: network of nerves, lymphatic vessels, or veins

popliteal: pertaining to the back of the knee

posterior: back or dorsal; the opposite of *anterior* or *ventral*

primary source: the patient

pronate: to turn the palm downward; the opposite of *supinate*

proximal: situated nearest the center of the body; the opposite of *distal*

pruritus: itching

pulse deficit: difference between the apical and radial pulse rates

pulse pressure: difference between the systolic blood pressure and diastolic blood pressure readings

purulent: pus producing or pus containing

range of motion: extent to which a person can move their joints or muscles

reflex: involuntary action

renal: pertaining to the kidney

respiration: exchange of carbon dioxide and oxygen in tissue and the lungs

restraint: device used to prevent a patient from moving or gaining access

role: expected function and behavior of a person

sanguineous: referring to or containing blood

secondary source: anyone other than the patient who supplies information

self-concept: mental image that a person has of self

serosanguineous: containing blood and serum

serous: serumlike, watery, and thin

spasticity: sudden, involuntary increase in muscle tone or contractions

standard precautions: set of infection control practices and guidelines developed by the Centers for Disease Control and Prevention to protect against infection transmission

sternum: long, flat bone that forms the middle portion of the thorax

striated: marked with parallel lines such as striated (skeletal) muscle

subcutaneous: related to the tissue layer under the dermis

sublingual: under the tongue

superior: higher; the opposite of *inferior*

supinate: to turn the palm of the hand upward; the opposite of *pronate*

surgical asepsis: sterile technique involving measures to keep an object free from all microorganisms

symphysis: growing together; a type of cartilaginous joint in which fibrocartilage firmly connects opposing surfaces

synapse: point of contact between adjacent neurons

tachycardia: rapid heart rate (greater than 100 beats/minute)

tachypnea: rapid respiratory rate (greater than 20 breaths/minute)

tendon: band of fibrous connective tissue that attaches a muscle to a bone

therapeutic communication: use of special techniques to interact with the patient, enabling them to express feelings and work out problems

thrombus: blood clot

total parenteral nutrition (TPN): administration of highly concentrated nutrient solutions via a central intravenous site

transfusion: administration of whole blood or blood products directly into a person's circulation

urinal: metal or plastic bottle used by patients assigned male at birth for urinary elimination

valve: structure that permits fluid to flow in only one direction

venipuncture: insertion of a needle or catheter into a vein

ventilation: movement of air in and out of the lungs

ventral: pertaining to the front or anterior; the opposite of *dorsal* or *posterior*

ventricle: small cavity, such as one of the two lower chambers of the heart or one of several cavities in the brain

viscera: internal organs

Z-track: technique of intramuscular injection that prevents medication from seeping into the tissue

Index

Note: Page numbers followed by f indicate figures, t indicates tables and b indicates boxes.